The Microbiology of Respiratory System Infections

The Microbiology of Respiratory System Infections

Editor: Tristen Johnston

AMERICAN
MEDICAL PUBLISHERS
www.americanmedicalpublishers.com

AMERICAN
MEDICAL PUBLISHERS
www.americanmedicalpublishers.com

Cataloging-in-Publication Data

The microbiology of respiratory system infections / edited by Tristen Johnston.
p. cm.
Includes bibliographical references and index.
ISBN 979-8-88740-582-7
1. Respiratory infections. 2. Respiratory infections--Diagnosis. 3. Respiratory infections--Treatment.
4. Respiratory infections--Prevention. 5. Respiratory organs—Diseases. I. Johnston, Tristen.
RC740 .R47 2023
616.2--dc23

American Medical Publishers,
41 Flatbush Avenue,
1st Floor, New York,
NY 11217, USA

ISBN 979-8-88740-582-7 (Hardback)

Contents

Preface

Every book is initially just a concept; it takes months of research and hard work to give it the final shape in which the readers receive it. In its early stages, this book also went through rigorous reviewing. The notable contributions made by experts from across the globe were first molded into patterned chapters and then arranged in a sensibly sequential manner to bring out the best results.

The respiratory system is a biological system comprising of particular structures and organs utilized for gas exchange. The voice box, nose, windpipe, mouth, lungs and throat are part of the respiratory system. It is negatively affected by infection, aging, allergies, asthma and other conditions causing inflammation. These infections can be further divided into lower respiratory tract infections (LRTI) or upper respiratory tract infections (URTI). A few of the upper respiratory tract infections are epiglottitis, common cold, laryngotracheitist and sinusitis. Major lower respiratory tract infections are bronchitis, pneumonia and bronchiolitis. The most common bacterial pathogens causing the lower and upper respiratory tract infections are Moraxella catarrhalis, Streptococcus pneumonia and Haemophilus influenza. This book contains some path-breaking studies on the topic of respiratory system infections. It presents researches and studies performed by experts across the globe on the microbiology of these infections. This book will help new researchers by foregrounding their knowledge in respiratory system infections.

It has been my immense pleasure to be a part of this project and to contribute my years of learning in such a meaningful form. I would like to take this opportunity to thank all the people who have been associated with the completion of this book at any step.

Editor

1

SHIP-1 Regulates Phagocytosis and M2 Polarization through the PI3K/Akt–STAT5–Trib1 Circuit in *Pseudomonas aeruginosa* Infection

Shugang Qin [1,2†], ***Jiaxin Li*** [1,3†], ***Chuanmin Zhou*** [1], ***Breanna Privratsky*** [1], ***Jacob Schettler*** [1], ***Xin Deng*** [4], ***Zhenwei Xia*** [4], ***Yong Zeng*** [2*], ***Hong Wu*** [2*] **and** ***Min Wu*** [1*]

[1] Department of Biomedical Sciences, School of Medicine and Health Sciences, University of North Dakota, Grand Forks, ND, United States, [2] State Key Laboratory of Biotherapy, West China Hospital, Sichuan University, Chengdu, China, [3] Department of Liver Surgery, West China Hospital, Sichuan University, Chengdu, China, [4] Department of Pediatrics and Department of Pulmonary & Critical Care Medicine, Ruijin Hospital Affiliated to Shanghai Jiao Tong University School of Medicine, Shanghai, China

***Correspondence:**
Yong Zeng
zengyong@medmail.com.cn
Hong Wu
wuhong7801@163.com
Min Wu
min.wu@med.und.edu

† These authors have contributed equally to this work

SHIP-1 is an inositol phosphatase that hydrolyzes phosphatidylinositol 3-kinase (PI3K) products and negatively regulates protein kinase B (Akt) activity, thereby modulating a variety of cellular processes in mammals. However, the role of SHIP-1 in bacterial-induced sepsis is largely unknown. Here, we show that SHIP-1 regulates inflammatory responses during Gram-negative bacterium *Pseudomonas aeruginosa* infection. We found that infected-SHIP-1$^{-/-}$ mice exhibited decreased survival rates, increased inflammatory responses, and susceptibility owing to elevated expression of PI3K than wild-type (WT) mice. Inhibiting SHIP-1 *via* sRNA silencing resulted in lipid raft aggregates, aggravated oxidative damage, and bacterial burden in macrophages after PAO1 infection. Mechanistically, SHIP-1 deficiency augmented phosphorylation of PI3K and nuclear transcription of signal transducer and activator of transcription 5 (STAT5) to induce the expression of Trib1, which is critical for differentiation of M2 but not M1 macrophages. These findings reveal a previously unrecognized role of SHIP-1 in inflammatory responses and macrophage homeostasis during *P. aeruginosa* infection through a PI3K/Akt–STAT5–Trib1 axis.

Keywords: ***Pseudomonas aeruginosa*, SHIP-1, PI3K, Akt, STAT5, M1 macrophages, M2 macrophage**

INTRODUCTION

The Src homology 2-containing inositol 5-phosphatase, SHIP-1, is a 145-kDa protein highly expressed in hematopoietic cells (1). SHIP-1 negatively regulates phosphatidylinositol 3-kinase (PI3K) activity through hydrolysis of the 5′-phosphate from the PI3K lipid product phosphatidylinositol 3,4,5-triphosphate [PI (3,4,5) P3] to phosphatidylinositol (3,4)-bisphosphate (PI (3,4) P2) (2). The PI3K–Akt pathway affects a spectrum of cellular functions including metabolism, growth, proliferation, survival, and adhesion (3). Mast cells and macrophages, which are essential for the negative regulation of type II immune responses to drive lung spontaneous inflammation and injury, are over-activated in SHIP-1$^{-/-}$ mice after *Candida albicans* infection (4). Pulmonary inflammation and M2-polarized macrophages were greatly exacerbated in SHIP-1$^{-/-}$ BALB/c mice (5). Other studies have also found that bacteria utilize lipid rafts to evade immune defense, indicating complex and intertwined signaling circuits in host defense (6, 7). Evaluating interactions between SHIP-1 and lipid rafts may help to understand their role in innate immunity during bacterial infection.

Macrophages, as an important component of the immune system to phagocytize and clear pathogens, are related to the control of inflammation (8). Macrophages are mainly composed of two functional subtypes, M1 and M2 (8, 9). Classically activated macrophages (M1) play a major role in defense against bacteria and viruses by activating inflammatory signaling pathways through secreting pro-inflammatory cytokines (IFN-γ, IL-1, IL-6, IL-12, IL-23, and TNFα) (10). Alternatively activated macrophages (M2) are activated by IL-4 and IL-13 and participate in tissue remodeling and fibrosis by regulation of anti-inflammatory response signal production through secreting IL-10 and TGF-β (11, 12). M2/M1 macrophage polarization is essential for maintaining macrophage phagocytosis and immune function (13, 14). Signal transducer and activator of transcription 5 (STAT5), which plays a critical role in the development of the hematopoietic system, can dominate the function of multiple cytokines by regulating the transcription of distinct target genes (15). Studies have shown that increased STAT5 activity in SHIP$^{-/-}$ mice may play a key role in promoting M2 macrophage polarization (16). The M2 phenotype is suppressed when STAT5($^{-/-}$) BM cells are used in response to IL-3 and granulocyte-macrophage colony-stimulating factor (GM-CSF) stimuli, which can skew murine macrophage progenitors toward an M2 phenotype in the absence of SHIP (17, 18). Tribbles homolog 1 (Trib1), as a member of the mammalian Tribbles homolog pseudokinase family, has been shown to be critical for the differentiation of tissue residence of M2-like macrophages (19). Trib1 induced macrophages to express M2 phenotype markers in prostate cancer (20), whereas Trib1 deficiency attenuated the expression of M2-marker genes upon IL-4 stimulation (21). M2 macrophages exhibited a selective depletion after myocardial infarction in Trib1$^{-/-}$ mice compared with wild-type (WT) mice (22). To date, no studies of the effects of Trib1, SHIP-1, and STAT5 on inflammatory response and subsequent sepsis induced by *Pseudomonas aeruginosa* infection have been reported.

Pseudomonas aeruginosa, an opportunistic bacterium, can infect almost any human organs and is particularly prevalent in immunocompromised individuals, such as patients with HIV-1, tuberculosis infection, cancer, and cystic fibrosis (23, 24). Whereas, antibiotic-resistant strains of PAO1 expand at an alarming pace, the development of effective anti-infectious measures including new antibiotics, chemical drugs, and vaccines has been disappointingly slow. SHIP is essential for endotoxin tolerance by suppressing the generation of M1 macrophages (25), suggesting that SHIP-1 is key for lung immune balance and suppression of inflammation disorders by controlling macrophage function. Nevertheless, the underlying mechanism of SHIP-1 for modulating macrophage function and inflammatory response remains largely elusive in bacterial infection. We herein studied the role of SHIP-1 in PAO1-induced cytokine responses and the underlying molecular mechanisms using SHIP-1$^{-/-}$ mice. Our research shows that SHIP-1 deficiency sabotaged phagocytosis by macrophages and M2 polarization by activating phosphorylation of PI3K/Akt and STAT5 to induce the expression of Trib1, which is critical for the differentiation of M2 as opposed to M1 macrophages. These findings reveal that SHIP-1 plays important roles in regulating macrophage differentiation and inflammatory responses following *P. aeruginosa* infection.

MATERIALS AND METHODS

Animals

SHIP-1$^{-/-}$ mice were graciously provided by Dr. Chris Baran of the Ohio State University and were backcrossed with the background C57BL/6N mice for seven generations (26). C57BL/6N mice (6–8 weeks) were purchased from the Harlan Laboratory. Both male and female were used and randomly grouped for assays (age of mice ranged from 6 to 8 weeks, body weight 22 $\pm$ 3 g) for both SHIP-1$^{-/-}$ mice and C57BL/6N mice. The mouse experiments have been approved by the University of North Dakota Institutional Animal Care and Use Committee (IACUC) and were performed following National Institutes of Health (NIH) guidelines. Mice were anesthetized using 45 mg/kg of ketamine and instilled intranasally with 2 $\times$ 10^7 colony-forming units (CFUs) of PAO1. The animals were dissected when they were moribund. Thereafter, bronchoalveolar lavage fluid (BALF) was performed, and the trachea and lung were excised for homogenization or inflated with 50% optical coherence tomography (OCT) in saline or 10% formalin fixation in phosphate-buffered saline (PBS) (27).

Cells

Murine alveolar macrophages (MH-S) cells were obtained from American Type Culture Collection (ATCC, Manassas, VA) and maintained following the manufacturer's instructions (28). Primary mouse alveolar macrophages (AM) cells and BALF were isolated by bronchoalveolar lavage as previously described (29). The AM obtained from lavage was centrifuged, and the precipitation (containing AM) was resuspended in Roswell Park Memorial Institute (RPMI) 1,640 medium containing 10% newborn bovine serum (HyClone Laboratories, Logan, UT), 100 U/ml of penicillin, and 100 g/ml of streptomycin (Life Technologies, Rockville, MD) and incubated in a 5% CO_2 incubator. For confocal studies, the MH-S cells were seeded on glass-bottomed dishes in order to enhance adherence.

Bacterial Strains

WT strain PAO1 was a gift from Steve Lory (Department of Molecular Genetics, Harvard Medical School). Green fluorescent protein (GFP)–PAO1 was obtained from Gerald Pier (Channing Laboratory, Harvard Medical School) and Dr. Shawn Lewenza (University of Calgary). Pseudomonas aeruginosa PAO1 Xen 41(PAO1 Xen 41) expressing bioluminescence was bought from PerkinElmer Caliper (Waltham, MA). Previous studies have shown that the virulence of these bacteria is consistent with that of PAO1 (30).

Infection Experiments

Bacteria were grown overnight in Luria–Bertani (LB) broth at 37°C with shaking. Then, the bacteria were pelleted by centrifugation at 5,000 g and resuspended in 10 ml of fresh LB broth. The mid-logarithmic phase of bacteria is determined by measuring the OD600 nm, and density was adjusted to OD600 = 0.5–0.6 (to ensure the same vitality) (1 OD = 1 × 10^9 cells/ml). Mammalian cells were counted and were washed once with PBS after overnight culture in RPMI 1,640 medium with 10% fetal bovine serum and changed to serum-free and antibiotic-free media immediately before infection. Cells were infected with 20 times the amount of bacteria (the amount of bacteria/the amount of cells = 20:1) for indicated time points; mice were infected with PAO1 (2 × 10^7 CFU/mouse) (31).

Bacterial Burden Assay

BALF obtained from mice was diluted to different gradients in PBS, and lung tissue was homogenized with PBS. They then were spread on LB dishes to evenly distribute bacteria. The dishes were cultured in a 37°C incubator overnight, and colonies were counted. Each experiment was performed in triplicates.

Cell Transfection

MH-S cells were transfected with SHIP-1 small interference RNA, STAT5 siRNA (sc-29496, Santa Cruz), and TRRB-1 siRNA (sc-154620, Santa Cruz) using Lipofectamine 3,000 reagent (Invitrogen, Carlsbad, CA) in serum-free RPMI 1640 medium following the manufacturer's instructions. The knockout efficiency was detected by western blotting after 48-h transfection.

Western Blotting

Following transfection and/or infection, the MH-S cells were lysed in radio-immunoprecipitation assay (RIPA) buffer containing a protease inhibitor cocktail (Thermo Fisher, Waltham, MA). The lysates were boiled for 10 min after adding loading dye. Equal amounts of each sample (30 μl) were loaded onto 10% sodium dodecyl sulfate (SDS)–polyacrylamide gel electrophoresis and electrophoresed to resolve proteins. The proteins were then transferred to nitrocellulose membranes (Santa Cruz) and blocked for 2 h at room temperature using 5% non-fat dry milk buffer in TBST. The membranes were then incubated with the first antibodies diluted 1:1,000 in 1% non-fat milk blocking buffer overnight at 4°C. After being washed four times with washing buffer, the membranes were incubated with horseradish peroxidase-conjugated secondary antibody (Amersham, St Louis, MO) diluted 1:2,000 for 2 h at room temperature. Signals were detected using enhanced chemiluminescence detection kit (SuperSignal West Pico, Pierce, Rockford, IL). Mouse monoclonal Abs against GAPDH (sc-29496), β-actin (sc-29496), Trib1 (sc-393536), STAT5 (sc-7442), p-STAT5 (sc-101806), SHIP-1 (sc-8425), NF-κB p50 (SC-372), p-NF-κB p50 (sc-271908), IL-4 (SC-32242), and IL-10 (SC-36585) were bought from Santa Cruz. p-Akt (4046s), Akt (2920s), TNF-α (11948S), IL-6 (12912S), IL-1β (12507S), and arginase-1 (93668) were purchased from Cell Signaling Technologies.

RNA Isolation and Real-Time Quantitative PCR Analysis

RNA was extracted from lung tissues by using TRIzol reagent (Invitrogen) and were reverse transcribed into DNA by using the reverse transcriptase kits (Invitrogen). For gene detection, real-time quantitative PCR reaction (RT-PCR) was performed using iTaq Universal SYBR Green Supermix (Bio-Rad), and the PCR primers used in the article are listed in **Supplemental Table 1.**

Nitroblue Tetrazolium Assay

This assay was used to determine the production of superoxide anion in phagocytic cells. BALF cells were obtained from WT mice and SHIP$^{-/-}$mice, then were grown in a 96-well plate in serum-containing medium at 37°C for 4 h, washed three times with PBS buffer, and subsequently infected with PAO1 for 2 h; and 1 μg/ml of nitroblue tetrazolium (NBT) dye (Sigma) was added to each well. The cells were incubated at 37°C for 1 h or until the color developed. The dye was yellow and gave a blue color formazan product upon reduction by superoxide. The reaction was terminated by adding 100 μl of stop solution (10% DMSO; 10% SDS in 50 mM HEPES buffer). The plate was left at room temperature overnight for complete dissolution of formazan product and read at 560-nm absorbance using a multiscan plate reader to quantify the dye conversion. Triplicates were done for each sample and control. Background was corrected by using blanks containing dye alone (32).

Quantitative Polymorphonuclear Neutrophils by HEMA-3 Staining

The infiltration level of polymorphonuclear neutrophils (PMNs) in the serum was used to assess the degree of inflammatory response as previously described (33). The animal blood was obtained by cardiac blood sampling on the sacrificed mouse and was stained on the smear by HEMA-3 staining (23-122929, Thermo Fisher), quantified by light microscopy at 400 × final magnification.

Dihydrodichlorofluorescein Diacetate Assay

Dihydrodichlorofluorescein diacetate (H_2DCF-DA) dye (Molecular Probes, Carlsbad, CA) does not normally fluoresce but emits green fluorescence upon reaction with cellular superoxides. AM cells were obtained from WT mice and SHIP$^{-/-}$ mice and were grown in a 96-well plate in serum-containing medium at 37°C for 4 h, washed three times with PBS buffer, and subsequently infected with PAO1 for 2 h; and an equal amount of dye was added. The plate fluorescence was measured by fluorescence plate reader (BioTek, Winooski, VT) after 1 h incubation using 485-nm excitation and 528-nm emission filter.

3-(4,5-Dimethylthiazol-2-yl)-2,5-diphenyltetrazolium Bromide Assay

The 3-(4,5-dimethylthiazol-2-yl)-2,5-diphenyltetrazolium bromide (MTT) assay was used to assess the viability of cells. Mice were anesthetized using 45 mg/kg of ketamine and instilled intranasally with 2×10^7 CFUs of PAO1 for 12 h. AM cells were obtained from infected mice and processed as above; 1 µg/ml of MTT dye was added to each well. The cells were incubated at 37°C for 1 h or until the color change occurred. The dye was reduced to form a purple formazan product inside living cells. Stop solution was added to dissolve the formazan product and quantified by absorbance measurement at 560 nm using a spectrometer plate reader.

Myeloperoxidase Assay

The myeloperoxidase (MPO) assay was performed as follows. Mice were anesthetized using 45 mg/kg of ketamine and instilled intranasally with 2×10^7 CFUs of PAO1 for 12 h. Lung tissues were obtained from infected mice and homogenized in 50 mM of hexadecyltrimethylammonium bromide, 50 mM of KH_2PO_4, pH 6.0, 0.5 mM of EDTA at 1 ml/100 mg of tissue and centrifuged for 15 min at 12,000 rpm at 4°C. Supernatants were decanted, and 100 µl of reaction buffer (0.167 mg/ml of *O*-dianisidine, 50 mM of KH_2PO_4, pH 6.0, and 0.0005% mM H_2O_2) was added to 100 µl of sample. Absorbance was read at 460 nm in 2-min intervals. Duplicates were done for each sample and control.

Lipid Peroxidation Assay

Malondialdehyde is an end product of the lipid peroxidation and was measured using a colorimetric assay (Calbiochem, Billerica, MA) according to the manufacturer's instructions. Mice were anesthetized using 45 mg/kg of ketamine and instilled intranasally with 2×10^7 CFUs of PAO1 for 12 h. Lung tissue was obtained from infected mice and homogenized in 62.5 mM of Tris–HCl (pH 6.8) supplemented with complete mini protease inhibitor (Roche Diagnostics, Indianapolis, IN) in equal protein amounts. Duplicates were done for each sample and control.

Phagocytosis Assays

Elimination of bacteria depends on many factors such as the phagocytosis of macrophages, which is closely related to macrophage polarization (34). GFP–PAO1 strain was used to determine the phagocytosis after infecting MH-S cell for 2 h and washing three times for PBS to remove the surface attached bacteria. The amounts of bacteria were counted by using bacterial burden assay. The amounts of intracellular bacteria were also determined by immunofluorescence, and cell nuclei were stained with DAPI. Then the amounts of intracellular bacteria (GFP–PAO1) were captured under the confocal microscope (Carl Zeiss, White Plains, NY).

Measurement of Inflammatory Cytokines

Cytokine concentrations were measured by an ELISA kit (eBioscience Co, Invitrogen, San Diego, CA). TNF-α (88-7324-22), IL-1β (88-7013-22), and IL-6 (BMS603-2) were used to represent inflammatory M1 macrophage markers and IL-10 (88-7105-22), IL-4 (BMS613), and TGF-β1 (BMS608-4) for M2 macrophage markers. Ninety-six-well plates (Corning Costar 9018) were coated with 100 µl/well of capture antibody in coating buffer and incubated overnight at 4°C. Cytokine concentrations were determined with corresponding detection horseradish peroxidase (HRP)-conjugated antibodies. Optical absorbance was read at 450 nm and analyzed (30).

Immunostaining

MH-S cells were grown either on coverslips in a 24-well plate or in glass-bottomed dishes (MatTek, Ashland, MA). For immunostaining, the cells were fixed in 4% paraformaldehyde and permeabilized with 0.5% Triton X-100 in PBS, then incubated with primary Abs at a 1:500 dilution in PBS for 1 h in the dark at room temperature, and then washed three times with PBS buffer. After incubation with the appropriate fluorescein-conjugated secondary Abs, DAPI (Sigma-Aldrich) was used to stain the nucleus for 10 min in the dark at room temperature. The coverslips were mounted on slides with VECTASHIELD mounting medium. The cholera toxin B (CTB) chain containing fluorescein (C34777, Thermo Fisher) was used to track lipid rafts, and arginase-1 (red, M2 type macrophage marker) (93668, CST) and TNF-α (green, M1 type macrophage marker) were visualized using indirect immunostaining. The images were captured on Zeiss Meta 510 confocal microscope (Carl Zeiss).

Flow Cytometry

MH-S cells were washed three times with PBS, and then the cells were centrifuged for 5 min in 1,500 rpm and resuspended in 500 µl of PBS. The untreated groups of cells were separately added with 0.5 µl of PBS, fluorescein isothiocyanate (FITC), and phycoerythrin (PE), which were used for calibration parameters. Other groups of cells were separately added 200 µl of CD38 antibody with PE (1:1,000 in PBS). Cells were incubated in the dark for 30 min at room temperature, washed two times with PBS, and then resuspended in 1 ml of PBS. Early growth response protein 2 (Egr2) was marked by Staining Intracellular Antigens for Flow Cytometry kit following the user guidelines provided by the company (00-5521-00, Thermo Fisher Scientific). The cells were filtered by using a 40-µm filter, and the macrophage type was tested by flow cytometry. M1 macrophages were marked by CD38 with FITC fluorescence (11038181, Thermo Fisher); and M2 macrophages were marked by early growth response protein 2 (Egr2) with PE fluorescence (12669182, Thermo Fisher) (35, 36). The percentages of M1 and M2 were recorded by flow cytometry. The ratio of M1 to M2 was calculated using the percentages of M1 divided by the percentages of M2.

In vivo Imaging

C57BL/6N and SHIP knockout mice were infected with bioluminescence-generating PAO1 (Xen 41) for 12 h, anesthetized by ketamine, and then imaged under an IVIS XRII system following the company's instructions (PerkinElmer-Caliper).

Statistical Analysis

All experiments were repeated at least three times. Data were presented as mean ± standard error of the mean (SEM). Statistical analysis was performed with GraphPad (GraphPad Software, La Jolla, CA) using one-way ANOVA plus Tukey *post hoc* test, and statistically significant differences are indicated as $^{*}p < 0.05$ and $^{**}p < 0.01$ (37).

RESULTS

SHIP-1$^{-/-}$ Mice Exhibited Increased Susceptibility and Severe Lung Injury After PAO1 Infection

To explore the roles of SHIP-1 in PAO1 infection, we challenged SHIP-1$^{-/-}$ and WT mice (on C57BL/6N background) with PAO1 (2×10^7 CFU/mouse) and performed a survival assay (uninfected group mice as control). We found that SHIP-1$^{-/-}$ mice exhibited markedly increased susceptibility to infection (approximately 66.7% SHIP-1$^{-/-}$ mice died within 48 h after infection, but just 16.7% WT mice died at this time point (**Figure 1A**). The outcome was presented with a Kaplan–Meier survival curve ($p = 0.043$). Lung injury dramatically increased in SHIP-1$^{-/-}$ mice compared with WT mice (**Figure 1B**). To better monitor the difference between SHIP-1$^{-/-}$ and WT mice, we set out to gauge the *in vivo* dynamics of infection with a bioluminescence bacterial strain Xen 41 (**Figure 1C**). This strain is derived from PAO1 and showed intense bioluminescence on both a dish and an Eppendorf tube (**Figure S1A**). We found a susceptible phenotype in SHIP-1$^{-/-}$ mice, compared with WT mice, with faster bacterial diffusion in the lung after instilling Xen 41 to mouse lungs for 12 h (**Figure 1C**). Importantly, the amount of Xen 41 in the lung and BALF were increased in the SHIP$^{-/-}$ mice as detected by CFU assay (**Figures 1D,E**). Concomitantly, we isolated alveolar macrophages (AM) to detect their viability after 12-h PAO1 infection in mice (**Figure 1F**). The viability of AM cells that were obtained from SHIP-1$^{-/-}$ mice was significantly reduced. Overall results suggest that SHIP-1 may be required for host defense against PAO1 infection in acute pneumonia models.

SHIP-1 Deficiency Aggravated Lipid Aggregates, Oxidative Damage, and Bacterial Dissemination Upon PAO1 Infection

We previously found that Lyn and membrane rafts were involved in phagocytosis and disease progression during *Pseudomonas aeruginosa* infection (6). To investigate the involvement of lipid rafts in the SHIP-1 model, we transfected AM cells with SHIP-1 siRNA (knocking down confirmed by western blotting) and then infected the cells with GFP–PAO1 at 20:1 of multiplicity of infection (MOI) to track lipid rafts using CTB conjugated with Alexa Fluor^{TM} 594. Lipid rafts aggregates were also evaluated using lipid rafts blocker MβCD, which significantly disrupted lipid raft platforms. Our data showed that aggregates significantly increased in SHIP-1 siRNA cells compared with negative control cells (**Figure 2A**). Furthermore, WT mice and SHIP-1$^{-/-}$ mice were anesthetized using 45 mg/kg of ketamine and instilled intranasally with 2×10^7 CFUs of PAO1 for 12 h; the lipid peroxidation was measured in the lung (**Figure 2B**), liver (**Figure S2A**), and spleen (**Figure S2B**). The oxidation state of the tissue and increased recruitment of PMNs and MPO activity are well-recognized for indicating the endpoints of acute lung injury (38, 39). To further assess the damage of lung tissue in

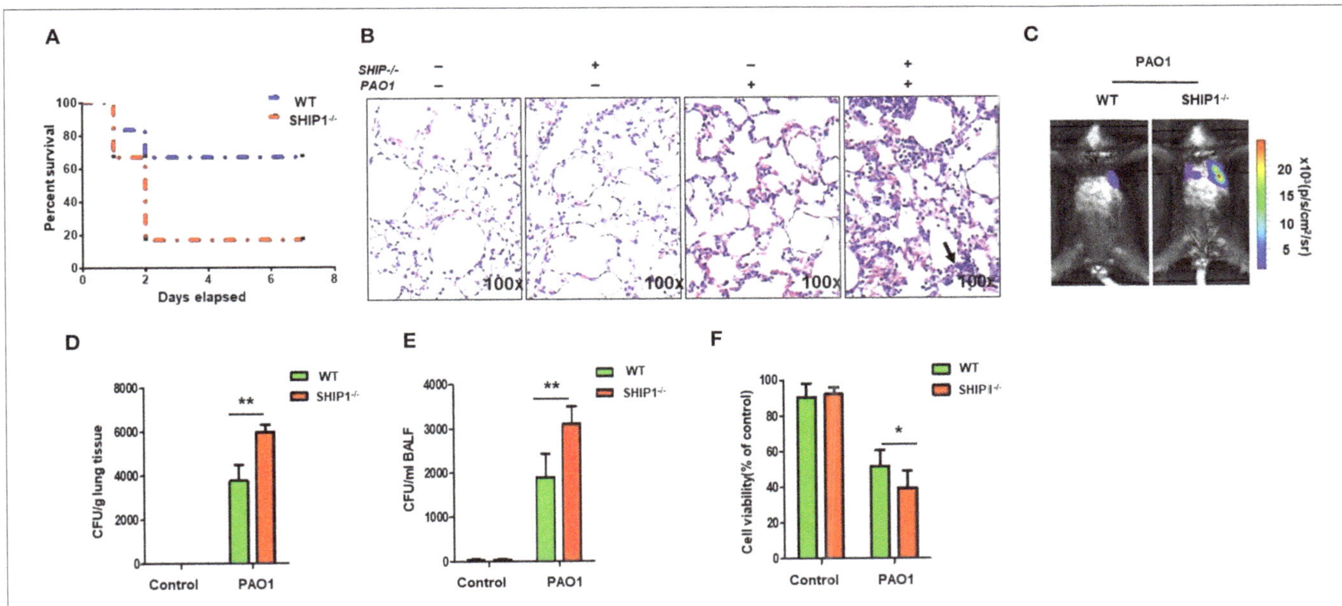

FIGURE 1 | SHIP-1$^{-/-}$ mice show increased susceptibility to PAO1 infection and severe disease. **(A)** Survival curves of SHIP-1$^{-/-}$ and wild-type (WT) mice infected by PAO1 with 2×10^7 colony-forming units (CFUs) per mouse. The survival test is represented by Kaplan–Meier survival curves (95% confidence interval, $n = 6$ for each group, $p = 0.043$). **(B)** Increased alveolar ruptures, thickened alveolar walls, and inflammatory cell infiltration were evaluated by H&E staining infected for 12 h. Arrows indicate the intensity of inflammation and disease progression. **(C)** Lung images were obtained using the bioluminescence in an IVIS XRII system after infection. Data are shown as mean ± SEM of three independent experiments. Bacterial burdens in the lungs **(D)** and bronchoalveolar lavage fluid (BALF) **(E)** were determined after PAO1 infection for 12 h. **(F)** Cell viability of AM were evaluated through the MTT assay after infection PAO1 for 2 h (data are displayed as mean ± SEM and are representative of three mice evaluated in each group, one-way ANOVA with Tukey *post hoc* test in **(D–F)**; $^*p < 0.05$, $^{**}p < 0.01$).

SHIP-1$^{-/-}$ mice, the amount of reactive oxygen species (ROS) released and cellular superoxide was measured by using NBT (**Figure 2C**) and H_2DCF assay (**Figure 2D**). Simultaneously, MPO activity and the amount of PMN infiltration into the blood smear were quantified using MPO Activity Assay Kit (ab105136, Cambridge, MA, USA) in the lung (**Figure 2E**), liver (**Figure S2C**), and spleen (**Figure S2D**) and by HEMA-3 staining assay (**Figure 2F**). Collectively, these data suggest that PAO1 SHIP-1 deficiency or knockdown aggregated lipid accumulation, oxidative damage, and bacterial dissemination after PAO1 infection.

SHIP-1 Deficiency Impeded Phagocytosis of Macrophages and Induced M2 Polarization

Macrophage phagocytosis is important for the immune response (40). To determine the impact of SHIP-1 on phagocytosis, CFU assay and immunofluorescence were performed in MH-S by using GFP–PAO1, which can be directly detected through confocal with a green fluorescent signal and has the same virulence as PAO1 (**Figures 3A,B**), which showed decreased phagocytosis in SHIP-1 siRNA-transfected MH-S cells. The ratio of proinflammatory (M1) to anti-inflammatory (M2) phenotypes often determines the immune response intensity (41). Appropriate polarization is essential to maintain the inflammatory balance and phagocytosis in response to different external environments (42, 43). Therefore, we believe that may be related to SHIP deficiency-induced macrophage polarization after PAO1 infection. To further analyze the role of macrophage polarization in infected SHIP-1$^{-/-}$ mice, we assessed macrophage types by ELISA (**Figure 3C**), western blotting (**Figure 3D**), and immunofluorescence (**Figure 3E**) using macrophage M1 markers (TNF-α, IL-1β, and IL-6) and M2 markers (IL-10, IL-4, arginase-1, and TGF-β1). Studies have shown that the ratio of CD38 and Egr2 (early growth response protein 2) can be used to characterize types of macrophage. M1 macrophages were labeled by CD38 with FITC fluorescence, and M2 macrophages were stained by Egr2 with PE fluorescence (35). The ratio of M2/M1 was determined by flow cytometry (**Figure 3F**). Our data displayed that M1 phenotype inflammatory factors were elevated in PAO1-infected MH-S cells (both PAO1-infected group and SHIP deficiency's PAO1 infected group). SHIP deficiency elicited a large number of expressions of the M2 phenotype inflammatory factors. Collectively, these findings imply that SHIP-1 deficiency hampered phagocytosis of macrophages, which may be associated with M2 polarization aggravation.

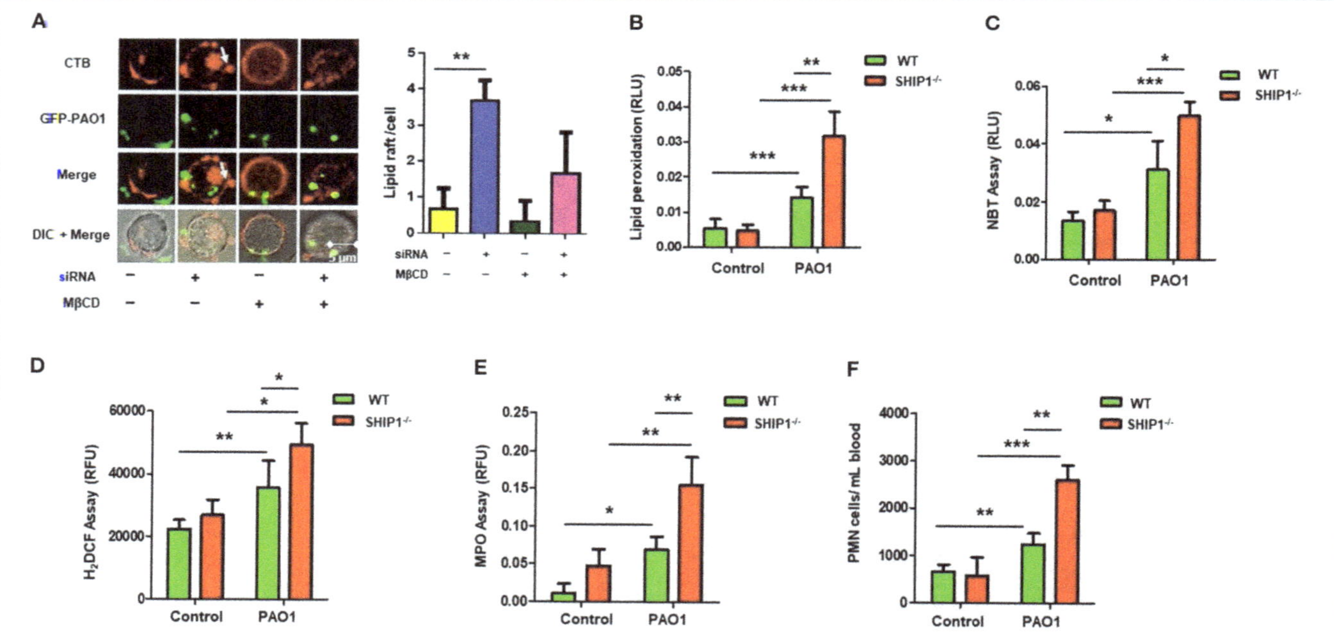

FIGURE 2 | SHIP-1 deficiency aggravates lipid raft aggregation, oxidative damage, and bacterial dissemination after PAO1 infection. **(A)** MH-S cells were transfected with SHIP-1 siRNA (or negative control siRNA) for 48 h or treated with lipid raft blocker MβCD at 10 mM, then infected with green fluorescent protein (GFP)–PAO1 for 30 min, and stained with lipid raft marker (TRITC-labeled cholera toxin B, CTB-red) at 1/10,000 dilution; images were captured using microscope and assessed using ImageJ software on the basis of minimal 100 cells; arrows indicate the extent of lipid raft aggregation. **(B)** Peroxidation product was measured by a colorimetric assay in the lung tissue lysate. **(C)** Superoxide production in bronchoalveolar lavage fluid (BALF) cells significantly increased in PAO1-infected SHIP-1$^{-/-}$ mice compared with WT mice using the nitroblue tetrazolium (NBT) assay (1 mg/ml) at 560-nm absorbance. **(D)** Oxidative stress was increased in SHIP-1$^{-/-}$ AM cells as determined by the H_2DCF fluorescence assay (5 μM) at 488 nm. **(E)** Myeloperoxidase (MPO) was measured from the lungs of SHIP$^{-/-}$ mice as compared with WT mice. **(F)** Polymorphonuclear neutrophils (PMNs) were significantly increased in infected SHIP-1$^{-/-}$ mice compared with WT mice (the data are mean ± SEM and are representative of three independent experiments, one-way ANOVA with Tukey *post hoc* test, $^*p < 0.05$, $^{**}p < 0.01$, $^{***}p < 0.001$).

SHIP-1 Deficiency Deucedly Activated Phosphorylation of PI3K/Akt–STAT5–Trib1 Circuit After PAO1 Infection

To further characterize the critical role of SHIP-1 and macrophage polarization during bacterial infection, we performed qPCR microarray to screen the genes that are involved in macrophage function and phagocytosis after transfection of SHIP siRNA and control siRNA in PAO1 infected MH-S cells (**Figure 4A**) (gene primers are shown in **Table S1**). We found that expression of STAT5 and Trib1 was significantly increased. STAT5, a transcription factor, has been shown to be related with regulation of M2 macrophage programming (16). Trib1 is also critical for the differentiation and tissue residence of M2-like macrophages (19). Therefore, we posit that STAT5 and Tribbles homolog 1 (Trib1) may play a crucial role in SHIP deficiency-associated impairment of macrophage phagocytosis and aggravating M2 polarization. Next, phosphorylation of STAT5 nuclear translocation is determined by immunofluorescence (**Figure 4B**); and PI3K, STAT5, and Trib1 protein levels were analyzed by western blotting (**Figure 4C**). These results revealed that SHIP-1 knockdown activated nuclear transfer of phosphorylation of STAT5, indicating a PI3K/Akt–STAT5–Trib1 circuit in PAO1-infected MH-S cells. We also found that Trib1 was significantly reduced after transfecting MH-S cells with STAT5 siRNA (**Figure 4D**). These findings demonstrate that SHIP-1 knockdown induced macrophage polarization, which is likely to be regulated by the PI3K/Akt–STAT5–Trib1 signal pathway.

Suppression of STAT5 Expression Reduced Polarization of M2 Macrophages and Impaired Phagocytosis

Previous studies have shown that M2 macrophage polarization is related to SHIP-1 deficiency and activation of STAT5 (16). To verify whether M2 macrophage polarization was regulated *via* activated STAT5, we evaluated the phagocytosis of macrophages by CFU and immunofluorescence after suppression of STAT5 expression using RNAi (**Figures 5A,B**) and found that MH-S cells with STAT5 siRNA transfection had increased phagocytosis. Moreover, the polarization of M2 macrophages was significantly decreased in STAT5 siRNA-transfected MH-S cells with PAO1 infection as measured by ELISA (**Figure 5C**), western blotting (**Figure 5D**), immunofluorescence (**Figure 5E**), and flow cytometry (**Figure 5F**). These results indicated that suppression of STAT5 expression reversed the over-activated M2 macrophage polarization and impaired phagocytosis that was mediated by hyperactivation of the PI3K/Akt–STAT5–Trib1 signal pathway due to SHIP-1 deficiency. Consistently, these

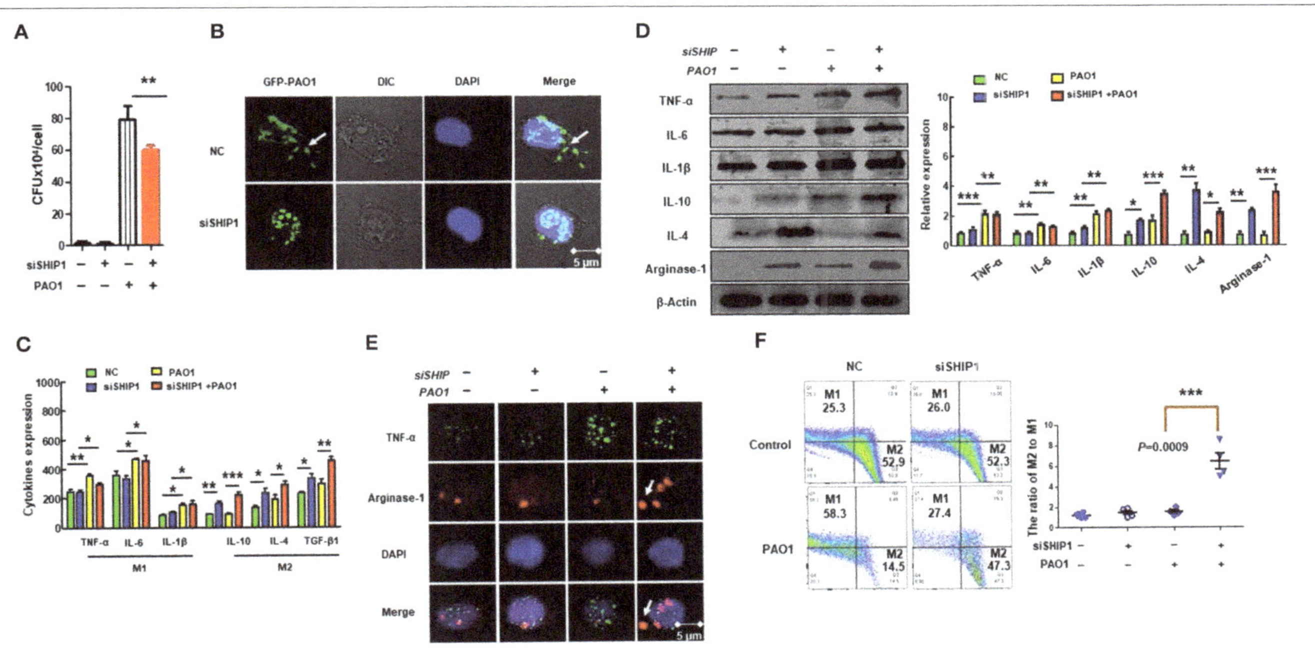

FIGURE 3 | SHIP-1 deficiency disrupts phagocytosis and M2 polarization. MH-S cells were transfected with SHIP-1 siRNA or negative siRNA for 48 h, followed by PAO1 infection for 2 h (uninfected group MH-S cells as control), knockout efficiency was detected by western blotting (**Figure S3**). **(A)** Phagocytosis in MH-S cells was measured by colony-forming units (CFU). **(B)** The number of bacteria engulfed by macrophages was observed by immunofluorescence by using green fluorescent protein (GFP)–PAO1, which can be directly detected through confocal with a green fluorescent signal and has the same virulence as PAO1 in MH-S cells. **(C)** The expression levels of inflammatory factors related to M1 macrophage markers (IL-6, INF-γ, and TNF-α) and M2 macrophage markers (IL-10, IL-4, and TGF-β1) were analyzed by ELISA in MH-S cells. **(D)** M1 macrophage type markers (TNF-α, IL-6, and IL-1β) and M2 macrophage markers (IL-10, IL-4, and arginase-1) were analyzed by western blotting in MH-S cells. **(E)** Representative M1 macrophages marker (TNF-α) and M2 macrophages marker (arginase-1) were analyzed by immunofluorescence in MH-S cells. **(F)** The percentage of M2 macrophages to M1 macrophages was analyzed by CD38/Egr2 by flow cytometry in MH-S cells (the data are mean ± SEM and are representative of three independent experiments, one-way ANOVA with Tukey *post hoc* test, $^{*}p < 0.05$, $^{**}p < 0.01$, $^{***}p < 0.001$).

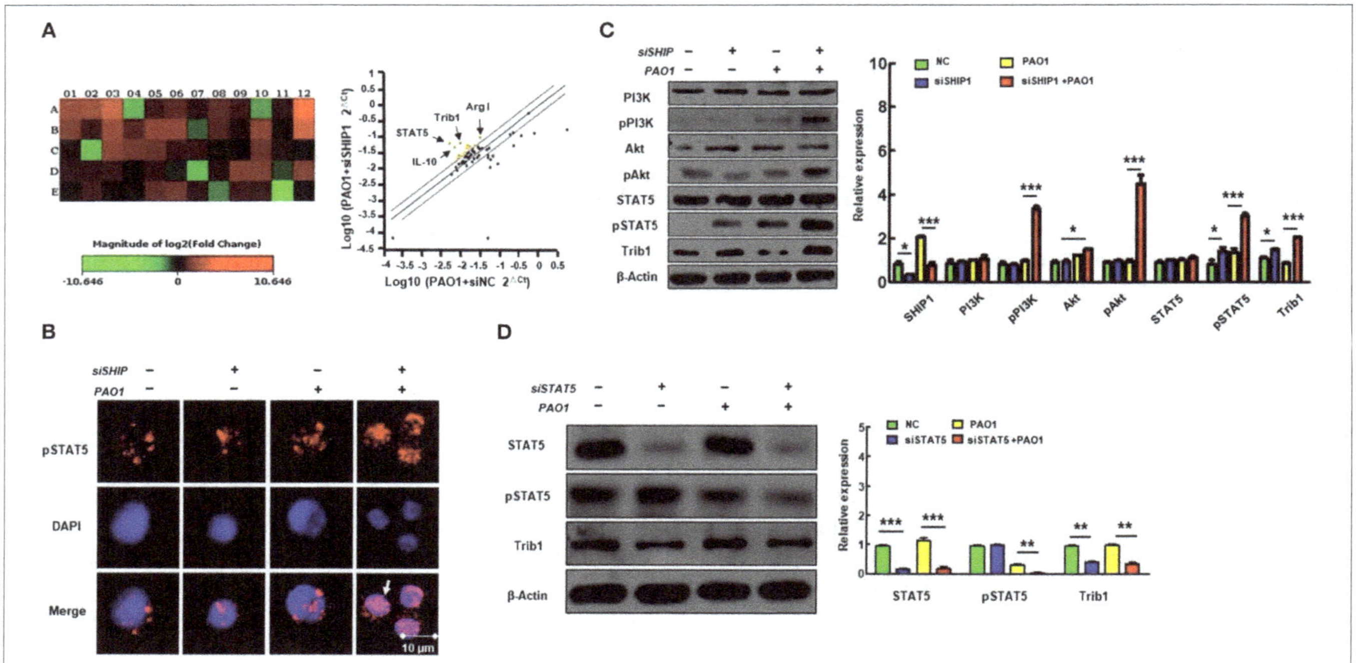

FIGURE 4 | SHIP-1 deficiency elevates phosphorylation of PI3K/Akt–STAT5–Trib1 after PAO1 infection in mice. MH-S cells were transfected with SHIP-1 siRNA or negative siRNA for 48 h, followed by PAO1 infection for 2 h (uninfected group MH-S cells as control); knockout efficiency was detected by western blotting (see **Figure S3**). **(A)** Sixty genes associated with macrophage function and phagocytosis were screened by qPCR. Relative expression of groups was normalized by the relative expression of housekeeping gene. The ratio of the relative expression of SHIP-1 siRNA to negative siRNA was counted. Heat maps are used to indicate differential expression of genes; each color of A1–E12 represents the expression level of a single gene. The corresponding gene names and primers are listed in **Supplemental Table 1**; yellow dots indicate increased expression of gene, and blue dots indicate decreased expression of genes in scatter plot (more than a 2-fold change and $p < 0.05$ by Student's *t*-test). **(B)** The phosphorylated STAT5 in the nucleus was analyzed by immunofluorescence. **(C)** Western blotting shows the activated PI3K/Akt–STAT5–Trib1 signaling proteins circuit of SHIP-1 siRNA in MH-S cells compared with control. **(D)** Western blotting shows reduced expression of Trib1 in STAT5 siRNA cells compared with controls (the data are mean ± SEM and are representative of two independent experiments, Student's *t*-test in **(B)**, one-way ANOVA with Tukey *post hoc* test in **(C,D)**, $^{*}p < 0.05$, $^{**}p < 0.01$, $^{***}p < 0.001$).

findings demonstrate that activated STAT5 is involved in the process of M2 macrophage polarization.

Trib1 Played Critical Roles in Polarization of M2-Like Macrophages and Phagocytosis

Trib1 has the potential to be regulated by MAPK and Akt signaling because it contains a unique pseudokinase C-tail, which can be targeted by MAPKK/MEK family. Importantly, it also contains a pseudokinase domain that can be modulated by Akt signaling (44). Research has shown that Trib1-deficient (Trib1$^{-/-}$) mice exhibited elevated phagocytic capacity and reduced M2-polarized macrophages in bone marrow-derived macrophages (BMDMs) (21). To clarify whether the excessive activation of Trib1 influences macrophage function, we evaluated the phagocytosis of macrophages by CFU (**Figure 6A**) and immunofluorescence (**Figure 6B**) after transfection of Trib1 siRNA into MH-S cells. We found that the phagocytosis of macrophages was increased after Trib1 RNAi. Furthermore, M1 and M2 macrophage-related markers were determined by ELISA (**Figure 6C**), western blotting (**Figure 6D**), immunofluorescence (**Figure 6E**), and flow cytometry (**Figure 6F**). Consistently, our data indicate that suppression of Trib1 expression reversed the over-activated M2 macrophage polarization and impaired phagocytosis that was mediated by hyperactivation of the PI3K/Akt–STAT5–Trib1 signal pathway due to SHIP-1 deficiency. Collectively, these data strongly support that SHIP-1 regulates phagocytosis and M2 polarization through the PI3K/Akt–STAT5–Trib1 circuit (**Figure 7**).

DISCUSSION

In this study, we investigated the role of SHIP-1 in PAO1 infection using SHIP-1$^{-/-}$ mice, which showed increased susceptibility and worsened infectious disease. Similarly, SHIP-1 deficiency aggravated lipid raft aggregates, oxidative damage, and bacterial dissemination. Importantly, our data elaborated a new mechanism that SHIP-1 deficiency activates PI3K/Akt–STAT5–Trib1 signal pathway to regulate phagocytosis of macrophages and promote M2-like polarization.

Previous studies have shown that SHIP-1 is an important regulator of immune cell function through the negative regulation of the PI3K–Akt pathway (45). SHIP-1$^{-/-}$ mice

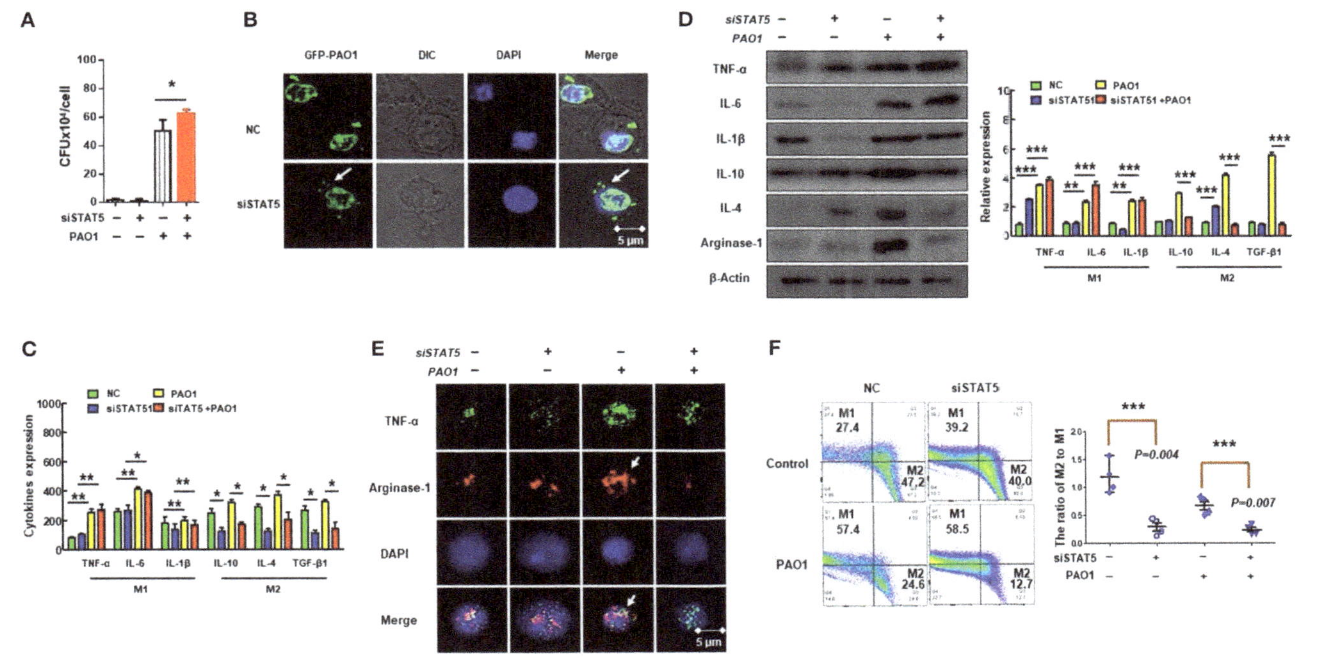

FIGURE 5 | Suppression of STAT5 expression improves polarization of M2 macrophages to impair phagocytosis. MH-S cells were transfected with STAT5 siRNA or negative siRNA for 48 h, followed by PAO1 infection for 2 h (uninfected group MH-S cells as control); knockout efficiency was detected by western blotting (see **Figure S3**). **(A)** Phagocytosis by MH-S was measured by colony-forming unit (CFU). **(B)** Immunofluorescence was performed to reveal the number of green fluorescent protein (GFP)–PAO1 engulfed by macrophages. **(C)** Markers of M1 macrophages (IL-6, INF-γ, and TNF-α) and M2 macrophages (IL-10, IL-4, and TGF-β1) were analyzed by ELISA. **(D)** M1 macrophage markers (TNF-α, IL-6, and IL-1β) and M2 macrophage markers (IL-10, IL-4, and arginase-1) were quantified by western blotting. **(E)** Typical marker for M1 (TNF-α) and M2 (arginase-1) was analyzed by immunofluorescence. **(F)** The ratio of M2 macrophages to M1 macrophages was measured using CD38 and Egr2 antibody by flow cytometry (the data are mean ± SEM and are representative of three independent experiments, one-way ANOVA with Tukey *post hoc* test, $^{*}p < 0.05$, $^{**}p < 0.01$, $^{***}p < 0.001$).

exhibited a myeloproliferative response, indicating that an increase of macrophages or monocytes was due to enhanced proliferation and survival of their progenitors (25, 46). SHIP-$1^{-/-}$ mice may have spontaneous inflammation in the lung, suggesting that SHIP-1 may be an important negative regulator of inflammatory responses (47). We evaluated the survival of SHIP-$1^{-/-}$ mice and lung injury. Our results demonstrate that SHIP-$1^{-/-}$ mice showed increased susceptibility and severe lung injury after PAO1 infection. These results indicate that SHIP-1 is essential for resistance to bacterial infection. Lipid rafts play important roles in innate and adaptive immunity by recruiting cellular signaling modifiers for T-cell activation, phagocytosis, and so on (48). The integrity of lipid rafts is implicated to be essential for LPS cellular activation owing to the presence of CD14, chemokine receptor 4, and toll-like receptor 4 on lipid microdomains of cell membrane following LPS stimulation (49). LPS stimulation can lead to lipid raft mobilization around SHIP-1, followed by activation of MAPK and release of TNF-α (50). Although the regulation of PI3K-Akt is not fully understood, our study reveals that gram-negative bacterial-mediated SHIP-1 mobilization to lipid rafts is related to PI3K-Akt (50, 51). Lipid rafts dynamic refers to the microdomain formation when membrane lipids and proteins intermingle, which may be a signal for cells to respond to acute infections. Our results showed that SHIP-1-deficient mice exhibited faster bacterial dissemination. Moreover, the penetration of PMN is increased in the lungs and increased ROS secretion that aggravates lung injury. Collectively, these observations indicate that SHIP-1 is critically involved in host inflammatory responses in *Pseudomonas aeruginosa* infection.

Macrophages are a type of white blood cells located in tissues derived from monocyte (52). Their main function is to phagocytize pathogens and activate lymphocytes or other immune cells to respond to pathogens, which is vital for innate immunity and adaptive immunity (53). Macrophages are divided into two subtypes according to their functions: proinflammatory M1 macrophages and anti-inflammatory M2 macrophages (54). The function of macrophages is regulated by multiple signaling pathways (55). Macrophage polarization is a process to adapt different functional programs in response to the signals from their microenvironment (42). We revealed that SHIP-$1^{-/-}$ mice displayed skewed M2 macrophages, which are hyporesponsive to proinflammatory stimuli and associated with tissue remodeling, wound healing, Th2 immunity promotion, and debris clearing, indicating that SHIP-1 is a negative regulator of M2 (56). SHIP-$1^{-/-}$ mice have the tendency to spontaneously develop chronic lung diseases with myeloid cell infiltration and

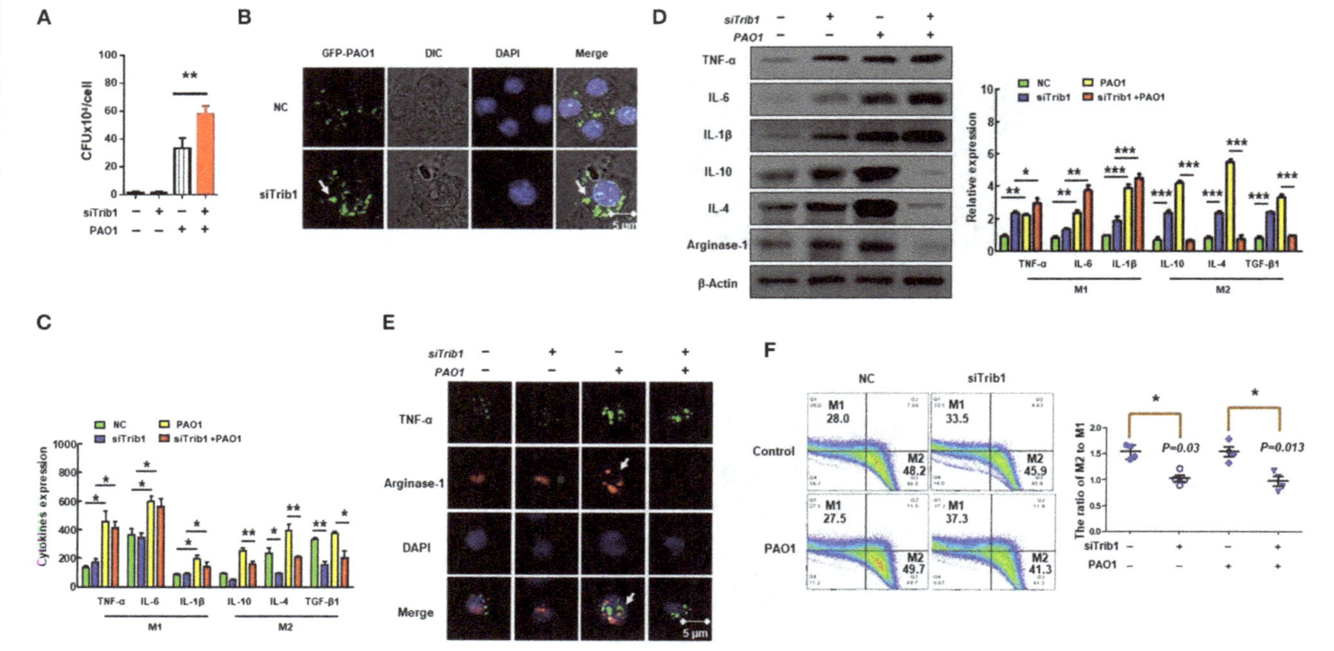

FIGURE 6 | Trib1 regulates polarization of M2-like macrophages. MH-S cells were transfected with Trib1 siRNA or negative siRNA for 48 h, followed by PAO1 infection for 2 h (uninfected group MH-S cells as control); knockout efficiency was detected by western blotting (**Figure S3**). **(A)** Phagocytosis was measured by colony-forming unit (CFU). **(B)** Immunofluorescence was used to show the number of intracellular green fluorescent protein (GFP)–PAO1. **(C)** ELISA determining the expression of M1 macrophage markers (IL-6, INF-γ, and TNF-α) and M2 macrophage markers (IL-10, IL-4, and TGF-β1). **(D)** Western blotting analyzing the expression of M1 macrophage markers (TNF-α, IL-6, and IL-1β) and M2 macrophages markers (IL-10, IL-4, and arginase-1). **(E)** TNF-α for M1 macrophage marker and arginase-1 for M2 macrophage marker analyzed by immunofluorescence. **(F)** The relative expression levels of M1 macrophages (CD38) and M2 macrophages (Egr2) were detected by flow cytometry. (The data are mean ± SEM and are representative of three independent experiments, one-way ANOVA with Tukey *post hoc* test, $^{*}p < 0.05$, $^{**}p < 0.01$, $^{***}p < 0.01$).

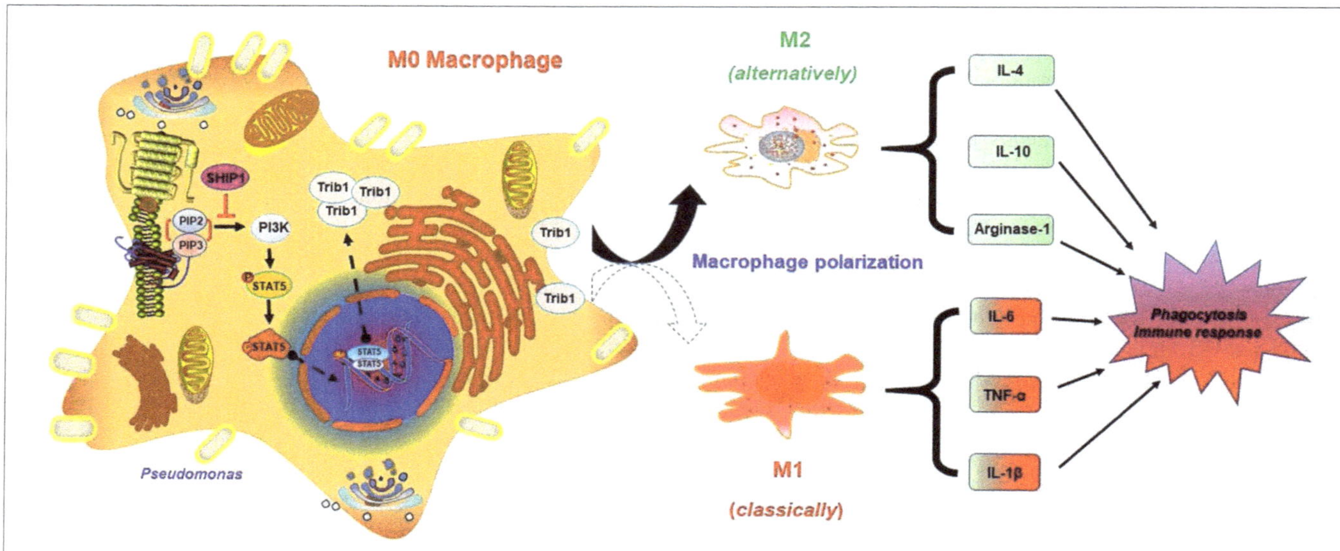

FIGURE 7 | Schematic illustration of the signaling pathways for SHIP-1 regulating phagocytosis and M2 polarization through the Akt–STAT5–Trib1 circuit. Infected macrophages inhibit the overexpression of PI3K by SHIP-1, preventing hyperactivation of STAT5, and Trib1, which is critical for maintaining the polarization balance of macrophages and resistance to bacteria by secreting diverse inflammatory factors and regulating phagocytosis. Depletion of SHIP-1 triggers the excessive activation of PI3K/Akt–STAT5–Trib1 signal pathway, causing macrophage polarization imbalance to superabundant switch to M2. M1 macrophage markers (TNF-α, IL-6, and IL-1β) and M2 macrophage markers (IL-10, IL-4, and arginase-1) were used to evaluate macrophage polarization. Both defect in phagocytosis and dysregulated cytokine production may cause the aggravated infection. Ultimately, impaired phagocytosis of macrophages leads to the expansion of infection.

macrophage subpopulation accumulation, and the number of M2 usually increased after infection (57, 58). However, the molecular mechanism of SHIP-1-mediated macrophage polarization during *P. aeruginosa* infection is still largely unclear. We evaluated the role of macrophage polarization and phagocytosis in SHIP-1 knockdown MH-S cells, and our results demonstrated that SHIP-1 deficiency impaired phagocytosis and M2 polarization. Trib1 proteins have also been reported to regulate the inflammation and macrophage polarization by activating MAPK (59, 60). We found that Trib1 is critically involved in macrophage polarization and phagocytosis by suppression of Trib1 expression in MH-S cells. These results indicate that SHIP-1 regulates M2 macrophage polarization and phagocytic function by activating the Akt–STAT5–Trib1 axis.

In summary, we have investigated the role of SHIP-1 in PAO1-challenged SHIP-1$^{-/-}$ mice and identified SHIP-1 as a negative regulator of inflammatory responses through a PI3K/Akt–STAT5–Trib1 circuit. The aggravated infectious phenotype is involved in macrophage polarization and phagocytosis following SHIP-1 deletion. Overall, this particular phenotype results from release of various proinflammatory cytokines that can be inhibited by SHIP-1. Mechanistically, SHIP-1 deficiency activates phosphorylation of PI3K and regulates STAT5 nuclear transcription to induce the expression of Trib1. These findings reveal that SHIP-1 plays important roles in regulating inflammatory responses and macrophage function during *P. aeruginosa* infection through the PI3K/Akt–STAT5–Trib1 axis. Our research is the first demonstration that SHIP can indirectly regulate the expression of Trib1 through altering STAT5 activation to mediate the function of macrophages, which may provide significant insight into development of novel therapeutics to conquer bacterial infection. These studies may have some limitations, as we have not gone back to investigate the M1/M2 polarization in cell-specific manners in SHIP-1$^{-/-}$ mice. In addition, studies with additional time points besides 12 (mice) and 2 h (cells) would provide holistic and dynamic mechanisms for strengthening our newly discovered role of SHIP-1. Hence, further study is warranted to understand how the M2 polarization caused by the SHIP deficiency in animals will affect the susceptibility to this bacterium in SHIP-1$^{-/-}$ mice.

ETHICS STATEMENT

The animal study was reviewed and approved by University of North Dakota Institutional Animal Care and Use Committee (IACUC).

AUTHOR CONTRIBUTIONS

SQ, YZ, HW, JL, and MW designed the project and wrote the manuscript. SQ, CZ, BP, HW, XD, and SQ designed and performed most of the experiments. JS, YZ, HW, MW, XD, ZX, and SQ analyzed the data.

ACKNOWLEDGMENTS

We thank the Imaging Core, Flow Cytometry Core, and Animal Center for excellent technical support.

REFERENCES

1. Lioubin MN, Algate PA, Tsai S, Carlberg K, Aebersold A, Rohrschneider LR. p150Ship, a signal transduction molecule with inositol polyphosphate-5-phosphatase activity. *Genes Dev.* (1996) 10:1084–95. doi: 10.1101/gad.10.9.1084
2. Ono M, Okada H, Boll S, Yanagi S, Kurosaki T, Ravetch JV. Deletion of SHIP or SHP-1 reveals two distinct pathways for inhibitory signaling. *Cell.* (1997) 90:293–301. doi: 10.1016/S0092-8674(00)80337-2
3. Ho L, Tan SY, Wee S, Wu Y, Tan SJ, Ramakrishna NB, et al. ELABELA is an endogenous growth factor that sustains hESC self-renewal via the PI3K/AKT pathway. *Cell Stem Cell.* (2015) 17:435–47. doi: 10.1016/j.stem.2015.09.018
4. Dobranowski P, Sly LM. SHIP negatively regulates type II immune responses in mast cells and macrophages. *J. Leukocyte Biol.* (2018) 103:1053–64. doi: 10.1002/JLB.3MIR0817-340R
5. Hamilton MJ, Halvorsen EC, LePard NE, Bosiljcic M, Ho VW, Lam V, et al. SHIP represses lung inflammation and inhibits mammary tumor metastasis in BALB/c mice. *Oncotarget.* (2016) 7:3677–91. doi: 10.18632/oncotarget.6611
6. Grassme H, Jendrossek V, Riehle A, von Kurthy G, Berger J, Schwarz H, et al. Host defense against *Pseudomonas aeruginosa* requires ceramide-rich membrane rafts. *Nat Med.* (2003) 9:322–30. doi: 10.1038/nm823
7. Kowalski MP, Pier GB. Localization of cystic fibrosis transmembrane conductance regulator to lipid rafts of epithelial cells is required for *Pseudomonas aeruginosa*-induced cellular activation. *J Immunol.* (2004) 172:418–25. doi: 10.4049/jimmunol.172.1.418
8. Biswas SK, Mantovani A. Macrophage plasticity and interaction with lymphocyte subsets: cancer as a paradigm. *Nat Immunol.* (2010) 11:889–96. doi: 10.1038/ni.1937
9. Martinez FO, Helming L, Gordon S. Alternative activation of macrophages: an immunologic functional perspective. *Ann Rev Immunol.* (2009) 27:451–83. doi: 10.1146/annurev.immunol.021908.132532
10. Yi-Hong C, Jing L, Lu H. [MicroRNA-155 induces macrophage polarization to M1 in Toxoplasma gondii infection]. *Zhongguo xue xi chong bing fang zhi za zhi Chin J Schistosomiasis Control.* (2019) 30:652–5. doi: 10.16250/j.32.1374.2018125
11. Suzuki K, Meguro K, Nakagomi D, Nakajima H. Roles of alternatively activated M2 macrophages in allergic contact dermatitis. *Allergol Int Offic J Japan Soc Allergol.* (2017) 66:392–7. doi: 10.1016/j.alit.2017.02.015
12. Ma PF, Gao CC, Yi J, Zhao JL, Liang SQ, Zhao Y, et al. Cytotherapy with M1-polarized macrophages ameliorates liver fibrosis by modulating immune microenvironment in mice. *J Hepatol.* (2017) 67:770–9. doi: 10.1016/j.jhep.2017.05.022
13. Lee PS, Teng CY, Hsieh KF, Chiou YS, Wu JC, Lu TJ, et al. Adzuki bean water extract attenuates obesity by modulating M2/M1 macrophage polarization and gut microbiota composition. *Mol Nutri Food Res.* (2019) 63:e1900626. doi: 10.1002/mnfr.201900626
14. Viola A, Munari F, Sanchez-Rodriguez R, Scolaro T, Castegna A. The metabolic signature of macrophage responses. *Front Immunol.* (2019) 10:1462. doi: 10.3389/fimmu.2019.01462
15. Wang Z, Bunting KD. STAT5 in hematopoietic stem cell biology and transplantation. *Jak Stat.* (2013) 2:e27159. doi: 10.4161/jkst.27159
16. Xiao W, Hong H, Kawakami Y, Lowell CA, Kawakami T. Regulation of myeloproliferation and M2 macrophage programming in mice by Lyn/Hck, SHIP, and Stat5. *J Clin Investig.* (2008) 118:924–34. doi: 10.1172/JCI34013
17. Kuroda E, Ho V, Ruschmann J, Antignano F, Hamilton M, Rauh MJ, et al. SHIP represses the generation of IL-3-induced M2 macrophages by inhibiting IL-4 production from basophils. *J Immunol.* (2009) 183:3652–60. doi: 10.4049/jimmunol.0900864

18. Meng Q, Liu J, Lin F, Bao L, Jiang Y, Zheng L, et al. IL-17 contributes to the pathogenesis of obliterative bronchiolitis via regulation of M1 macrophages polarization in murine heterotopic trachea transplantation models. *Int Immunopharmacol.* (2017) 52:51–60. doi: 10.1016/j.intimp.2017.08.022
19. Wilson DM, Kool ET. Ultrafast oxime formation enables efficient fluorescence light-up measurement of DNA base excision. *J Am Chem Soc.* (2013) 141:19379–88. doi: 10.1021/jacs.9b09812
20. Liu ZZ, Han ZD, Liang YK, Chen JX, Wan S, Zhuo YJ, et al. TRIB1 induces macrophages to M2 phenotype by inhibiting IKB-zeta in prostate cancer. *Cell Signal.* (2019) 59:152–62. doi: 10.1016/j.cellsig.2019.03.017
21. Arndt L, Dokas J, Gericke M, Kutzner CE, Muller S, Jeromin F, et al. Tribbles homolog 1 deficiency modulates function and polarization of murine bone marrow-derived macrophages. *J Biol Chem.* (2018) 293:11527–36. doi: 10.1074/jbc.RA117.000703
22. Shiraishi M, Shintani Y, Shintani Y, Ishida H, Saba R, Yamaguchi A, et al. Alternatively activated macrophages determine repair of the infarcted adult murine heart. *J Clin Investig.* (2016) 126:2151–66. doi: 10.1172/JCI85782
23. Pu Q, Gan C, Li R, Li Y, Tan S, Li X, et al. Atg7 deficiency intensifies inflammasome activation and pyroptosis in *Pseudomonas sepsis. J Immunol.* (2017) 198:3205–13. doi: 10.4049/jimmunol.1601196
24. Li X, He S, Li R, Zhou X, Zhang S, Yu M, et al. *Pseudomonas aeruginosa* infection augments inflammation through miR-301b repression of c-Myb-mediated immune activation and infiltration. *Nat Microbiol.* (2016) 1:16132. doi: 10.1038/nmicrobiol.2016.132
25. Rauh MJ, Ho V, Pereira C, Sham A, Sly LM, Lam V, et al. SHIP represses the generation of alternatively activated macrophages. *Immunity.* (2005) 23:361–74. doi: 10.1016/j.immuni.2005.09.003
26. Baran CP, Tridandapani S, Helgason CD, Humphries RK, Krystal G, Marsh CB. The inositol 5'-phosphatase SHIP-1 and the Src kinase Lyn negatively regulate macrophage colony-stimulating factor-induced Akt activity. *J Biol Chem.* (2003) 278:38628–36. doi: 10.1074/jbc.M305021200
27. Li R, Fang L, Pu Q, Bu H, Zhu P, Chen Z, et al. MEG3-4 is a miRNA decoy that regulates IL-1beta abundance to initiate and then limit inflammation to prevent sepsis during lung infection. *Sci Signal.* (2018) 11:eaao2387. doi: 10.1126/scisignal.aao2387
28. Mbawuike IN, Herscowitz HB. MH-S, a murine alveolar macrophage cell line: morphological, cytochemical, and functional characteristics. *J Leukocyte Biol.* (1989) 46:119–27. doi: 10.1002/jlb.46.2.119
29. Li R, Fang L, Pu Q, Lin P, Hoggarth A, Huang H, et al. Lyn prevents aberrant inflammatory responses to Pseudomonas infection in mammalian systems by repressing a SHIP-1-associated signaling cluster. *Signal Trans Target Therap'* (2016) 1:16032. doi: 10.1038/sigtrans.2016.32
30. Li R, Tan S, Yu M, Jundt MC, Zhang S, Wu M. Annexin A2 regulates autophagy in *Pseudomonas aeruginosa* infection through the Akt1-mTOR-ULK1/2 signaling pathway. *J Immunol.* (2015) 195:3901–11. doi: 10.4049/jimmunol.1500967
31. Kipnis E, Guery BP, Tournoys A, Leroy X, Robriquet L, Fialdes P, et al. Massive alveolar thrombin activation in *Pseudomonas aeruginosa*-induced acute lung injury. *Shock.* (2004) 21:444–51. doi: 10.1097/00024382-200405000-00008
32. Ye Y, Lin P, Zhang W, Tan S, Zhou X, Li R, et al. DNA repair interacts with autophagy to regulate inflammatory responses to pulmonary hyperoxia. *J. Immunol.* (2017) 198:2844–53. doi: 10.4049/jimmunol.1601001
33. Vijayasekaran S, Fitton JH, Hicks CR, Chirila TV, Crawford GJ, Constable IJ. Cell viability and inflammatory response in hydrogel sponges implanted in the rabbit cornea. *Biomaterials.* (1998) 19:2255–67. doi: 10.1016/S0142-9612(98)00128-8
34. Vergadi E, Ieronymaki E, Lyroni K, Vaporidi K, Tsatsanis C. Akt signaling pathway in macrophage activation and M1/M2 polarization. *J Immunol.* (2017) 198:1006–14. doi: 10.4049/jimmunol.1601515
35. Jablonski KA, Amici SA, Webb LM, D. Ruiz-Rosado Jde, Popovich PG, Partida-Sanchez S, et al. Novel markers to delineate murine M1 and M2 macrophages. *PLoS ONE.* (2015) 10:e0145342. doi: 10.1371/journal.pone.0145342
36. Li R, Fang L, Tan S, Yu M, Li X, He S, et al. Type I CRISPR-cas targets endogenous genes and regulates virulence to evade mammalian host immunity. *Cell Res.* (2016) 26:1273–87. doi: 10.1038/cr.2016.135
37. He YH, Wu M, Kobune M, Xu Y, Kelley MR, Martin WJ. Expression of yeast apurinic/apyrimidinic endonuclease (APN1) protects lung epithelial cells from bleomycin toxicity. *Am J Respir Cell Mol Biol.* (2001) 25:692–8. doi: 10.1165/ajrcmb.25.6.4550
38. Nicu EA, Loos BG. Polymorphonuclear neutrophils in periodontitis and their possible modulation as a therapeutic approach. *Periodontol 2000.* (2016) 71:140–63. doi: 10.1111/prd.12113
39. Piacenza L, Trujillo M, Radi R. Reactive species and pathogen antioxidant networks during phagocytosis. *J Exp Med.* (2019) 216:501–16. doi: 10.1084/jem.20181886
40. Shlyakhover E, Shklyar B, Hakim-Mishnaevski K, Levy-Adam F, Kurant E. Drosophila GATA factor serpent establishes phagocytic ability of embryonic macrophages. *Front Immunol.* (2018) 9:266. doi: 10.3389/fimmu.2018.00266
41. Krausgruber T, Blazek K, Smallie T, Alzabin S, Lockstone H, Sahgal N, et al. IRF5 promotes inflammatory macrophage polarization and TH1-TH17 responses. *Nat Immunol.* (2011) 12:231–8. doi: 10.1038/ni.1990
42. Satoh T, Takeuchi O, Vandenbon A, Yasuda K, Tanaka Y, Kumagai Y, et al. The Jmjd3-Irf4 axis regulates M2 macrophage polarization and host responses against helminth infection. *Nat Immunol.* (2010) 11:936–44. doi: 10.1038/ni.1920
43. Lv R, Bao Q, Li Y. Regulation of M1type and M2type macrophage polarization in RAW264.7 cells by Galectin9. *Mol Med Rep.* (2017) 16:9111–9. doi: 10.3892/mmr.2017.7719
44. Eyers PA, Keeshan K, Kannan N. Tribbles in the 21st century: the evolving roles of tribbles pseudokinases in biology and disease. *Trends Cell Biol.* (2017) 27:284–98. doi: 10.1016/j.tcb.2016.11.002
45. Gold MJ, Antignano F, Hughes MR, Zaph C, McNagny KM. Dendritic-cell expression of ship1 regulates Th2 immunity to helminth infection in mice. *Eur J Immunol.* (2016) 46:122–30. doi: 10.1002/eji.201545628
46. Sly LM, Rauh MJ, Kalesnikoff J, Song CH, Krystal G. LPS-induced upregulation of SHIP is essential for endotoxin tolerance. *Immunity.* (2004) 21:227–39. doi: 10.1016/j.immuni.2004.07.010
47. Oh SY, Zheng T, Bailey ML, Barber DL, Schroeder JT, Kim YK, et al. Src homology 2 domain-containing inositol 5-phosphatase 1 deficiency leads to a spontaneous allergic inflammation in the murine lung. *J Allergy Clin Immunol.* (2007) 119:123–31. doi: 10.1016/j.jaci.2006.08.029
48. Nakayama H, Nagafuku M, Suzuki A, Iwabuchi K, Inokuchi JI. The regulatory roles of glycosphingolipid-enriched lipid rafts in immune systems. *FEBS Lett.* (2018) 592:3921–42. doi: 10.1002/1873-3468.13275
49. Triantafilou M, Miyake K, Golenbock DT, Triantafilou K. Mediators of innate immune recognition of bacteria concentrate in lipid rafts and facilitate lipopolysaccharide-induced cell activation. *J Cell Sci.* (2002) 115:2603–11.
50. Cuschieri J, Bulger E, Biligren J, Garcia I, Maier RV. Vitamin E inhibits endotoxin-mediated transport of phosphatases to lipid rafts. *Shock.* (2007) 27:19–24. doi: 10.1097/01.shk.0000238060.61955.f8
51. Antignano F, Ibaraki M, Ruschmann J, Jagdeo J, Krystal G. SHIP negatively regulates Flt3L-derived dendritic cell generation and positively regulates MyD88-independent TLR-induced maturation. *J Leukocyte Biol.* (2010) 88:925–35. doi: 10.1189/jlb.1209825
52. Varol C, Mildner A, Jung S. Macrophages: development and tissue specialization. *Ann Rev Immunol.* (2015) 33:643–75. doi: 10.1146/annurev-immunol-032414-112220
53. Russell DG, Huang L, VanderVen BC. Immunometabolism at the interface between macrophages and pathogens. *Nat Rev Immunol.* (2019) 19:291–304. doi: 10.1038/s41577-019-0124-9
54. Leopold Wager CM, Arnett E, Schlesinger LS. Macrophage nuclear receptors: emerging key players in infectious diseases. *PLoS Pathog.* (2019) 15:e1007585. doi: 10.1371/journal.ppat.1007585
55. Abdullah Z, Knolle PA. Liver macrophages in healthy and diseased liver. *Pflugers Archiv Eur J Physiol.* (2017) 469:553–60. doi: 10.1007/s00424-017-1954-6
56. Sha H, Zhang D, Zhang Y, Wen Y, Wang Y. ATF3 promotes migration and M1/M2 polarization of macrophages by activating tenascinC via Wnt/betacatenin pathway. *Mol Med Rep.* (2017) 16:3641–7. doi: 10.3892/mmr.2017.6992

57. Nahrendorf M, Swirski FK. Abandoning M1/M2 for a network model of macrophage function. *Circul Res.* (2016) 119:414–7. doi: 10.1161/CIRCRESAHA.116.309194
58. Keeler DM, Grandal MK, McCall JR. Brevenal, a marine natural product, is anti-inflammatory and an immunomodulator of macrophage and lung epithelial cells. *Marine Drugs.* (2019) 17:184. doi: 10.3390/md17030184
59. Eder K, Guan H, Sung HY, Francis SE, Crossman DC, Kiss-Toth E. LDL uptake by monocytes in response to inflammation is MAPK dependent but independent of tribbles protein expression. *Immunol Lett.* (2008) 116:178–83. doi: 10.1016/j.imlet.2007.12.011
60. Guan C, Xiao Y, Li K, Wang T, Liang Y, Liao G. MMP-12 regulates proliferation of mouse macrophages via the ERK/P38 MAPK pathways during inflammation. *Exp Cell Res.* (2019) 378:182–90. doi: 10.1016/j.yexcr.2019.03.018

2

Mechanisms of Epithelial Immunity Evasion by Respiratory Bacterial Pathogens

*Lokesh Sharma[1], Jingjing Feng[1,2], Clemente J. Britto[1] and Charles S. Dela Cruz[1]**

[1] Section of Pulmonary, Critical Care and Sleep Medicine, Yale University School of Medicine, New Haven, CT, United States,
[2] Department of Respiratory Medicine, The Fifth People's Hospital of Shanghai, Fudan University, Shanghai, China

***Correspondence:**
Charles S. Dela Cruz
charles.delacruz@yale.edu

Bacterial lung infections are major healthcare challenges killing millions of people worldwide and resulting in a huge economic burden. Both basic and clinical research have elucidated host mechanisms that contribute to the bacterial clearance where an indispensable role of immune cells has been established. However, the role of respiratory epithelial cells in bacterial clearance has garnered limited attention due to their weak inflammatory or phagocytic ability compared to immune cells such as macrophages and neutrophils. These studies often underappreciate the fact that epithelial cells are the most abundant cells in the lung, not only serving as building blocks but also providing immune protection throughout the lung. Epithelial cells function either independently to eradicate the pathogen or communicate with immune cells to orchestrate pathogen clearance. The epithelial cells have multiple mechanisms that include mucus production, antimicrobial peptide production, muco-ciliary clearance, and phagocytosis, all of which contribute to their direct antibacterial function. Secretion of cytokines to recruit immune cells and potentiate their antimicrobial activities is a pathway by which the epithelium contributes to bacterial clearance. Successful pathogens outsmart epithelial resistance and find a way to replicate in sufficient numbers to establish infections in the airway or lung epithelial surfaces. In this mini-review, we discuss evidences that establish important roles for epithelial host defense against invading respiratory bacterial pathogens and demonstrate how pathogens outsmart these epithelial immune mechanisms to successfully establish infection. Finally, we discuss briefly how to boost epithelial immunity to improve outcomes in bacterial lung infections.

Keywords: bacterial dissemination, host pathogen interaction, epithelial immunity, pathogen evolution, lung epithelium

EPITHELIAL IMMUNITY IN THE LUNG

The lung surface area of more than 50 m^2 consists of epithelial monolayers which cover the upper and lower airways as well as lung alveoli (1). The large epithelial surfaces are continuously exposed to particles, pollutants, and microbes. It is not surprising that the lung epithelium has a well-developed immunity to fend off these microbes. Different subsets of lung epithelium are equipped with their unique antimicrobial mechanisms (2–4). While nasal epithelium is known to secrete large amounts of antimicrobial peptides (AMPs) and type II pneumocytes secrete surfactant proteins, both of these are host protective mechanisms against bacterial infections. Ciliated airway epithelium mechanically removes invading pathogens with the help of mucus secreted by the secretory epithelium. If the epithelium fails to limit the invading pathogens itself, the epithelium signals to seek the help of resident immune cells such as alveolar macrophages or to recruit immune cells to help eradicate the invading pathogen, which often comes at a cost of tissue injury, including to the epithelium (5, 6). Lung epithelium also contributes to the removal of dead inflammatory cells to ensure restoration of lost lung function post infection. However, pathogens have developed multiple mechanisms to avoid various epithelial resistance mechanisms. Respiratory pathogens discussed here include clinically relevant pathogens such as *Pseudomonas aeruginosa* (infects patients with chronic lung diseases such as cystic fibrosis and COPD) (7), *Streptococcus pneumoniae* (affects healthy people and causes post-viral bacterial infections) (8), *Staphylococcus aureus* (major cause of hospital-acquired pneumonia) (9), and *Klebsiella pneumoniae* (opportunistic pathogen with high antimicrobial resistant) (10).

Antimicrobial functions of the lung epithelium can be divided into two main categories: direct killing and indirect control of lung infections.

Direct Killing

Killing of the invading pathogen is the most effective strategy to remove the invading pathogen, however the primary aim of the epithelium is to survive the infection (**Figure 1**). To avoid unnecessary inflammatory damage, which may be unavoidable consequence of the pathogen killing, the host epithelium tolerates commensal microbes or colonizing pathogens, which are present at higher density especially in the upper respiratory tract (11). However, an appropriate level of active epithelial immunity is required to maintain the colonization status of these pathogens. Any impairment in the epithelial immunity can lead to infection from colonizing pathogens, as seen during influenza infection, where nasally colonized *Streptococcus* invades and establishes a lower respiratory tract infection (12). Multiple mechanisms have been attributed to influenza enhanced susceptibility including a damaged epithelial barrier, increased micronutrition due to cell death and decreased surfactant proteins (13). Other colonizing pathogens such as *Staphylococcus aureus* show similar infecting mechanisms post influenza, where colonizing pathogens are often associated with the disease. The detailed mechanisms of colonization are discussed in other reviews (14). The epithelium has multiple tools to limit the growth of pathogens or to remove them completely from the host.

Phagocytosis

Phagocytosis is the main mechanism of bacterial killing used by professional phagocytes such as macrophages and neutrophils. However, epithelial cells also possess significant phagocytic ability, which is often referred to as "internalization" against a wide range of bacterial pathogens (15, 16). There are major differences in the capacity and mechanisms of phagocytosis among the professional phagocytes and epithelial cells. Professional phagocytes like macrophages actively phagocytose the pathogens by recognizing them using its pattern recognition receptors, where antibody mediated opsonization plays a major role in the process (17). On the other hand, epithelial phagocytosis is relatively low and often initiated by the pathogen. Pathogens use two distinct mechanisms to enter the epithelial cells: "zipper" and "trigger" mechanisms (18). In the "zipper" mechanism, pathogen attachment induces rearrangement of actin cytoskeleton and the resultant internalization. In the "trigger" method, the pathogen secretes soluble factors that cause actin fiber rearrangement to form a phagocytic cup and subsequent internalization of the pathogen. However, the epithelium expresses various pattern recognition receptors that actively recognize the invading pathogen and allow them to respond to the pathogen by releasing cytokines and chemokines. A wide range of TLRs and nod like receptors have been detected on lung epithelium on both the surfaces as well as within the cell (19–21). Although epithelial cells have lower phagocytic activity per cell compared to the professional phagocytes, given the number of epithelial cells in the lung compartment and the surface area covered by these cells, their phagocytic activity provides significant contribution to pathogen clearance.

Phagocytosis allows digestion of the bacterial components within the cell and thus limits inflammatory signaling arising from extracellular bacterial killing. Antibiotic induced bacterial killing has been shown to be highly inflammatory (22). Phagocytic ability of the epithelium also helps maintain the homeostatic lung environment, which is disrupted in the aftermath of an infectious injury by an abundance of dead cells and cellular debris from various cells, including the epithelium. Epithelial phagocytosis of apoptotic cells is dependent on small GTPase Rac-1, which allows the epithelium to secrete anti-inflammatory cytokines upon phagocytosis of cell debris to inhibit inflammatory recruitment and restore homeostasis (23).

How pathogens circumvent phagocytic ability

Epithelial-mediated phagocytosis is dependent on various host and pathogen factors. Pathogens often harbor structures on their surface to evade epithelial phagocytosis as seen in *Klebsiella*, where the amount of capsular polysaccharide is inversely related to epithelial internalization. As expected, bacterial strains lacking capsular polysaccharides are effectively cleared by the lung epithelium (24). *Pseudomonas* forms multicellular complexes known as biofilms, which are enormous in size, to prevent phagocytosis (25, 26). Avoiding epithelial phagocytosis may even provide *Pseudomonas* an advantage by dysregulating the inflammatory response and causing systemic sepsis that is detrimental to the host but supports bacterial growth (27). Some pathogens have developed ways to reside within the epithelium, such as *Bordetella* which uses host tubulin activity to enter the epithelial cells. This entry provides protection not only against antibiotic treatment but also against host antimicrobial peptides (28). Pathogens also avoid fusion with acidic lysosomes, which are filled with enzymes that can lyse the bacterial cell wall by manipulating cellular trafficking. Similarly, highly pathogenic strains of *Legionella* reside and replicate in the lung epithelium in addition to replicating within macrophages, which are normal targets of *Legionella* (29). Pathogens also alter their phenotype to adjust themselves within the epithelium to cause chronic

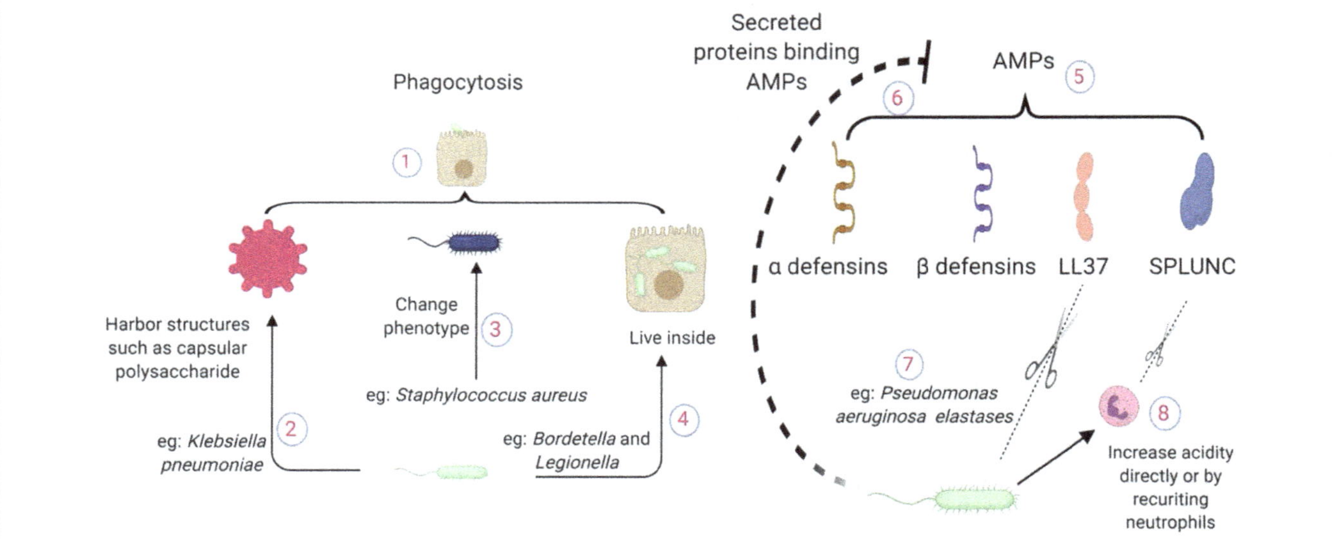

FIGURE 1 | Pathogen mechanisms to circumvent direct killing of bacteria by lung epithelial cells. (1) Epithelial cells possess phagocytic ability. (2) Bacteria harbor structures to evade epithelial phagocytosis, such as capsular polysaccharides of *Klebsiella pneumoniae.* (3) Altered phenotypes in pathogens cause chronic infections e.g., small colony variant of *Staphylococcus aureus*. (4) Pathogens can live inside the lung epithelium e.g., *Bordetella or Legionella.* (5) Epithelium releases antimicrobial peptides during lung infections, which bind to the pathogen surface and neutralize the pathogen. (6) During inflammation, a large number of proteins are accumulated in the lung. AMPs interact with other proteins and lose their antimicrobial potency. (7) *P. aeruginosa* elastase breaks down human LL37 in a dose dependent manner. (8) Pathogen recruited neutrophils contribute to the acidity. SPLUNC loses its function in an acidic environment; also, neutrophil elastases can break down SPLUNC. AMPs, antimicrobial proteins and peptides; SPLUNC, short palate lung and nasal epithelium clone 1.

infections. A small colony variant of *Staphylococcus aureus* often persists intracellularly including in the epithelium due to its ability to exert minimal inflammatory response compared to wild type strains (30). These examples demonstrate a wide array of pathogen mechanisms to outsmart epithelial phagocytosis, which contributes to the disease pathogenesis.

Antimicrobial Proteins and Peptides (AMPs)

The lung epithelium is a primary source of many AMPs released during lung infection. AMPs are charged peptides that can bind to the pathogen surface and kill them. These AMPs are separate from complement pathways, which primarily "tag" the pathogen to be identified by professional phagocytes, although some evidences of direct killing of pathogens by complements has been reported (31).

Defensins are a group of AMPs, of which β-defensins are almost exclusively secreted by the lung epithelium (32). Inflammatory cytokines produced during infection can lead to the release of AMPs (33, 34). The role of AMPs has been well established whereby they kill a wide range of pathogens including *E. coli*, *Pseudomonas* and *Haemophilus influenzae* in a salt dependent manner (34, 35). These antibacterial effects are confirmed in a mouse model of *H. influenzae,* where β-defensin deficiency impaired bacterial clearance (36). Over-expression of β-defensin 2 in a porcine model has been shown to increase the clearance of *Actinobacillus pleuropneumoniae* (37).

Cathelicidins, another important epithelial AMPs, are cleaved into their mature form LL37. Unlike β-defensins, only a single cathelicidin peptide has been found in the lungs of various species, including humans. The positively charged LL37 is secreted by lung epithelial cells (38) and has bactericidal activity against a variety of lung pathogens such as *P. aeruginosa* and *S. aureus* (39, 40). Besides direct antibacterial activity, LL37 also promotes bacterial phagocytosis in macrophages (41), indicating AMPs serve as important communicators between the epithelial and immune cells.

More recently, short palate lung and nasal epithelium clone 1 (SPLUNC) has been identified as an important AMP expressed in the upper airways and has a binding affinity for lipopolysaccharides (LPS) (42). SPLUNC has been shown to protect mice from infection with respiratory pathogens such as *P. aeruginosa* and *Mycoplasma* (43, 44). Furthermore, this study demonstrated that there might be a positive feedback mechanism between various AMPs since deficiency of SPLUNC1 led to decreased expression in LL37.

How pathogens evade AMP mediated death

Successful pathogens often develop strategies to overcome AMP-mediated host defense. These strategies include cleavage of AMPs by secreted proteases such as aureolysin and V8 protease from *S. aureus* (45). *P. aeruginosa* elastase can effectively break down LL37 (46) and SPLUNC (47). Given the wide substrate range, it is very likely that various AMPs are susceptible to host neutrophil elastase mediated cleavage and subsequent loss of antibacterial activity, as neutrophil elastase levels are significantly increased during bacterial infections (48).

During inflammation, a large number of host and pathogen proteins/products are accumulated in the lung airspace. Given

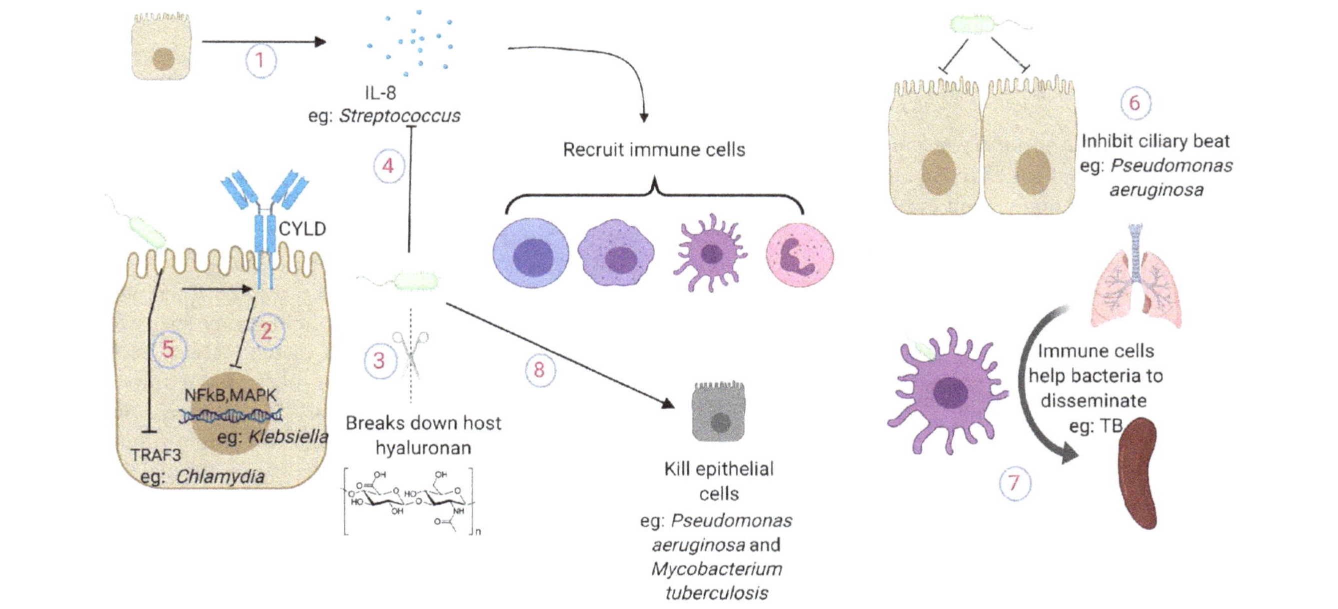

FIGURE 2 | Pathogen tactics to avoid indirect killing during lung infections. (1) Lung epithelium secrete cytokines and chemokines to recruit immune cells in the lung. (2) Klebsiella inhibits the activation of NFkB and MAPK pathway by promoting the expression of ubiquitinating enzyme CYLD in lung epithelial cells. (3) Gram positive pathogens break down host hyaluronan. (4) *Streptococcus* cleaves and inactivates IL-8. (5) Chlamydia targets TRAF3 in the epithelial cells. (6) *Pseudomonas aeruginosa* inhibits ciliary beat function. (7) Macrophages and dendritic cells carry TB from the lung to secondary lymphoid organs. (8) Pathogens induce damage to lung cells or to the extracellular matrix. IL-8, interleukin-8; NFkB, nuclear factor kappa B; MAPK, mitogen activated protein kinase; TRAF3, TNF receptor-associated factor 3.

the charged nature of AMPs, they easily interact with other charged molecules and lose their antimicrobial potency (49). Pathogens also modulate the lung environment to decrease the toxicity of AMPs. For example, the antimicrobial properties of SPLUNC are lost in the airways in cystic fibrosis due to its acidic environment. Pathogens can directly create an acidic environment by changing their metabolic activity or by recruiting metabolically active immune cells such as neutrophils (50).

Pathogens also shed components that actively bind to AMPs and prevent their binding to the bacterial surface to avoid AMP mediated toxicity. LPS, a part of the bacterial outer membrane in gram negative pathogens, are shed during infection. β-defensin binds to LPS and blocks its signaling. At the same time, LPS effectively block the antimicrobial activity of AMPs by direct binding (51). The capsule polysaccharide from *K. pneumoniae* has been shown to act as a bacterial decoy for AMPs secreted by the host to abrogate antimicrobial capacity (52).

Indirect Control of Lung Infections

Despite having well-developed mechanisms to prevent bacterial invasion, the epithelium often fails to completely eradicate the pathogens. In these situations, the epithelium often collaborates with other cells to ensure proper removal of invading pathogens. In cases where removing the pathogen completely seems impossible, the epithelium ensures that the infection remains localized and does not spread systemically. To perform these indirect functions, the epithelium communicates with other cells either by direct contact or by releasing soluble factors like cytokines and chemokines. Mechanisms of indirect pathogens control include the following: (see **Figure 2**).

Recruitment of Immune Cells

If the lung epithelium fails to control the growth of invading pathogens, it recruits immune cells to participate in the bacterial removal process. To sense pathogen, pattern recognition receptors are expressed on both apical and basolateral surfaces of the epithelium (20). Upon recognition of the pathogens, these cells secrete cytokines and chemokines to increase the expression of complementary adhesion molecules on the vascular endothelium and immune cells. The epithelium itself also expresses adhesion molecules such as ICAM-1 and VCAM1 (53) to facilitate the recruitment of immune cells in the lung. Epithelial-macrophage interactions can further amplify the secretion of cytokines to mount a robust inflammatory response; for example, epithelial release of CXCL8 can be enhanced by incubation with macrophages or macrophage supernatants (54). Upon recruitment, immune cells eliminate the pathogens by phagocytosis or extracellular killing by neutrophils and macrophage extracellular traps (55–57). Immune cells are highly effective in pathogen clearance but may cause lung injury by proteolytic enzymes contained within the immune cells. Upon pathogen clearance, the epithelium also contributes to clearance of the infiltrated immune cells. Conventionally, macrophages have been credited to clear the dead cells present in the lung post inflammatory response; however, recent studies have also implicated important roles of the lung epithelium in clearing the dead cells and cellular debris from the lung and preventing persistent inflammation (58). Blocking epithelial phagocytosis by inducible mutation of small GTPase Rac1 leads to persistent lung inflammation (23).

How pathogens blunt inflammatory responses

As inflammation is essential for effective clearance of invading bacterial pathogens, the pathogens can evade this inflammation by either suppressing the inflammatory response or by causing excessive inflammatory response. *K. pneumoniae* lung infections often induce very limited early inflammatory response, and it successfully disseminates across organs before inducing a robust inflammatory response (59). *Klebsiella* inhibits the activation of NFkB and MAPK pathway by promoting the expression of ubiquitinating enzyme CYLD in lung epithelial cells (60). *Streptococcus* secretes hyaluronidases that break down host hyaluronan into small components that inhibit not only inflammatory host hyaluronan fragments but also other TLR ligands such as LPS (61). Epithelial cells can recognize the pathogens and secrete IL-8, which is a potent chemokine in the lungs (62). *Streptococcus* species that cause aggressive disseminating disease have developed mechanisms by which they can cleave and inactivate IL-8 to blunt the inflammatory response through cell envelope proteinase (63). *Chlamydia pneumoniae* manipulates epithelial immunity by targeting TRAF3 in the epithelial cells and thus impairing TRAF3 mediated immunity (64). In contrast, some pathogens can use the presence of inflammatory cytokines as growth factors and survive excessive inflammation (65).

Prevent Bacterial Dissemination

The lung epithelium is a continuous barrier between the environment and circulation. This barrier ensures that pathogens in the lung do not achieve access to the circulation. Pathogens often strive to reach the blood circulation, likely due to the high amount of nutrients present in the blood. It is well documented that systemic spread of lung infection results in higher mortality compared to localized lung infection (66, 67).

The tight junctions between the lung epithelium are maintained by various junction proteins such as occludin family members and ZO-1 (68). Various enhancements in the lung epithelium increases the effectiveness of the barrier. These include muco-ciliary clearance in the upper airways (69) and surfactant proteins secreted by type II pneumocytes, which can promote bacterial killing including *Klebsiella* (70). Together these physical and biochemical structures ensure that lung infections do not extend outside the lung compartment.

How pathogens circumvent the epithelial immunity to disseminate

Ciliary beat function serves as one of the first physical defenses to prevent the pathogen from reaching the lung and subsequently causing systemic infection. It has been shown that virulence factors from *P. aeruginosa* can significantly inhibit ciliary beat, possibly allowing the bacteria to stick to the lung epithelium (71). Despite maintaining the uniform monolayer with sealed tight junctions, the epithelium provides regulated passage to immune cells such as those recruited during infections. This passage is provided by expression of complementary adhesion molecules on both immune and epithelial cells (72). Pathogens often take advantage of this host mechanism to spread by hiding within the immune cells. Antigen presenting cells such as macrophages and dendritic cells are well known to sense the pathogen and leave the lung compartment to present the antigen to lymphoid organs. However, recent evidence suggests that neutrophils also leave the lung and return to the bone marrow through the circulation once the inflammation is resolved (73). Macrophages and dendritic cells are believed to carry *Mycobacteria tuberculosis* from the lung to secondary lymphoid organs such as spleen (74). Other mechanisms of bacterial dissemination across the lung epithelium such as "ejectosomes" observed in amoeba have not yet been described in mammals (75). Pathogens also use TLR pathways to downregulate expression of tight junction protein claudins 7 and 10, which are essential to maintain intercellular junctions (76). Inhibition of claudins allows the pathogen to escape the lung by increasing epithelial permeability and causing systemic disease.

Various pathogens also induce damage to the lung structure by either directly killing epithelial cells or by digesting the extracellular matrix. These effects can be directly caused by pathogens or by pathogen induced host responses (77). *P. aeruginosa* has been shown to inject Exos, a potent toxin, using its type III secretion system to induce localized epithelial cell death to facilitate bacterial dissemination (78). Pore forming toxins secreted by a wide range of pathogens have also been shown to cause necroptotic cell death in the lung epithelium (79). Damage to the lung epithelium by other exposures such as hyperoxia or exposure to environmental particles increases the bacterial dissemination for *P. aeruginosa* (80). *M. tuberculosis* can directly cause epithelial death by secreting virulence factors such as ESAT6, leading to its dissemination (81).

BOOSTING EPITHELIAL IMMUNITY

Antibiotics remain the current first line therapy for bacterial infections, but their efficacy is being challenged with current rising of antimicrobial resistance (82). Given the urgency, it is essential to develop alternatives to treat lung infections. As the epithelium provides important host defense, it is logical to boost their function to improve outcomes during infections. Boosting the epithelial host defense can provide an important immunomodulatory strategy, especially in patients who have either a limited number of immune cells (genetic or acquired immunodeficiency, chemotherapy), a defect in immunity derived particularly from defects in the lung epithelium (such as CF), a recipient of lung transplant (where immunosuppression is required to prevent lung rejection) or those with extremes of the age. Boosting epithelial immunity can not only prevent the collateral damage that can be caused by recruited immune cells but also circumvent the need to remove the immune cells from tissue once the invading bacteria is cleared.

A large number of mouse studies have demonstrated the usefulness of promoting epithelial resistance to help the host clear

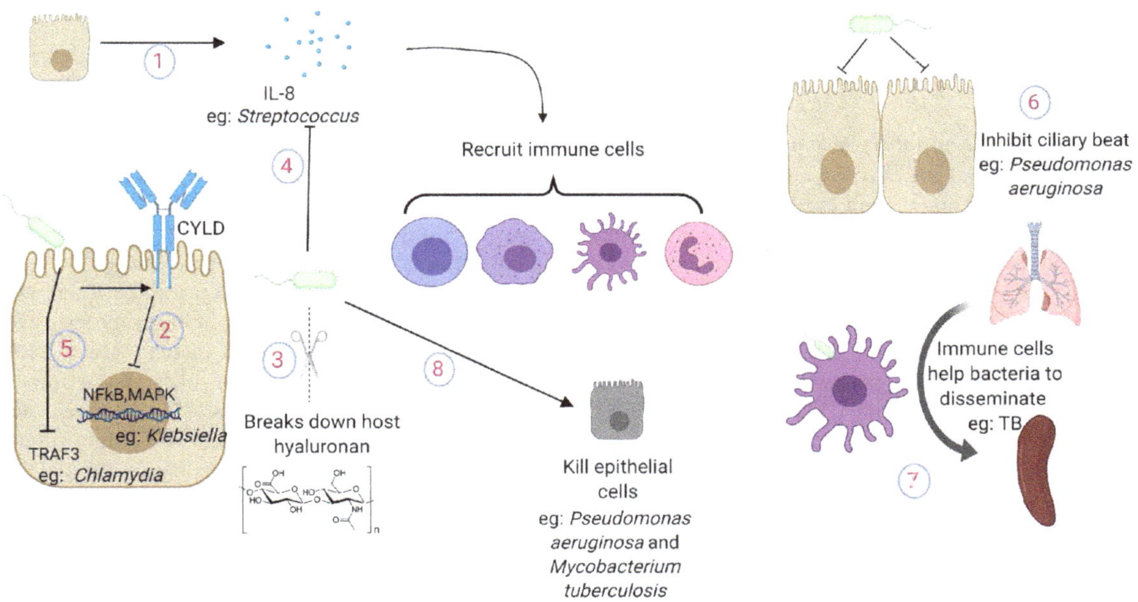

FIGURE 2 | Pathogen tactics to avoid indirect killing during lung infections. (1) Lung epithelium secrete cytokines and chemokines to recruit immune cells in the lung. (2) Klebsiella inhibits the activation of NFkB and MAPK pathway by promoting the expression of ubiquitinating enzyme CYLD in lung epithelial cells. (3) Gram positive pathogens break down host hyaluronan. (4) *Streptococcus* cleaves and inactivates IL-8. (5) Chlamydia targets TRAF3 in the epithelial cells. (6) *Pseudomonas aeruginosa* inhibits ciliary beat function. (7) Macrophages and dendritic cells carry TB from the lung to secondary lymphoid organs. (8) Pathogens induce damage to lung cells or to the extracellular matrix. IL-8, interleukin-8; NFkB, nuclear factor kappa B; MAPK, mitogen activated protein kinase; TRAF3, TNF receptor-associated factor 3.

the charged nature of AMPs, they easily interact with other charged molecules and lose their antimicrobial potency (49). Pathogens also modulate the lung environment to decrease the toxicity of AMPs. For example, the antimicrobial properties of SPLUNC are lost in the airways in cystic fibrosis due to its acidic environment. Pathogens can directly create an acidic environment by changing their metabolic activity or by recruiting metabolically active immune cells such as neutrophils (50).

Pathogens also shed components that actively bind to AMPs and prevent their binding to the bacterial surface to avoid AMP mediated toxicity. LPS, a part of the bacterial outer membrane in gram negative pathogens, are shed during infection. β-defensin binds to LPS and blocks its signaling. At the same time, LPS effectively block the antimicrobial activity of AMPs by direct binding (51). The capsule polysaccharide from *K. pneumoniae* has been shown to act as a bacterial decoy for AMPs secreted by the host to abrogate antimicrobial capacity (52).

Indirect Control of Lung Infections

Despite having well-developed mechanisms to prevent bacterial invasion, the epithelium often fails to completely eradicate the pathogens. In these situations, the epithelium often collaborates with other cells to ensure proper removal of invading pathogens. In cases where removing the pathogen completely seems impossible, the epithelium ensures that the infection remains localized and does not spread systemically. To perform these indirect functions, the epithelium communicates with other cells either by direct contact or by releasing soluble factors like cytokines and chemokines. Mechanisms of indirect pathogens control include the following: (see **Figure 2**).

Recruitment of Immune Cells

If the lung epithelium fails to control the growth of invading pathogens, it recruits immune cells to participate in the bacterial removal process. To sense pathogen, pattern recognition receptors are expressed on both apical and basolateral surfaces of the epithelium (20). Upon recognition of the pathogens, these cells secrete cytokines and chemokines to increase the expression of complementary adhesion molecules on the vascular endothelium and immune cells. The epithelium itself also expresses adhesion molecules such as ICAM-1 and VCAM1 (53) to facilitate the recruitment of immune cells in the lung. Epithelial-macrophage interactions can further amplify the secretion of cytokines to mount a robust inflammatory response; for example, epithelial release of CXCL8 can be enhanced by incubation with macrophages or macrophage supernatants (54). Upon recruitment, immune cells eliminate the pathogens by phagocytosis or extracellular killing by neutrophils and macrophage extracellular traps (55–57). Immune cells are highly effective in pathogen clearance but may cause lung injury by proteolytic enzymes contained within the immune cells. Upon pathogen clearance, the epithelium also contributes to clearance of the infiltrated immune cells. Conventionally, macrophages have been credited to clear the dead cells present in the lung post inflammatory response; however, recent studies have also implicated important roles of the lung epithelium in clearing the dead cells and cellular debris from the lung and preventing persistent inflammation (58). Blocking epithelial phagocytosis by inducible mutation of small GTPase Rac1 leads to persistent lung inflammation (23).

How pathogens blunt inflammatory responses

As inflammation is essential for effective clearance of invading bacterial pathogens, the pathogens can evade this inflammation by either suppressing the inflammatory response or by causing excessive inflammatory response. *K. pneumoniae* lung infections often induce very limited early inflammatory response, and it successfully disseminates across organs before inducing a robust inflammatory response (59). *Klebsiella* inhibits the activation of NFkB and MAPK pathway by promoting the expression of ubiquitinating enzyme CYLD in lung epithelial cells (60). *Streptococcus* secretes hyaluronidases that break down host hyaluronan into small components that inhibit not only inflammatory host hyaluronan fragments but also other TLR ligands such as LPS (61). Epithelial cells can recognize the pathogens and secrete IL-8, which is a potent chemokine in the lungs (62). *Streptococcus* species that cause aggressive disseminating disease have developed mechanisms by which they can cleave and inactivate IL-8 to blunt the inflammatory response through cell envelope proteinase (63). *Chlamydia pneumoniae* manipulates epithelial immunity by targeting TRAF3 in the epithelial cells and thus impairing TRAF3 mediated immunity (64). In contrast, some pathogens can use the presence of inflammatory cytokines as growth factors and survive excessive inflammation (65).

Prevent Bacterial Dissemination

The lung epithelium is a continuous barrier between the environment and circulation. This barrier ensures that pathogens in the lung do not achieve access to the circulation. Pathogens often strive to reach the blood circulation, likely due to the high amount of nutrients present in the blood. It is well documented that systemic spread of lung infection results in higher mortality compared to localized lung infection (66, 67).

The tight junctions between the lung epithelium are maintained by various junction proteins such as occludin family members and ZO-1 (68). Various enhancements in the lung epithelium increases the effectiveness of the barrier. These include muco-ciliary clearance in the upper airways (69) and surfactant proteins secreted by type II pneumocytes, which can promote bacterial killing including *Klebsiella* (70). Together these physical and biochemical structures ensure that lung infections do not extend outside the lung compartment.

How pathogens circumvent the epithelial immunity to disseminate

Ciliary beat function serves as one of the first physical defenses to prevent the pathogen from reaching the lung and subsequently causing systemic infection. It has been shown that virulence factors from *P. aeruginosa* can significantly inhibit ciliary beat, possibly allowing the bacteria to stick to the lung epithelium (71). Despite maintaining the uniform monolayer with sealed tight junctions, the epithelium provides regulated passage to immune cells such as those recruited during infections. This passage is provided by expression of complementary adhesion molecules on both immune and epithelial cells (72). Pathogens often take advantage of this host mechanism to spread by hiding within the immune cells. Antigen presenting cells such as macrophages and dendritic cells are well known to sense the pathogen and leave the lung compartment to present the antigen to lymphoid organs. However, recent evidence suggests that neutrophils also leave the lung and return to the bone marrow through the circulation once the inflammation is resolved (73). Macrophages and dendritic cells are believed to carry *Mycobacteria tuberculosis* from the lung to secondary lymphoid organs such as spleen (74). Other mechanisms of bacterial dissemination across the lung epithelium such as "ejectosomes" observed in amoeba have not yet been described in mammals (75). Pathogens also use TLR pathways to downregulate expression of tight junction protein claudins 7 and 10, which are essential to maintain intercellular junctions (76). Inhibition of claudins allows the pathogen to escape the lung by increasing epithelial permeability and causing systemic disease.

Various pathogens also induce damage to the lung structure by either directly killing epithelial cells or by digesting the extracellular matrix. These effects can be directly caused by pathogens or by pathogen induced host responses (77). *P. aeruginosa* has been shown to inject Exos, a potent toxin, using its type III secretion system to induce localized epithelial cell death to facilitate bacterial dissemination (78). Pore forming toxins secreted by a wide range of pathogens have also been shown to cause necroptotic cell death in the lung epithelium (79). Damage to the lung epithelium by other exposures such as hyperoxia or exposure to environmental particles increases the bacterial dissemination for *P. aeruginosa* (80). *M. tuberculosis* can directly cause epithelial death by secreting virulence factors such as ESAT6, leading to its dissemination (81).

BOOSTING EPITHELIAL IMMUNITY

Antibiotics remain the current first line therapy for bacterial infections, but their efficacy is being challenged with current rising of antimicrobial resistance (82). Given the urgency, it is essential to develop alternatives to treat lung infections. As the epithelium provides important host defense, it is logical to boost their function to improve outcomes during infections. Boosting the epithelial host defense can provide an important immunomodulatory strategy, especially in patients who have either a limited number of immune cells (genetic or acquired immunodeficiency, chemotherapy), a defect in immunity derived particularly from defects in the lung epithelium (such as CF), a recipient of lung transplant (where immunosuppression is required to prevent lung rejection) or those with extremes of the age. Boosting epithelial immunity can not only prevent the collateral damage that can be caused by recruited immune cells but also circumvent the need to remove the immune cells from tissue once the invading bacteria is cleared.

A large number of mouse studies have demonstrated the usefulness of promoting epithelial resistance to help the host clear the invading pathogens. These strategies involve stimulation with TLR ligands. These include single reagents such as flagellin (for TLR5) (83), poly I:C (84), aminoalkyl glucosaminide phosphate (synthetic TLR4 ligand) (85), CpG ODN (TLR 9 ligand) (86) or a combination of two or more ligands such as Pam2CSK4 + ODNM62 (87). Possible mechanisms of this trained immunity include early recruitment of immune cells (88) and promoting epithelial resistance by epigenetic changes (89) or promoting reactive oxygen species production (90).

Although these strategies have been highly successful in the mouse models, their use in susceptible human populations still needs to be confirmed. Major challenges in their success remain to be their tolerability in subjects and their provision of sufficient protection in the lungs against these infections.

In summary, the epithelium provides an array of host defense mechanisms to prevent and control bacterial lung infections. However, pathogens often circumvent these mechanisms to establish successful infections. Our aim should be to improve the epithelial host defense to boost host immunity and improve survival in lung infections.

AUTHOR CONTRIBUTIONS

LS drafted the manuscript. JF prepared the figures. CB Provided critical comments. CD revised the manuscript and provided critical comments.

REFERENCES

1. Hasleton PS. The internal surface area of the adult human lung. *J Anat.* (1972) 112(Pt 3):391–400.
2. Knowles MR, Boucher RC. Mucus clearance as a primary innate defense mechanism for mammalian airways. *J Clin Invest.* (2002) 109:571–7. doi: 10.1172/JCI0215217
3. Mason RJ. Biology of alveolar type II cells. *Respirology.* (2006) 11:S12–5. doi: 10.1111/j.1440-1843.2006.00800.x
4. Leiva-Juárez MM, Kolls JK, Evans SE. Lung epithelial cells: therapeutically inducible effectors of antimicrobial defense. *Mucosal Immunol.* (2018) 11:21–34. doi: 10.1038/mi.2017.71
5. Moldoveanu B, Otmishi P, Jani P, Walker J, Sarmiento X, Guardiola J, Saad M, Yu J. Inflammatory mechanisms in the lung. *J Inflamm Res.* (2009) 2:1–11.
6. Grommes J, Soehnlein O. Contribution of neutrophils to acute lung injury. *Mol Med.* (2011) 17:293. doi: 10.2119/molmed.2010.00138
7. Gellatly SL, Hancock RE. *Pseudomonas aeruginosa*: new insights into pathogenesis and host defenses. *Pathog Dis.* (2013) 67:159–73. doi: 10.1111/2049-632X.12033
8. van der Poll T, Opal SM. Pathogenesis, treatment, and prevention of pneumococcal pneumonia. *Lancet.* (2009) 374:1543–56. doi: 10.1016/S0140-6736(09)61114-4
9. Jones RN. Microbial etiologies of hospital-acquired bacterial pneumonia and ventilator-associated bacterial pneumonia. *Clin Infect Dis.* (2010) 51(Suppl_1):S81–7. doi: 10.1086/653053
10. Munoz-Price LS, Poirel L, Bonomo RA, Schwaber MJ, Daikos GL, Cormican M, et al. Clinical epidemiology of the global expansion of *Klebsiella pneumoniae* carbapenemases. *Lancet Infect Dis.* (2013) 13:785–96. doi: 10.1016/S1473-3099(13)70190-7
11. Kirst ME, Baker D, Li E, Abu-Hasan M, Wang GP. Upper versus lower airway microbiome and metagenome in children with cystic fibrosis and their correlation with lung inflammation. *PLoS ONE.* (2019) 14:e0222323. doi: 10.1371/journal.pone.0222323
12. Small CL, Shaler CR, McCormick S, Jeyanathan M, Damjanovic D, Brown EG, et al. Influenza infection leads to increased susceptibility to subsequent bacterial superinfection by impairing NK cell responses in the lung. *J Immunol.* (2010) 184:2048–56. doi: 10.4049/jimmunol.0902772
13. McCullers JA. The co-pathogenesis of influenza viruses with bacteria in the lung. *Nat Rev Microbiol.* (2014) 12:252. doi: 10.1038/nrmicro3231
14. Siegel SJ, Weiser JN. Mechanisms of bacterial colonization of the respiratory tract. *Annu Rev Microbiol.* (2015) 69:425–44. doi: 10.1146/annurev-micro-091014-104209
15. Plotkowski MC, de Bentzmann S, Pereira SHM, Zahm J, Bajolet-Laudinat O, Roger P, et al. *Pseudomonas aeruginosa* internalization by human epithelial respiratory cells depends on cell differentiation, polarity, and junctional complex integrity. *Am J Respir Cell Mol Biol.* (1999) 20:880–90. doi: 10.1165/ajrcmb.20.5.3408
16. Fumagalli O, Tall BD, Schipper C, Oelschlaeger TA. N-glycosylated proteins are involved in efficient internalization of *Klebsiella pneumoniae* by cultured human epithelial cells. *Infect Immun.* (1997) 65:4445–51. doi: 10.1128/IAI.65.11.4445-4451.1997
17. Mosser DM, Zhang X. Measuring opsonic phagocytosis via fcγ receptors and complement receptors on macrophages. *Curr Protoc Immunol.* (2011) 95:14.27. doi: 10.1002/0471142735.im1427s95
18. Günther J, Seyfert H. The first line of defence: insights into mechanisms and relevance of phagocytosis in epithelial cells. *Semin Immunopathol.* (2018) 40:555–65. doi: 10.1007/s00281-018-0701-1
19. Fukata M, Vamadevan AS, Abreu MT. Toll-like receptors (TLRs) and nod-like receptors (NLRs) in inflammatory disorders. *Semin Immunol.* (2009) 21:242–53. doi: 10.1016/j.smim.2009.06.005
20. Ioannidis I, Ye F, McNally B, Willette M, Flano E. Toll-like receptor expression and induction of type I and type III interferons in primary airway epithelial cells. *J Virol.* (2013) 87:3261–70. doi: 10.1128/JVI.01956-12
21. Ritter M, Mennerich D, Weith A, Seither P. Characterization of toll-like receptors in primary lung epithelial cells: strong impact of the TLR3 ligand poly (I: C) on the regulation of toll-like receptors, adaptor proteins and inflammatory response. *J Inflamm.* (2005) 2:16. doi: 10.1186/1476-9255-2-16
22. Silverstein R, Wood JG, Xue Q, Norimatsu M, Horn DL, Morrison DC. Differential host inflammatory responses to viable versus antibiotic-killed bacteria in experimental microbial sepsis. *Infect Immun.* (2000) 68:2301–8. doi: 10.1128/IAI.68.4.2301-2308.2000
23. Juncadella IJ, Kadl A, Sharma AK, Shim YM, Hochreiter-Hufford A, Borish L, et al. Apoptotic cell clearance by bronchial epithelial cells critically influences airway inflammation. *Nature.* (2013) 493:547. doi: 10.1038/nature11714
24. Cortes G, Alvarez D, Saus C, Alberti S. Role of lung epithelial cells in defense against *Klebsiella pneumoniae* pneumonia. *Infect Immun.* (2002) 70:1075–80. doi: 10.1128/IAI.70.3.1075-1080.2002
25. Høiby N, Ciofu O, Bjarnsholt T. *Pseudomonas aeruginosa* biofilms in cystic fibrosis. *Future Microbiol.* (2010) 5:1663–74. doi: 10.2217/fmb.10.125
26. Murray TS, Egan M, Kazmierczak BI. *Pseudomonas aeruginosa* chronic colonization in cystic fibrosis patients. *Curr Opin Pediatr.* (2007) 19:83–8. doi: 10.1097/MOP.0b013e3280123a5d
27. Grassme H, Jendrossek V, Riehle A, Von Kürthy G, Berger J, Schwarz H, et al. Host defense against *Pseudomonas aeruginosa* requires ceramide-rich membrane rafts. *Nat Med.* (2003) 9:322. doi: 10.1038/nm823
28. Lamberti Y, Gorgojo J, Massillo C, Rodriguez ME. *Bordetella pertussis* entry into respiratory epithelial cells and intracellular survival. *Pathog Dis.* (2013) 69:194–204. doi: 10.1111/2049-632X.12072
29. Maruta K, Miyamoto H, Hamada T, Ogawa M, Taniguchi H, Yoshida S. Entry and intracellular growth of *Legionella dumoffii* in alveolar epithelial cells.

Am J Respir Crit Care Med. (1998) 157:1967–74. doi: 10.1164/ajrccm.157.6.9710108
30. Ou JJ, Drilling AJ, Cooksley C, Bassiouni A, Kidd SP, Psaltis AJ, et al. Reduced innate immune response to a *Staphylococcus aureus* small colony variant compared to its wild-type parent strain. *Front Cell Infect Microbiol.* (2016) 6: 187. doi: 10.3389/fcimb.2016.00187
31. Nordahl EA, Rydengard V, Nyberg P, Nitsche DP, Morgelin M, Malmsten M, et al. Activation of the complement system generates antibacterial peptides. *Proc Natl Acad Sci USA.* (2004) 101:16879–84. doi: 10.1073/pnas.0406678101
32. Fellermann K, Stange EF. Defensins–innate immunity at the epithelial frontier. *Eur J Gastroenterol Hepatol.* (2001) 13:771–6. doi: 10.1097/00042737-200107000-00003
33. Scharf S, Zahlten J, Szymanski K, Hippenstiel S, Suttorp N, N'Guessan PD. *Streptococcus pneumoniae* induces human β-defensin-2 and-3 in human lung epithelium. *Exp Lung Res.* (2012) 38:100–10. doi: 10.3109/01902148.2011.652802
34. Singh PK, Jia HP, Wiles K, Hesselberth J, Liu L, Conway BA, et al. Production of beta-defensins by human airway epithelia. *Proc Natl Acad Sci USA.* (1998) 95:14961–6. doi: 10.1073/pnas.95.25.14961
35. Morrison G, Kilanowski F, Davidson D, Dorin J. Characterization of the mouse beta defensin 1, Defb1, mutant mouse model. *Infect Immun.* (2002) 70:3053–60. doi: 10.1128/IAI.70.6.3053-3060.2002
36. Moser C, Weiner DJ, Lysenko E, Bals R, Weiser JN, Wilson JM. Beta-defensin 1 contributes to pulmonary innate immunity in mice. *Infect Immun.* (2002) 70:3068–72. doi: 10.1128/IAI.70.6.3068-3072.2002
37. Yang X, Cheng YT, Tan MF, Zhang HW, Liu WQ, Zou G, et al. Overexpression of porcine beta-defensin 2 enhances resistance to actinobacillus pleuropneumoniae infection in pigs. *Infect Immun.* (2015) 83:2836–43. doi: 10.1128/IAI.03101-14
38. Rivas-Santiago B, Hernandez-Pando R, Carranza C, Juarez E, Contreras JL, Aguilar-Leon D, et al. Expression of cathelicidin LL-37 during mycobacterium tuberculosis infection in human alveolar macrophages, monocytes, neutrophils, and epithelial cells. *Infect Immun.* (2008) 76:935–41. doi: 10.1128/IAI.01218-07
39. Bals R, Wang X, Zasloff M, Wilson JM. The peptide antibiotic LL-37/hCAP-18 is expressed in epithelia of the human lung where it has broad antimicrobial activity at the airway surface. *Proc Natl Acad Sci USA.* (1998) 95:9541–6. doi: 10.1073/pnas.95.16.9541
40. Dürr UH, Sudheendra U, Ramamoorthy A. LL-37, the only human member of the cathelicidin family of antimicrobial peptides. *Biochim Biophys Acta.* (2006) 1758:1408–25. doi: 10.1016/j.bbamem.2006.03.030
41. Wan M, van der Does, Anne M, Tang X, Lindbom L, Agerberth B, et al. Antimicrobial peptide LL-37 promotes bacterial phagocytosis by human macrophages. *J Leukoc Biol.* (2014) 95:971–81. doi: 10.1189/jlb.0513304
42. Walton WG, Ahmad S, Little MS, Kim CS, Tyrrell J, Lin Q, et al. Structural features essential to the antimicrobial functions of human SPLUNC1. *Biochemistry.* (2016) 55:2979–91. doi: 10.1021/acs.biochem.6b00271
43. Gally F, Di YP, Smith SK, Minor MN, Liu Y, Bratton DL, et al. SPLUNC1 promotes lung innate defense against mycoplasma pneumoniae infection in mice. *American J Pathol.* (2011) 178:2159–67. doi: 10.1016/j.ajpath.2011.01.026
44. Lukinskiene L, Liu Y, Reynolds SD, Steele C, Stripp BR, Leikauf GD, et al. Antimicrobial activity of PLUNC protects against *Pseudomonas aeruginosa* infection. *J Immunol.* (2011) 187:382–90. doi: 10.4049/jimmunol.1001769
45. Sieprawska-Lupa M, Mydel P, Krawczyk K, Wojcik K, Puklo M, Lupa B, et al. Degradation of human antimicrobial peptide LL-37 by *Staphylococcus aureus*-derived proteinases. *Antimicrob Agents Chemother.* (2004) 48:4673–9. doi: 10.1128/AAC.48.12.4673-4679.2004
46. Schmidtchen A, Frick I, Andersson E, Tapper H, Björck L. Proteinases of common pathogenic bacteria degrade and inactivate the antibacterial peptide LL-37. *Mol Microbiol.* (2002) 46:157–68. doi: 10.1046/j.1365-2958.2002.03146.x
47. Jiang D, Wenzel SE, Wu Q, Bowler RP, Schnell C, Chu HW. Human neutrophil elastase degrades SPLUNC1 and impairs airway epithelial defense against bacteria. *PLoS ONE.* (2013) 8:e64689. doi: 10.1371/journal.pone.0064689
48. Domon H, Nagai K, Maekawa T, Oda M, Yonezawa D, Takeda W, et al. Neutrophil elastase subverts the immune response by cleaving toll-like receptors and cytokines in pneumococcal pneumonia. *Front Immunol.* (2018) 9:732. doi: 10.3389/fimmu.2018.00732
49. Burris D, Sharma L, Mantell L. Effects of bacterial endotoxins on the toxicity of extracellular histones to mammalian cells. *FASEB J.* (2015) 29(1_Suppl):718.3.
50. Ahmad S, Gilmore RC, Alexis NE, Tarran R. SPLUNC1 loses its antimicrobial activity in acidic cystic fibrosis airway secretions. *Am J Respir Crit Care Med.* (2019) 200:633–6. doi: 10.1164/rccm.201812-2303LE
51. Liu H, Yu H, Gu Y, Xin A, Zhang Y, Diao H, et al. Human beta-defensin DEFB126 is capable of inhibiting LPS-mediated inflammation. *Appl Microbiol Biotechnol.* (2013) 97:3395–408. doi: 10.1007/s00253-012-4588-9
52. Llobet E, Tomas JM, Bengoechea JA. Capsule polysaccharide is a bacterial decoy for antimicrobial peptides. *Microbiology.* (2008) 154:3877–86. doi: 10.1099/mic.0.2008/022301-0
53. Atsuta J, Sterbinsky SA, Plitt J, Schwiebert LM, Bochner BS, Schleimer RP. Phenotyping and cytokine regulation of the BEAS-2B human bronchial epithelial cell: demonstration of inducible expression of the adhesion molecules VCAM-1 and ICAM-1. *Am J Respir Cell Mol Biol.* (1997) 17:571–82. doi: 10.1165/ajrcmb.17.5.2685
54. Marriott HM, Gascoyne KA, Gowda R, Geary I, Nicklin MJ, Iannelli F, et al. Interleukin-1beta regulates CXCL8 release and influences disease outcome in response to *Streptococcus pneumoniae*, defining intercellular cooperation between pulmonary epithelial cells and macrophages. *Infect Immun.* (2012) 80:1140–9. doi: 10.1128/IAI.05697-11
55. Byrne AJ, Mathie SA, Gregory LG, Lloyd CM. Pulmonary macrophages: key players in the innate defence of the airways. *Thorax.* (2015) 70:1189–96. doi: 10.1136/thoraxjnl-2015-207020
56. Chow OA, von Köckritz-Blickwede M, Bright AT, Hensler ME, Zinkernagel AS, Cogen AL, et al. Statins enhance formation of phagocyte extracellular traps. *Cell Host Microbe.* (2010) 8:445–54. doi: 10.1016/j.chom.2010.10.005
57. Brinkmann V, Reichard U, Goosmann C, Fauler B, Uhlemann Y, Weiss DS, et al. Neutrophil extracellular traps kill bacteria. *Science.* (2004) 303:1532–5. doi: 10.1126/science.1092385
58. Penberthy KK, Juncadella IJ, Ravichandran KS. Apoptosis and engulfment by bronchial epithelial cells. Implications for allergic airway inflammation. *Ann Am Thorac Soc.* (2014) 11(Suppl. 5):S259–62. doi: 10.1513/AnnalsATS.201405-200AW
59. Sharma L, Amick AK, Vasudevan S, Lee SW, Marion CR, Liu W, et al. Regulation and role of chitotriosidase during lung infection with *Klebsiella pneumoniae*. *J Immunol.* (2018) 201:615–26. doi: 10.4049/jimmunol.1701782
60. Regueiro V, Moranta D, Frank CG, Larrarte E, Margareto J, March C, et al. *Klebsiella pneumoniae* subverts the activation of inflammatory responses in a NOD1-dependent manner. *Cell Microbiol.* (2011) 13:135–53. doi: 10.1111/j.1462-5822.2010.01526.x
61. Kolar SL, Kyme P, Tseng CW, Soliman A, Kaplan A, Liang J, et al. Group B *Streptococcus* evades host immunity by degrading hyaluronan. *Cell Host Microbe.* (2015) 18:694–704. doi: 10.1016/j.chom.2015.11.001
62. Eckmann L, Kagnoff MF, Fierer J. Epithelial cells secrete the chemokine interleukin-8 in response to bacterial entry. *Infect Immun.* (1993) 61:4569–74. doi: 10.1128/IAI.61.11.4569-4574.1993
63. Edwards RJ, Taylor GW, Ferguson M, Murray S, Rendell N, Wrigley A, et al. Specific C-terminal cleavage and inactivation of interleukin-8 by invasive disease isolates of *Streptococcus* pyogenes. *J Infect Dis.* (2005) 192:783–90. doi: 10.1086/432485
64. Wolf K, Fields KA. Chlamydia pneumoniae impairs the innate immune response in infected epithelial cells by targeting TRAF3. *J Immunol.* (2013) 190:1695–701. doi: 10.4049/jimmunol.1202443
65. Meduri GU, Kanangat S, Stefan J, Tolley E, Schaberg D. Cytokines IL-1 β, IL-6, and TNF-α enhance *in vitro* growth of bacteria. *Am J Respir Crit Care Med.* (1999) 160:961–7. doi: 10.1164/ajrccm.160.3.9807080
66. Borer A, Saidel-Odes L, Riesenberg K, Eskira S, Peled N, Nativ R, et al. Attributable mortality rate for carbapenem-resistant *Klebsiella pneumoniae* bacteremia. *Infect Control Hosp Epidemiol.* (2009) 30:972–6. doi: 10.1086/605922
67. Tsay R, Siu L, Fung C, Chang F. Characteristics of bacteremia between community-acquired and nosocomial *Klebsiella pneumoniae* infection: risk factor for mortality and the impact of capsular serotypes as a herald for community-acquired infection. *Arch Intern Med.* (2002) 162:1021–7. doi: 10.1001/archinte.162.9.1021

68. Brune K, Frank J, Schwingshackl A, Finigan J, Sidhaye VK. Pulmonary epithelial barrier function: some new players and mechanisms. *Am J Physiol Lung Cell Mol Physiol.* (2015) 308:L731–745. doi: 10.1152/ajplung.00309.2014
69. Munkholm M, Mortensen J. Mucociliary clearance: pathophysiological aspects. *Clin Physiol Funct Imaging.* (2014) 34:171–7. doi: 10.1111/cpf.12085
70. Ofek I, Mesika A, Kalina M, Keisari Y, Podschun R, Sahly H, et al. Surfactant protein D enhances phagocytosis and killing of unencapsulated phase variants of *Klebsiella pneumoniae. Infect Immun.* (2001) 69:24–33. doi: 10.1128/IAI.69.1.24-33.2001
71. Wilson R, Pitt T, Taylor G, Watson D, MacDermot J, Sykes D, et al. Pyocyanin and 1-hydroxyphenazine produced by *Pseudomonas aeruginosa* inhibit the beating of human respiratory cilia *in vitro. J Clin Invest.* (1987) 79:221–9. doi: 10.1172/JCI112787
72. Rosseau S, Selhorst J, Wiechmann K, Leissner K, Maus U, Mayer K, et al. Monocyte migration through the alveolar epithelial barrier: adhesion molecule mechanisms and impact of chemokines. *J Immunol.* (2000) 164:427–35. doi: 10.4049/jimmunol.164.1.427
73. Wang J, Hossain M, Thanabalasuriar A, Gunzer M, Meininger C, Kubes P. Visualizing the function and fate of neutrophils in sterile injury and repair. *Science.* (2017) 358:111–16. doi: 10.1126/science.aam9690
74. Krishnan N, Robertson BD, Thwaites G. The mechanisms and consequences of the extra-pulmonary dissemination of mycobacterium tuberculosis. *Tuberculosis.* (2010) 90:361–6. doi: 10.1016/j.tube.2010.08.005
75. Hagedorn M, Rohde KH, Russell DG, Soldati T. Infection by tubercular mycobacteria is spread by nonlytic ejection from their amoeba hosts. *Science.* (2009) 323:1729–33. doi: 10.1126/science.1169381
76. Clarke TB, Francella N, Huegel A, Weiser JN. Invasive bacterial pathogens exploit TLR-mediated downregulation of tight junction components to facilitate translocation across the epithelium. *Cell Host Microbe.* (2011) 9:404–14. doi: 10.1016/j.chom.2011.04.012
77. Rosendahl A, Bergmann S, Hammerschmidt S, Goldmann O, Medina E. Lung dendritic cells facilitate extrapulmonary bacterial dissemination during pneumococcal pneumonia. *Front Cell Infect Microbiol.* (2013) 3:21. doi: 10.3389/fcimb.2013.00021
78. Rangel SM, Diaz MH, Knoten CA, Zhang A, Hauser AR. The role of ExoS in dissemination of *Pseudomonas aeruginosa* during pneumonia. *PLoS Pathog.* (2015) 11:e1004945. doi: 10.1371/journal.ppat.1004945
79. González-Juarbe N, Bradley KM, Shenoy AT, Gilley RP, Reyes LF, Hinojosa CA, et al. Pore-forming toxin-mediated ion dysregulation leads to death receptor-independent necroptosis of lung epithelial cells during bacterial pneumonia. *Cell Death Differ.* (2017) 24:917. doi: 10.1038/cdd.2017.49
80. Kikuchi Y, Tateda K, Fuse ET, Matsumoto T, Gotoh N, Fukushima J, et al. Hyperoxia exaggerates bacterial dissemination and lethality in *Pseudomonas aeruginosa* pneumonia. *Pulm Pharmacol Ther.* (2009) 22:333–9. doi: 10.1016/j.pupt.2008.12.021
81. Kinhikar AG, Verma I, Chandra D, Singh KK, Weldingh K, Andersen P, et al. Potential role for ESAT6 in dissemination of *M. tuberculosis*via human lung epithelial cells. *Mol Microbiol.* (2010) 75:92–106. doi: 10.1111/j.1365-2958.2009.06959.x
82. *Ten Threats to Global Health in 2019.* (2019). Available online at: https://www.who.int/emergencies/ten-threats-to-global-health-in-2019 (accessed September 26, 2019).
83. Porte R, Fougeron D, Munoz-Wolf N, Tabareau J, Georgel AF, Wallet F, et al. A toll-like receptor 5 agonist improves the efficacy of antibiotics in treatment of primary and influenza virus-associated pneumococcal mouse infections. *Antimicrob Agents Chemother.* (2015) 59:6064–72. doi: 10.1128/AAC.01210-15
84. Davis CG, Chang K, Osborne D, Walton AH, Ghosh S, Dunne WM, et al. TLR3 agonist improves survival to secondary pneumonia in a double injury model. *J Surg Res.* (2013) 182:270–6. doi: 10.1016/j.jss.2012.09.039
85. Lembo A, Pelletier M, Iyer R, Timko M, Dudda JC, West TE, et al. Administration of a synthetic TLR4 agonist protects mice from pneumonic tularemia. *J Immunol.* (2008) 180:7574–81. doi: 10.4049/jimmunol.180.11.7574
86. Wu CC, Sabet M, Hayashi T, Tawatao R, Fierer J, Carson DA, et al. *In vivo* efficacy of a phosphodiester TLR-9 aptamer and its beneficial effect in a pulmonary anthrax infection model. *Cell Immunol.* (2008) 251:78–85. doi: 10.1016/j.cellimm.2008.04.001
87. Duggan JM, You D, Cleaver JO, Larson DT, Garza RJ, Guzman Pruneda FA, et al. Synergistic interactions of TLR2/6 and TLR9 induce a high level of resistance to lung infection in mice. *J Immunol.* (2011) 186:5916–26. doi: 10.4049/jimmunol.1002122
88. Jean D, Rezaiguia-Delclaux S, Delacourt C, Leclercq R, Lafuma C, Brun-Buisson C, et al. Protective effect of endotoxin instillation on subsequent bacteria-induced acute lung injury in rats. *Am J Respir Crit Care Med.* (1998) 158:1702–8. doi: 10.1164/ajrccm.158.6.9709122
89. Bigot J, Guillot L, Guitard J, Ruffin M, Corvol H, Chignard M, et al. Respiratory epithelial cells can remember infection: a proof-of-concept study. *J Infect Dis.* (2019) jiz569. doi: 10.1093/infdis/jiz569
90. Ware HH, Kulkarni VV, Wang Y, García JP, Juarez ML, Kirkpatrick CT, et al. Inducible lung epithelial resistance requires multisource reactive oxygen species generation to protect against bacterial infections. *PLoS ONE.* (2019) 14:e0208216. doi: 10.1371/journal.pone.0208216

3

Mycobacterium tuberculosis Infection-Driven Foamy Macrophages and their Implications in Tuberculosis Control as Targets for Host-Directed Therapy

Dahee Shim [1,2], Hagyu Kim [1] and Sung Jae Shin [1*]

[1] Department of Microbiology, Institute for Immunology and Immunological Diseases, Brain Korea 21 Program for Leading Universities and Students (PLUS) Project for Medical Science, Yonsei University College of Medicine, Seoul, South Korea,
[2] Department of Life Science, Research Institute for Natural Sciences, College of Natural Sciences, Hanyang University, Seoul, South Korea

***Correspondence:**
Sung Jae Shin
sjshin@yuhs.ac

Tuberculosis (TB) is a leading cause of death worldwide following infection with *Mycobacterium tuberculosis* (Mtb), with 1.5 million deaths from this disease reported in 2018. Once the bacilli are inhaled, alveolar and interstitial macrophages become infected with Mtb and differentiate into lipid-laden foamy macrophages leading to lung inflammation. Thus, the presence of lipid-laden foamy macrophages is the hallmark of TB granuloma; these Mtb-infected foamy macrophages are the major niche for Mtb survival. The fate of TB pathogenesis is likely determined by the altered function of Mtb-infected macrophages, which initiate and mediate TB-related lung inflammation. As Mtb-infected foamy macrophages play central roles in the pathogenesis of Mtb, they may be important in the development of host-directed therapy against TB. Here, we summarize and discuss the current understanding of the alterations in alveolar and interstitial macrophages in the regulation of Mtb infection-induced immune responses. Metabolic reprogramming of lipid-laden foamy macrophages following Mtb infection or virulence factors are also summarized. Furthermore, we review the therapeutic interventions targeting immune responses and metabolic pathways, from *in vitro*, *in vivo*, and clinical studies. This review will further our understanding of the Mtb-infected foamy macrophages, which are both the major Mtb niche and therapeutic targets against TB.

Keywords: *Mycobacterium tuberculosis*, foamy macrophage, tuberculosis, immune responses, lipid metabolism, lung inflammation, host-directed therapy

INTRODUCTION

Tuberculosis (TB) is a chronic inflammatory disease caused by a *Mycobacterium tuberculosis* (Mtb) infection (1). When the Mtb bacilli become inhaled into alveoli, the bacilli are phagocytosed by alveolar macrophages in the lung (2). Phagocytosed Mtb uses various approaches to avoid host defense mechanisms, such as inhibition of phagosome maturation, expression of virulence-associated factors, inhibition of phagolysosomal fusion, and protection from reactive oxidative radicals (3, 4).

Following infection with Mtb, alveolar macrophages migrate to the interstitium and induce inflammatory responses, resulting in the extravasation of dendritic cells, neutrophils, natural killer cells, T cells, and B cells (2). These infiltrated immune cells surround the infected alveolar macrophages, which are reservoirs of Mtb, to construct TB granulomas (5–7). Thus, understanding the fate of alveolar macrophages at the initial infectious phase is critical for preventing TB pathogenesis.

During the construction of TB granulomas, Mtb-infected macrophages accumulate lipid bodies in their cytosolic area, differentiating into foamy macrophages, which are hallmarks of TB lesions (8, 9). The accumulated bubble-like lipid bodies contain cholesteryl esters and triglycerides (10). Mtb-infected foamy macrophages play central roles in granuloma development, maintenance, and infection dissemination (9). In advanced granulomas, the core region is characterized by caseous necrosis, which further leads to the formation of a lipid-rich environment (6, 8, 9, 11). In granulomas, Mtb can grow and persist in foamy macrophages and the necrotic core (7). When foamy macrophages leave the original granuloma, a secondary granuloma is established, promoting dissemination (11). As the primary niche for Mtb, determining the features of Mtb-infected foamy macrophages is essential for investigating and controlling TB pathogenesis. This review describes the current understanding of foamy macrophages infected with Mtb.

MACROPHAGES

Differentiation and General Features of Lung Macrophages

Macrophages are well-classified by their ontogeny (12–14). The functions and phenotypes of macrophages are influenced by their developmental origins and locations. Macrophages are generally formed as three major precursors: embryonic yolk sac precursor, fetal liver precursors, and bone-marrow derived blood monocytes (13, 14). In the steady state lungs, macrophages consist of alveolar macrophages and interstitial macrophages (15). The alveolar macrophages originate from fetal liver macrophages and fetal monocytes under the control of granulocyte/macrophage colony-stimulating factor (GM-CSF), peroxisome proliferator-activated receptors-gamma (PPAR-γ), and the lung microenvironment (16–19). To maintain homeostatic regulation, alveolar macrophages have a unique enhancer repertoire, including *Spi-C* and *Car4*, which are induced by the macrophage lineage-determining factor PU.1 in the lung-specific microenvironment (20, 21). A recent study demonstrated that mammalian target of rapamycin (mTOR) signaling is also required for the self-renewing ability of alveolar macrophages, accompanied by a distinctive metabolic signature based on the expression of sterol regulatory binding protein (SREBP) target genes (22). While undergoing tissue imprinting in the lungs, alveolar macrophages generally express immunosuppressive genes, including tumor growth factor-β (TGF-β) and interleukin-10 (IL-10) (17, 23). Alveolar macrophages have unique phenotypic features; they are loosely adherent, round-shaped cells expressing high levels of cluster of differentiation 206 (CD206), which detects microbial carbohydrates and high levels of scavenger receptors, such as macrophage scavenger receptor class A and macrophage receptor with collagenous structure (23). Notably, alveolar macrophages also express high levels of CD11c and CD170; moreover, their expression of F4/80 and CR3 is low or absent compared with that in other parts of the lung or peripheral tissue-resident macrophages (17).

In contrast, interstitial macrophages originate from primitive yolk sac macrophages and bone marrow monocytes (15). These cells are smaller and have monocyte-like morphology, which is characterized by a high nuclear/cytoplasm ratio with cytosolic vacuoles compared to alveolar macrophages (24). Interstitial macrophages express high levels of CD11b, CD64, F4/80, and the proto-oncogene tyrosine-protein kinase MER (25). Following invasion by microorganisms, interstitial macrophages play a role in the second-line defense via their phagocytosis and antigen presentation abilities (26). These interstitial macrophages have diverse immune responses depending on the activation stimulus, explained by the concepts of M1 and M2 macrophages. The activated spectrums and concepts for the M1 and M2 macrophages are further described below.

General Functions and Metabolic Programing of M1 and M2 Macrophages and Their Distinct Roles in Lung Inflammation by Mtb Infection

Overall, when macrophages are infected with bacteria or viruses, they elicit pro-inflammatory responses by releasing anti-microbial proteins and cytokines, such as complement proteins, tumor necrosis factor α, IL-1β, IL-6, IL-12, and IL-23 (27–29). These pro-inflammatory macrophages can activate endothelial cells in the blood vessels to support extravasation of other immune cells into inflamed areas (28, 29). Macrophages also trigger T cell responses through their antigen presenting abilities via major histocompatibility complex II molecules (30). *In vitro*, macrophages can be classically activated by lipopolysaccharide or interferon γ (IFN-γ) to mimic bacterial infection or pro-inflammatory activation, respectively. These classically activated macrophages are named as M1 macrophages (31). From the perspective of immunometabolism, M1 macrophages are well-known to drive pro-inflammatory responses during the metabolic switch for glycolysis with a broken tricarboxylic acid (TCA) cycle (32, 33). The pentose phosphate pathway and NAD^+ salvage pathway are essential for generation of mitochondrial reactive oxygen species (ROS), which induces DNA damage following M1 macrophage activation (34). In addition to massive glycolysis with an impaired TCA cycle, glucose-derived carbons are incorporated into fatty acids or sterol via lipogenesis in activated M1 macrophages (35).

Macrophages also play pro-resolving or anti-inflammatory roles that depend on signal transducer and activator of transcription-6 (STAT-6) and IL-10 release (27–29). These macrophages are involved in the phagocytosis of apoptotic cells, induction of collagen deposition, and coordination of tissue integrity to reinforce tissue repair, regeneration, and fibrosis (27, 36). There is also a method to polarize anti-inflammatory macrophages through the activation of IL-4/IL-13 or IL-10 *in vitro*; these alternatively activated macrophages are generally named as M2 macrophages (31). M2 macrophages preferentially utilize oxidative phosphorylation and fatty acid oxidation (FAO) to drive anti-inflammatory responses (37). In M2 macrophage activation with IL-4 treatment, mitochondrial metabolism is regulated by polyamine biosynthesis to regulate the integrity of the TCA cycle and electron transport chain (38). Collectively, M1 and M2 macrophages may undergo distinct lipid metabolic reprogramming, followed by their differential immune responses.

When infected with Mtb, both alveolar and interstitial macrophages play important roles in defending against TB and modulate immune responses (39). Mtb-infected alveolar macrophages exhibit enrichment in gene sets such as those involved in lipid uptake, oxidative phosphorylation and fatty acid oxidation, similar to M2 macrophages (39, 40). Mtb-infected alveolar macrophages express an antioxidant transcriptional signature via NRF2-dependent pathways, resulting in impaired control of Mtb growth with reduced inflammatory responses in the early stage of infection (40, 41). Mtb enhances the expression of genes in alveolar macrophages that are involved in Mtb division, growth, ribosomal protein synthesis, cell wall synthesis, fatty acid import, mycolic acid biosynthesis, the TCA cycle, and β-oxidation (40). Because the features of interstitial macrophages are determined by immunological stimuli, TB lesions have been investigated using M1 and M2 macrophages to dissect the immune responses occurring during TB progression (42, 43). In the early stage of Mtb infection, interstitial macrophages are typically differentiated to M1 macrophages. Mtb-infected interstitial macrophages express gene sets for cell adhesion, chemotaxis, ROS biosynthesis, nuclear factor-κB responses, hypoxia, and glycolysis *in vivo* (39, 40). In M1-like interstitial macrophages, Mtb shows a gene signature related to the response to environmental stresses and a non-replicative state (40). Mtb-infected M1 macrophages are transformed into M2 macrophages over time by the 6-kDa early secretory antigenic target (ESAT-6), which is a major virulence factor of Mtb (43). In addition to controlling the bacterial burden, modulating granuloma formation, and immune responses, Mtb-infected macrophages contribute to TB dissemination (44, 45). Mtb was shown to translocate from the phagolysosome to the cytosol, thereby eliciting host cell apoptosis in an ESAT-6–dependent manner (44). Apoptotic cells are then phagocytosed by newly infiltrating macrophages to generate the primary granuloma, and Mtb-infected macrophages egress to the distal tissues, contributing to the initiation of secondary granuloma formation (45) (**Figure 1A**).

From the perspective of immunometabolism, the Warburg effect in M1 macrophages generates pro-inflammatory responses, such as the secretion of IL-1β, which is known as a beneficial cytokine against Mtb (46, 47). Induced Warburg effects in the early phase of Mtb infection also generate ROS with the activation of hypoxia inducible factor 1α, which is necessary to induce Mtb specific IFN-γ dependent immunity (48, 49). IL-12, another cytokine secreted by M1 macrophages, can generate protective immune responses against Mtb (50). In contrast, M2 macrophages possess less bactericidal activities compared to M1 macrophages against Mtb infection (42). IL-10, a representative cytokine secreted from M2 macrophages, suppresses antimycobacterial immunity and promotes Mtb survival (51). It has been reported that another M2 macrophage-secreted cytokine, TGF-β, suppresses IFN-γ responses from T cells against Mtb in the lungs of mice and humans infected with TB; deletion of TGF-β signaling decreases the bacterial burden via the generation of cytotoxic T cell responses in TB granulomas (52).

Collectively, these investigations suggest the dynamic activation status of Mtb-infected macrophages (**Figure 1A**). Alveolar macrophages show enhanced lipid metabolism via PPAR-γ and inflammatory properties that facilitate infection and persistence of Mtb bacilli (18). In the progression of TB granulomas, blood monocyte-derived macrophages infiltrate and polarize to M1 macrophages. In the early phase of Mtb infection, excessive glycolysis with increasing lipids drives fatty acid synthesis in M1 macrophages. Further differentiation to M2 macrophages by ESAT-6 is closely linked to FAO with anti-inflammatory responses, providing favorable environments for Mtb survival (43). Therefore, these lipid metabolic reprogramming pathways may be considered targets for supporting host-directed therapy (HDT) to elicit anti-TB immune responses.

INTERACTION BETWEEN MTB AND MTB–DRIVEN FOAMY MACROPHAGES

Characteristics of Mtb-Infected Foamy Macrophages and the Utilization of Their Lipids by Mtb

Alterations of metabolic pathways are involved not only in the inflammatory responses of macrophages but also in the transformation of Mtb-infected macrophages into foamy macrophages, which are the major contributors to TB pathogenesis (**Figure 1B**), as previously described (5, 6). Foamy macrophages are named based on their morphology as they contain bubble-like lipid bodies in their cytoplasm (53). Mtb-infected foamy macrophages have different features compared to non-foamy macrophages (**Table 1**, upper). Specifically, Mtb-infected foamy macrophages express higher levels of MHCII, CD11c, CD40, and CD205, similar to dendritic cells, but show reduced capacity for antigen processing (54). Moreover, Mtb-infected foamy macrophages induce nitric oxide with elevated secretion of TGF-β to suppress T cell responses (55–57).

Upon infection, intracellular Mtb is located in the phagosomes, and the membrane of Mtb-containing phagosomes is enclosed and interacts with lipid bodies (58). A recent study demonstrated that the phagosome–lipid body interaction is regulated by the mycobacterial cell wall components lipoarabinomannan and phosphatidylinositol mannoside mediated by the late endosome marker Rab7 (59). After the phagosomes surrounded lipid bodies, Mtb translocated to lipid bodies for the utilization of lipids, such as cholesterols, fatty acids, and triglycerides, as carbon sources for survival. Mtb takes advantage of cholesterol and fatty acids in foamy macrophages to

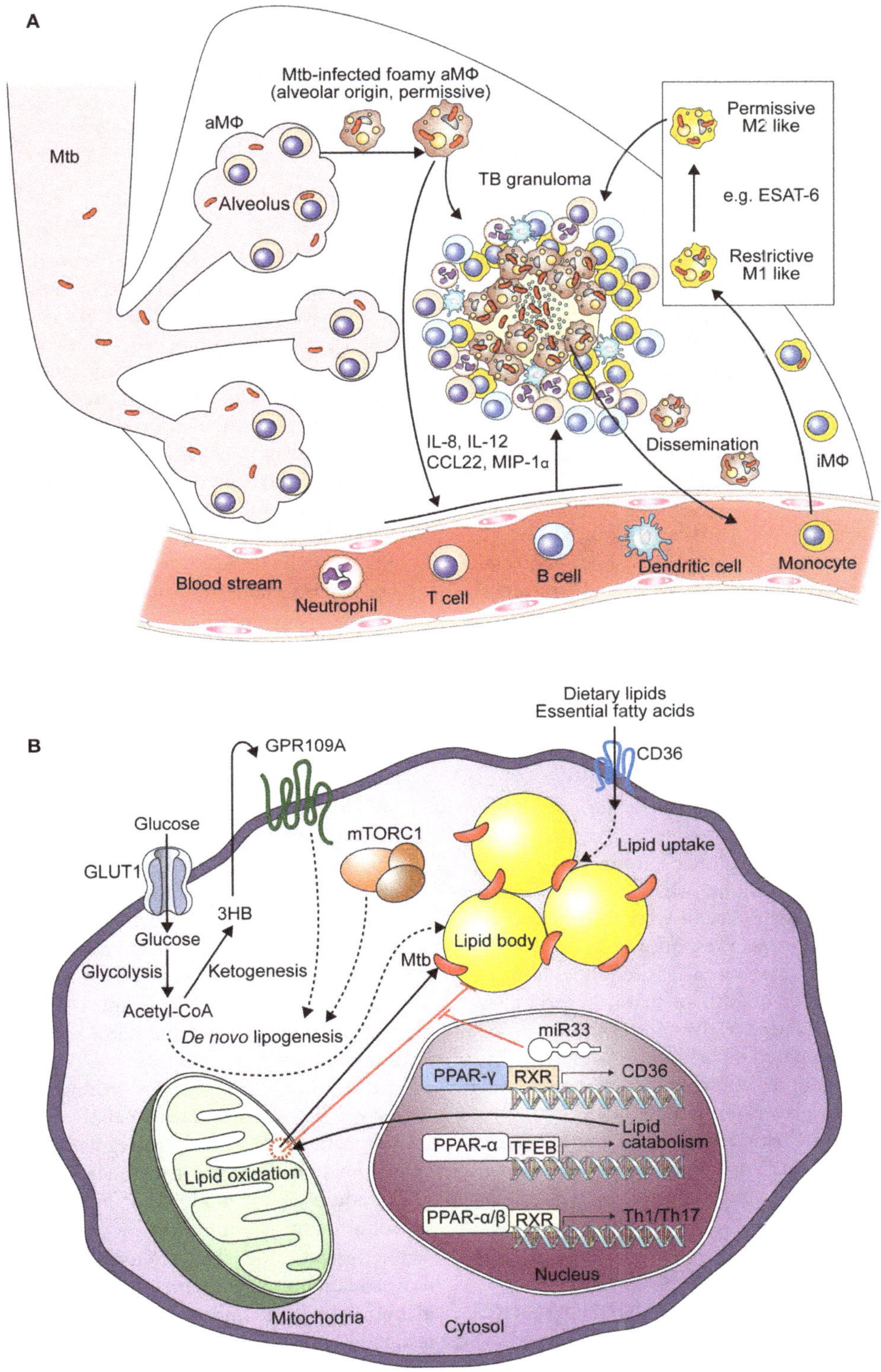

FIGURE 1 | Generation of Mtb-infected foamy macrophages during the formation of TB granulomas. **(A)** Composition of Mtb-infected foamy macrophages during TB pathogenesis. Alveolar macrophages initially infected by Mtb and translocated into the interstitial space to generate immune responses. With the extravasation of immune cells Mtb-infected alveolar macrophages differentiate into foamy macrophages. Infiltrated interstitial macrophages are also infected with Mtb and further differentiate into foamy macrophages. In the early stage of Mtb infection, macrophages show pro-inflammatory responses like M1 macrophages contributing to the restriction of Mtb survival. ESAT-6, a representative virulence factor of Mtb, polarizes these M1 macrophages into M2 macrophages to induce permissive responses in

(Continued)

FIGURE 1 | Mtb survival in the chronic stage of TB. These Mtb-infected foamy macrophages are hallmarks of TB granulomas; translocation of Mtb-infected foamy macrophages induces dissemination of Mtb. "aMΦ" and "iMΦ" indicate "alveolar macrophage" and "interstitial macrophage," respectively. **(B)** Metabolic perturbation by Mtb infection to generate foamy macrophages with Mtb infection, lipid accumulation leads to the generation foamy macrophages via metabolic reprogramming. In the early stage of Mtb infection, excessive glycolysis with defective mitochondrial respiration contributes to *de novo* lipogenesis. Acetyl-CoA, a product of glycolysis, is metabolized to 3-hydroxybutyrate (3-HB) by ketogenesis to induce GPR109A signaling. *De novo* lipogenesis is also induced by signal transduction of GPR109A and mTORC1 signaling, which is induced by macrophage activation. Nuclear receptors, such as those in the PPAR and LXR family, also contribute to both metabolic reprogramming and immune responses. The expression of miR33 is induced by Mtb and miR33 inhibits lipid catabolism, supporting Mtb survival. Direct and indirect processes are indicated by arrows and dotted arrows, respectively.

generate energy and metabolic intermediates via the expression of isocitrate lyases for the glyoxylate cycle (60). To utilize lipids, Mtb contains abundant genes encoding lipid transporters and lipolytic enzymes. It has been reported that LucA and Mcel are expressed in Mtb to import fatty acids (61). Rv0200/OmamB, Rv0172/Mce1D, Rv0655/MceG, and Rv0966c are also known as fatty acid transporters of Mtb in foamy macrophages (62). Rv2672 is the membrane-associated Mtb protein mycobacterial secreted hydrolase 1 and is required for Mtb persistence via utilization of host lipids under hypoxic conditions (63). In addition to Mtb survival, fatty acids are required for the synthesis of virulence-associated lipids, including polyketide lipids phiocerol-dimycoseroic acid, poly-acylated trehaloses, sulfolipids, and mycolic acids (60). Increased accumulation of triglycerides and elevated levels of triglyceride synthetase 2 have been reported in the modern Mtb Beijing strain compared to the ancient Mtb Beijing strain. Moreover, these elevated levels of triglyceride are associated with rapid disease development (64).

Furthermore, it has been suggested the use of lipids in host cells is related to dormancy of Mtb (58, 65–67). It is reported that Mtb persists in a dormant non-replicative state in foamy macrophages compared to infect non-foamy macrophages (58). Mtb utilize fatty acids from host cells to generate intracellular lipid inclusions, which are lipid bodies in the cytoplasm of mycobacteria. Bacilli with these inclusions show persistently arrested growth in response to stress (65, 66). Particularly, utilization of host triglycerides is required to obtain the dormancy-like phenotypes of Mtb in foamy macrophages (68). The Mtb mutant with reduced triglyceride synthesis is more sensitive to antibiotics compared to wild-type Mtb (65). The region of difference 1 protein in Mtb contributes to increasing the levels of intracellular triglycerides in Mtb by enhancing the expression of diacylglycerol *O*-acyltransferase, a key enzyme in triglyceride synthesis (67). Therefore, reducing lipid bodies in Mtb-infected foamy macrophages may control the intracellular survival of Mtb.

Mechanism of Lipid Accumulation of Foamy Macrophages by Mtb Infection and Their Implications for HDT

Recently, it has been reported that several bacterial factors of Mtb have additive modulatory effects on the lipid metabolism of host cells (**Figure 1B**). For example, ESAT-6 stimulates the translocation of glucose transporter GLUT-1, resulting in the active transport of glucose with the perturbation of metabolic flux (69, 70). Enhanced glucose metabolism leads to increased *de novo* lipid synthesis, which elevates the accumulation of lipids in foamy macrophages (69). It has been reported that activation of the G protein-coupled receptor GPR109A, an anti-lypolytic receptor, by ESAT-6 leads to the accumulation of lipid bodies in foamy macrophages, contributing to Mtb survival (70). In contrast, blockage of glycolysis with 2-deoxyglucose is detrimental to defense against Mtb infection because it disturbs M1-like activation in interstitial macrophages (39). Overall, glycolysis has contradictory roles against Mtb infection. By inducing pro-inflammatory immune responses, glycolysis with a broken TCA cycles supports anti-microbial responses in macrophages (39). However, excessive glycolysis is associated with elevated lipid accumulation by bacterial factors, including ESAT-6, to generate a niche that is suitable for Mtb (69, 70). Therefore, metabolic links between excessive glycolysis and lipogenesis are potential targets for reducing bacterial burdens with effective immune responses (**Table 1**).

Mtb also modulates nuclear transcription receptors of host cells involved in metabolic reprogramming and immune responses (71, 72). The Mtb-induced PPAR-γ pathway, which is a prominent signaling pathway that induces the activation of M2 macrophages, leads lipid accumulation to support the intracellular survival of Mtb. In this processes, PPAR-γ, with testicular receptor 4, increases the level of CD36 to contribute to lipid uptake (71). Another PPAR family member, PPAR-α, is a transcriptional inducer of FAO that prevents lipid accumulation in Mtb-infected foamy macrophages and promotes autophagy with transcription factor EB to reduce intracellular Mtb growth (73). Liver X-receptor (LXR)-α and LXR-β are also critical regulators of oxysterol metabolism that modulate immune responses in Mtb infection (74, 75). In mice with Mtb infection, LXR-α and LXR-β signaling is required to generate protective T cell responses (74). It has been reported that LXR signaling plays a role in regulating antimicrobial peptide expression to restrict Mtb growth via IL-36 (75).

In addition to modulating nuclear transcription factor signaling pathways, infection by Mtb induces tumor necrosis factor receptor signaling, followed by the activation of its downstream mTOR complex 1 (mTORC1) and caspase pathways in human primary macrophages (10). Activation of mTORC1 results in the accumulation of triglycerides in Mtb-infected macrophages. Mtb also induces miR-33 expression in foamy macrophages to inhibit lipid catabolism and autophagy, enabling intracellular survival and persistence (76).

Additionally, accumulating evidence has suggested that the disruption of lipid homeostasis, including hypercholesterolemia, leads to increased TB susceptibility. It is reported that apolipoprotein E-deficient mice have an increased susceptibility

TABLE 1 | Comparison of general characteristics between foamy and non-foamy macrophages, and metabolic interventions of Mtb-infected foamy macrophages for host-directed therapy.

Cell type	Mtb states	Features	Surface marker	Immune responses	References
Non-foamy macrophages	Replicative	Highly-phagocytic	$CD11b^{+}$ $CD64^{+}$ $F4/80^{+}$ $MertK^{+}$	Not reported	(25, 58)
Foamy macrophages	Dormant, non-replicative (after 6 days of infection)	Less-bactericidal Less-phagocytic	$CD11b^{+}CD11c^{hi}$ $MHCII^{hi}$ $CD40^{hi}$ $CD205^{hi}$	Reduced antigen processing capacity	(54, 58)
				Suppressive effects on effector T cells via higher level of nitric oxide	(55, 56)
				Reduced TNF-α and IL-1α secretion Elevated TGF-β secretion	(57)
Metabolic perturbation	**Reported conditions**	**Experimental type**	**Mtb strain**	**Effect on TB control**	**References**
Glycolysis boosting	Treatment with metformin	Type 2 diabetes patients (cohort study)	NA*	Beneficial effects on prevention and treatment against TB	(88–90)
Glycolysis inhibition	Treatment with 2-deoxyglucose	BMDMs from C57BL/6	Erdman	Increased Mtb burdens	(39)
Increased lipid uptake via CD36	Genetic ablation of PPAR-γ using shRNA transfection	THP-1 cells with PPAR-γ knockdown	H37Ra, H37Rv	Decreased both Mtb burden and lipids	(71)
Increased lipid efflux by ATP-binding cassette transporter	Genetic ablation of LXR-α using shRNA transfection	THP-1 cells with LXR-α knockdown	H37Ra, H37Rv	Increased Mtb burden and intracellular lipids	(71)
De novo fatty acid synthesis inhibition	C75 treatment	THP-1 cells and human MDM	H37Rv	Lowering bacterial burden and lipid accumulation	(91)
De novo triacyglyceride synthesis inhibition	Rapamycin treatment for blocking mTORC1	Human MDM	H37Rv	Reduced both Mtb burden and lipid accumulation	(10)
	Everolimus and temsirolimus treatment for blocking mTORC1	Patients with metastatic renal cell carcinoma (cohort study)	NA*	Aggravation of TB progression by their immunosuppressive activities	(92, 93)
De novo cholesterol synthesis inhibition	Treatment with simvastatin in combination with rifampicin, pyrazinamide, and isoniazid	THP-1 cells and BALB/c mice	H37Rv	Beneficial effects on anti-TB therapy	(79)
	Treatment with simvastatin in combination with rifampicin, pyrazinamide, and isoniazid	J774 cells and BALB/c mice	CDC1551	Increased first-line anti-TB drug efficacy	(82)
	Treatment with atorvastatin	THP-1 cells and human MDM	H37Rv	Decreased both Mtb survival and intracellular lipids	(91)
	Treatment with seven different statins	Patients with metabolic syndrome (cohort study)	NA*	Lowering risk of active TB progression	(83)
	Treatment with statins in combination with anti-TB drugs	Patients with pulmonary TB (cohort study)	NA*	Not associated with improved outcomes of pulmonary TB	(81)
	Treatment with seven different statins in combination with anti-TB drugs or not	Type 2 diabetes patients (cohort study)	NA*	Not associated with decreased TB development	(80)
Fatty acid oxidation	Treatment of etomoxir, as CPT1a inhibitor	BMDMs from C57BL/6	Erdman	Decreased bacterial burdens	(39)

NA, not applicable; BMDM, bone marrow-derived macrophage; CPT1a, carnitine palmitoyltransferase 1a; LXR-α, liver X receptor-alpha; MDM, monocyte-derived macrophage; Mtb, Mycobacterium tuberculosis; mTORC1, mammalian target of rapamycin complex 1; PPAR-γ, peroxisome proliferator-activated receptor-gamma; shRNA, short hairpin RNA; TB, tuberculosis.*

to hypercholesterolemia, showing defective priming of IFN-γ responses (77). Oxidized low-density lipoproteins, which are modified under hyperlipidemic conditions, also contribute to enhancing TB susceptibility via lysosomal dysfunction, impairing the control of Mtb survival (78). Statins, the 3-hydroxy-3-methylglutaryl-CoA reductase inhibitors for reducing cholesterol synthesis, have been attempted to treat Mtb infection (79–82). Clinically, treatment with statins has been reported to elicit improved outcomes for patients with TB (82, 83), but showed no additional effects in some cases (80, 81). By considering the characteristics of each patient, it is necessary for novel HDT approaches to modulate the immune response and/or cholesterol metabolism to be effective against TB. Collectively, these observations suggest that lipid metabolism and/or homeostatic pathways are promising targets for HDT against TB (**Table 1**, lower).

FUTURE DIRECTION AND PERSPECTIVES

To discover new therapeutic strategies against TB, many researches have attempted to alleviate Mtb infection through HDT. Foamy macrophages provide a niche for bacilli survival, maintenance, and persistence using their enriched cytosolic lipids. Even worse, necrosis of Mtb-infected foamy macrophages results in the generation of the necrotic core of TB granulomas, causing extracellular growth of Mtb. As Mtb actively utilizes lipids to generate energy and virulent factors from host cells, the regulation of host lipid metabolism pathways is a potential therapeutic strategy for alleviating TB by preventing vicious cycles between Mtb and macrophages.

In summary, alveolar and interstitial macrophages exert opposite roles against Mtb infection; therefore, understanding these macrophages is important for establishing strategies against TB pathogenesis. In TB pathogenesis, alveolar macrophages are susceptible to Mtb with elevated fatty acid uptake and FAO. In contrast, interstitial macrophages show resistance features like M1 macrophages in the early stage of Mtb infection. Pro-inflammatory M1 macrophages exhibit massively increased glycolysis and fatty acid synthesis with bactericidal activities. M2 macrophages show elevated lipid catabolism with suppressive activities in their antibacterial responses against Mtb. Thus, the Mtb-induced transformation processes from M1 to M2 macrophages are potential immunological targets of TB. Some recent revolutionary investigations have been conducted using *in vitro* granuloma and organoid culture systems to gain further insights into TB (42, 84–86). Using *in vitro* granuloma culture systems, M1 macrophages were shown to transform into M2 macrophages following Mtb infection (42). Although these techniques have only provided limited information of Mtb-infected macrophages to date, they have potential for further detailed investigations of Mtb-infected foamy macrophages to suggest more promising targets of HDT. Moreover, the metabolic pathways of Mtb-infected foamy macrophages perturbed by Mtb infection are important targets of HDT against TB. A recent study indicated that Mtb-infected foamy macrophages could uptake more fluoroquinolones compared to non-foamy macrophages *in vivo* (87), suggesting that it is important to consider the functions of foamy macrophages for anti-TB drug treatment. With consideration of the physiology of macrophages, it is expected that HDT strategy targeting immunological functions and/or metabolic perturbation of Mtb-infected foamy macrophages can be developed.

AUTHOR CONTRIBUTIONS

DS, HK, and SS wrote and revised the manuscript. SS conceptualized and edited the manuscript. All authors read and gave final approval of the manuscript.

ACKNOWLEDGMENTS

The authors thank MID (Medical Illustration & Design), a part of the Medical Research Support Services of Yonsei University College of Medicine, for all artistic support related to this work.

REFERENCES

1. The Lancet. End the tuberculosis emergency: a promise is not enough. *Lancet.* (2019) 394:1482. doi: 10.1016/S0140-6736(19)32459-6
2. Cohen SB, Gern BH, Delahaye JL, Adams KN, Plumlee CR, Winkler JK, et al. Alveolar macrophages provide an early *Mycobacterium tuberculosis* niche and initiate dissemination. *Cell Host Microbe.* (2018) 24:439–46.e4. doi: 10.1016/j.chom.2018.08.001
3. Bussi C, Gutierrez MG. *Mycobacterium tuberculosis* infection of host cells in space and time. *FEMS Microbiol Rev.* (2019) 43:341–61. doi: 10.1093/femsre/fuz006
4. Meena LS, Rajni. Survival mechanisms of pathogenic *Mycobacterium tuberculosis* H37Rv. *FEBS J.* (2010) 277:2416–27. doi: 10.1111/j.1742-4658.2010.07666.x
5. Ehlers S, Schaible UE. The granuloma in tuberculosis: dynamics of a host-pathogen collusion. *Front Immunol.* (2012) 3:411. doi: 10.3389/fimmu.2012.00411
6. Orme IM, Basaraba RJ. The formation of the granuloma in tuberculosis infection. *Semin Immunol.* (2014) 26:601–9. doi: 10.1016/j.smim.2014.09.009
7. Cadena AM, Fortune SM, Flynn JL. Heterogeneity in tuberculosis. *Nat Rev Immunol.* (2017) 17:691–702. doi: 10.1038/nri.2017.69
8. Russell DG, Cardona PJ, Kim MJ, Allain S, Altare F. Foamy macrophages and the progression of the human tuberculosis granuloma. *Nat Immunolgy.* (2009) 10:943–8. doi: 10.1038/ni.1781
9. Ramakrishnan L. Revisiting the role of the granuloma in tuberculosis. *Nat Rev Immunol.* (2012) 12:352–66. doi: 10.1038/nri3211
10. Guerrini V, Prideaux B, Blanc L, Bruiners N, Arrigucci R, Singh S, et al. Storage lipid studies in tuberculosis reveal that foam cell biogenesis is disease-specific. *PLoS Pathog.* (2018) 14:e1007223. doi: 10.1371/journal.ppat.1007223

11. McClean CM, Tobin DM. Macrophage form, function, and phenotype in mycobacterial infection: lessons from tuberculosis and other diseases. *Pathog Dis.* (2016) 74:ftw068. doi: 10.1093/femspd/ftw068
12. Gentek R, Molawi K, Sieweke MH. Tissue macrophage identity and self-renewal. *Immunol Rev.* (2014) 262:56–73. doi: 10.1111/imr.12224
13. Ginhoux F, Guilliams M. Tissue-Resident macrophage ontogeny and homeostasis. *Immunity.* (2016) 44:439–49. doi: 10.1016/j.immuni.2016.02.024
14. Ginhoux F, Schultze JL, Murray PJ, Ochando J, Biswas SK. New insights into the multidimensional concept of macrophage ontogeny, activation and function. *Nat Immunol.* (2016) 17:34–40. doi: 10.1038/ni.3324
15. Tan SY, Krasnow MA. Developmental origin of lung macrophage diversity. *Development.* (2016) 143:1318–27. doi: 10.1242/dev.129122
16. Malur A, McCoy AJ, Arce S, Barna BP, Kavuru MS, Malur AG, et al. Deletion of PPAR gamma in alveolar macrophages is associated with a Th-1 pulmonary inflammatory response. *J Immunol.* (2009) 182:5816–22. doi: 10.4049/jimmunol.0803504
17. Hussell T, Bell TJ. Alveolar macrophages: plasticity in a tissue-specific context. *Nat Rev Immunol.* (2014) 14:81–93. doi: 10.1038/nri3600
18. Schneider C, Nobs SP, Kurrer M, Rehrauer H, Thiele C, Kopf M. Induction of the nuclear receptor PPAR-gamma by the cytokine GM-CSF is critical for the differentiation of fetal monocytes into alveolar macrophages. *Nat Immunol.* (2014) 15:1026–37. doi: 10.1038/ni.3005
19. Guilliams M, De Kleer I, Henri S, Post S, Vanhoutte L, De Prijck S, et al. Alveolar macrophages develop from fetal monocytes that differentiate into long-lived cells in the first week of life via GM-CSF. *J Exp Med.* (2013) 210:1977–92. doi: 10.1084/jem.20131199
20. Gosselin D, Link VM, Romanoski CE, Fonseca GJ, Eichenfield DZ, Spann NJ, et al. Environment drives selection and function of enhancers controlling tissue-specific macrophage identities. *Cell.* (2014) 159:1327–40. doi: 10.1016/j.cell.2014.11.023
21. Lavin Y, Winter D, Blecher-Gonen R, David E, Keren-Shaul H, Merad M, et al. Tissue-resident macrophage enhancer landscapes are shaped by the local microenvironment. *Cell.* (2014) 159:1312–26. doi: 10.1016/j.cell.2014.11.018
22. Sinclair C, Bommakanti G, Gardinassi L, Loebbermann J, Johnson MJ, Hakimpour P, et al. mTOR regulates metabolic adaptation of APCs in the lung and controls the outcome of allergic inflammation. *Science.* (2017) 357:1014–21. doi: 10.1126/science.aaj2155
23. Allard B, Panariti A, Martin JG. Alveolar macrophages in the resolution of inflammation, tissue repair, and tolerance to infection. *Front Immunol.* (2018) 9:1777. doi: 10.3389/fimmu.2018.01777
24. Fathi M, Johansson A, Lundborg M, Orre L, Skold CM, Camner P. Functional and morphological differences between human alveolar and interstitial macrophages. *Exp Mol Pathol.* (2001) 70:77–82. doi: 10.1006/exmp.2000.2344
25. Yu YR, O'Koren EG, Hotten DF, Kan MJ, Kopin D, Nelson ER, et al. A Protocol for the comprehensive flow cytometric analysis of immune cells in normal and inflamed murine non-lymphoid tissues. *PLoS ONE.* (2016) 11:e0150606. doi: 10.1371/journal.pone.0150606
26. Gibbings SL, Thomas SM, Atif SM, McCubbrey AL, Desch AN, Danhorn T, et al. Three unique interstitial macrophages in the murine lung at steady state. *Am J Respir Cell Mol Biol.* (2017) 57:66–76. doi: 10.1165/rcmb.2016-0361OC
27. Arango Duque G, Descoteaux A. Macrophage cytokines: involvement in immunity and infectious diseases. *Front Immunol.* (2014) 5:491. doi: 10.3389/fimmu.2014.00491
28. Ley K. M1 Means Kill; M2 Means Heal. *J Immunol.* (2017) 199:2191–3. doi: 10.4049/jimmunol.1701135
29. Orecchioni M, Ghosheh Y, Pramod AB, Ley K. Macrophage polarization: different gene signatures in M1(LPS+) vs. classically and M2(LPS-) vs. alternatively activated macrophages. *Front Immunol.* (2019) 10:1084. doi: 10.3389/fimmu.2019.01084
30. Hume DA. Macrophages as APC and the dendritic cell myth. *J Immunol.* (2008) 181:5829–35. doi: 10.4049/jimmunol.181.9.5829
31. Murray PJ. Macrophage polarization. *Ann Rev Physiol.* (2017) 79:541–66. doi: 10.1146/annurev-physiol-022516-034339
32. O'Neill LA, Kishton RJ, Rathmell J. A guide to immunometabolism for immunologists. *Nat Rev Immunol.* (2016) 16:553–65. doi: 10.1038/nri.2016.70
33. Wculek SK, Khouili SC, Priego E, Heras-Murillo I, Sancho D. Metabolic control of dendritic cell functions: digesting information. *Front Immunol.* (2019) 10:775. doi: 10.3389/fimmu.2019.00775
34. Cameron AM, Castoldi A, Sanin DE, Flachsmann LJ, Field CS, Puleston DJ, et al. Inflammatory macrophage dependence on NAD(+) salvage is a consequence of reactive oxygen species-mediated DNA damage. *Nat Immunol.* (2019) 20:420–32. doi: 10.1038/s41590-019-0336-y
35. Feingold KR, Shigenaga JK, Kazemi MR, McDonald CM, Patzek SM, Cross AS, et al. Mechanisms of triglyceride accumulation in activated macrophages. *J Leukoc Biol.* (2012) 92:829–39. doi: 10.1189/jlb.1111537
36. Watanabe S, Alexander M, Misharin AV, Budinger GRS. The role of macrophages in the resolution of inflammation. *J Clin Invest.* (2019) 129:2619–28. doi: 10.1172/JCI124615
37. Russell DG, Huang L, VanderVen BC. Immunometabolism at the interface between macrophages and pathogens. *Nat Rev Immunol.* (2019) 19:291–304. doi: 10.1038/s41577-019-0124-9
38. Puleston DJ, Buck MD, Klein Geltink RI, Kyle RL, Caputa G, O'Sullivan D, et al. Polyamines and eIF5A hypusination modulate mitochondrial respiration and macrophage activation. *Cell Metab.* (2019) 30:352–63.e8. doi: 10.1016/j.cmet.2019.05.003
39. Huang L, Nazarova EV, Tan S, Liu Y, Russell DG. Growth of *Mycobacterium tuberculosis in vivo* segregates with host macrophage metabolism and ontogeny. *J Exp Med.* (2018) 215:1135–52. doi: 10.1084/jem.20172020
40. Pisu D, Huang L, Grenier JK, Russell DG. Dual RNA-Seq of Mtb-infected macrophages *in vivo* reveals ontologically distinct host-pathogen interactions. *Cell Rep.* (2020) 30:335–50.e4. doi: 10.1016/j.celrep.2019.12.033
41. Rothchild AC, Olson GS, Nemeth J, Amon LM, Mai D, Gold ES, et al. Alveolar macrophages generate a noncanonical NRF2-driven transcriptional response to *Mycobacterium tuberculosis in vivo. Sci Immunol.* (2019) 4:eaaw6693. doi: 10.1126/sciimmunol.aaw6693
42. Huang Z, Luo Q, Guo Y, Chen J, Xiong G, Peng Y, et al. *Mycobacterium tuberculosis*-induced polarization of human macrophage orchestrates the formation and development of tuberculous granulomas *in vitro. PLoS ONE.* (2015) 10:e0129744. doi: 10.1371/journal.pone.0129744
43. Refai A, Gritli S, Barbouche MR, Essafi M. *Mycobacterium tuberculosis* virulent factor ESAT-6 drives macrophage differentiation toward the pro-inflammatory M1 phenotype and subsequently switches it to the anti-inflammatory M2 phenotype. *Front Cell Infect Microbiol.* (2018) 8:327. doi: 10.3389/fcimb.2018.00327
44. van der Wel N, Hava D, Houben D, Fluitsma D, van Zon M, Pierson J, et al. *M. tuberculosis* and M. leprae translocate from the phagolysosome to the cytosol in myeloid cells. *Cell.* (2007) 129:1287–98. doi: 10.1016/j.cell.2007.05.059
45. Davis JM, Ramakrishnan L. The role of the granuloma in expansion and dissemination of early tuberculous infection. *Cell.* (2009) 136:37–49. doi: 10.1016/j.cell.2008.11.014
46. Huang SC, Everts B, Ivanova Y, O'Sullivan D, Nascimento M, Smith AM, et al. Cell-intrinsic lysosomal lipolysis is essential for alternative activation of macrophages. *Nat Immunol.* (2014) 15:846–55. doi: 10.1038/ni.2956
47. Mayer-Barber KD, Andrade BB, Oland SD, Amaral EP, Barber DL, Gonzales J, et al. Host-directed therapy of tuberculosis based on interleukin-1 and type I interferon crosstalk. *Nature.* (2014) 511:99–103. doi: 10.1038/nature13489
48. Shi L, Salamon H, Eugenin EA, Pine R, Cooper A, Gennaro ML. Infection with *Mycobacterium tuberculosis* induces the Warburg effect in mouse lungs. *Sci Rep.* (2015) 5:18176. doi: 10.1038/srep18176
49. Braverman J, Sogi KM, Benjamin D, Nomura DK, Stanley SA. HIF-1α Is an essential mediator of IFN-γ-dependent immunity to *Mycobacterium tuberculosis. J Immunol.* (2016) 197:1287–97. doi: 10.4049/jimmunol.1600266
50. Cooper AM, Solache A, Khader SA. Interleukin-12 and tuberculosis: an old story revisited. *Curr Opin Immunol.* (2007) 19:441–7. doi: 10.1016/j.coi.2007.07.004
51. Abdalla AE, Lambert N, Duan X, Xie J. Interleukin-10 family and tuberculosis: an old story renewed. *Int J Biol Sci.* (2016) 12:710–7. doi: 10.7150/ijbs.13881
52. Warsinske HC, Pienaar E, Linderman JJ, Mattila JT, Kirschner DE. Deletion of TGF-β1 increases bacterial clearance by cytotoxic T cells in a tuberculosis granuloma model. *Front Immunol.* (2017) 8:1843. doi: 10.3389/fimmu.2017.01843
53. Mori M, Itabe H, Higashi Y, Fujimoto Y, Shiomi M, Yoshizumi M, et al. Foam cell formation containing lipid droplets enriched with free cholesterol by hyperlipidemic serum. *J Lipid Res.* (2001) 42:1771–81.
54. Ordway D, Henao-Tamayo M, Orme IM, Gonzalez-Juarrero M. Foamy macrophages within lung granulomas of mice infected with *Mycobacterium*

tuberculosis express molecules characteristic of dendritic cells and antiapoptotic markers of the TNF receptor-associated factor family. *J Immunol.* (2005) 175:3873–81. doi: 10.4049/jimmunol.175.6.3873

55. Ríos-Barrera VA, Campos-Peña V, Aguilar-León D, Lascurain LR, Meraz-Ríos MA, Moreno J, et al. Macrophage and T lymphocyte apoptosis during experimental pulmonary tuberculosis: their relationship to mycobacterial virulence. *Eur J Immunol.* (2006) 36:345–53. doi: 10.1002/eji.200535202
56. Nabeshima S, Nomoto M, Matsuzaki G, Kishihara K, Taniguchi H, Yoshida S, et al. T-Cell hyporesponsiveness induced by activated macrophages through nitric oxide production in mice infected with *Mycobacterium tuberculosis*. *Infect Immun.* (1999) 67:3221–6. doi: 10.1128/IAI.67.7.3221-3226.1999
57. Hernandez-Pando R, Orozco H, Arriaga K, Sampieri A, Larriva-Sahd J, Madrid-Marina V. Analysis of the local kinetics and localization of interleukin-1 alpha, tumour necrosis factor-alpha and transforming growth factor-beta, during the course of experimental pulmonary tuberculosis. *Immunology.* (1997) 90:607–17. doi: 10.1046/j.1365-2567.1997.00193.x
58. Peyron P, Vaubourgeix J, Poquet Y, Levillain F, Botanch C, Bardou F, et al. Foamy macrophages from tuberculous patients' granulomas constitute a nutrient-rich reservoir for *M. tuberculosis* persistence. *PLoS Pathog.* (2008) 4:e1000204. doi: 10.1371/journal.ppat.1000204
59. Roque NR, Lage SL, Navarro R, Fazolini N, Maya-Monteiro CM, Rietdorf J, et al. Rab7 controls lipid droplet-phagosome association during mycobacterial infection. *Biochim Biophys Acta Mol Cell Biol Lipids.* (2020) 1865:158703. doi: 10.1016/j.bbalip.2020.158703
60. Munoz-Elias EJ, Upton AM, Cherian J, McKinney JD. Role of the methylcitrate cycle in *Mycobacterium tuberculosis* metabolism, intracellular growth, and virulence. *Mol Microbiol.* (2006) 60:1109–22. doi: 10.1111/j.1365-2958.2006.05155.x
61. Nazarova EV, Montague CR, La T, Wilburn KM, Sukumar N, Lee W, et al. Rv3723/LucA coordinates fatty acid and cholesterol uptake in *Mycobacterium tuberculosis*. *ELife.* (2017) 6:e26969. doi: 10.7554/eLife.26969.019
62. Nazarova EV, Montague CR, Huang L, La T, Russell D, VanderVen BC. The genetic requirements of fatty acid import by *Mycobacterium tuberculosis* within macrophages. *ELife.* (2019) 8:e43621. doi: 10.7554/eLife.43621.015
63. Singh KH, Jha B, Dwivedy A, Choudhary E, N AG, Ashraf A, et al. Characterization of a secretory hydrolase from *Mycobacterium tuberculosis* sheds critical insight into host lipid utilization by M. tuberculosis. *J Biol Chem.* (2017) 292:11326–35. doi: 10.1074/jbc.M117.794297
64. Tong J, Liu Q, Wu J, Jiang Y, Takiff HE, Gao Q. *Mycobacterium tuberculosis* strains of the modern Beijing sublineage excessively accumulate triacylglycerols *in vitro*. *Tuberculosis.* (2019) 120:101892. doi: 10.1016/j.tube.2019.101892
65. Baek SH, Li AH, Sassetti CM. Metabolic regulation of mycobacterial growth and antibiotic sensitivity. *PLoS Biol.* (2011) 9:e1001065. doi: 10.1371/journal.pbio.1001065
66. Rodriguez JG, Hernandez AC, Helguera-Repetto C, Aguilar Ayala D, Guadarrama-Medina R, Anzola JM, et al. Global adaptation to a lipid environment triggers the dormancy-related phenotype of *Mycobacterium tuberculosis*. *mBio.* (2014) 5:e01125-14. doi: 10.1128/mBio.01125-14
67. Jaisinghani N, Dawa S, Singh K, Nandy A, Menon D, Bhandari PD, et al. Necrosis driven triglyceride synthesis primes macrophages for inflammation during *Mycobacterium tuberculosis* infection. *Front Immunol.* (2018) 9:1490. doi: 10.3389/fimmu.2018.01490
68. Daniel J, Maamar H, Deb C, Sirakova TD, Kolattukudy PE. *Mycobacterium tuberculosis* uses host triacylglycerol to accumulate lipid droplets and acquires a dormancy-like phenotype in lipid-loaded macrophages. *PLoS Pathog.* (2011) 7:e1002093. doi: 10.1371/journal.ppat.1002093
69. Singh V, Kaur C, Chaudhary VK, Rao KV, Chatterjee S. M. tuberculosis secretory protein ESAT-6 induces metabolic flux perturbations to drive foamy macrophage differentiation. *Sci Rep.* (2015) 5:12906. doi: 10.1038/srep12906
70. Singh V, Jamwal S, Jain R, Verma P, Gokhale R, Rao KV. *Mycobacterium tuberculosis*-driven targeted recalibration of macrophage lipid homeostasis promotes the foamy phenotype. *Cell Host Microbe.* (2012) 12:669–81. doi: 10.1016/j.chom.2012.09.012
71. Mahajan S, Dkhar HK, Chandra V, Dave S, Nanduri R, Janmeja AK, et al. *Mycobacterium tuberculosis* modulates macrophage lipid-sensing nuclear receptors PPARgamma and TR4 for survival. *J Immunol.* (2012) 188:5593–603. doi: 10.4049/jimmunol.1103038
72. Arnett E, Weaver AM, Woodyard KC, Montoya MJ, Li M, Hoang KV, et al. PPARγ is critical for *Mycobacterium tuberculosis* induction of Mcl-1 and limitation of human macrophage apoptosis. *PLoS Pathog.* (2018) 14:e1007100. doi: 10.1371/journal.ppat.1007100
73. Kim YS, Lee HM, Kim JK, Yang CS, Kim TS, Jung M, et al. PPAR-α activation mediates innate host defense through induction of TFEB and lipid catabolism. *J Immunol.* (2017) 198:3283–95. doi: 10.4049/jimmunol.1601920
74. Korf H, Vander Beken S, Romano M, Steffensen KR, Stijlemans B, Gustafsson JA, et al. Liver X receptors contribute to the protective immune response against *Mycobacterium tuberculosis* in mice. *J Clin Invest.* (2009) 119:1626–37. doi: 10.1172/JCI35288
75. Ahsan F, Maertzdorf J, Guhlich-Bornhof U, Kaufmann SHE, Moura-Alves P. IL-36/LXR axis modulates cholesterol metabolism and immune defense to *Mycobacterium tuberculosis*. *Sci Rep.* (2018) 8:1520. doi: 10.1038/s41598-018-19476-x
76. Ouimet M, Koster S, Sakowski E, Ramkhelawon B, van Solingen C, Oldebeken S, et al. *Mycobacterium tuberculosis* induces the miR-33 locus to reprogram autophagy and host lipid metabolism. *Nat Immunol.* (2016) 17:677–86. doi: 10.1038/ni.3434
77. Martens GW, Arikan MC, Lee J, Ren F, Vallerskog T, Kornfeld H. Hypercholesterolemia impairs immunity to tuberculosis. *Infect Immun.* (2008) 76:3464–72. doi: 10.1128/IAI.00037-08
78. Vrieling F, Wilson L, Rensen PCN, Walzl G, Ottenhoff THM, Joosten SA. Oxidized low-density lipoprotein (oxLDL) supports *Mycobacterium tuberculosis* survival in macrophages by inducing lysosomal dysfunction. *PLoS Pathog.* (2019) 15:e1007724. doi: 10.1371/journal.ppat.1007724
79. Dutta NK, Bruiners N, Pinn ML, Zimmerman MD, Prideaux B, Dartois V, et al. Statin adjunctive therapy shortens the duration of TB treatment in mice. *J Antimicrob Chemother.* (2016) 71:1570–7. doi: 10.1093/jac/dkw014
80. Kang YA, Choi NK, Seong JM, Heo EY, Koo BK, Hwang SS, et al. The effects of statin use on the development of tuberculosis among patients with diabetes mellitus. *Int J Tuberc Lung Dis.* (2014) 18:717–24. doi: 10.5588/ijtld.13.0854
81. Chen YT, Kuo SC, Chao PW, Chang YY. Use of lipid-lowering agents is not associated with improved outcomes for tuberculosis patients on standard-course therapy: a population-based cohort study. *PLoS ONE.* (2019) 14:e0210479. doi: 10.1371/journal.pone.0210479
82. Skerry C, Pinn ML, Bruiners N, Pine R, Gennaro ML, Karakousis PC. Simvastatin increases the *in vivo* activity of the first-line tuberculosis regimen. *J Antimicrob Chemother.* (2014) 69:2453–7. doi: 10.1093/jac/dku166
83. Lai CC, Lee MT, Lee SH, Hsu WT, Chang SS, Chen SC, et al. Statin treatment is associated with a decreased risk of active tuberculosis: an analysis of a nationally representative cohort. *Thorax.* (2016) 71:646–51. doi: 10.1136/thoraxjnl-2015-207052
84. Kapoor N, Pawar S, Sirakova TD, Deb C, Warren WL, Kolattukudy PE. Human granuloma *in vitro* model, for TB dormancy and resuscitation. *PLoS ONE.* (2013) 8:e53657. doi: 10.1371/journal.pone.0053657
85. Fonseca KL, Rodrigues PNS, Olsson IAS, Saraiva M. Experimental study of tuberculosis: from animal models to complex cell systems and organoids. *PLoS Pathog.* (2017) 13:e1006421. doi: 10.1371/journal.ppat.1006421
86. Elkington P, Lerm M, Kapoor N, Mahon R, Pienaar E, Huh D, et al. *In vitro* granuloma models of tuberculosis: potential and challenges. *J Infect Dis.* (2019) 219:1858–66. doi: 10.1093/infdis/jiz020
87. Blanc L, Daudelin IB, Podell BK, Chen PY, Zimmerman M, Martinot AJ, et al. High-resolution mapping of fluoroquinolones in TB rabbit lesions reveals specific distribution in immune cell types. *ELife.* (2018) 7:e41115. doi: 10.7554/eLife.41115.025
88. Tseng CH. Metformin decreases risk of tuberculosis infection in type 2 diabetes patients. *J Clin Med.* (2018) 7:264. doi: 10.3390/jcm7090264
89. Lin SY, Tu HP, Lu PL, Chen TC, Wang WH, Chong IW, et al. Metformin is associated with a lower risk of active tuberculosis in patients with type 2 diabetes. *Respirology.* (2018) 23:1063–73. doi: 10.1111/resp.13338
90. Zhang M, He JQ. Impacts of metformin on tuberculosis incidence and clinical outcomes in patients with diabetes: a systematic review and meta-analysis. *Eur J Clin Pharmacol.* (2019) 76:149–59. doi: 10.1007/s00228-019-0 2786-y
91. Mehrotra P, Jamwal SV, Saquib N, Sinha N, Siddiqui Z, Manivel V, et al. Pathogenicity of *Mycobacterium tuberculosis* is expressed by regulating metabolic thresholds of the host macrophage.

PLoS Pathog. (2014) 10:e1004265. doi: 10.1371/journal.ppat.1004265

92. Coriat R, Mir O, Ropert S, Loulergue P, Billemont B, Goldwasser F. Reactivation of tuberculosis during temsirolimus therapy. *Invest New Drugs.* (2011) 29:1494–6. doi: 10.1007/s10637-010-9487-2
93. Jeon SY, Yhim HY, Lee NR, Song EK, Kwak JY, Yim CY. Everolimus-induced activation of latent *Mycobacterium tuberculosis* infection in a patient with metastatic renal cell carcinoma. *Korean J Intern Med.* (2017) 32:365–8. doi: 10.3904/kjim.2015.121

4

Competitive Cell Death Interactions in Pulmonary Infection: Host Modulation Versus Pathogen Manipulation

Ethan S. FitzGerald†*, Nivea F. Luz*†* and Amanda M. Jamieson**

Division of Biology and Medicine, Department of Molecular Microbiology and Immunology, Brown University, Providence, RI, United States

***Correspondence:**
Amanda M. Jamieson
Amanda_Jamieson@brown.edu

†*These authors have contributed equally to this work*

In the context of pulmonary infection, both hosts and pathogens have evolved a multitude of mechanisms to regulate the process of host cell death. The host aims to rapidly induce an inflammatory response at the site of infection, promote pathogen clearance, quickly resolve inflammation, and return to tissue homeostasis. The appropriate modulation of cell death in respiratory epithelial cells and pulmonary immune cells is central in the execution of all these processes. Cell death can be either inflammatory or anti-inflammatory depending on regulated cell death (RCD) modality triggered and the infection context. In addition, diverse bacterial pathogens have evolved many means to manipulate host cell death to increase bacterial survival and spread. The multitude of ways that hosts and bacteria engage in a molecular tug of war to modulate cell death dynamics during infection emphasizes its relevance in host responses and pathogen virulence at the host pathogen interface. This narrative review outlines several current lines of research characterizing bacterial pathogen manipulation of host cell death pathways in the lung. We postulate that understanding these interactions and the dynamics of intracellular and extracellular bacteria RCD manipulation, may lead to novel therapeutic approaches for the treatment of intractable respiratory infections.

Keywords: bacterial pathogen, regulated cell death, lung, macrophages and neutrophils, pulmonary epithelium

INTRODUCTION

Pulmonary Immune Response to Infection Overview

At homeostasis, the pulmonary system remains a tightly regulated environment with resident cell types performing highly specialized functions to maintain a pathogen-free space with unimpeded respiratory function. The immune response to respiratory pathogens requires carefully regulated processes to prevent uncontrolled pathogen replication and lethal tissue destruction (1–3). Such tissue destruction may be mediated by the pathogen virulence factors, the host response, or a combination of the two. Limiting such pathology requires precise orchestration of tissue cells, tissue resident immune cells, and infiltrating immune cells when responding to infections. Constant coordination between these cell types is orchestrated by secreted and intracellular signals, many of which are generated as byproducts or effectors of regulated cell death (RCD). Both tissue cells and immune cells undergo RCD processes during infections, with dysregulation of these complex

RCD signaling networks often underlying the pathogenesis of pulmonary infectious disease. Below we provide a brief primer on the innate immune defenses of the lung and their status during homeostasis, before exploring the interplay of RCD signaling at the interface of bacterial pulmonary pathogens and host immunity.

Respiratory epithelial cells form a barrier between the outside environment and sterile zones in the body such as the blood (4). This is accomplished through a range of biophysical defenses, including the production of mucus by goblet or club cells and expulsion by ciliated epithelial cells (5). The composition of mucus also contains many antimicrobial peptides which impede bacterial translocation and effect bactericide (6). Furthermore, the physical barrier of tight cell-cell junctions formed between epithelial cells and underlying stroma is critical to barrier integrity (7). There is slow but constant turnover of respiratory epithelial cells via programmed cell death at homeostasis, with cells completely renewed every 30–50 days (8). Respiratory epithelial basal cells are stem cell-like cells which are long-lived and slowly dividing. They serve as progenitors for other subtypes of respiratory epithelial cells. The role and maintenance of the lung epithelium is reviewed extensively elsewhere (9).

Additionally, diverse lung resident innate immune cells patrol the lung (10). The majority of tissue resident phagocytes at steady state are alveolar macrophages (AMs). They reside in close proximity to respiratory epithelia and are responsible for immune surveillance. They recognize and are activated by pathogen-associated molecular patterns (PAMPs) and damage-associated molecular patterns (DAMPs). AMs serve as critical first responders that are required to both regulate signaling and carry out effector functions necessary to control bacterial infections of the lung. They are responsible for clearance of dead cells, debris, pathogens and inhaled particulates (10). In addition, AMs play important functions in maintaining homeostasis of the lung and promoting tissue repair through paracrine cell signaling (11). Other innate immune cells that are important in the lung immune response are interstitial macrophages and dendritic cells (DCs) (12). DCs in particular are sentinels throughout the lung epithelium and interstitium, where they serve as important early responders while helping to coordinate immunity to lung infections via antigen presentation (13). In addition to myeloid cells there are small numbers of lymphocytes that are found at steady state in the lung (14). If lung resident phagocytes cannot clear the infection, then other innate immune cells quickly infiltrate from circulation, and homing to secreted cytokines mediating immune cell recruitment (15). This includes neutrophils and inflammatory monocytes. Many of these resident and infiltrating innate immune cells are important replicative niches for distinct intracellular pulmonary pathogens. In addition, they are often targeted by cytocidal virulence factors from extracellular and intracellular pathogens, given their importance in initiating the sterilizing immune response. The pulmonary immune response is reviewed in greater detail elsewhere (10–15).

Respiratory epithelial cells and lung resident immune cells perform immune surveillance with a diverse repertoire of pattern recognition receptors (PRRs), such as Toll-like receptors (TLR), C-type lectin receptors (CLR), cytoplasmic retinoic acid-inducible gene-I-like receptors (RLR), and NOD-like receptors (NLR) (16). These PRRs are responsible for the detection of microbes in the respiratory system via the binding of PAMPs and DAMPs (17). Downstream signaling coordinated by PAMP/DAMP sensing cells includes the induction of bactericidal effector functions in immune cells such as reactive oxygen species (ROS) production, phagocytosis, or the secretion of mucus and bactericidal proteins in epithelial cells (18). PAMP-sensing cells that become overburdened by pathogens will also induce RCD processes (19). This can range from quiet apoptotic cell death to restrict pathogens within apoptotic bodies, or a pro-inflammatory pyroptotic cell death driving immune activity. Phagocytes responsible for engulfing pathogens also engulf dead or dying host cells via efferocytosis (20). Finally, upon clearing the infection, respiratory epithelial cells and immune cells in the lung coordinate the resolution of the inflammatory response and transition efforts from bacterial clearance to repair and remodeling in order to restore pulmonary homeostasis (21, 22).

Cell Death Mechanisms

Cell death is intricately connected with life in multicellular organisms. The balance between cell death, proliferation, and differentiation is crucial for the maintenance of tissue homeostasis, and particularly in response to infectious disease. RCD is essential for many physiological processes, including cancer, neurodegeneration, autoimmune diseases, and response to infection (23, 24). This narrative review focuses specifically on the types of cell death that are modulated by bacteria during pulmonary infection that impact infection pathogenesis. All the cell types described above that are essential to the maintenance of a healthy lung are also targets of infection by bacterial pathogens. After infection, various types of RCD can be triggered by the host in an effort to control the pathogen, or by the pathogen in an effort to manipulate the host response to promote bacterial fitness. This is particularly relevant in the pulmonary epithelium, which provides a barrier that separates the air-filled compartment of the respiratory system from the aqueous interstitial compartment (25). Phagocytes, which are often a target of pathogen infection, have also evolved many adaptations to orchestrate diverse RCD pathways to promote resolution of infections (19, 26). Below, we will provide brief overviews of the cell death pathways activated during the pulmonary bacterial infections described in this review. We categorize the cell death types as those that do not cause significant disruption of the cellular membrane (membrane non-permeabilizing), and those that cause a lytic and inflammatory form of cell death (membrane permeabilizing). We classify apoptosis, autophagy, and anoikis as generally non-permeabilizing, and pyroptosis, necroptosis, and ferroptosis as generally permeabilizing (**Figure 1**). This classification was largely informed by recommendations from the Nomenclature Committee on Cell Death (24). Classically, forms cell death which resulted in membrane rupture were classified as "necrosis" and were thought to occur through an unregulated process. However, many recent works have determined that lytic cell death often occurs via regulated processes dependent on molecular signal transduction. Contemporarily and in this

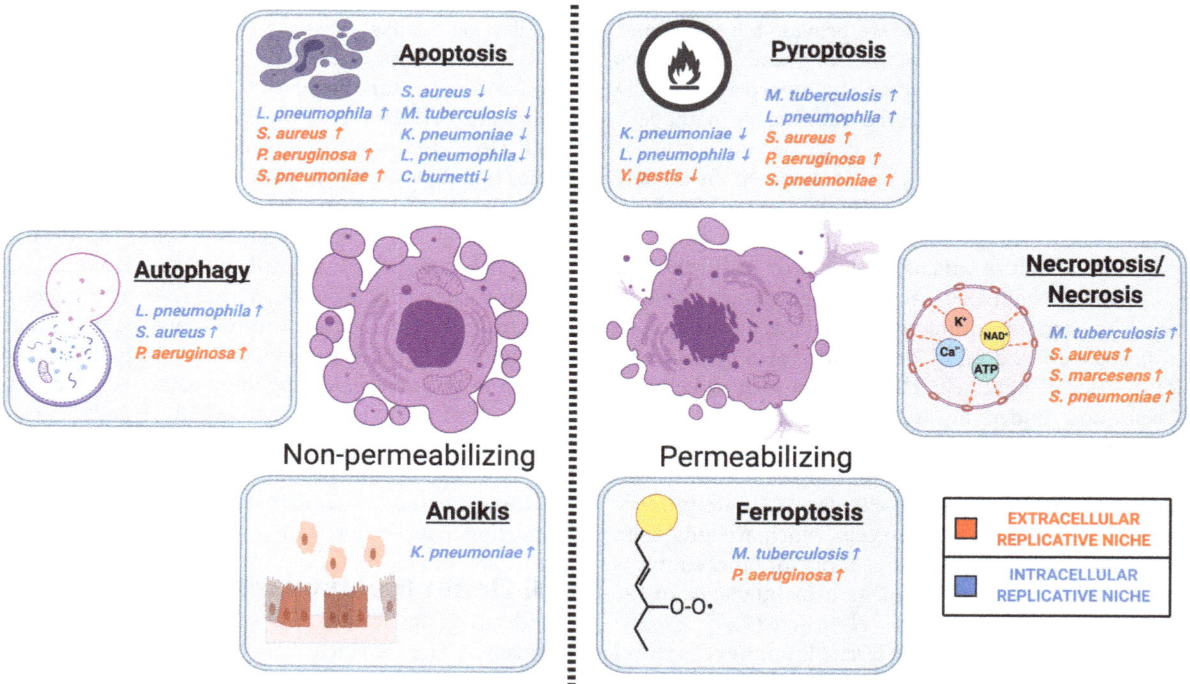

FIGURE 1 | Regulated cell death in host-pulmonary bacterial interactions. Major cell death pathways are shown in the figure according to their membrane permeabilization status. Pulmonary bacteria induce or inhibit host cell death through several distinct modalities, including apoptosis, autophagy, anoikis, ferroptosis, necrosis/necroptosis, and pyroptosis. ↑ Indicates that the bacteria induces the indicated cell death pathway, while ↓ indicates that the bacteria inhibits the indicated cell death pathway. Intracellular or extracellular bacteria are labeled according to the legend. Image created with BioRender.com.

review, the term necrosis is used to describe the morphological loss of membrane integrity occurring as a result of regulated and non-RCD. It is important to note that this review is not meant to be a review on all aspects of cell death, but only how bacterial pathogens interact with cell death pathways in the lung. The underlying mechanisms of RCD are well described in other literature, which we have cited throughout the manuscript for further reference. However, this section on cell death mechanisms should serve as a brief primer on the subject.

Apoptosis is a form of RCD characterized by a distinct morphological phenotype in which cells shrink and undergo nuclear condensation, form outer membrane blebs, and fragment into apoptotic bodies (27). Throughout this process, cells maintain cytoplasmic membrane integrity, which serves to limit inflammation mediated by DAMPs, prevent the dissemination of intracellular pathogens, and enable efficient efferocytic clearance and recycling of cytoplasmic contents by phagocytes (28). The canonical forms of apoptosis are differentiated based on the extracellular or intracellular nature of the stimulus inducing RCD (29). Extrinsic apoptosis is mediated by the activation of membrane-bound extracellular receptors such as Fas Death Receptor 4/5, or TNFR1 (30). These receptors bind to cytokine signaling molecules produced by epithelial cells and immune cells that are sensing proximal pathogens, DAMPs from infected cells, or their own intracellular infection (30). Activation of these receptors by their ligand results in the assembly of the death-inducing signaling complex (DISC) (31). DISC assembly serves to promote caspase-8 activity, which proteolytically activates many proteins that mark the cells as actively undergoing apoptosis such as cFLIP, as well as caspase-3 and caspase-7 (31). The activity of caspase-3 and -7 effect the terminal progression of apoptosis (32). Intrinsic apoptosis is initiated by the sensing of a broad range of intracellular damage and stressors (33). However, with regards to bacterial pulmonary infections, intrinsic apoptosis is commonly induced by intracellular infections, genomic damage mediated by reactive free radicals, ER stress, or inactivation of inhibitory signals suppressing apoptosis (24, 34). Intrinsic apoptosis is terminally effected by the induction of mitochondrial outer membrane permeabilization when the correct combination of pro-apoptotic regulators are activated and anti-apoptotic signals are suppressed (35). Many of these regulators are members of the BCL protein family (35). Intrinsic apoptosis is also marked by the activity of caspase-3 and -7; however, they are activated by caspase-9 rather than caspase-8 (36). Both extrinsic and intrinsic apoptosis play critical roles in the control of pulmonary infectious diseases mediated by cell death signaling.

Autophagy has an important homeostatic role, mediating the removal of dysfunctional or damaged organelles through the action of lysosomes, which effects the recycling of diverse cellular components. Autophagy contributes to the maintenance of cellular homeostasis as part of many cell autonomous stress responses, including nutrient and growth factor deprivation, oxidative stress or hypoxia, the restriction of intracellular pathogens, and the resolution of immune responses (37, 38).

Autophagy takes place in a series of steps. Autophagy initiation happens under starvation conditions when the unc-51-like kinase 1 (ULK1) complex dissociates from mTORC1 and becomes activated to initiate the formation of a phagophore. This is followed by a nucleation step driven by the PI3K complex. Phagophore elongation is then mediated by the Atg5-Atg 12-Atg16L and LC3II-PE conjugates. This results in the formation of autophagosomes. The autophagosomes then fuse to the lysosomes to form autophagolysosomes. The content present within the autophagosome is then delivered into the lysosomes where it gets degraded by the lysosomal enzymes (39). However, unrestrained autophagy can result in cell death. Based on guidelines published by the Nomenclature Committee on Cell Death, autophagy-dependent cell death is a type of RCD that relies on components of the autophagic machinery and takes place when the induction of autophagy coincides with the induction of apoptosis (24). Autophagic responses can play a key role in host defense to bacterial infections of the lung by reducing pathogen burden, but some pulmonary pathogens have evolved adaptions to benefit from such autophagic host responses or impede its execution (38, 40).

Anoikis is a form of regulatory cell death resulting from loss of cell anchorage to the basal membrane (41). Anoikis results in the loss of microtubule organization and basal cell junctions required for adherence to the extracellular matrix (41). Cellular escape from anoikis signal transduction is critical for the establishment of metastatic tumors, and anoikis has been implicated in bacterial and viral infections targeting cell anchorage (42). Further work is required to characterize the induction of anoikis RCD in the context of infectious disease.

Pyroptosis is a form of pro-inflammatory RCD that triggers mature IL-1β production and membrane permeabilization via gasdermins, which are host-derived pore-forming proteins (43). Pyroptotic signaling is triggered by recognition of PAMPs by NLRs. The PAMP-mediated activation of NLRs induces the assembly of multi-protein complexes called inflammasomes (44). There are many sub-types of inflammasomes, carrying out varying responses to unique pathogens (45). PAMPs from a given pathogen can trigger multiple inflammasome species (45). Generally, an activated inflammasome carries out the proteolytic maturation of caspase-1, which processes gasdermins, IL-1β, and IL-18 into their mature/active forms (46). Mature gasdermin proteins rapidly assemble into multimeric pore complexes that insert into the cell's cytoplasmic membrane, resulting in cytoplasmic efflux and membrane-permeabilizing cell death (47). IL-1β and IL-18 are cytokines released during this process which promote inflammation and immune cell recruitment/effector function (46). Outcomes of pyroptosis induction vary from infection to infection, with pyroptosis having the capacity to both promote pathogen clearance and/or drive tissue damage and immunopathology.

The term "necroptosis" was originally introduced by Yuan et al., to delineate a specific form of regulated necrosis that is triggered by death receptor ligation and blockage of caspase-8 (48). One of the most intensively investigated subroutines of regulated membrane-permeabilizing cell death is necroptosis. The molecular pathway of tumor necrosis factor alpha (TNF-α)-induced necroptosis involves activation of Receptor-interacting serine/threonine protein kinase 1 (RIPK1)/Receptor-interacting serine/threonine protein kinase 3 (RIPK3)/mixed lineage kinase domain-like (MLKL) (49). Necroptosis is negatively regulated by caspase-8 and inhibitor of apoptosis proteins (IAPs), with the inactivation of caspase-8 resulting in the phosphorylation and activation of RIPK1, RIPK3, and MLKL which complex together to form the necrosome. To date, the only known kinase that is capable of phosphorylating MLKL is RIPK3, likely to reduce spurious induction of necroptosis. After becoming phosphorylated, MLKL oligomerizes into a membrane pore structure and inserts itself into the cell membrane, resulting in cytoplasmic leak (49). The unique molecular structure of MLKL oligomers enabling it to bind lipid bilayers is required for its pore forming properties (50). Insertion of sufficient amounts of oligomerized MLKL ultimately effects necroptosis al through lytic cell death (50, 51). The execution of necroptosis results in the disruption of ion homeostasis and the release of molecules that are recognized as DAMPs when in the extracellular environment (52).

Ferroptosis is a membrane-permeabilizing RCD dependent on iron in which glutathione, oxidative stress and lipid hyper-peroxidation play crucial roles. Suppression of glutathione antioxidant defense via inactivation of glutathione peroxidase 4 (GPX4) drives the hyper-peroxidation of lipids (53). Enrichment of membranes with polyunsaturated fatty acids, such as arachidonic acid (AA) esterified in phosphatidylethanolamines (PE), provides possible substrates for lipid hydroperoxides (54). The accumulation of hyper-peroxidized lipids within the cell results in a membrane-permeabilizing form of lytic cell death.

Role of Cell Death During Bacterial Lung Infection Overview

The precise regulation of programmed cell death by respiratory epithelial cells and immune cells is a key determinant of morbidity and mortality (**Table 1**, 55). Hosts rely on infected cells initiating the appropriate programmed cell death response to prompt responding immune cells and proximal epithelial cells to restrict infections. In addition, uninfected immune cells must avoid cell death to carry out their functions. However, due to the evolutionary competition underlying every host-pathogen relationship, pulmonary pathogens have evolved amazingly diverse means to disrupt or redirect host cell death signaling toward cell death modalities that are beneficial to bacterial fitness. We argue that the specific modalities which bacteria aim to induce are primarily determined by the need to maintain a hospitable replicative niche for the bacteria. As such, bacterial tropism can be considered as an organizing principle when classifying the different cell death modalities bacteria seek to induce in hosts. The citations in this review evidence the claim that pulmonary bacteria have focused on modulating aspects of host cell death to better mold a replicative niche within the lung (**Table 1**). Interestingly, bacteria rely on both suppression and induction of RCD to accomplish these ends. This narrative review focuses on pulmonary bacterial pathogens where RCD plays an important role in their disease pathogenesis.

TABLE 1 | RCD directionality through diverse pulmonary bacterial infections.

Bacteria	RCD direction	Host target	Bacterial effector	Cell type
P. aeruginosa	Apoptosis – ↑	TNFR1 (caspase-8–caspase-3 axis activation)	Quorum-sensing (N-3-oxo-dodecanoyl) (67)	Neutrophils from C57BL/6 mice and *in vivo* murine model
	Intrinsic apoptosis – ↑	Caspase-9 and effector caspase-3	ExoS (58)	Epithelial cells
	Apoptosis – ↑	Mitochondrial acid sphingomyelinase	Pyocyaninman (72)	Neutrophil (*ex vivo*), Jurkat T cells and HL-60 neutrophils
	Ferroptosis – ↑	15-hydroperoxy-AA-PE (15-HOO-AA-PE)	Lipoxygenase (pLoxA) (69)	HBE (human bronchial epithelial cell line)
	Pyroptosis – ↑	NLRC4 inflammasome	Type III secretion system	Phagocytes (THP-1 macrophages)
	Autophagy – ↑	unfolded protein response (UPR)	Type VI secretion system (71)	Human epithelial cells
S. marcescens	Necroptosis – ↑	RIPK1, RIPK3, and MLKL	ShlA (51)	Macrophages, neutrophil (*in vivo* murine model)
	Necroptosis – ↑	RIPK1, RIPK3, and MLKL	Pore-forming toxin (75)	Mouse bronchial epithelial cells (*in vivo* murine model)
S. pneumoniae	Intrinsic Apoptotis – ↑	Genomic DNA	Pyruvate oxidase produced ROS (84)	A549 human alveolar epithelial cell line and *in vivo* murine models
	Necroptosis – ↑	Cytoplasmic membrane	Pneumolysin (54)	A549 Human Alveolar Epithelial cell line and *in vivo* murine models
	Pyroptosis – ↑	Diverse inflammasomes	S. pneumoniae PAMPs (90)	Epithelial cells and immune cells
S. aureus	Apoptosis – ↑	Cell membrane and other Structures	Enterotoxins and α-toxin (52)	Leukocytes
	Apoptosis – ↑	Deoxyadenosine	S nuclease and adenosine synthase (103)	U937 (human lung macrophage cell line)
	Necroptosis – ↑	Mixed lineage kinase-like protein (MLKL)	Phenol-soluble modulines (PSMs) (103)	Neutrophil (*in vivo* murine model)
	Necroptosis – ↑	RIPK1, RIPK3, and MLKL	Pore forming toxins (99)	Human peripheral blood neutrophils and mouse bone marrow neutrophil
	Pyroptosis – ↑	NLRP3	agr, hla, lukAB, and PSMs (93)	Neutrophil (*in vivo* murine model)
		↑ Extracellular bacteria ↑ | ↓ Intracellular bacteria ↓		
S. aureus	Apoptosis – ↓	iNOS	Arginine deaminase (110)	16HBE14o- Cell Line
	Apoptosis – ↓	MCL-1 (116)	Unknown Effector	Human marrow derived macrophages and RAW264.7 cell line
	Autophagy – ↑	Unc-51–like autophagy-activating kinase 1	agr quorum-sensing system (113)	Epithelial cells
	Autophagy – ↓	MAPK14 (114)	Unknown Effector	NIH/3T3 and mouse embryonic fibroblasts
M. tuberculosis	Apoptosis – ↓	iNOS activity/TLR Signaling	Esx-1 effector EspR (119)	RAW264.7 murine macrophage cell line
	Apoptosis – ↓	iNOS activity/MAPK-P53 Signaling	Esx-1 effector MptpB (120)	RAW264.7 murine macrophage cell line
	Apoptosis – ↓	ROS production/jnk signaling	AcpM Acyl carrier protein (121)	Murine bone marrow derived macrophages
	Apoptosis – ↓	IL10 mediated expression of TNFR2	HSP60 (124)	Differentiated Thp-1 human macrophage cell line
	Apoptosis – ↓	PPARg – MCL-1 signaling	Mannosylated lipoarabinomannan (125)	Human primary alveolar and monocyte derived macrophages
	Necrosis – ↑	Cytoplasmic membrane/phosphotidyl serine	Esx-1 effector ESAT-6 (126)	Human primary Neutrophils
	Pyroptosis – ↑	Unknown Effector	RD1 locus expression of Esx-1 and ESAT-6 (128)	Differentiated Thp-1 human macrophage cell line
	Necroptosis – ↑	NAD + Depletion	Tuberculosis necrotizing toxin (TNT) (129)	Differentiated Thp-1 human macrophage cell line
	Necrosis – ↑	PGE2 synthesis	Phospholipase C (132)	Rat primary alveolar macrophages
	Ferroptosis – ↑	Gpx4 peroxidase activity (133)	Unknown Effector	Murine bone marrow-derived macrophages and human monocyte derived macrophages
K. pneumoniae	Apoptosis – ↓	Bax-BCL2	*K. pneumoniae* capsule components (137)	Human primary neutrophils
	Apoptosis – ↓	Flippase regulation of phosphotidyl serine (139)	Unknown Effector	Murine peritoneal macrophages and neutrophils and *in vivo* murine models
	Pyroptosis – ↑	Diverse inflammasomes	*K. pneumoniae* PAMPs (141)	Murine bone marrow-derived macrophages and *in vivo* murine models

(Continued)

TABLE 1 | Continued

Bacteria	RCD direction	Host target	Bacterial effector	Cell type
	Anoikis – ↑	Microtubule disassembly via KATNAL1 and KATNB1	YtfL (142)	A549 human alveolar epithelial cell line and *in vivo* murine models
Y. pestis	Pyroptosis – ↓	NLR pattern recognition receptors	YopK (146)	Bone marrow derived-macrophages and *in vivo* murine models
	Pyroptosis – ↓	Caspase-1	YopM (148)	Bone marrow derived-macrophages and *in vivo* murine models
	Pyroptosis – ↓	IQGAP1 Caspase-1 scaffolding protein	YopM (149)	Bone marrow derived-macrophages and *in vivo* murine models
	Pyroptosis – ↓	Pyrin inflammasome	YopM (150)	Bone marrow derived macrophages and *in vivo* murine models
	Pyroptosis – ↓	TAK1 – IKK IL1B activity	YopJ (151)	Bone marrow derived-macrophages
	Necrosis – ↑	Gasdermin D	YopK (151)	Bone marrow derived-macrophages
	Extrinsic apoptosis – ↓	FasL	Plasminogen activator (Pla) (146)	A549 human alveolar epithelial cell line, Jurkat cells, and *in vivo* murine models
C. burnetti	Intrinsic apoptosis – ↓	p32 transcription factor/Importin-alpha 1	AnkG (155)	Murine bone marrow-derived dendridic cells, CHO, HEK293T, and MEF cell lines
	Intrinsic apoptosis – ↓	p32 transcription factor	AnkG (155)	Murine bone marrow-derived dendridic cells, HELA, and HEK293T cell lines
	Intrinsic apoptosis – ↓	PARP cleavage	CaeA/CaeB (154)	Differentiated Thp-1 human macrophage cell line
	Intrinsic apoptosis – ↓	Bcl-1 and Bcl-2	Type IV secretion effectors (158)	HeLa cell line
L. pneumophila	Parthanatos – ↑	PARP	RpsL (173)	Bone marrow-derived macrophages
	Pyroptosis – ↑	NAIP5/NLRC4 (Birc1e/IPAF)	FlaA (171)	Bone marrow-derived macrophages
	Apoptosis – ↓	Caspase 3/7	Lipophosphoglycans (166, 169)	HeLa cell line, HEK293T cell line, and murine bone marrow-derived dendridic cells
	Apoptosis – ↓	BNIP3, Bcl-rambo	SidF (168)	Bone marrow-derived macrophages and U937 cell line
	Apoptosis – ↓	NF-kb	LegK1 and LnaB (169)	Bone marrow-derived macrophages
	Apoptosis – ↓	Caspase 3, 8,9, and 1	Dot/Icm, strain dependent (170)	Bone marrow-derived macrophages
	Pyroptosis – ↑	Caspase-11	Dot/Icm flaA-independent (166)	Bone marrow-derived macrophages and *in vivo* murine models
	Autophagy – ↑	Atg7, Atg, and MDC	Dot/Icm (169)	Bone marrow-derived macrophages

Diverse pulmonary bacteria are listed in the table along with the RCD that the host cells undergo, host protein targeted by the bacteria, the bacterial effector used to manipulate cell death, and the cell type the finding was observed in. Intracellular bacteria are listed above the red line, and extracellular bacteria are listed below. ↑ Indicates that the bacteria induce the indicated cell death pathway, while ↓ indicates that the bacteria inhibits the indicated cell death pathway.

Much experimental work has been conducted to elucidate cell death pathways implicated in the pathogenesis of pneumonia caused by diverse etiological agents. The application of small molecule inhibitors of key signal transducers for RCD pathways has shown that bacterial manipulation of RCD is often necessary for their survival *in vivo*. While there is much diversity in how pathogens manipulate RCD, we suggest that pathogens can be categorized based on: (1) intracellular or extracellular bacterial tropism and (2) whether pathogens can be regarded as inducers or suppressors of the inflammatory response. Briefly, we find that intracellular pathogens tend to manipulate RCD to promote the maintenance of the intracellular niche. Intracellular pathogens that induce the inflammatory response and immune cell recruitment rely on membrane-permeabilizing cell death to release bacteria from infected cells, rather than having them sequestered in membrane integral apoptotic bodies. Intracellular pathogens that suppress the inflammatory response seek to establish minimally immunogenic and chronic infections that evade recognition and clearance by the immune system. Many intracellular pathogens have evolved the ability to suppress RCD signal transduction by directly binding and inhibiting host factors.

Bacteria with extracellular tropism tend to aggravate the inflammatory response to promote tissue damage that speeds bacterial dissemination from the lung and releases crucial cytoplasmic nutrients into the comparatively nutrient poor extracellular space. They suppress the activity of immune effector cells and destroy epithelial barrier integrity by driving RCD through the secretion of toxins and other cytotoxic agents. Recent findings have determined that pore-forming toxins expressed by many pulmonary pathogens such as *Serratia marcescens*, *Staphylococcus aureus*, and *Streptococcus pneumoniae* stimulate necroptotic programmed cell death (56). Recombinant pore-forming toxins and bacteria-synthesized pore-forming toxins have been shown to induce necroptosis in both alveolar epithelial cells and in AMs, due to cytoplasmic dysbiosis resultant from loss of membrane integrity. These include ATP and metal ion efflux, mitochondrial damage, and ROS production. Necroptotic cell death can also be induced independent of PRR activation, through the activation of host proteins RIPK1, RIPK3, and

MLKL, after sensing changes in the cytoplasmic environment such as ion and nutrient availability (57).

Given the centrality of RCD in determining pneumonia disease outcomes, it is clear that the pharmacologic or genetic manipulation of RCD during infection could represent a novel therapeutic strategy for the treatment of complicated or drug-resistant bacterial pneumonia (58). However, further study of the ways that pulmonary pathogens manipulate host RCD signaling during infection is required to design effective therapeutic strategies for validation. This review aims to provide a survey of pneumonia-causing bacterial manipulation of RCD and begin defining classifications of bacterial pulmonary pathogens based on their manipulation of RCD. By aggregating such information of diverse pathogens, trends regarding bacterial pathogenesis mechanisms can be elucidated to inform future work investigating bacterial manipulation of RCD and host-targeted therapeutic strategies.

PATHOGEN-SPECIFIC REGULATED CELL DEATH RESPONSES

Extracellularly Replicative Bacteria

Pseudomonas aeruginosa

Pseudomonas aeruginosa is an extracellular, Gram-negative pathogen (59). While considered primarily an extracellular pathogen, Bajmoczi et al., have reported that *P. aeruginosa* can be found in epithelial cells (60). However, we will focus on its primary extracellular tropism. *P. aeruginosa* opportunistically causes serious infections and is a leading cause of nosocomial pneumonia. It also contributes to morbidity and mortality due to respiratory failure and sepsis in immunocompromised patients, particularly in cystic fibrosis patients (59, 61). It is noteworthy that there has been a significant increase in the incidence of multi-drug resistant isolates of *P. aeruginosa* in hospital settings, making complementary therapeutic approaches to augment immune clearance and control RCD in epithelial and endothelial pulmonary tissue more essential (62).

The antibacterial host response initiated during *P. aeruginosa* infection is multifaceted and includes the activation of RCD pathways including apoptosis, necroptosis, and pyroptosis. *P. aeruginosa* induces endothelial cells to undergo apoptosis, through mechanisms that are partially dependent on the oxidative stress response (63). The production of ROS is classically known to be an essential mechanism for the immune cell mediated killing of *Pseudomonas* (64). Such apoptosis induction is likely a byproduct of these bactericidal activities. *P. aeruginosa*-infected endothelial cell death via apoptosis has been adapted to contribute host elimination of *P. aeruginosa* because apoptotic cells and associated bacteria are readily efferocytosed by professional phagocytes, particularly AMs (65). *P. aeruginosa* adhesion receptors fail to distinguish between adherence of apoptotic epithelial cells and epithelial cell apoptotic bodies, similarly allowing *P. aeruginosa* to be internalized through efferocytosis (65). However, due to the importance of endothelial barrier integrity, death and the elimination of infected cells from the endothelium lining can also provide a route for dissemination of *P. aeruginosa* to distal sites where metastatic infections can be established.

Given the restrictive effects of such epithelial or endothelial tissue cell apoptosis on these infections, it stands to reason that *P. aeruginosa* and other bacteria may have developed strategies to counteract this RCD. However, *P. aeruginosa*, as an extracellular pathogen, has mainly evolved protein effectors, which agonize cell death. This is consistent with the trend that extracellular bacteria prioritize activities that are detrimental to pulmonary barrier integrity as opposed to modulating cell death to inhibit bacterial clearance. For instance, *P. aeruginosa* derived LPS is sufficient to induce human alveolar morphological changes, inflammation, and apoptosis in A549 and human bronchial BEAS-2B cells (64). Exotoxins from the type III secretion system (T3SS), once in the cytoplasm of host epithelial cells, also have been shown to induce cell death by programmed necrosis or apoptosis, thus favoring disruption of epithelial barriers (66).

Some *P. aeruginosa* quorum-sensing metabolites also function to induce host immune cell death through cell surface lipid domain dissolution (67). Bacterial quorum-sensing auto-inducers are small chemicals released to control microbial community behaviors. Interestingly, one of these quorum sensing metabolites, N-(3-oxo-dodecanoyl)-L-homoserine lactone, was found to integrate into host cell membranes and induce RCD in responding immune cells through dissolution of the lipid bilayer. The effect of this membrane disruption resulted in host cells expelling tumor necrosis factor receptor 1 (TNFR1) associated with its membrane into the disordered lipid phase. There it trimerized into its active form and drove caspase-3–caspase-8-mediated apoptosis. Thus, *P. aeruginosa* gains a survival advantage by inducing RCD in responding leukocytes which suppresses bacterial clearance. Song et al., noted that the suppression of caspase activity effecting apoptotic RCD, was able to diminish pathogenicity by inhibiting this effect.

Pseudomonas aeruginosa also utilizes secreted exotoxins such as ExoS and ExoT, two homologous T3SS virulence factors that induce apoptosis in target host epithelial cells through toxin associated stress responses relating to cytoskeletal regulation (68). A recent work showed that T3SS also activates the cytosolic nucleotide-binding domain, leucine-rich repeat-containing caspase activation and recruitment domain CARD_ containing 4 (NLRC4) inflammasome, which activates caspase-1 and induces gasdermin-mediated cytotoxicity and the release of mature IL-1β (68). ExoU-producing isolates of *P. aeruginosa* caused massive cell death *in vitro* in THP-1 human monocytes but drove minimal release of IL-1β. In contrast, those expressing T3SS but not ExoU induced caspase-1 activation and IL-1β release, the level of which was correlated with cytotoxicity. Both effects were prevented by a specific caspase-1 inhibitor; however, further forms of cell death have not been examined in this model. Thus, T3SS cytotoxicity is mediated partially through the modification of inflammasome regulated cytokine production for *P. aeruginosa* clinical isolates that do not express ExoU.

Pseudomonas aeruginosa have also been found to induce ferroptosis, which is a cell death program executed via selective oxidation of arachidonic acid–phosphatidylethanolamines

(AA-PE) by 15-lipoxygenases (69). *P. aeruginosa* can express lipoxygenase (pLoxA), which oxidizes host AA-PE to 15-hydroperoxy-AA-PE (15-HOO-AA-PE), and triggers ferroptosis in human bronchial epithelial cells. A biofilm of *P. aeruginosa* is capable of inducing ferroptosis in human bronchial epithelial cells via enhanced expression of pLoxA and oxidation of host cell AA-PE to 15-HOO-AA-PE (69). To date, the majority of work on *P. aeruginosa*-phagocyte interactions has focused on apoptosis, and to a lesser extent, pro-inflammatory/membrane-permeabilizing forms of cell death, such as ferroptosis. Further research is required to determine whether ferroptosis induction is an effective strategy employed by *P. aeruginosa* to promote disruption of the epithelial barrier and immune-regulatory functions.

Pseudomonas aeruginosa also utilizes a type VI secretion system (T6SS) to secrete numerous virulence effectors that can both interfere with competing microbes and manipulate host cells (70). *P. aeruginosa* infection induces autophagy in epithelial cells and this response plays a vital role in clearing intracellular bacteria. In addition to epithelial cells, neutrophils also play a pivotal role in the host's early acute defense against pulmonary *P. aeruginosa*. Pyocyanin is a membrane-permeable pigment that also functions as an exotoxin when released by *P. aeruginosa* by inducing neutrophil apoptosis (71). Pyocyanin interacts with components of the mitochondrial electron transport chain, driving the dysregulated release of ROS, activation of mitochondrial acid sphingomyelinase, synthesis of mitochondrial ceramide, and the release of pro-apoptotic cytochrome c from the intermembrane space (71). This mechanism is associated with neutrophil depletion, an event that can sensitize the host to *P. aeruginosa* infections and colonization, since neutrophils are key elements of the host defense against infection (71).

Summary – *P. aeruginosa* largely conforms to the expected behaviors of pulmonary extracellular bacterial pathogens by inducing RCD in tissue and immune cells, rather than suppressing restrictive RCD mechanisms. *Pseudomonas* utilizes the secretion of exotoxins to damage cellular structures and tissues while coordinating colony behavior. Toxins also act to suppress the activity of host immune cells. Like many pyrogenic infections, PAMP and DAMP signaling are necessary for bacterial clearance, but also drive tissue damages through the induction of stress responses. Therapeutic strategies augmenting the cytoprotection of immune cells through suppression of their apoptotic signaling while driving tissue cell efferocytic clearance and phagocytic activities, may serve as critical measures in the context of antibiotic-resistant nosocomial infections. Designing and validating such RCD modulating therapeutic strategies could significantly improve clinical options for immunosuppressed and cystic fibrosis patients who often suffer from these infections.

Serratia marcescens

Serratia marcescens is an opportunistic Gram-negative bacteria classified in the order Enterobacteriaceae and the family *Yersiniaceae*. *Serratia* species are not typical constituents of human microbiomes, more commonly residing in environmental niches such as fresh water, soil, and the fecal flora of many animals (72). However, *S. marcescens* has also been identified a nosocomial pathogen causing diseases including severe bacterial pneumonia, in part due to its ability to persist on abiotic substrates for extended periods and the emergence of antibiotic resistant strains (73).

Limited data exists characterizing Serratia infections in pulmonary model systems. For instance, *S. marcescens* was show to produce ShlA, a pore-forming toxin that effects macrophages by inducing necroptosis, damaging mitochondrial membranes, inducing ATP depletion via cytoplasmic leak, and driving ROS production (74). Recent work found that the activity of ShlA was dependant on its activity as a calcium channel disrupting Ca^{2+} ion homeostasis, and that the effects ShlA toxicity could be inhibited *in vitro* through the direct application of Ni^{2+} ions (75). In an *in vivo murine* model of hemorrhagic pneumonia caused by *S. marcescens*, inhibition of necroptosis via RIPK1 and MLKL inhibition resulted in decreased morbidity and mortality (56). A previous study has also shown that *S. marcescens* is able to induce apoptosis in human lung adenocarcinoma A549 cells (76). In addition, Krzymińska et al., reported that hospital-isolated strains of *S. marcescens* produce toxins that contribute to its virulence and are essentials for the bacteria to adhere and invade to epithelial cells and induce hemolysis, cytotoxicity, and apoptosis of human epithelial cells and macrophages (77).

While very few mechanistic details characterizing *S. marcescens* pathogenesis and host cell death modulation in pulmonary system are available, significant *in vitro* data illustrates how *S. marcescens* also targets host RCD signaling known to exacerbate pneumonia and manipulates RCD signaling that is useful for defense against pulmonary infections. Such RCD manipulation strategies likely play key roles in the pathogenesis of *S. marcescens* in the clinic. For instance, direct injection of *S. marcesens* into the hemolymph of silkworms agonized c-Jun NH2-terminal kinase signaling which eventually resulted in the caspase mediated apoptosis of blood cells (75). This effect was also observed during *in vitro* infection of mouse peritoneal macrophages (78). Using a transposon library for forward genetic screening, Ischii et al., found that apoptosis induction was inhibited with the loss of genes necessary for lipopolysaccharide and flagellin synthesis (78).

Additionally, work performed in a Chinese Hamster Ovary epithelial cells, HeLa cells, *Atg* 5+/+ Mouse Embryonic Fibroblasts, and T24 cells revealed that *S. marcescens* is capable of manipulating autophagy to establish an intracellular niche in diverse cell types (73). During *in vitro* infection, approximately 20% of bacteria were able to induce endocytic uptake in these cells and form intracellular replicative niches in Rab7 and LC3 positive vesicles in a Atg5 dependent manner. Despite these autophagic markers, *S. marcescens* containing vesicles failed to acidify and restrict bacterial growth (73). Fedrigo et al., hypothesized that cell wall components of *S. marcescens* may play a key role in the induction of this process. Such manipulation of epithelial cell autophagy in the pulmonary environment, could significantly agonize respiratory epithelial cell death due to the induction of intracellular stress responses that may help shield the bacteria from responding host immune cells and phagocytes. Further investigation of *S. marcescens*' ability to manipulate autophagy in the context of pulmonary infection capacities is required.

In vitro data also suggests specific bacterial proteins and peptides that are able to manipulate RCD. For instance, non-pore forming toxin produced by *S. marcescens* was shown to induce cytolysis (79). Ectopic expression of *S. marcescens* PhlA was found to induce cytolysis in HeLa cells via the direct hydrolysis of phospholipids to lysophosphoylipids, which effected membrane permeabilization after they are incorporated into the cytoplasmic membrane (79). Hydrolyzed lysophospholipids generated by PlaA are capable of triggering both hemolysis and cytolysis. Another Serratia derived peptide, AT514 or serratamolide, was also found to strongly induce apoptosis in typically apoptosis resistant B cell chronic lymphocytic leukemia cells (80). Administration of the peptide to tumor cells cancerous B cells effected the induction of intrinsic apoptosis through the release of cytochrome c from mitochondria and the activation of caspase-9 and caspase-3 (80). AT514 was also found to inhibit the pro-survival signals of Bcl2, phosphatidylinositol-3 kinase, and protein kinase C. Also, the *S. marcescens* derived metabolic compound prodigiosin was found to agonize p53-induced apoptosis and suppress the activity of survivin in acute lymphoblastic leukemia. This is accomplished by driving the synthesis of ROS, that damage dsDNA, RNA, and other cell components (81). The observation of multiple apoptosis inducing compounds and cellular components produced by *S. marcescens*, lends credibility to the hypothesis that the induction of apoptosis aggravates *S. marcescens* pneumonia and other forms of nosocomial infections.

Summary - Generally, *S. marcescens* induces cell death to disrupt epithelial cells–extracellular matrix adhesions in airway epithelial cells, which allows for bacteria invasion into the submucosal tissues. Alternatively, when *S. marcescens* induces necroptosis through pore-forming toxins this leads to enhanced disease severity. Induction of cell death within cells of the immune system may contribute to the spread of infection and prolonged disease manifestation. One of the most catastrophic of *S. marcescens*' strategies is the induction of necroptosis in AMs. This not only abolishes a critical element of the early immune response, but also results in inflammation and tissue damage, which intensifies disease. Thus, targeting necroptosis may provide an important therapeutic strategy to block both cell death and inflammation for the treatment of human hemorrhagic pneumonia triggered by *S. marcescens*.

Streptococcus pneumoniae

Streptococcus pneumoniae is a Gram-positive bacteria commonly causing pulmonary infections with a preferred extracellular tropism (82). *S. pneumoniae* effects much of their virulence through direct killing of responding immune cells and respiratory epithelial cells via ROS production and the secretion of pore-forming toxins. While these effector functions do not directly manipulate or suppress host proteins regulating cell death to promote their survival, their activity has been shown to drive several host RCD pathways which underlie much of the pathogenesis of *S. pneumoniae* infection and impede host clearance efforts.

The *S. pneumoniae* enzyme SpxB, a pyruvate oxidase, acts upon bacterial intracellular pyruvate to generate H_20_2 ROS that are secreted into the pulmonary microenvironment. Elevated ROS has been shown to induce double-strand breaks in the host's genome and result in a p53-dependent apoptotic cell death that can exacerbate tissue damage (83). However, this induction of apoptosis can be pro-resolving in the context of *S. pneumoniae* that have already been engulfed by phagocytes, particularly macrophages. In murine infection models, inhibiting the activity of caspases that cause apoptosis was shown to increase pathogen burden (84). Apoptotic death of some AMs during *S. pneumoniae* infection has also been proposed to limit hyper-inflammatory damage associated with severe bacterial infection and promote efferocytic clearance of bacteria-laden phagocytes. It has recently been observed that inhibition of TNF-induced AM apoptosis via TNF-related apoptosis-inducing ligand (TRAIL) knockout significantly inhibited bacterial clearance and survival in a murine *S. pneumoniae* infection model. The inhibition of TNF-induced apoptosis drove AMs toward a necrotic cell death phenotype, which was able to be rescued through TRAIL add back and an application of anti-DR5 antibodies to drive apoptosis without an upstream TNF signal. They also determined that dying neutrophils served as a major source of TRAIL, and hypothesized that an inability to induce macrophage apoptosis during early pneumococcal infection may explain the severe pathology of neutropenic hosts during pulmonary bacterial infection (85). Other factors inhibiting macrophage apoptosis, such as host-derived MIF or bacterial PcpA, have also been shown to be detrimental to the host during pneumococcal infection (86, 87). For instance, recent research has demonstrated that AM-specific expression of the anti-apoptotic protein MCL-1 in mice inhibited the cells' capacity to kill phagocytosed *S. pneumoniae*. Researchers generated a transgenic mouse line constitutively overexpressing human MCL-1 protein in AMs. The researchers found that wild-type AMs would phagocytose *S. pneumoniae* and carry out killing through the phagolysosome. However, prolonged uptake of bacteria over 12 h eventually overwhelms the phagocytic clearance pathway, resulting in the activation of macrophage apoptosis which drives the release of mitochondrial-derived ROS and nitric oxide production to enhance killing of intracellular bacteria. While MCL-1 overexpressing AMs were able to successfully uptake *S. pneumoniae* and activate nitric oxide synthesis after becoming overwhelmed with intracellular bacteria, they were unable to release mitochondrial-derived ROS to kill bacteria (88).

Many independent research groups have demonstrated the induction of regulated membrane-permeabilizing cell death via pyroptotic or necroptotic signaling to be detrimental to the host response to pneumococcal pneumonia, primarily due to the hyper-inflammatory response these modes of cell death promote. For instance, recent work demonstrated that nucleotide-binding domain, leucine-rich repeat-containing, and pyrin domain-containing 3 (NLRP3) and apoptosis-associated speck-like protein containing a caspase recruitment domain (ASC) knockout mice had improved host defense in a lethal infection model with *S. pneumoniae* (89). The inhibition of pyroptosis is thought to improve host defense to pneumococcal pneumoniae by suppressing hyper-inflammation that is detrimental to pulmonary barrier integrity without inhibiting bacterial clearance by phagocytes.

Like many other pulmonary bacterial pathogens *S. pneumoniae* produces pore-forming toxins leading to necroptosis (56). The pore-forming toxin pneumolysin (Ply) is one of the most well characterized virulence factors produced by *S. pneumoniae*. *S. pneumoniae* Ply (like many bacterial pore-forming toxins) drives necroptotic cell death signaling in diverse cell types, including alveolar epithelial cells and macrophages. *S. pneumoniae* species that induce lower degrees of NF-kB activity have been associated with more severe pneumonia (90). Lower NF-kB activity has also been shown to drive macrophages away from an active state focused on bacterial clearance and toward pro-inflammatory necroptosis (90).

Summary – *S. pneumoniae* are bacteria that prefer to replicate extracellularly on the surface of respiratory epithelium. They primarily induce host cell death in responding immune cells and respiratory epithelial cells through the secretion of protein or chemical toxins that damage cellular structures. These include pneumolysin, which damage cell membranes by forming pores, and bacteria-synthesized ROS, which induce genomic damage to drive apoptosis. In the context of engulfing macrophages, bacterial surface proteins have been shown to inhibit pro-resolving macrophage apoptosis. Host-directed therapeutic strategies augmenting phagocyte or respiratory epithelial cell resistance to the cytocidal effect of *S. pneumoniae*-derived protein or chemical toxins may help ameliorate the burden of pneumococcal pneumonia, in conjunction with current antibiotic therapies and vaccination strategies. These could include inhibitors of membrane permeabilizing RCD or strategies to limit the impact of ROS.

Staphylococcus aureus

Staphylococcus aureus has been classically identified as extracellular pyrogenic bacteria, but it has also been recognized to have facultative intracellular tropism during infection (91). Below we explore the behavior of *Staphylococci* as an extracellular bacteria in the pulmonary space, and we will discuss the intracellular ramifications in the section "Intracellularly Replicative Bacteria." An array of the *S. aureus* proteins function as virulence factors that worsen the pathogenicity of infection. For instance, *S. aureus* produces potent toxins, such as staphylococcal enterotoxins (SEs) and α-toxin (α-hemolysin), which have been shown to induce biological membranes disruption (92). In spite of several toxin-mediated cytotoxic properties, only α-toxin (α-hemolysin) and Panton-Valentine leukocidin (PVL) have been reported to promote exhibit pro-apoptosis-like death in host cells (93). Apoptosis induced by membrane-damaging toxins is characterized by caspase-3 and caspase-9 activation, as well as activation of intrinsic mitochondrial-mediated apoptotic signaling pathway (93, 94). This apoptosis induction is primarily associated with host phagocytes and induces stress responses. By targeting these important immune cells, the host immune response is suppressed and this allows *S. aureus* to maintain extracellular colonization of host tissues in necrotizing biofilms.

Extracellular *S. aureus* also impart much of their characteristic necrotic tissue damage, via the expression of secreted toxins as a major mechanism to induce lung damage through necroptosis induction through RIPK1/RIPK3/MLKL (92). *S. aureus* mutants lacking pore-forming toxins, such as Psms, agr, and hla are less effective at inducing cytotoxicity in human and murine immune cells. Host directed perturbations of necroptosis by inhibition of either RIPK1 or MLKL were also shown to decrease *S. aureus*-mediated cytotoxicity in immune cells *ex vivo*, but this RCD activity may be pro-resolving *in vivo* (92). These secreted factors from extracellular *S. aureus* biofilms impart necrotic tissue damage by destroying both epithelial and endothelial cells in the lung, which also promotes severe lung barrier disruption and pulmonary edema (95). Also, secreted toxins will act as leukocidins to dampen the effectiveness of responding phagocytes by inducing RCD and disrupting phagocytic clearance activity (96).

These observations are characterized particularly well in neutrophils. Neutrophil recruitment and activity is necessary to eradicate *S. aureus* from the lung. In a mouse model of *S. aureus*-induced pneumonia, NLRC4-associated necroptosis was observed in infiltrating neutrophils. This RCD was shown to drive interleukin-18 (IL-18), which results in the suppression of IL-17A signaling from T cells. This suppression of IL-17A results in decreased neutrophil recruitment to the lung which in turn exacerbates *S. aureus* pneumonia by inhibiting successive waves of neutrophil recruitment required to clear the infection (97). The induction of neutrophil necroptosis also triggers the release of neutrophil extracellular traps (NETs), which typically restrict extracellular pathogens such as extracellular *S. aureus*. In neutrophils, MLKL translocates to the plasma membrane and binds phosphatidylinositol phosphates, which activates NADPH oxidase-derived ROS production to trigger the breakdown of the nuclear membrane and extrusion of bacteriostatic NETs (98). This process is known to require RIPK1, as RIPK1 inhibition or kinase deficiency inhibits NET generation by mouse and human neutrophils (98). 98 have also reported that peptidylarginine deiminase 4 (PAD4) is essential for anti-Staphylococcus innate immunity mediated by NET extrusion (27). It is also important to note that NET release can also be necroptosis independent (98). Alternative mechanisms of NET release include ligation of adhesion receptors, including CD11b, CD18, and CD15 or paracrine signaling downstream of lipopolysaccharide (LPS) detection (99, 100). It has also reported that the induction of necroptosis can limit excessive inflammation that worsens *S. aureus* infection, in part by limiting the expression of IL-1. MLKL knockout mice that were unable to execute necroptosis, were shown to redirect RCD to a pyroptotic and hyper-inflammatory cell death phenotype during *S. aureus* infection (101). The effect of MLKL activity and necroptosis in neutrophils was reported to be pro-resolving in this model.

However, *S. aureus* has been shown to subvert the host immune response mediated by neutrophil necroptosis and NET release by secreting nuclease and adenosine synthase A, which convert NETs to deoxyadenosine (dAdo). This also drives dATP formation that can induce caspase-3–dependent apoptotic RCD in phagocytes. Disruption of this signaling pathway rescues macrophages that had taken up dAdo from caspase-3–induced cell death (102). The induction of apoptosis in responding host immune cells, helps to promote the maintenance of the extracellular niche and the defense of *S. aureus* biofilms from the activity of innate immune phagocytes. The activity of *S. aureus* alpha toxin has also been found to suppress the efferocytic clearance of apoptotic phagocytes, particularly dead neutrophils by AMs *ex vivo* and *in vivo* (103). The lingering of apoptotic cells activity resulted in higher degrees of cell lysis, likely via secondary necrosis. This would tend to drive greater DAMP sensing in the pulmonary space during *in vivo* infection. This DAMP sensing may agonize pyroptosis induction, which has been associated with worse *S. aureus* infection outcomes. However, more research is required to elucidate these potential disease mechanisms.

Summary – Extracellular *S. aureus* causes acute pyrogenic infections in the lung by forming biofilms around colonies that induce severe tissue damage and impede phagocytic clearance. Tissue damage is imparted by the activity of extracellular toxins on tissue cells, which induce necroptotic cell death. PAMP and DAMP sensing also induces pyroptosis in tissue cells. The induction of these membrane permeabilizing RCDs in tissue cells release nutrients for the colony and diminish lung barrier and respiratory function. Dying tissue cells and sentinel cells recruit phagocytes which are similarly targeted by secreted toxins to impede their immune effector functions. Secondary metabolic effectors generated by *S. aureus* also trigger stress responses in immune cells resulting in apoptotic RCD and impaired function. The dual intracellular and extracellular tropisms of *S. aureus* make the design of host directed therapeutics very challenging. Suppression of the immune response to ameliorate tissue damage may promote bacterial cell growth while agonizing the immune response may promote tissue damage. Immune cell or tissue cell targeted drug delivery strategies may be required for effective therapeutic design in order to strike the balance between required inflammation and cytoprotection, particularly when antibiotics are not an effective option.

Intracellularly Replicative Bacteria

Staphylococcus aureus

Staphylococcus aureus is a Gram-positive bacteria that is a facultative intracellular pathogen. The behavior of the bacteria and their cell death manipulation strategies post-engulfment or intracellular invasion differ starkly different from their activity extracellularly. In the intracellular context, they commonly replicate within the autophagosomes or cytoplasm of diverse host cell types (104). Modulation of RCD from the intracellular niche is one of the main strategies utilized by *S. aureus* against epithelial and endothelial cells that comprise pulmonary tissue and macrophages, neutrophils, and monocytes that mediate immune clearance. These strategies for intracellular RCD manipulation enable *S. aureus* to establish chronic pulmonary infections by avoiding phagocytic and efferocytic clearance and interaction with therapeutic antibiotics (105). The ability to escape the intracellular niche, and re-establish acute pyrogenic extracellular infection further exacerbates *S. aureus* infections and complicates clinical treatment strategies (105). Intracellular *staphylococci* within tissue cells, tend have a small colony morphology and downregulate batteries of genes required for virulence. Downregulated genes particularly include α-hemolysin and other secreted toxins that would induce RCD stress responses that would deny the intracellular niche (106, 107). Suppression of the agr quorum sensing system during intracellular infection contributes to induction of this phenotype by limiting secreted protein production and upregulating cell wall associated proteins (106).

Intracellular *S. aureus* must not only suppress their own cytotoxic activities, but also must subvert RCD mechanisms to restrict intracellular pathogens, such as autophagy and apoptosis, partially through the induction of anti-apoptotic and pro-survival pathways (108). A recent study by Medina et al., investigated the dynamic interactions between 16HBE14o- lung epithelial cells and intracellular *S. aureus*, up to 4 days after infection by a time-resolved analysis of both the bacteria and the host cells by mass spectrometry. Proteomic analysis revealed significant modulation of RCD regulating and effector proteins within bronchial epithelial cells by *S. aureus* up to 4 days post-infection. Specifically, internalized *S. aureus* were found to activate pathways required for the sequestration and utilization of arginine from the host cytosol (109). This metabolic activity has several effects that impede host defense via RCD, including limiting ROS production by iNOS to prevent apoptosis induction that promotes efferocytic clearance of intracellular bacteria. The deamination of sequestered arginine by *S. aureus* also releases ammonia into the cell, which increases cytosolic pH and inhibits pH gradient dependent fusion of bacteria containing endosomes with lysosomes and autophagosomes (109). Arginine starvation is known to induce autophagy, making this manipulation of RCD useful for preventing autophagic clearance of intracellular *S. aureus* (110). Other research has also shown that the induction of autophagy favors *Staphylococcus* intracellular survival (111). Lipidated autophagy-related protein (LC3B-II) conjugates are greatly enriched in epithelial cells infected with *Staphylococcus*. Inhibition of the autophagy-activating kinase 1 (ULK1) suppresses *Staphylococcus*-induced autophagy and *Staphylococcus intracellular replication* (112). *S. aureus* also is also able to escape from LC3B labeled autophagosomes, in part by impeding the maturation of autophagosomes. This is accomplished by the activation of MAPK14, which has been reported to block autophagosome maturation (113). This effect was most prominently observed in the vicinity of *S. aureus* containing autophagosomes, implying that unidentified bacterial factors are likely responsible for such activation (114). In sum, these findings provides further evidence that while intracellular *S. aureus* induces host cell autophagy pathways, it also manipulates the execution of autophagy to promote its intracellular niche.

A well-defined feature of *S. aureus* is its capacity to induce apoptosis through α-toxin activity, which is also required for phagosomal escape intracellularly (108). Medina et al., also found that host regulators of p53 apoptosis including BAG6 and DDX5 were upregulated during early infection. However, in addition to the downregulation of secreted toxins and virulence factors described previously, they also observed that intracellular *S. aureus* promoted the expression of anti-apoptotic proteins which suppressed the expression of apoptotic effectors and proteins known to correlate with the execution of apoptosis (109). Like many intracellular pathogens, the induction of cytoprotection to prevent RCD mediated restriction of the intracellular niche is an essential activity for intracellular *S. aureus*. Intracellular infection of human monocyte derived macrophages led to increased expression and stability of the key anti-apoptotic regulator MCL-1 (115). This upregulation of MCL-1 was also associated with increased secretion of interleukin-6 and activation of NfκB, both of which are pro-inflammatory, but also necessary for MCL-1 dependent cytoprotection (115). Interestingly, suppression of MCL-1 via siRNA in this system abrogated the cytoprotection and interleukin-6 secretion induced by intracellular *S. aureus* (115). Such cytoprotective activities by intracellular staphylococci may contribute to the establishment of chronic pulmonary infections *in vivo*. Further elucidation of these mechanisms could lead to promising therapeutic approaches modulating apoptotic RCD could help clinicians restrict the viability of intracellular *S. aureus*.

Summary – *S. aureus* infection and treatment are both profoundly complicated by the bacteria's ability to act as an extracellular pyrogenic pathogen inducing RCD and its capacity to invade cells and adopt a RCD suppressive intracellular phenotype. Intracellularly, *S. aureus* has evolved the capacity to induce anti-apoptotic phenotypes that promote the maintenance of an intracellular niche. The capacity to invade immune cells, while inhibiting their effector functions and paracrine signaling, suppresses immune clearance. Their ability to invade tissue cells promotes chronic infections by shielding intracellular bacteria from patrolling immune cells, as well as endogenous and exogenous antibiotic compounds. *S. aureus*-induced suppression of phagosome and autophagosome vesicle maturation is essential for its cell invasive tropism. Therapeutic strategies restoring autophagic and phagocytic functions in host cells could significantly diminish the clinical burden of chronic *S. aureus* infections by denying the intracellular niche, as well as promoting *S. aureus* susceptibility to therapeutic antibiotics and immune clearance.

Mycobacterium tuberculosis

Mycobacterium, including *Mycobacterium tuberculosis*, are intracellular pathogens which form pulmonary lesions consisting of a core of necrotic cells and free extracellular bacteria (116). This necrotic core is surrounded by immune cells such as macrophages and neutrophils, which *mycobacterium* infect to enable intracellular division (116). To promote the stability of their intracellular replicative niche, *mycobacterium* have evolved host-interacting proteins that interfere with host signaling driving apoptosis (117). This inhibition of apoptosis effectively shunts infected cells toward a necrotic cell death morphology when the intracellular bacterial burden becomes too severe. This results in the expansion of the tubercular lesion and exacerbates the morbidity and mortality of mycobacterial infections by interfering with lung function. *M. tuberculosis* has struck a delicate balance between inducing the immune cell recruitment and pro-inflammatory response necessary to induce the formation of a granuloma with a necrotic core, without succumbing to the immune response and being cleared.

Mycobacterium tuberculosis employs components of its ESX-1 secretion system to inhibit macrophages' ability to execute apoptosis and deny *M. tuberculosis* the intracellular replicative niche. For instance, overexpression of the EspR protein in a macrophage cell line increases intracellular *M. tuberculosis* bacterial burdens. This effect was elicited via suppression of iNOS activity and targeted inhibition of MyD88-mediated TLR signaling that promotes apoptosis and cytokine expression (118). The same research team also identified the secreted bacterial protein MptpB as a mycobacterial virulence factor similarly suppressing iNOS and apoptosis, but via the inhibition of MAPK and p53 signaling (119). This suggests that *M. tuberculosis* is under selective pressure to evolve diverse and redundant mechanisms to modulate host cell death by limiting host apoptosis to promote intracellular replication and driving cells toward a necrotic phenotype that promotes the formation of tubercular lesions.

Another mycobacterium, *M. smegmatis*, also has direct effectors that inhibit cellular apoptosis signal transduction. The overexpression of recombinant *M. smegmatis* protein AcpM, an acyl carrier protein, significantly reduces the degree of ROS production and JNK signaling in infected bone marrow-derived macrophages (BMDMs). This promotes a significant increase in the survival of infected macrophages, which contributes to the pathogenesis of mycobacterial infections by also improving the intracellular survival and replication of the pathogen. *M. tuberculosis* also expresses similar acyl carrier proteins which exert similar effects (120).

Virulent strains of *M. tuberculosis* have also long been known for their ability to inhibit apoptosis via the manipulation of host cytokine responses. For instance, the avirulent strain H37Ra was found to induce significantly more apoptosis relative to a virulent strain H37Rv (121). Later work found that H37Rv induces greater IL-10 secretion relative to the avirulent strain H37Ra. AMs infected with H37Rv are found to be secreting TNF-α in an attempt to drive apoptosis, but this is subverted by IL-10-mediated expression of TNFR2, a soluble TNF receptor which inhibits TNF signaling via direct binding (122). This activity is dependent on the endocytic uptake of mycobacterial heat shock protein 60 interacting with TLR2 (123). Another major pro-survival regulator that is driven by *M. tuberculosis* during infection is PPARγ. *M. tuberculosis* synthesized mannosylated lipoarabinomannan, has been shown to enhance PPARγ activity by activating upstream mannose receptors. This induction of PPAR activity drives the expression of the pro-survival protein MCL-1, as shown by the gene expression analysis during infection and the loss of MCL-1 expression during infection in a PPAR knockout model. The expression of MCL-1, when a phagocyte is attempting to control an intracellular infection, significantly impairs the host's ability to restrict infection (124).

In addition to suppressing host apoptotic signaling, Mycobacteria also have several means through which they promote immune cell necrosis to expand the necrotic core of tubercular lesions. They have evolved diverse effector mechanisms to inhibit phagocyte activity in the granuloma, including through direct killing by leukocidin effectors targeting both neutrophils and macrophages. One such mechanism targeting neutrophils is the ESX-1 type VII secretion system, which induces the necrosis of neutrophils. One bacterial effector protein carrying out this induction is ESAT-6, which induces a calcium influx into the host cell that activates the protease calpain. Hyperactivity of ESAT-6 in a calcium-rich environment induces a secondary necrotic phenotype characterized by the exposure of phosphotidylserine on the outer leaflet of the cell membrane and loss of membrane permeability (125).

Utilizing its ESX-1 secretion system, *M. tuberculosis* has been shown to induce potassium efflux and calcium influx in infected macrophage cell lines. The loss of ion homeostasis subsequently drives the activation of the NLRP3 inflammasome, which results in gasdermin D (GSDMD)-mediated pyroptosis. Visualization of this effect by TIRF microscopy found the induction of pyroptosis to be dependent on bacterial proximity to the plasma membrane (126). This effect could be elicited by both extracellular and intracellular bacteria. The mechanism through which the ESX-1 secretion system disrupts membrane permeability and ion homeostasis remains poorly understood, but evidence across the field indicates that pyroptotic signaling likely contributes significantly to the formation of the necrotic core of tubercular lesions. *M. tuberculosis* also employs its type IV secretion system to inhibit uptake and phagosome maturation in neutrophils, while also driving neutrophils to induce a necrotic phenotype which promotes extracellular release of the bacteria. This enables sustained infection of other immune cells without being killed during efferocytic clearance. *M. tuberculosis* accomplishes this by inducing hyper-production of neutrophil ROS that drives necrotic cell death and through effector proteins expressed off the RD1 genomic region, such as PPE68 and RV2626c. Human primary neutrophils infected with PPE68 and RV2626c knockout *M. tuberculosis* strains more often die through apoptotic signaling, which promotes subsequent clearance *ex vivo* by uninfected human BMDMs (127). Conversely, wild-type *M. tuberculosis* is able to induce ROS-mediated necrosis in neutrophils through the activity of its ESX-1 secretion system, and subsequently infect the BMDMs in this model (128). Many other mycobacterial proteins that are structurally similar to ESAT-6 that are also secreted through the type VII secretion system seem to function in similar pathways. Such redundancies occurring through evolution strongly support the centrality of pathogen-directed cell death in the survival of mycobacterial species (127, 128).

Mycobacterium tuberculosis benefits from driving the pro-necroptotic signaling to push infected cells away from classical apoptosis. Similar to many other bacterial pathogens, *M. tuberculosis* produces a secreted toxin known as tuberculosis necrotizing toxin (TNT) that promotes necroptosis. However, this induction of necroptosis is not mediated by the direct formation of membrane pores; rather, TNT-mediated necroptosis is induced in macrophages by depleting NAD+ through its NAD+ glycohydrolase activity. The depletion of cellular pools of NAD+ triggers necroptosis via RIPK3- and MLKL-dependent signaling through the necrosome, without requiring the typical TNF-(or RIPK1 propagation signal for necroptosis (129). Unfortunately, the deletion or inhibition of MLKL was not found to improve disease outcomes in vivo (130). While many would argue that this result suggests that the contribution of the necroptotic pathway to the progression of M. tuberculosis infection is minimal, we would caution that this is more likely evidence of the redundant mechanisms through which mycobacterium induce necrosis in responding phagocytes.

Mycobacterium tuberculosis also drives the induction of necrotic cell death by antagonizing the activity of anti-necrotic/pro-survival host responses and metabolites. One example of this antagonism is the suppression of prostaglandin E2 (PGE2) synthesis by the bacterial enzyme phospholipase C (PLC). Pharmacologic inhibition of mycobacterial PLCs was found to restore the production of PGE2 and significantly inhibit the induction of necrosis in *M. tuberculosis*-infected macrophages (131). Recent data indicate that ferroptosis, is implicated in the formation of tubercular lesions. *M. tuberculosis*-induced cell death is significantly suppressed by ferroptosis inhibition and iron chelation. The role of metal homeostasis and metabolism in infectious disease, particularly with regards to RCD, requires further investigation (132).

The centrality of modulating host cell death responses to mycobacterial pathogenesis also shows the promise of host-directed therapeutic strategies in modulating cell death for the treatment of *Mycobacterium* infections. For instance, the activity of HIF-1α is critical for the host to restrict the growth of necrotic cores in tubercular lesions. As immune cells aggregate into granulomas to restrict bacterial dissemination, the middle of the granuloma becomes increasingly hypoxic. This tends to drive cells toward a necrotic phenotype, but the activity of HIF-1α antagonizes the induction of necrosis. A model of *M. avian* infection in mice lacking HIF-1α in myeloid cells rapidly formed granulomas with a necrotic core through this mechanism (133). Promoting macrophage re-programming to survive in a hypoxic environment by driving HIF-1α expression may help to restrict the expansion of necrotic cores in mycobacterial granulomas in the lung. Additionally, dexamethasone inhibits necrotic cell death by promoting the dephosphorylation of p38 MAPK. While the basic cellular phenotype characterizing this protection is the inhibition of mitochondrial outer membrane permeabilization (MOMP)-induced cell death, the underlying molecular signals mediating this inhibition of necrotic cell death remains under-characterized (134). Diverse stimuli that induce apoptosis have also been shown to promote resilience to tuberculosis infection across many diverse model systems. For instance, crude plant extracts from Rubiaceae species that are known to induce apoptosis demonstrated antimicrobial effects *in vitro* (135). However, the induction of apoptosis restricting bacterial burdens in an *in vitro* system cannot necessarily be assumed to have a therapeutic effect when translated to an *in vivo* system. Further validation and testing of host-targeted therapeutics is required.

Summary – *M. tuberculosis* deploys secreted effector proteins from their niche inside phagocytes to inhibit microbicidal functions. Inhibited pathways include MyD88/TLR pattern recognition, ROS production mediated by apoptosis, and JNK/p53-mediated apoptosis. Pathways agonized by mycobacterial effectors secreted within phagocytes include IL-10-mediated anti-inflammatory signaling, PPARγ-mediated

MCL-1 expression that inhibits apoptosis, and secreted leukecidal toxins that induce diverse necrotizing RCD modalities to form the necrotic core of tubercular lesions. Host-targeted therapeutics inhibiting necrotic RCD in host phagocytes and/or agonizing apoptotic/efferocytic effector functions downstream of MyD88/TLR pattern recognition may help resolve clinically challenging multidrug-resistant tuberculosis infections.

Klebsiella pneumoniae

Klebsiella pneumoniae is a facultative intracellular pathogen. It causes complicated pulmonary infections, which are frequently antibiotic resistant. *Klebsiella* aims to promote an amenable intracellular niche by inhibiting phagocyte apoptosis, phagosome maturation, and the acceleration of bactericidal effector functions. Many phagocytes, but particularly neutrophils, will undergo apoptosis as a means of denying this niche to intracellular pathogens like *K. pneumoniae*. Recently, researchers have found that the components of the *K. pneumoniae* capsule are able to delay constitutive neutrophil apoptosis up to 2 times the normal time span, allowing for extended intracellular survival and replication. This was accomplished through bacterial inhibition of the Bax-BCL2 signaling axis, which prevented caspase-3 activation and induced anti-inflammatory IL-8 production (136). This delay in constitutive apoptosis may be critical for *Klebsiella* species to establish infections in the lung and in newly colonized metastatic infection sites after breaching the respiratory epithelial barrier.

Klebsiella pneumoniae also inhibits the maturation of endosomes after engulfment into phagolysosomes. These *Klebsiella*-containing vacuoles become acidified (which benefits bacterial survival), but do not contain cathepsin D protease, indicating that the bacterial- vacuoles never successfully fuse with the lysosome. This interference with lysosomal maturation prevents the efficient clearance of bacteria from the intracellular niche of macrophages, ultimately leading to the induction of programmed cell death in infected macrophages, and enabling the spread of the pathogen to new cells via apoptotic bodies or release from membrane-permeabilized cells (137).

Klebsiella infection has also been observed to modify the exposure of "eat me" signals to promote the longevity of cells that eventually execute apoptosis. Particularly, *Klebsiella* was observed to inhibit the exposure of phosphatidylserine by agonizing flippases that invert phosphatidylserine from the outer to the inner leaflet of the plasma membrane. This inhibition of apoptosis in neutrophils was shown to drive neutrophils toward caspase-independent cell death via the necroptosis machinery (138). Preventing the containment of cytoplasmic contents in apoptotic bodies and inhibiting debris removal via efferocytic phagocytes are other means through which *Klebsiella* maintains a suitable intracellular niche during infection.

The centrality of pyroptotic cell death as a cell autonomous response required to restrict *K. pneumoniae* pulmonary infections has been well established in the field over the past decade. For instance, researchers demonstrated that effective induction of macrophage and monocyte pyroptotic cell death through the NLRP3 inflammasome is required for restriction of *K. pneumoniae* in an *in vivo* murine model. They found that the restriction of *K. pneumoniae* infection required the activity of ASC and NLRP3, as *Nlrp3*$^{-/-}$ *and Asc*$^{-/-}$ mice show significantly greater mortality. Histology also demonstrates severely attenuated inflammatory response to infection in *Nlrp3*$^{-/-}$ mice (139). However, some clinically isolated strains of *K. pneumoniae* have also demonstrated diverse means through which they subvert the host's pyroptotic cell death response to maintain the intracellular niche and limit bactericidal effector function. For instance, one strain of *K. pneumoniae* was reported to induce high IL-1β production, leading to a pyroptotic cell death phenotype in responding macrophages. This resulted in effective bacterial clearance via hydrogen peroxide release and efficient efferocytic clearance of pyroptotic cells. However, a second strain has evolved means to limit the induction of IL-1β, which subverts the propagation of pyroptotic cell death mediated DAMP signaling that promotes immune clearance (140). This results in bacterial survival within phagocytic macrophages and ultimately permits dissemination into the host. Particularly given the antibiotic-resistant nature of *Klebsiella* spp., an improved understanding of their methods of host immune evasion is critical in developing new therapeutic approaches. Also, the possible benefit of pyroptotic cell death induction in bacteria-laden macrophages should also be explored.

Finally, *Klebsiella* promote its dissemination from the lung to metastatic infection sites by manipulating the RCD of respiratory epithelial cells required to maintain barrier integrity. One of the ways in which *K. pneumoniae* promotes the loss of barrier integrity is through the targeted disassembly of microtubules in host epithelial cells, likely promoting anoikis-mediated epithelial cell death. The bacterial gene ytfL was found to contribute to the microtubule disassembly phenotype via random screening of genomic segments trans-expressed in *E. coli*, although complete knockout of the gene did not ablate microtubule disassembly during infection (141). This suggests that other *Klebsiella* proteins contribute significantly to the induction of microtubule disassembly and anchorage dependent cell death of epithelial cells during infection. Host factors relating to microtubule disassembly such as KATNAL1 and KATNB1 contribute to this observed phenotype, indicating a probable axis of direct host-pathogen interaction at the protein level. *Klebsiella* infection of A549 cells was also shown to upregulate transcription factors, which trigger the induction of EMT. This sort of host-pathogen interaction could be critical to the observed anoikis-like cell death phenotype due to the disassembly of epithelial cell microtubules (142). However, further work is required to confirm that such microtubule dissociation by *K. pneumoniae* terminally results in anoikis cell death.

Summary – *K. pneumoniae* are obligate intracellular pathogens that reside within phagocytes post-engulfment. They hijack phagolysosomes by inhibiting proteolytic lysosomal effectors such as cathepsin D, while allowing endosome acidification. Unlike tubercular pathogens, *K. pneumoniae* has evolved to inhibit both apoptotic and necrotizing RCD pathways, which requires further study to elucidate diverse bacterial effectors. They also are capable of inhibiting efferocytic clearance of dead cells that may contain bacteria-laden vacuoles by suppressing the exposure of "eat me" signals. Given the stealthy and RCD-suppressive nature of *K. pneumoniae* infections, host-targeted therapeutics agonizing phagocyte cell death and efferocytic clearance may prove effective clinically. Such therapeutics would be highly desirable in the context of treating antibiotic-resistant strains often observed in nosocomial infections.

Yersinia pestis

Yersinia pestis is a facultative intracellular bacteria primarily infecting responding phagocytes during pneumonic infections (143, 144). To promote clearance, infected phagocytes induce pyroptotic cell death via inflammasome signaling to deny *Y. pestis* an intracellular niche and promote immune clearance via pro-inflammatory IL-1β signaling (144). At the same time, *Y. pestis* interferes with the caspase-1-mediated inflammasome signaling by inhibiting pyroptosis using diverse effector molecules targeting signal transduction steps from pathogen recognition to cytokine secretion (145). *Y. pestis* also acts to inhibit apoptotic RCD through the caspase-3/7 signaling axis to prevent cellular condensation into easily-cleared apoptotic bodies. The inhibition of these regulated mechanisms of cell death results in caspase-8 activity along with dysregulated GSDMD-mediated cell death and inflammation through non-canonical pathways that do not promote an effective immune response and enable bacterial outgrowth (146). *Y. pestis* ultimately aims to survive the process of phagocyte engulfment and escape the phagocyte in order to resume extracellular division, while subverting the pro-inflammatory process associated with phagocytic clearance (143).

Like many intracellular pathogens, *Y. pestis* utilizes a secretion system to export virulence factors into the cytoplasm of infected cells (145). The various components of this type 3 secretion system (T3SS) are identified by the host cell as PAMPs, which trigger inflammasome activation via the activity of caspase-1 when recognized. Caspase-1 activation and inflammasome activity is commonly associated with the progression of pyroptotic cell death, which in this context promotes efficient clearance of *Y. pestis* infections. However, one of the effector proteins exported via the T3SS is YopK, which prevents inflammasome activation by inhibiting the cellular recognition of the T3SS (145). The inhibition of the inflammasome and its downstream cell death pathways greatly exacerbates the severity of *Y. pestis* infection. Other Yop proteins, including YopM, have been found to inhibit caspase-1 activation as well. YopM can inhibit caspase-1 via direct binding interactions, preventing its maturation and association with the inflammasome. The inhibition of inflammasome activity through this mechanism significantly antagonizes macrophage pyroptosis and decreases host resilience to infection (147). YopM also binds to and inhibits IQGAP1, a scaffolding protein that is central to the downstream activity of caspase-1 (148). Lastly, YopM not only restricts the traditional caspase-1-NLRP3 inflammasome, it also inhibits the pyrin-activated inflammasome (149). *Yersinia* species target the activity of RhoA by inhibiting RhoA GTPases through the activity of YopE and YopT (T3SS). This activity prevents effective bacterial clearance by macrophages, by preventing RhoA signaling from modulating cytoskeletal dynamics necessary for effective phagocytosis. To mitigate the negative effects of *Yersinia* RhoA inhibition, the host activates the pyrin inflammasome which activates caspase-1 through non-pyroptotic signaling to drive additional immune cell recruitment to the infection site. YopM inhibition of caspase-1 activity also inhibits the downstream effect of pyrin-mediated inflammasomes, exacerbating the infection (149).

Gasdermin D is normally processed by inflammasome-activated caspase-1 or caspase-11, which enables it to carry out its effector functions generating pyroptotic pores in the cell membrane. However, the *Yersinia* effector protein YopJ triggers non-canonical activation of GSDMD through the function of RIPK1 and caspase-8. This is caused by YopK inhibiting the phosphorylation/activation of TAK1 and IKK, which blocks apoptosis in response to infection, and enables GSDMD-mediated cell death to predominate while other Yop proteins inhibit the activity of IL-1β and its proinflammatory function (150).

To inhibit apoptotic cell death by infected phagocytes, *Y. pestis* also produces a cell surface-bound protease known as Pla (plasminogen activator). The Pla protein inhibits Fas-mediated apoptosis by cleaving soluble and membrane bound FasL, preventing the assembly of the DISC and the activation of caspase-3 and -7 dependent apoptosis. This inhibition of apoptosis also indirectly inhibits the host immune response, by limiting the production of cytokines and the recruitment of immune cells typically coordinated by caspase-3 and -7 dependent cell death (146). This host-pathogen interaction synergizes with the T3SS to inhibit the RCD-initiated host response to both pyroptotic and apoptotic cell death, while bacteria continue to impart direct tissue damage as a result of their outgrowth in the lung (146).

Summary – *Y. pestis* are facultative intracellular pathogens that prefer to divide extracellularly but have evolved means of surviving within engulfing phagocytes, particularly macrophages. They aim to suppress apoptosis-supporting phagolysosomal clearance by subverting DISC assembly via plasminogen activation. They also antagonize the induction of inflammasome signaling driving pyroptosis and IL-1β secretion via the direct interference by Yop family proteins and other secreted effectors. The end result of *Y. pestis* RCD interference is the induction of non-canonical GSDMD-mediated necrosis, which does not produce an effective IL-1β-mediated inflammatory response required for efficient clearance and resolution. Host-targeted therapeutics driving pro-resolving apoptotic signaling in infected cells downstream of suppressed DISC assembly, or the restoration of pro-resolving pyroptotic cytokine signaling could help resolve *Y. pestis* infections. While the clinical impact of *Y. pestis* has declined in the modern age, the development of such host-directed therapies against pathogens defined as select agents remains a critical public interest.

Coxiella Burnettii

Coxiella burnetii is an obligate intracellular pathogen that is the etiological agent of Q-fever (151). It primarily infects host phagocytes by residing in bacteria-laden parasitophorous vacuoles, relying on its anti-apoptotic activity effected through its Dot/Icm Type IV secretion system (T4SS) to maintain its replicative niche in the host (151, 152). Even during TNF-α treatment to provide a strong induction of extrinsic apoptosis, *C. burnettii* infection was observed to offer strong protection from pro-apoptotic signaling. *C. burnettii*-infected cells were observed to upregulate expression of anti-apoptotic effectors such as A1/Bfl-1 and c-IAP2 in THP-1 cells and non-human primate primary AMs. *C. burnettii*-infected cells are often characterized by stark reductions in caspase proteolytic activity with increased expression of pro-survival mediators (153). One of the many anti-apoptotic effector proteins of *C. burnetii*, is the protein AnkG. Studies ectopically expressing AnkG in CHO cells found that AnkG initially associates with the mitochondria before directly binding with p32 during early apoptotic signaling. The direct binding of AnkG to p32 results in their colocalization in the nucleus where p32's transcriptional regulatory activity is restrained (154). Ectopic expression of *C. burnetii* AnkG in *Legionella pneumophila* was also shown to suppress pathogen-induced apoptosis in DCs, which are normally highly restrictive host cells for these intracellular bacteria (154). Recent work has also shown that AnkG requires association with both p32 and the nuclear localization protein importin α1 to carry out its anti-apoptotic function (155).

While AnkG is the most studied anti-apoptotic component of the *C. burnetii* T4SS, it is not singly responsible for carrying out the bacteria's anti-apoptotic effector functions. Ectopic expression of two other T4SS products from *C. burnetti*, CaeA and CaeB, in CHO cells were also found to significantly inhibit intrinsic apoptosis signal transduction. CaeA was found to localize to the nucleus, while CaeB was found to localize to mitochondria and was a more effective inhibitor of apoptosis. Cells overexpressing CaeB have a significant reduction in PARP cleavage downstream of Bax activation (156). *C. burnetii* also effects its anti-apoptotic functions through interference with vesicle trafficking and the autophagic machinery. Beclin-1 (necessary for regulated maturation of the autophagosome) and BCL-2 are both recruited to *C. burnetii*-containing vacuoles and augment the replicative capacity of the bacteria by inhibiting RCD and autophagic recycling (157).

Coxiella burnettii also has been found to manipulate the regulation of host regulatory kinases to inhibit macrophage apoptosis. For instance, *C. burnettii* agonizes cAMP-dependent protein kinase (PKA). Studies found that pharmacologic inhibition of PKA in THP-1 cells and human AMs resulted in significantly more apoptotic cell death than untreated cells. They found that PKA propagates anti-apoptotic/pro-survival signals in the infected macrophage via phosphorylation and inactivation of Bad. *C. burnettii* was observed to direct the localization of Bad to bacteria-laden vacuoles to carry out this kinase activity (158). Avirulent *C. burnetii* was also found to inhibit caspase-3 cleavage while agonizing pro-survival MAPK p38, Erk, and PI3k signaling. Caspase-3 inhibition by *Coxiella* is effected through the activity of the pro-survival protein MCL-1, which is stabilized by Erk1 phosphorylation. Knockout studies found that the T4SS in *Coxiella* was necessary for this inhibition (159).

Summary – *C. brunettii* are obligate intracellular pathogens that reside within host phagocytes in bacteria-laden vacuoles. From these vacuoles, *C. brunettii* secrete a diverse range of anti-apoptotic effectors designed to prevent the appropriate induction and execution of apoptosis due to phagocyte pattern recognition of bacteria-laden vacuoles. Host-targeted therapeutic strategies aimed at restoring apoptosis in infected phagocytes to deny *C. brunettii* its intracellular niche could be useful in treating chronic Q-fever in patients at risk of acute infection.

Legionella pneumophila

Legionella pneumophila is an intracellular Gram-negative bacteria that infects the lungs and causes a severe pneumonia known as Legionnaires disease. Its natural hosts are free-living freshwater protozoa; however, aerosolizations of contaminated water supplies enable the bacteria to infect the human lung (160). AMs are the primary site of bacterial replication but neutrophils can also be infected (161, 162). Upon infection, *Legionella* replicates within a *Legionella*-containing vacuole (LCV). There is also evidence that it can infect lung epithelial cells, although the formation of a replicative vacuole is distinct (163). *L. pneumophila* has a T4SS, which is essential for bacterial virulence. Virulence factors of *Legionella* control many aspects of the cellular machinery including cell death pathways (164). Cells infected with *L. pneumophila* undergo a variety of types of RCD (165). Much of this is dependent on the cell type, and to some extent the strain of *L. pneumophila*.

Apoptosis is triggered in many myeloid cell types, including DCs and macrophages. Interestingly DCs undergo rapid apoptosis upon infection with *L. pneumophila*, while macrophages are relatively resistant to infection-induced apoptosis (166). Suppression of apoptosis in DCs allows for the replication of bacteria. *L. pneumophila* uses several effector molecules and strategies to avoid undergoing apoptosis upon infection. This includes the bacterial protein SidF, which interferes with the pro-apoptotic proteins BNIP3 and Bcl-rambo (167). In addition, LegK1 and LnaB increase activation of NF-b, which induces a pro-survival/anti-apoptotic phenotype. When apoptosis in suppressed even further in myeloid cells there is an increase in pulmonary inflammation, which suggests that the regulation of apoptosis is important for decreasing inflammation in the host (168).

While *L. pneumophila* has many mechanisms to decrease apoptosis, other types of cell death are increased upon infection. This includes pyroptosis, necrosis, and autophagic cell death (169, 170). Pyroptosis is triggered by both a flagellin-dependent and flagellin-independent mechanism (166, 171). Flagellin-dependent signaling through the NAIP5/NLRC4 inflammasome causes pyroptosis in macrophages from some mouse lines. This is dependent on the T4SS. Pyroptosis induced by caspase-11 signaling is also dependent on the T4SS, but independent of flagellin. Autophagy also requires virulence factors secreted by the T4SS to be induced in macrophages following infection. There is also evidence in human monocyte cell lines and primary mouse macrophages that cathepsin-dependent necrosis can be triggered through the recognition of RpsL (172).

Summary – Similar to many intracellular pathogens, *L. pneumophila* uses a variety of mechanisms to suppress apoptosis, and thus insure a niche for replication. However, the mechanisms that *L. pneumophila* takes to survive are counteracted by the host response. Given that *Legionella* is a relatively new human pathogen, the interactions with the host may still be evolving.

DISCUSSION

In this review, we have summarized the recent studies that have shown the impact that cell death-mediated host-pathogen interactions on pulmonary infections. We suggest that cell death inhibition, induction, and recovery function synchronously to maintain host homeostasis. Having aggregated data from diverse research teams regarding the targeted manipulation of host RCD by pulmonary bacterial pathogens, several clear trends and functional groupings can be identified. It is clear that the overall strategies of intracellular and extracellular pathogens vary greatly regarding how they use host cell death programs to promote the establishment and maintenance of infection. Generally, extracellular pathogens are primarily agonizers of RCD, triggering the induction of regulated host-programmed cell death via direct cytocidal effectors. While many extracellular pathogens also induce apoptotic cell death, the secretion of such direct effectors (including pore-forming toxins, exotoxins, and ROS), likely induces membrane permeabilization in apoptotic cells as well (often referred to as secondary necrosis). The less discriminating nature of extracellular pathogens to target cell types is due to their mechanism of action being effected through direct physical disruption or destruction of cellular organelles and proteins, rather than targeted inhibition via binding. As such, extracellular pulmonary pathogens impact respiratory epithelial cell mucociliary defenses and barrier integrity, along with immune cell effector functions and maintenance using the same biologic activities. The direct and less discriminate damage imparted by extracellular pathogens establishes a pulmonary niche for the bacteria that is analogous to a cellular war zone bathed in pro-inflammatory mediators in the form of cellular debris, cytoplasmic nutrients, and PAMPs. This environment is uniquely conducive to bacterial dissemination to distal infection sites due to bacterial translocation from the lung to the bloodstream.

Antibiotics are the primary intervention for such bacterial infections. However, understanding that extracellular pulmonary pathogens rely on the induction of such membrane-permeabilizing RCD modalities for their pathogenesis allows us to consider novel therapeutic approaches that target the host to treat pneumonia. The inhibition of membrane-permeabilizing cell death that these bacteria rely on to form an amenable pulmonary niche could hold significant advantages relative to pathogen-targeted therapeutic strategies. Firstly, by targeting host factors to augment tolerance to infection, pathogens will be less likely to escape the therapy by evolving resistance to pathogen-targeted therapeutics, which rely on binding inhibition of specific bacterial targets. Improving the host response to infection will also provide clinicians with alternative approaches for treating antibiotic-resistant infections under the same rationale. Understanding that diverse extracellular pathogens induce the same forms of cell death using similarly evolved mechanisms of action also allows us to consider how one might develop a class of host-directed therapeutics targeting a range of extracellular pathogens. Compounds and gene therapies limiting the induction of membrane-permeabilizing cell deaths via secondary necrosis, pyroptosis, necroptosis, and ferroptosis may inhibit the formation of pulmonary niches conducive to the progression of extracellular bacterial pneumonia. The simultaneous inhibition of several cell death pathways may be required to design effective therapeutics, as inhibiting one form of membrane-permeabilizing cell death may simply push cells toward another membrane-permeabilizing cell death modality. Such approaches to controlling the inflammatory environment by limiting environmental DAMPs would also avoid key pitfalls of many host-targeted therapies such as corticosteroids, which directly suppress immune effector functions to limit immunopathology. Inhibition of membrane-permeabilizing RCD, the promotion of membrane integral cell death, the promotion of barrier integrity or epithelial cell autonomous defenses, and many other host factors should be considered for investigation in designing host-directed therapeutic approaches leveraging cell death.

With regards to intracellular bacterial pathogens' manipulation of RCD, they generally aim to promote an amenable intracellular niche for bacterial replication within phagocytic cells or cells that may endocytose pathogens. This typically requires targeted inhibition of apoptotic signal transduction, but the mechanisms employed by specific bacteria to accomplish such inhibition varies widely. With this in mind, intracellular pathogens can also be further divided into two functional categories. One class of intracellular pathogens are pro-inflammatory and generally present an acute pneumonia with necrotic cell phenotypes driven in responding immune cells. Such pathogens will often rely on the induction of necrosis in bacteria-burdened cells, which both promotes the release of bacteria to infect new cells and drives further immune cell recruitment and tissue damage. Often, these bacteria will utilize the immunopathology-induced damage to the lung epithelial barrier to cross over into the bloodstream and colonize metastatic infection sites, which contributes significantly to morbidity and mortality. Such pathogens, including *K. pneumoniae* and *M. tuberculosis*, are serious clinical threats, which are often greatly complicated by the existence of multiple drug resistant serotypes. Designing host-targeted therapeutic strategies against these bacteria might rely on the induction of non-permeabilizing cell death to trap bacteria in apoptotic bodies or the promotion of "eat me" signals on apoptotic cells to more efficiently clear them via efferocytosis. Pharmacologic suppression of membrane-permeabilizing cell death during such infections also might promote non-permeabilizing RCD that restricts bacterial growth. However, it is important to note the overlapping complexities of RCD may require combinatorial inhibition of permeabilizing cell death pathways to elicit therapeutic effects. Further work determining underlying mechanisms through which intracellular bacteria manipulate pro-inflammatory cell death is required, alongside the design and testing of novel therapeutic strategies modulating cell death.

The other classes of intracellular pathogens are primarily focused on suppressing pattern recognition signaling, inflammation, and immune effector functions associated with the induction of both membrane-permeable and non-permeable RCD. They also tend to drive the upregulation of host factors promoting cellular survival and replication, which would normally be rapidly inactivated upon sensing an intracellular pathogen. These intracellular bacteria tend to establish chronic infections and rely on stealth to maintain an amenable pulmonary niche for replication. For instance, *C. brunettii* infection can develop into chronic Q-fever months or even years after initial infection (173). These infections can often persist, even after aggressive treatment with broad-spectrum antibiotics (173). Difficulty clearing such infections, even with the application of typical antibiotic therapies, lends support to the hypothesis that pharmacologic control of RCD dynamics could be used to promote clearance. Applying therapeutic compounds to promote the induction of apoptotic death or subvert pathogen blockade of RCD signals should be investigated in this context. Some researchers have investigated such approaches *in vitro*, but research aimed at translating positive findings inducing cell death to restrict bacterial pneumonia is required (135). Such approaches could be used in conjunction with traditional antibiotic therapeutics to eliminate stealthy and stubborn pulmonary infections by direct killing and denial of an amenable intracellular niche.

Conclusion and Open Questions

Pulmonary bacterial infection triggers diverse host cell responses that include activation of cell death and/or survival signaling, inflammatory responses, and the immune system. Cell death is now recognized by the work of multiple labs as an important, druggable target which controls the degree of inflammatory injury in many pathologies, including ischemia–reperfusion injuries (heart, brain, kidney, and liver), brain trauma, eye diseases, and pulmonary bacterial infections (174). Because barrier disruption not only depends on cell death but also on the capacity of the remaining cells to proliferate and keep the barrier sealed, it is important to also study whether different forms of necrosis regulate key barrier-related properties of neighboring pulmonary epithelial cells such as proliferation, migration, and adhesion. The host's regulation and bacterial manipulation of RCD is a critical determinant of outcomes during bacterial pneumonia. The literature cited in this article shows that pulmonary bacteria can induce a vicious circle of cell death, pore-forming toxin release, activation of immune-cell, and the release of death-inducing cytokines and toxins that may fuel prolonged non-resolving inflammatory responses and contribute to the pathogenesis of chronic lung inflammatory diseases.

Cell death is now established as an important strategy to control bacterial infection and/or promote host tolerance, but many questions remain to be addressed. Is cell death a primary driver or secondary mechanism manipulated by bacterial pathogens to successfully establish within the host? Can targeting cell death-related proteins be an effective strategy as anti-bacterial therapeutics? What is the relative contribution of cell death-dependent functions of bacteria-infected phagocytes in inflammation? How does cell death contribute to the initiation, amplification, and chronicity of lung inflammation? On a mechanistic level, what are the different bacterial effectors involved with cell death manipulation and why do some bacteria selectively induce membrane non-permeabilizing death pathways? Which therapeutic strategy would be the most effective against cell death-associated lung injury in clinical settings? Can we predict and interfere with host outcomes whether a species of bacteria is more or less prone to induce cell death? How does infection with multiple pathogens influence RCD? We posit that current progress in the field suggests that therapeutics modulating host RCD signaling to treat infectious disease may soon be a reality, but further investigations into pulmonary host-pathogen interactions governing cell death are required in the interim to meet this goal.

AUTHOR CONTRIBUTIONS

EF, NL, and AJ designed all the research, wrote the manuscript, and contributed data to the table. EF finalized the table. EF and NL made the figure.

ACKNOWLEDGMENTS

The authors would like to thank Meredith Crane and Kayla Marie Campbell for their thoughtful comments and editing advice.

REFERENCES

1. Crane MJ, Lee KM, FitzGerald ES, Jamieson AM. Surviving deadly lung infections: innate host tolerance mechanisms in the pulmonary system. *Front Immunol.* (2018) 9:1421. doi: 10.3389/fimmu.2018.01421
2. Hartl D, Tirouvanziam R, Laval J, Greene CM, Habiel D, Sharma L, et al. Innate immunity of the lung: from basic mechanisms to translational medicine. *J Innate Immun.* (2018) 10:487–501. doi: 10.1159/000487057
3. Riches DWH, Martin TR. Overview of innate lung immunity and inflammation. *Methods Mol Biol.* (2018) 1809:17–30. doi: 10.1007/978-1-4939-8570-8_2

4. Yuksel H, Turkeli A. Airway epithelial barrier dysfunction in the pathogenesis and prognosis of respiratory tract diseases in childhood and adulthood. *Tissue Barriers.* (2017) 5:e1367458. doi: 10.1080/21688370.2017.1367458
5. Leiva-Juárez MM, Kolls JK, Evans SE. Lung epithelial cells: therapeutically inducible effectors of antimicrobial defense. *Mucosal Immunol.* (2018) 11:21-34. doi: 10.1038/mi.2017.71
6. Bals R. Epithelial antimicrobial peptides in host defense against infection. *Respir Res.* (2000) 1:141–50.
7. Brune K, Frank J, Schwingshackl A, Finigan J, Sidhaye VK. Pulmonary epithelial barrier function: some new players and mechanisms. *Am J Physiol Lung Cell Mol Physiol.* (2015) 308:L731–45.
8. Crystal RG, Randell SH, Engelhardt JF, Voynow J, Sunday ME. Airway epithelial cells. *Proc Am Thorac Soc.* (2008) 5:772–7.
9. Rock JR, Randell SH, Hogan BLM. Airway basal stem cells: a perspective on their roles in epithelial homeostasis and remodeling. *Dis Models Mech.* (2010) 3:545–56.
10. Ardain A, Marakalala MJ, Leslie A. Tissue-resident innate immunity in the lung. *Immunology.* (2020) 159:245–56.
11. Allard B, Panariti A, Martin JG. Alveolar macrophages in the resolution of inflammation, tissue repair, and tolerance to infection. *Front Immunol.* (2018) 9:1777. doi: 10.3389/fimmu.2018.01777
12. Kim TH, Lee HK. Differential roles of lung dendritic cell subsets against respiratory virus infection. *Immune Netw.* (2014) 14:128–37.
13. Vermaelen K, Pauwels R. Pulmonary dendritic cells. *Am J Respir Crit Care Med.* (2005) 172:530–51.
14. Fan X, Rudensky AY. Hallmarks of tissue-resident lymphocytes. *Cell.* (2016) 164:1198–211.
15. Eddens T, Kolls JK. Host defenses against bacterial lower respiratory tract infection. *Curr Opin Immunol.* (2012) 24:424–30.
16. Hiemstra PS, McCray PB, Bals R. The innate immune function of airway epithelial cells in inflammatory lung disease. *Eur Respir J.* (2015) 45:1150–62.
17. Parker D, Prince A. Innate immunity in the respiratory epithelium. *Am J Respir Cell Mol Biol.* (2011) 45:189–201. doi: 10.1165/rcmb.2011-0011rt
18. Hippenstiel S, Opitz B, Schmeck B, Suttorp N. Lung epithelium as a sentinel and effector system in pneumonia – molecular mechanisms of pathogen recognition and signal transduction. *Respir Res.* (2006) 7:97.
19. Ashida H, et al. Cell death and infection: a double-edged sword for host and pathogen survival. *J Cell Biol.* (2011) 195:931–42.
20. Elliott MR, Koster KM, Murphy PS. Efferocytosis signaling in the regulation of macrophage inflammatory responses. *J Immunol.* (2017) 198:1387–94.
21. Robb CT, Regan KH, Dorward DA, Rossi AG. Key mechanisms governing resolution of lung inflammation. *Semin Immunopathol.* (2016) 38:425–48.
22. Uddin M, Levy BD. Resolvins: natural agonists for resolution of pulmonary inflammation. *Prog Lipid Res.* (2011) 50:75–88. doi: 10.1016/j.plipres.2010.09.002
23. Tang D, Kang R, Berghe TV, Vandenabeele P, Kroemer G. The molecular machinery of regulated cell death. *Cell Res.* (2019) 29:347–64.
24. Galluzi M, Vitale I, Aaronson S, Abrams J, Adam D, Agostinis P, et al. Molecular mechanisms of cell death: recommendations of the nomenclature committee on cell death. *Cell Death Differ.* (2018) 25:486–541.
25. Wittekindt OH. Tight junctions in pulmonary epithelia during lung inflammation. *Pflugers Arch Eur J Physiol.* (2017) 469:135–47.
26. Lamkanfi M, Dixit VM. Manipulation of host cell death pathways during microbial infections. *Cell Host Microbe.* (2010) 8:44–54. doi: 10.1016/j.chom.2010.06.007
27. Saraste A, Pulkki K. Morphologic and biochemical hallmarks of apoptosis. *Cardiovasc Res.* (2000) 45:528–37.
28. Sánchez-Alcázar JA, Rodríguez-Hernández A, Cordero MD, Fernández-Ayala DJ, Brea-Calvo G, Garcia K, et al. The apoptotic microtubule network preserves plasma membrane integrity during the execution phase of apoptosis. *Apoptosis.* (2007) 12:1195–208.
29. Elmore S. Apoptosis: a review of programmed cell death. *Toxicol Pathol.* (2007) 35:495–516.
30. Nair P, Lu M, Petersen S, Ashkenazi A. Apoptosis initiation through the cell-extrinsic pathway. *Meth Enzymol.* (2014) 544:99–128. doi: 10.1016/b978-0-12-417158-9.00005-4
31. Dickens LS, Boyd RS, Jukes-Jones R, Hughes MA, Robinson GL, Fairall L, et al. A Death Effector domain chain DISC model reveals a crucial role for caspase-8 chain assembly in mediating apoptotic cell death. *Mol Cell.* (2012) 47:291–305. doi: 10.1016/j.molcel.2012.05.004
32. Julien O, Wells JA. Caspases and their substrates. *Cell Death Differ.* (2017) 24:1380–9.
33. Jendrossek V. The intrinsic apoptosis pathways as a target in anticancer therapy. *Curr Pharm Biotechnol.* (2012) 13:1426–38.
34. Bock FJ, Tait SWG. Mitochondria as multifaceted regulators of cell death. *Nat Rev Mol Cell Biol.* (2019) 21:85–100. doi: 10.1038/s41580-019-0173-8
35. Kalkavan H, Green DR. MOMP, cell suicide as a BCL-2 family business. *Cell Death Differ.* (2018) 25:46–55. doi: 10.1038/cdd.2017.179
36. Brentnall M, Rodriguez-Menocal L, De Guevara RL, Cepero E, Boise LH. Caspase-9, caspase-3 and caspase-7 have distinct roles during intrinsic apoptosis. *BMC Cell Biol.* (2013) 14:32. doi: 10.1186/1471-2121-14-32
37. Mizushima N. Autophagy: process and function. *Genes Dev.* (2007) 21:2861–73.
38. Mizumura K, Cloonan S, Choi M, Hashimoto S, Nakahira K, Ryter S, et al. Autophagy: friend or foe in lung disease. *Ann Am Thorac Soc.* (2016) 13 (Suppl. 1):S40–7.
39. Ravanan P, Srikumar IF, Talwar P. Autophagy: the spotlight for cellular stress responses. *Life Sci.* (2017) 188:53–67. doi: 10.1016/j.lfs.2017.08.029
40. Rao L, Eissa NT. Autophagy in pulmonary innate immunity. *JIN.* (2020) 12:21–30. doi: 10.1159/000497414
41. Taddei ML, Giannoni E, Fiaschi T, Chiarugi P. Anoikis: an emerging hallmark in health and diseases. *J Pathol.* (2012) 226:380–93.
42. Guadamillas MC, Cerezo A, Pozo MA. Overcoming anoikis – pathways to anchorage-independent growth in cancer. *J Cell Sci.* (2011) 124:3189–97.
43. Bergsbaken T, Fink SL, Cookson BT. Pyroptosis: host cell death and inflammation. *Nat Rev Microbiol.* (2009) 7:99–109. doi: 10.1038/nrmicro2070
44. Yuan Y-Y, Xie K-X, Wang S-L, Yuan L-W. Inflammatory caspase-related pyroptosis: mechanism, regulation and therapeutic potential for inflammatory bowel disease. *Gastroenterol Rep (Oxf).* (2018) 6:167–76.
45. Platnich JM, Muruve DA. NOD-. like receptors and inflammasomes: a review of their canonical and non-canonical signaling pathways. *Arch Biochem Biophys.* (2019) 670:4–14. doi: 10.1016/j.abb.2019.02.008
46. Franchi L, Eigenbrod T, Muñoz-Planillo R, Nuñez G. The inflammasome: a caspase-1-activation platform that regulates immune responses and disease pathogenesis. *Nat. Immunol.* (2009) 10:241–7.
47. Kovacs SB, Miao EA. Gasdermins: effectors of pyroptosis. *Trends Cell Biol.* (2017) 27:673–84.
48. Ahn D, Prince A. Participation of necroptosis in the host response to acute bacterial pneumonia. *J Unnate Immun.* (2017) 9:262–70.
49. Murphy JM, Czabotar PE, Hildebrand JM, Lucet IS, Zhang JG, Alvarez-Diaz S, et al. The pseudokinase MLKL mediates necroptosis via a molecular switch mechanism. *Immunity.* (2013) 39:443–53.
50. Wang H, Sun L, Su L, Rizo J, Liu L, Wang LF, et al. Mixed lineage kinase domain-like protein MLKL causes necrotic membrane disruption upon phosphorylation by RIP3. *Mol Cell.* (2014) 54:133–46.
51. Ros U, Pena-Blanco A, Hanggi K, Kunzendorf U, Kratwald S, Wong WW, et al. Necroptosis execution is mediated by plasma membrane nanopores independent of calcium. *Cell Rep.* (2017) 19:175–87.
52. Zhang Y, Chen X, Gueydan C, Han J. Plasma membrane changes during programmed cell deaths. *Cell Res.* (2018) 28:9–21. doi: 10.1038/cr.2017.133
53. Fearnhead HO, Vandenabeele P, Vanden Berghe T. How do we fit ferroptosis in the family of regulated cell death? *Cell Death Differ.* (2017) 24:1991–8.
54. Maiorino M, Conrad M, Ursini F. GPx4, lipid peroxidation, and cell death: discoveries, rediscoveries, and open issues. *Antioxidants Redox Signaling.* (2017) 29:61–74. doi: 10.1089/ars.2017.7115
55. Jorgensen I, Rayamajhi M, Miao EA. Programmed cell death as a defence against infection. *Nat Rev Immunol.* (2017) 17:151–64.
56. González-Juarbe N, Gilley RP, Hinojosa CA, Bradley KM, Kamei A, Gao G, et al. Pore-forming toxins induce macrophage necroptosis during acute bacterial pneumonia. *PLoS Pathog.* (2015) 11:e1005337. doi: 10.1371/journal.ppat.1005337
57. González-Juarbe N, Bradley KM, Shenoy AT, Gilley RP, Reyes LF, Hinojosa CA, et al. Pore-forming toxin-mediated ion dysregulation leads to death

receptor-independent necroptosis of lung epithelial cells during bacterial pneumonia. *Cell Death Differ.* (2017) 24:917–28.

58. Kaminskyy VO, Zhivotovsky B. Cell death-based treatment of various diseases: a fifty-year journey. *Cell Death Dis.* (2018) 9:1–3.
59. Migiyama Y, Yanagihara K, Kaku N, Harada Y, Yamada K, Nagaoka K, et al. *Pseudomonas aeruginosa* bacteremia among immunocompetent and immunocompromised patients: relation to initial antibiotic therapy and survival. *Jpn J Infect Dis.* (2016) 69:91–6.
60. Bajmoczi M, Gadjeva M, Alper SL, Pier GB, Golan DE. Cystic fibrosis transmembrane conductance regulator and caveolin-1 regulate epithelial cell internalization of *Pseudomonas aeruginosa*. *Am J Physiol Cell Physiol.* (2009) 297:C263–77.
61. Lyczak JB, Cannon CL, Pier GB. Lung infections associated with cystic fibrosis. *Clin Microbiol Rev.* (2002) 15:194–222.
62. Ruffin M, Brochiero E. Repair process impairment by *Pseudomonas aeruginosa* in epithelial tissues: major features and potential therapeutic avenues. *Front Cell Infect Microbiol.* (2019) 9:182. doi: 10.3389/fcimb.2019.00182
63. Valente E, Assis MC, Alvim IMP, Pereira GMB, Plotkowski MC. *Pseudomonas aeruginosa* induces apoptosis in human endothelial cells. *Microb Pathog.* (2000) 29:345–56.
64. Mizgerd JP, Brain JD. Reactive oxygen species in the killing of *Pseudomonas aeruginosa* by human leukocytes. *Curr Microbiol.* (1995) 31:124–8.
65. Capasso D, Pepe M, Rossello J, Lepanto P, Arias P, Salzman V, et al. Elimination of *Pseudomonas aeruginosa* through efferocytosis upon binding to apoptotic cells. *PLoS Pathog.* (2016) 12:e1006068.
66. Rangel SM, Diaz MH, Knoten CA, Zhang A, Hauser AR. The role of ExoS in dissemination of *Pseudomonas aeruginosa* during pneumonia. *PLoS Pathog.* (2015) 11:e1004945. doi: 10.1371/journal.ppat.1004945
67. Song D, Meng J, Cheng J, Fan Z, Ruan H. *Pseudomonas aeruginosa* quorum-sensing metabolite induces host immune cell death through cell surface lipid domain dissolution. *Nat Microbiol.* (2019) 4:97–111.
68. Anantharajah A, Buyck J, Faure E, Glupczynski Y, Rodriguez-Villalobos H, De Vos D, et al. Correlation between cytotoxicity induced by *Pseudomonas aeruginosa* clinical isolates from acute infections and IL-1β secretion in a model of human THP-1 monocytes. *Pathog Dis.* (2015) 73:ftv049. doi: 10.1093/femspd/ftv049
69. Dar H, Tyurina Y, Mikulska-Ruminska K, Shrivastava I, Ting H, Tyurin V, et al. *Pseudomonas aeruginosa* utilizes host polyunsaturated phosphatidylethanolamines to trigger theft-ferroptosis in bronchial epithelium. *J Clin Invest.* (2019) 128:4639–53.
70. Jiang F, Wang X, Wang B, Chen L, Zhao Z, Waterfield NR, et al. The *Pseudomonas aeruginosa* Type VI secretion PGAP1-like effector induces host autophagy by activating endoplasmic reticulum stress. *Cell Rep.* (2016) 16:1502–9.
71. Managò A, Becker K, Carpinteiro A, Wilker B, Soddemann M, Seitz A, et al. *Pseudomonas aeruginosa* pyocyanin induces neutrophil death via mitochondrial reactive oxygen species and mitochondrial acid sphingomyelinase. *Antioxidants Redox Signal.* (2015) 22:1097–110.
72. Mahlen SD. Serratia infections: from military experiments to current practice. *Clin Microbiol Rev.* (2011) 24:755–91.
73. Fedrigo GV, Campoy EM, Venanzio GD, Colombo MI, Véscovi EG. *Serratia marcescens* is able to survive and proliferate in autophagic-like vacuoles inside non-phagocytic cells. *PLoS One.* (2011) 6:e24054.
74. Gonzalez-Juarbe N, Bradley K, Riegler A, Reyes L, Brissac T, Park S, et al. Bacterial pore-forming toxins promote the activation of caspases in parallel to necroptosis to enhance alarmin release and inflammation during pneumonia. *Sci Rep.* (2018) 8:5846.
75. Lazzaro M, Krapf D, Véscovi EG. Selective blockage of *Serratia marcescens* ShlA by nickel inhibits the pore-forming toxin-mediated phenotypes in eukaryotic cells. *Cell Microbiol.* (2019) 21:e13045.
76. Zhou W, Jin Z-X, Wan Y-J. Apoptosis of human lung adenocarcinoma A549 cells induced by prodigiosin analogue obtained from an entomopathogenic bacterium *Serratia marcescens*. *Appl Microbiol Biotechnol.* (2010) 88:1269–75.
77. Krzymińska S, Ochocka K, Kaznowski A. Apoptosis of epithelial cells and macrophages due to nonpigmented *Serratia marcescens* strains. *Hindawi Sci World J.* (2012) 2012:679639.
78. Ishii K, Adachi T, Imamura K, Takano S, Usui K, Suzuki K, et al. *Serratia marcescens* induces apoptotic cell death in host immune cells via a lipopolysaccharide- and flagella-dependent mechanism. *J Biol Chem.* (2012) 287:36582–92.
79. Shimuta K, Ohnishi M, Iyoda S, Gotoh N, Koizumi N, Watanabe H. The hemolytic and cytolytic activities of *Serratia marcescens*phospholipase A (PhlA) depend on lysophospholipid production by PhlA. *BMC Microbiol.* (2009) 9:261. doi: 10.1186/1471-2180-9-261
80. Escobar-Díaz E, Lopez-Martin EM, Hernandez del Cerro M, Puig-Kroger A, Soto-Cerrato V, Montaner B, et al. AT514, a cyclic depsipeptide from *Serratia marcescens*, induces apoptosis of B-chronic lymphocytic leukemia cells: interference with the Akt/NF- κ B survival pathway. *Leukemia.* (2005) 19:572–9.
81. Kimyon Ö, Das T, Ibugo A, Kutty S, Ho K, Tebben J, et al. serratia secondary metabolite prodigiosin inhibits *Pseudomonas aeruginosa* biofilm development by producing reactive oxygen species that damage biological molecules. *Front Microbiol.* (2016) 7:972. doi: 10.3389/fmicb.2016.00972
82. Henriques-Normark B, Tuomanen EI. The pneumococcus: epidemiology, microbiology, and pathogenesis. *Cold Spring Harb Perspect Med.* (2013) 3:a010215. doi: 10.1101/cshperspect a010215
83. Rai P, Parrish M, Tay I, Li N, Ackerman S, He F, et al. Streptococcus pneumoniae secretes hydrogen peroxide leading to DNA damage and apoptosis in lung cells. *Proc Natl Acad Sci USA.* (2015) 112:E3421–30.
84. Dockrell DH, Whyte MKB, Mitchell TJ. Pneumococcal pneumonia: mechanisms of infection and resolution. *Chest.* (2012) 142:482–91.
85. Steinwede K, Henken S, Bohling J, Maus R, Ueberberg B, Brumshagen C, et al. TNF-related apoptosis-inducing ligand (TRAIL) exerts therapeutic efficacy for the treatment of pneumococcal pneumonia in mice. *J Exp Med.* (2012) 209:1937–52.
86. Weiser J, Roche A, Hergott C, LaRose M, Connolly T, Jorgensen W, et al. Macrophage migration inhibitory factor is detrimental in pneumococcal pneumonia and a target for therapeutic immunomodulation. *J Infect Dis.* (2015) 212:1677–82.
87. Walker M, Novak L, Widener R, Grubbs J, King J, Hale J, et al. PcpA promotes higher levels of infection and modulates recruitment of myeloid-derived suppressor cells during pneumococcal pneumonia | the journal of immunology. *J Immunol.* (2016) 196:2239–48.
88. Preston J, Bewley M, Marriott H, McGarry Houghton A, Mohasin M, Jubrail J, et al. Alveolar macrophage apoptosis–associated bacterial killing helps prevent murine pneumonia. *Am J Respir Crit Care Med.* (2019) 200:84–97. doi: 10.1164/rccm.201804-0646oc
89. De Vos AF, Dessing MC, de Porto APNA, de Boer OJ, de Beer R, Terpstra S, et al. ASC and NLRP3 impair host defense during lethal pneumonia caused by serotype 3 Streptococcus pneumoniae in mice. *Eur J Immunol.* (2018) 48:66–79. doi: 10.1002/eji.201646554
90. Coleman F, Blahna M, Kamata H, Yamamoto K, Zabinski M, Kramnik I, et al. Capacity of pneumococci to activate macrophage nuclear factor κb: influence on necroptosis and pneumonia severity. *J Infect Dis.* (2017) 216:425–35.
91. Kobayashi SD, Malachowa N, DeLeo FR. Pathogenesis of *Staphylococcus aureus* abscesses. *Am J Pathol.* (2015) 185:1518–27.
92. Kitur K, Parker D, Nieto P, Ahn D, Cohen T, Chung S, et al. Toxin-induced necroptosis is a major mechanism of *Staphylococcus aureus* lung damage. *PLoS Pathog.* (2015) 11:e1004820. doi: 10.1371/journal.ppat.1004820
93. Zhang X, Hu X, Rao X. Apoptosis induced by *Staphylococcus aureus* toxins. *Microbiological Research* (2017) 205:19–24. doi: 10.1016/j.micres.2017.08.006
94. Suliman H, Kraft B, Bartz R, Chen L, Welty-Wolf K, Piantadosi C, et al. Mitochondrial quality control in alveolar epithelial cells damaged by S. aureus pneumonia in mice. *Am J Physiol Lung Cell Mol Physiol.* (2017) 313:L699–709.
95. Wang J, Zhou X, Li W, Deng X, Deng Y, Niu X, et al. Curcumin protects mice from *Staphylococcus aureus* pneumonia by interfering with the self-assembly process of α-hemolysin. *Sci Rep.* (2016) 6:1–12.
96. Berends E, Zheng X, Zwack E, Ménager M, Cammer M, Shopsin B, et al. *Staphylococcus aureus* impairs the function of and kills human dendritic cells via the LukAB toxin. *mBio.* (2019) 10:e1918–1918.
97. Paudel S, Ghimire L, Jin L, Baral P, Cai S, Jeyaseelan S. NLRC4 suppresses IL-17A-mediated neutrophil-dependent host defense through upregulation of

IL-18 and induction of necroptosis during Gram-positive pneumonia. *Muc Immunol.* (2019) 12:247–57.

98. D'Cruz A, Speir M, Bliss-Moreau M, Dietrich S, Wang S, Chen A, et al. The pseudokinase MLKL activates PAD4-dependent NET formation in necroptotic neutrophils. *Sci Signal.* (2018) 11:eaao1716. doi: 10.1126/scisignal.aao1716
99. Pieterse E, Rother N, Yanginlar C, Hilbrands LB, van der Vlag J. Neutrophils discriminate between lipopolysaccharides of different bacterial sources and selectively release neutrophil extracellular traps. *Front Immunol.* (2016) 7:484.
100. Li RHL, Tablin FA. Comparative review of neutrophil extracellular traps in sepsis. *Front Vet Sci.* (2018) 5:291. doi: 10.3389/fvets.2018.00291
101. Kitur K, Wachtel S, Brown A, Wickersham M, Paulino F, Pealoza H, et al. Necroptosis promotes *Staphylococcus aureus* clearance by inhibiting excessive inflammatory signaling. *Cell Rep.* (2016) 16:2219–30.
102. Thammavongsa V, Missiakas DM, Schneewind O. *Staphylococcus aureus* degrades neutrophil extracellular traps to promote immune cell death. *Science.* (2013) 342:863–6.
103. Cohen TS, Hilliard JJ, Jones-Nelson O, Keller AE, O'Day T, Tkaczyk C, et al. *Staphylococcus aureus* α toxin potentiates opportunistic bacterial lung infections. *Sci Transl Med.* (2016) 8:329ra31.
104. Qazi SNA, Harrison SE, Self T, Williams P, Hill PJ. Real-time monitoring of intracellular *Staphylococcus aureus* replication. *J Bacteriol.* (2004) 186:1065–77.
105. Tan X, Coureuil M, Ramond E, Euphrasie D, Dupuis M, Tros F, et al. Chronic *Staphylococcus aureus* lung infection correlates with proteogenomic and metabolic adaptations leading to an increased intracellular persistence. *Clin Infect Dis.* (2019) 69:1937–45.
106. Kahl B, Belling G, Becker P, Chatterjee I, Wardecki K, Hilgert K, et al. Thymidine-dependent *Staphylococcus aureus* small-colony variants are associated with extensive alterations in regulator and virulence gene expression profiles. *Infect Immun.* (2005) 73:4119–26.
107. Kahl B, Becker K, Löffler B. Clinical significance and pathogenesis of staphylococcal small colony variants in persistent infections. *Clin Microbiol Rev.* (2016) 29:401–27.
108. Fraunholz M, Sinha B. Intracellular *Staphylococcus aureus*: live-in and let die. *Front. Cell. Infect. Microbiol.* (2012) 2:43. doi: 10.3389/fcimb.2012.00043
109. Palma Medina L, Becker A, Michalik S, Yedavally H, Raineri E, Hildebrandt P, et al. Metabolic cross-talk between human bronchial epithelial cells and internalized *Staphylococcus aureus* as a driver for infection. *Mol. Cell Proteomics.* (2019) 18:892–908. doi: 10.1074/mcp.ra118.001138
110. Savaaraj N, You M, Wu C, Wangpaichitr M, Kuo MT, Feun LG. Arginine deprivation, autophagy, apoptosis (AAA) for the treatment of melanoma. *Curr Mol Med.* (2010) 10:405–12.
111. Mestre MB, Colombo MI. *Staphylococcus aureus* promotes autophagy by decreasing intracellular cAMP levels. *Autophagy.* (2012) 8:1865–7.
112. Radhi O, Davidson S, Scott F, Zeng R, Jones D, Tomkinson N, et al. Inhibition of the ULK1 protein complex suppresses *Staphylococcus*-induced autophagy and cell death. *J Biol Chem.* (2019) 2019:8923.
113. Höcker R, Walker A, Schmitz I. Inhibition of autophagy through MAPK14-mediated phosphorylation of ATG5. *Autophagy.* (2013) 9:426–8.
114. Neumann Y, Bruns S, Rohde M, Prajsnar T, Foster S, Schmitz I. Intracellular *Staphylococcus aureus* eludes selective autophagy by activating a host cell kinase. *Autophagy.* (2016) 12:2069–84.
115. Koziel J, Kmiecik K, Chmiest D, Maresz K, Mizgalska D, Maciag-Gudowska A, et al. The role of Mcl-1 in S. aureus-induced cytoprotection of infected macrophages. *Med Inflam.* (2013) 2013:427021.
116. Amaral EP, Lasunskaia EB, D'Império-Lima MR. Innate immunity in tuberculosis: how the sensing of mycobacteria and tissue damage modulates macrophage death. *Microb Infect.* (2016) 18:11–20. doi: 10.1016/j.micinf.2015.09.005
117. Korb VC, Chuturgoon AA, Moodley D. Mycobacterium tuberculosis: manipulator of protective immunity. *Int J Mol Sci.* (2016) 17:131. doi: 10.3390/ijms17030131
118. Jin C, Wu X, Dong C, Li F, Fan L, Xiong S, et al. EspR promotes mycobacteria survival in macrophages by inhibiting MyD88 mediated inflammation and apoptosis. *Tuberculosis.* (2019) 116:22–31. doi: 10.1016/j.tube.2019.03.010
119. Fan L, Wu X, Jin C, Li F, Xiong S, Dong Y. MptpB promotes mycobacteria survival by inhibiting the expression of inflammatory mediators and cell apoptosis in macrophages. *Front Cell Infect Microbiol.* (2018) 8:171. doi: 10.3389/fcimb.2018.00171
120. Paik S, Choi S, Lee KI, Back YW, Son YJ, Jo EK, et al. Mycobacterium tuberculosis acyl carrier protein inhibits macrophage apoptotic death by modulating the reactive oxygen species/c-Jun N-terminal kinase pathway. *Microb Infect.* (2019) 21:40–9.
121. Keane J, Balcewicz-Sablinska MK, Remold HG, Chupp GL, Meek BB, Fenton MJ, et al. Infection by Mycobacterium tuberculosis promotes human alveolar macrophage apoptosis. *Infect Immun.* (1997) 65:298–304. doi: 10.1128/iai.65.1.298-304.1997
122. Balcewicz-Sablinska MK, Keane J, Kornfeld H, Remold HG. Pathogenic Mycobacterium tuberculosis evades apoptosis of host macrophages by release of TNF-R2, resulting in inactivation of TNF-alpha. *J Immunol.* (1998) 161:2636–41.
123. Parveen N, Varman R, Nair S, Das G, Ghosh S, Mukhopadhyay S. Endocytosis of Mycobacterium tuberculosis heat shock protein 60 is required to induce interleukin-10 production in macrophages. *J Biol Chem.* (2013) 288:24956–71.
124. Arnett E, Weaver A, Woodyard K, Montoya M, Li M, Hoang K, et al. PPARγ is critical for Mycobacterium tuberculosis induction of Mcl-1 and limitation of human macrophage apoptosis. *PLoS Pathog.* (2018) 14:e1007100. doi: 10.1371/journal.ppat.1007100
125. Francis RJ, Butler RE, Stewart GR. *Mycobacterium tuberculosis* ESAT-6 is a leukocidin causing Ca^{2+} influx, necrosis and neutrophil extracellular trap formation. *Cell Death Dis.* (2014) 5:e1474.
126. Beckwith KS, Beckwith MS, Ullmann S, Saetra R, Kim H, Marstad A, et al. Plasma membrane damage causes NLRP3 activation and pyroptosis during *Mycobacterium tuberculosis* infection. *bioRxiv.* (2019). [Preprint]. bioRxiv:747014.
127. Danelishvili L, Everman J, Bermudez LE. Mycobacterium tuberculosis PPE68 and Rv2626c genes contribute to the host cell necrosis and bacterial escape from macrophages. *Virulence.* (2016) 7:23–32. doi: 10.1080/21505594.2015.1102832
128. Dallenga T, Repnik U, Corleis B, Eich J, Reimer R, Griffiths G, et al. *M. tuberculosis*-induced necrosis of infected neutrophils promotes bacterial growth following phagocytosis by macrophages. *Cell Host Microbe.* (2017) 22:519–30.
129. Pajuelo D, Gonzalez-Juarbe N, Tak U, Sun J, Orihuela C, Niederweis M. NAD. + depletion triggers macrophage necroptosis, a cell death pathway exploited by *Mycobacterium tuberculosis*. *Cell Rep.* (2018) 24:429–40.
130. Stutz M, Ojaimi S, Allison C, Preston S, Arandjelovic P, Hildebrand J, et al. Necroptotic signaling is primed in Mycobacterium tuberculosis -infected macrophages, but its pathophysiological consequence in disease is restricted. *Cell Death Differ.* (2018) 25:951–65.
131. Assis P, Espíndola M, Paula-Silva F, Rios W, Pereira P, Leão S, et al. Mycobacterium tuberculosis expressing phospholipase C subverts PGE2 synthesis and induces necrosis in alveolar macrophages. *BMC Microbiol.* (2014) 14:128. doi: 10.1186/1471-2180-14-128
132. Amaral E, Costa D, Namasivayam S, Riteau N, Kamenyeva O, Mittereder L, et al. A major role for ferroptosis in Mycobacterium tuberculosis–induced cell death and tissue necrosis. *J Exp Med.* (2019) 216:556–70.
133. Cardoso MS, Silva TM, Resende M, Appelberg R, Borges M. Lack of the transcription factor hypoxia-inducible factor 1α (HIF-1α) in macrophages accelerates the necrosis of mycobacterium avium-induced granulomas. *Infect Immun.* (2015) 83:3534–44.
134. Gräb J, Suárez I, van Gumpel E, Winter S, Schreiber F, Esser A, et al. Corticosteroids inhibit Mycobacterium tuberculosis -induced necrotic host cell death by abrogating mitochondrial membrane permeability transition. *Nat Commun.* (2019) 10:1–14.
135. Aro A, Dzoyem J, Goddard A, Fonteh P, Kayoka-Kabongo P, McGaw L. In vitro antimycobacterial, apoptosis-inducing potential, and immunomodulatory activity of some *Rubiaceae Species. Front Pharmacol.* (2019) 10:185. doi: 10.3389/fphar.2019.00185
136. Lee C-H, Chuah S-K, Tai W-C, Chang C-C, Chen F-J. Delay in human neutrophil constitutive apoptosis after infection with *Klebsiella pneumoniae*

Serotype K1. *Front Cell Infect Microbiol.* (2017) 7:87. doi: 10.3389/fcimb. 2017.00087

137. Cano V, Moranta D, Llobet-Brossa E, Bengoechea JA, Garmendia J. *Klebsiella pneumoniae* triggers a cytotoxic effect on airway epithelial cells. *BMC Microbiol.* (2009) 9:156.
138. Jondle CN, Gupta K, Mishra BB, Sharma J. *Klebsiella pneumoniae* infection of murine neutrophils impairs their efferocytic clearance by modulating cell death machinery. *PLoS Pathog.* (2018) 14:e1007338. doi: 10.1371/journal. ppat.1007338
139. Willingham S, Allen I, Bergstralh D, Brickey W, Huang M, Taxman D, et al. NLRP3 (NALP3, Cryopyrin) facilitates in vivo caspase-1 activation, necrosis, and HMGB1 release via inflammasome-dependent and -independent pathways. *J Immunol.* (2009) 183:2008–15.
140. Codo A, Saraiva A, dos Santos L, Visconde M, Gales A, Zamboni D, et al. Inhibition of inflammasome activation by a clinical strain of *Klebsiella pneumoniae* impairs efferocytosis and leads to bacterial dissemination. *Cell Death Dis.* (2018) 9:1182.
141. Chua MD, Liou CH, Bogdan AC, Law HT, Yeh KM, Lin JC, et al. *Klebsiella pneumoniae* disassembles host microtubules in lung epithelial cells. *Cell Microbiol.* (2019) 21:e12977.
142. Leone L, Mazzetta F, Martinelli D, Valente S, Alimandi M, Raffa S, et al. *Klebsiella pneumoniae* is able to trigger epithelial-mesenchymal transition process in cultured airway epithelial cells. *PLoS One.* (2016) 11:e0146365.
143. Ke Y, Chen Z, Yang R. Yersinia pestis: mechanisms of entry into and resistance to the host cell. *Front Cell Infect Microbiol.* (2013) 3:106. doi: 10.3389/fcimb.2013.00106
144. Price PA, Jin J, Goldman WE. Pulmonary infection by Yersinia pestis rapidly establishes a permissive environment for microbial proliferation. *Proc Natl Acad Sci USA.* (2012) 109:3083–8.
145. Brodsky I, Palm N, Sadanand S, Ryndak M, Sutterwala F, Flavell R, et al. A Yersinia secreted effector protein promotes virulence by preventing inflammasome recognition of the type III secretion system. *Cell Host Microbe.* (2010) 7:376–87.
146. Caulfield AJ, Walker ME, Gielda LM, Lathem WW. The pla protease of yersinia pestis degrades fas ligand to manipulate host cell death and inflammation. *Cell Host Microbe.* (2014) 15:424–34.
147. LaRock CN, Cookson BT. The Yersinia virulence effector YopM binds caspase-1 to arrest inflammasome assembly and processing. *Cell Host Microbe.* (2012) 12:799–805. doi: 10.1016/j.chom.2012.10.020
148. Chung L, Philip N, Schmidt V, Koller A, Strowig T, Flavell R, et al. IQGAP1 Is Important for Activation of Caspase-1 in Macrophages and Is Targeted by Yersinia pestis Type III Effector YopM. *mBio.* (2014) 5:e1402–14.
149. Chung L, Park Y, Zheng Y, Brodsky I, Hearing P, Kastner D, et al. The yersinia virulence factor YopM hijacks host kinases to inhibit type III effector-triggered activation of the pyrin inflammasome. *Cell Host Microbe.* (2016) 20:296–306. doi: 10.1016/j.chom.2016.07.018
150. Orning P, Weng D, Starheim K, Ratner D, Best Z, Lee B, et al. Pathogen blockade of TAK1 triggers caspase-8-dependent cleavage of gasdermin D and cell death. *Science.* (2018) 362:1064–9.
151. Eldin C, Mélenotte C, Mediannikov O, Ghigo E, Million M, Edouard S, et al. From Q Fever to *Coxiella burnetii* infection: a paradigm change. *Clin Microbiol Rev.* (2017) 30:115–90.
152. Cordsmeier A, Wagner N, Lührmann A, Berens C. Defying death – how *Coxiella burnetii* copes with intentional host cell suicide. *Yale J Biol Med.* (2019) 92:619–28.
153. Voth DE, Howe D, Heinzen RA. *Coxiella burnetii* inhibits apoptosis in human THP-1 cells and monkey primary alveolar macrophages. *Infect Immun.* (2007) 75:4263–71.
154. Eckart R, Bisle S, Schulze-Luehrmann J, Wittmann I, Jantsch J, Schmid B, et al. Antiapoptotic activity of *Coxiella burnetii* effector protein AnkG is controlled by p32-dependent trafficking. *Infect Immun.* (2014) 82:2763–71.
155. Schäfer W, Eckart RA, Schmid B, Cagkoylu H, Hof K, Muller YA, et al. Nuclear trafficking of the anti-apoptotic *Coxiella burnetii* effector protein AnkG requires binding to p32 and Importin-α1. *Cell Microbiol.* (2017) 19:e12634.
156. Klingenbeck L, Eckart RA, Berens C, Lührmann A. The *Coxiella burnetii* type IV secretion system substrate CaeB inhibits intrinsic apoptosis at the mitochondrial level. *Cell Microbiol.* (2013) 15:675–87.
157. Vázquez CL, Colombo MI. *Coxiella burnetii* modulates Beclin 1 and Bcl-2, preventing host cell apoptosis to generate a persistent bacterial infection. *Cell Death Differ.* (2010) 17:421–38.
158. MacDonald LJ, Graham JG, Kurten RC, Voth DE. *Coxiella burnetii* exploits host cAMP-dependent protein kinase signalling to promote macrophage survival. *Cell Microbiol.* (2014) 16:146–59.
159. Cherla R, Zhang Y, Ledbetter L, Zhang G. *Coxiella burnetii* inhibits neutrophil apoptosis by exploiting survival pathways and antiapoptotic protein Mcl-1. *Infect Immun.* (2018) 86:e504–17.
160. Sherwood RK, Roy CR. Autophagy evasion and endoplasmic reticulum subversion: the yin and yang of legionella intracellular infection. *Ann Rev Microbiol.* (2016) 70:413–33.
161. Copenhaver A, Casson C, Nguyen H, Fung T, Duda M, Roy C, et al. Alveolar macrophages and neutrophils are the primary reservoirs for *Legionella pneumophila* and mediate cytosolic surveillance of type IV secretion. *Infect Immun.* (2014) 82:4325–36.
162. Massis LM, Zamboni DS. Innate immunity to *Legionella Pneumophila*. *Front Microbiol.* (2011) 2:109. doi: 10.3389/fmicb.2011.00109
163. Prashar A, Bhatia S, Tabatabaeiyazdi Z, Duncan C, Garduno RA, Tang P, et al. Mechanism of invasion of lung epithelial cells by filamentous *Legionella pneumophila*. *Cell Microbiol.* (2012) 14:1632–55.
164. Vance RE. Immunology taught by bacteria. *J Clin Immunol.* (2010) 30:507–11.
165. Speir M, Vince JE, Naderer T. Programmed cell death in Legionella infection. *Fut Microb.* (2014) 9:107–18.
166. Nogueira C, Lindsten T, Jamieson A, Case C, Shin S, Thompson C, et al. Rapid pathogen-induced apoptosis: a mechanism used by dendritic cells to limit intracellular replication of *Legionella pneumophila*. *PLoS Pathog.* (2009) 5:e1000478. doi: 10.1371/journal.ppat.1000478
167. Banga S, Gao P, Shen X, Fiscus V, Zong W, Chen L, et al. *Legionella pneumophila* inhibits macrophage apoptosis by targeting pro-death members of the Bcl2 protein family. *Proc Natl Acad Sci USA.* (2007) 104:5121–6.
168. Gamradt P, Xu Y, Gratz N, Duncan K, Kobzik L, Högler S, et al. The influence of programmed cell death in myeloid cells on host resilience to infection with *Legionella pneumophila* or *Streptococcus pyogenes*. *PLoS Pathog.* (2016) 12:e1006032. doi: 10.1371/journal.ppat.1006032
169. Tao L, Zhu W, Hu B-J, Qu J-M, Luo Z-Q. Induction of rapid cell death by an environmental isolate of *Legionella pneumophila* in mouse macrophages. *Infect Immun.* (2013) 81:3077–88.
170. Akhter A, Gavrilin M, Frantz L, Washington S, Ditty C, Limoli D, et al. Caspase-7 activation by the Nlrc4/Ipaf inflammasome restricts *Legionella pneumophila* infection. *PLoS Pathog.* (2009) 5:e1000361. doi: 10.1371/journal. ppat.1000361
171. Casson CN, Shin S. Inflammasome-mediated cell death in response to bacterial pathogens that access the host cell cytosol: lessons from *legionella pneumophila*. *Front Cell Infect Microbiol.* (2013) 3:111. doi: 10.3389/fcimb. 2013.00111
172. Zhu W, Tao L, Quick M, Joyce J, Qu J, Luo Z. Sensing cytosolic RpsL by macrophages induces lysosomal cell death and termination of bacterial infection. *PLoS Pathog.* (2015) 11:e1004704. doi: 10.1371/journal.ppat. 1004704
173. Karakousis PC, Trucksis M, Dumler JS. Chronic Q fever in the United States. *J Clin Microbiol.* (2006) 44:2283–7.
174. Riegler AN, Brissac T, Gonzalez-Juarbe N, Orihuela CJ. Necroptotic cell death promotes adaptive immunity against colonizing pneumococci. *Front Immunol.* (2019) 10:615. doi: 10.3389/fimmu.2019.00615

5

Harnessing the Immunomodulatory Properties of Bacterial Ghosts to Boost the Anti-Mycobacterial Protective Immunity

Jieling Lim [1,2], Vanessa Hui Qi Koh [1,2], Sharol Su Lei Cho [1,2], Balamurugan Periaswamy [3], Dawn Poh Sum Choi [3], Maurizio Vacca [1,2], Paola Florez De Sessions [3], Pavol Kudela [4], Werner Lubitz [4], Giorgia Pastorin [5] and Sylvie Alonso [1,2]*

*[1] Department of Microbiology and Immunology, Yong Loo Lin School of Medicine, National University of Singapore, Singapore, Singapore, [2] Immunology Programme, Life Sciences Institute, National University of Singapore, Singapore, Singapore, [3] Genome Institute of Singapore, Agency for Science, Technology and Research (A*STAR), Singapore, Singapore, [4] Biotech Innovation Research Development & Consulting (BIRD-C), Vienna, Austria, [5] Department of Pharmacy, Faculty of Science, National University of Singapore, Singapore, Singapore*

***Correspondence:**
Sylvie Alonso
micas@nus.edu.sg

Tuberculosis (TB) pathogenesis is characterized by inadequate immune cell activation and delayed T cell response in the host. Recent immunotherapeutic efforts have been directed at stimulating innate immunity and enhancing interactions between antigen presenting cells and T cells subsets to improve the protective immunity against TB. In this study, we investigated the immunostimulatory properties of bacterial ghosts (BG) as a novel approach to potentiate the host immunity against mycobacterial infection. BG are intact cytoplasm-free *Escherichia coli* envelopes and have been developed as bacterial vaccines and adjuvant/delivery system in cancer immunotherapy. However, BG have yet to be exploited as immunopotentiators in the context of infectious diseases. Here, we showed that BG are potent inducers of dendritic cells (DC), which led to enhanced T cell proliferation and differentiation into effector cells. BG also induced macrophage activation, which was associated with enhanced nitric oxide production, a key anti-mycobacterial weapon. We further demonstrated that the immunostimulatory capability of BG far exceeds that of LPS and involves both TLR4-dependent and independent pathways. Consistently, BG treatment, but not LPS treatment, reduced the bacterial burden in infected mice, which correlated with increased influx of innate and adaptive effector immune cells and increased production of key cytokines in the lungs. Finally and importantly, enhanced bacilli killing was seen in mice co-administered with BG and second-line TB drugs bedaquiline and delamanid. Overall, this work paves the way for BG as potent immunostimulators that may be harnessed to improve mycobacteria killing at the site of infection.

Keywords: bacterial ghosts, tuberculosis, host-directed therapy, drug resistance, adjunct immune therapy

INTRODUCTION

Tuberculosis (TB) remains one of the most persistent diseases of the modern world, despite steady improvement in TB mortality and incidence rates in 2017 (1). Many factors contribute to the high burden of disease including poverty, HIV co-infection, limited vaccine efficacy and drug resistance (2, 3). As the development of vaccines with improved protective efficacy (4) and drugs with novel modes of action (5) has proven to be challenging and expensive, alternative solutions are urgently needed.

The main causative agent of TB, *Mycobacterium tuberculosis* (Mtb) is an intracellular pathogen that is capable of infecting a variety of cell types including epithelial, myeloid and lymphoid cell lineages. This pathogen has evolved numerous strategies to counteract, escape, subvert or delay the host protective immune responses. In innate immune cells, such as macrophages and dendritic cells (DC), Mtb hinders phago-lysosomal fusion (6), limits MHC antigen presentation (7), inhibits apoptosis (8), and dampens the migratory potential of DC (9). At the adaptive immunity level, Mtb-specific CD8 T cells were found to exhibit suppressed cytotoxic activity and proliferative ability due to impaired differentiation (10, 11). Importantly, Mtb also skews the protective Th1-mediated immunity toward Th2 responses by perturbing IFNγ signaling and inducing high IL-4 levels, which results in reduced iNOS activity, impaired apoptosis of infected cells, increased regulatory T cell numbers and greater iron availability to intracellular Mtb (12, 13).

Host-directed therapies (HDT) have been increasingly explored as alternative or adjunct TB treatment that focus on potentiating the host (immune) responses to improve mycobacterial killing (14, 15). Some notable examples include interferon (IFN) α or γ therapy (16–18), antibody-based therapy (19–21), metabolic pathways targeting approaches (22, 23) and therapeutic vaccination with non-pathogenic mycobacteria or Mtb fragments (24–26).

Here, we investigated the therapeutic potential of *Escherichia coli* bacterial ghosts (BG) against TB. BG are cytoplasm-free, intact bacterial cell envelopes that are obtained through the conditional expression of plasmid-encoded gene E from the bacteriophage ΦX174 (27). Integration of the 91 amino-acid polypeptide E in the bacterial envelope triggers a fusion process of the inner and outer membranes to form a transmembrane tunnel structure through which the cytoplasmic content is expelled driven by a proton-motive force (28, 29). To date, BG have been made from a variety of pathogens including *Escherichia coli* K12 (30), enterotoxigenic and enterohemaorrhagic *E. coli* (EHEC, ETEC) (31), *Helicobacter pylori* (32), *Salmonella typhimurium* (33), *S. enteritidis* (34), and *Vibrio cholerae* (35) for both veterinary and clinical vaccine purposes. BG have also been evaluated as drug delivery (36) and adjuvant (37) systems. Additionally, mucosal routes, including oral, aerosol and intranasal, have been deemed suitable for BG administration (38–41). The presence of various pathogen associated molecular patterns (PAMPs) in the cell wall of BG—lipopolysaccharide (LPS), peptidoglycan, glycolipids, flagellin, and lipoproteins—makes them potent activators of innate immune cells, which leads to the production of pro-inflammatory cytokines and bactericidal elements, such as reactive oxygen and nitrogen intermediates (ROIs and RNIs) (37, 42, 43). Furthermore, through their ability to activate DC, BG have also been shown to promote greater pathogen-specific antibody responses (40), increased T lymphocytes recruitment and proliferation with their associated cytokine production (39, 41, 44, 45).

In this study, the immunostimulatory properties of BG were assessed in the context of mycobacterial infection and our data demonstrate that BG can enhance mycobacterial killing and improve the efficacy of second-line TB drugs. With greater development to further boost the extent of killing, BG may represent a promising option for HDT.

METHODS

Bacteria, BG, and Mammalian Cell Culture

Cultures of *M. bovis* BCG Pasteur strain (ATCC, 35734) were cultured in standing T25 flasks in Middlebrook 7H9 broth (Becton Dickinson Difco™, NJ, USA) at 37°C until OD_{600nm} 0.5–0.7 and then stored at −80°C in 7H9 and 25% glycerol (1st Base, Singapore). Mtb H37Rv were cultivated in 50 mL 7H9 rolling culture and processed as described above.

Bacterial ghosts (BG) prepared from *Escherichia coli* NM522, as previously described (30), were obtained from Biotech Innovation Research Development & Consulting (BIRD-C, Austria).

Bone marrow cells flushed out from femurs and tibia of 7–8 weeks-old female WT or TLR4 KO C57BL/6 mice were differentiated into macrophages (BMMO) over 6–8 days at 37°C, under 5% CO_2 in complete differentiation medium containing DMEM (Gibco), 1X penicillin-streptomycin (Gibco), 1 mM sodium pyruvate (Gibco), 10% heat-inactivated fetal bovine serum (FBS) (Gibco), and 20 ng/mL murine M-CSF (R&D Systems) in HEPES (Gibco). Bone marrow derived dendritic cells (BMDC) were cultured in complete differentiation medium—RPMI (Gibco), 10% FBS, 0.05 mM β-mercaptoethanol (Gibco), 1× glutamax (Gibco) with 20 ng/mL murine GM-CSF (Peprotech)—over 10–12 days. Media changes were conducted on 3rd, 6th, 8th, and 10th day of culture. BMMO and BMDC were maintained in antibiotic-free, complete medium containing 10 ng/mL murine M-CSF and 5 ng/mL murine GM-CSF, respectively after differentiation.

In vitro M. bovis BCG Infection

BMMO and BMDC (5×10^4 cells) were infected with *M. bovis* BCG at a multiplicity of infection (MOI) of 2 for 1 h at 37°C and 5% CO_2. The cells were then washed once with 1 X PBS to remove extracellular bacteria. At indicated time points, cells were lysed by vigorous flushing with 0.1% Triton X-100 (USB Corporation). Cell lysates were serially diluted in Middlebrook 7H9 broth before plating onto 7H11 agar plates (Difco, BD) for colony forming unit (CFU) enumeration after 16–19 days incubation at 37°C and 5% CO_2.

LPS Extraction From BG and Quantification

BG (10^9) lyophilized particles (17.8 mg) were resuspended in 2 mL of millicule water and pelleted by centrifugation. BG pellet was resuspended and lysed, before total LPS was extracted using the LPS Extraction Kit from iNtRON Biotechnology (South Korea), according to the manufacturer's instructions. Extracted LPS was then washed using 70% EtOH, before reconstitution in 10 mM Tris-HCl. The amount of LPS extracted from BG was quantified using Pierce™ Limulus Amebocyte Lysate Chromogenic Endotoxin Kit (Thermofisher Scientific, MA, USA). Results indicated a total LPS content of 7.5×10^{-5} EU/BG particle.

BG, LPS, and IFNγ Treatments of Macrophages and DC

BMMO and BMDC were treated with BG at MOI 40 and 5, respectively or as indicated in the figure legends. Treatment with TLR4-specific lipopolysaccharide (LPS) from *E. coli* 0111:B4 strain (LPS-EB Ultrapure) (Invivogen; CA, USA), murine recombinant IFNγ (Gibco) were done at a concentration indicated in the figure legends.

Mouse Experiments

Animal experiments were approved by the Institutional Animal Care and Use Committee of National University of Singapore (NUS) under protocol R15-1030 and were performed in the AALAAC-accredited animal facilities at NUS. 7–8 weeks old female Jackson C57BL/6 mice were purchased from InVivos (Singapore) and were intratracheally (IT) infected with $\sim 10^6$ CFU of *M. bovis* BCG or 10^3 CFU of Mtb H37Rv. Starting day 7 p.i. or as indicated in the figure legends, BG (10^6 particles/mouse), normalized LPS treatment (75 EU/mouse corresponding to 75 ng) or vehicle (millicule water) were administered IT once weekly up to 4 consecutive weeks. Drug treatments started on day 7 p.i. INH was incorporated in drinking water of mice at 0.05 mg/mL for daily consumption. All other drugs were formulated in 20% D-α-tocopherol polyethylene glycol 1000 succinate (TPGS, Sigma-Aldrich) + 1% DMSO and were administered by oral gavage thrice weekly for 4 consecutive weeks at the following doses: Q203 (10 mg/kg), bedaquiline (BDQ; 15 mg/kg), delamanid (DLM; 15 mg/kg) and linezolid (LZD; 50 mg/kg). For combined therapy, mice were treated by oral gavage or IT on separate days to prevent excessive handling. Mice were monitored daily for weight loss. At specified time points, lungs from euthanized mice were harvested and homogenized on ice in PBS + 0.1% Triton X-100 with Halt protease inhibitor cocktail (Thermofisher Scientific). Appropriate dilutions of the lung homogenates were plated onto 7H11 agar (Difco, BD) for CFU determination after 16–19 days incubation at 37°C and 5% CO_2. Alternatively, lung homogenates were spun down and the supernatants were collected for cytokine quantification. For lung histology, lungs from euthanized mice were inflated with 4% paraformaldehyde (PFA) and kept at 4°C overnight before H&E staining. For flow cytometry analyses, mice were euthanized at the indicated time points and harvested lungs were treated with collagenase D (Roche, Germany) for 1 h at 37°C and gently mashed through a cell strainer to obtain single cell suspensions before quenching with FACS buffer, containing 2% FBS, 2 mM EDTA in PBS.

Flow Cytometry

Single cell suspensions from murine lungs were treated with red blood cell (RBC) lysis buffer and blocked with mouse Fc block (BD Pharmingen, Germany). Cells were stained for 30 min with Live/Dead eFluor780 Fixable Viability Dye (ThermoFisher Scientific) and the following panel of antibodies were used: (i) myeloid cells: CD45 BUV395 (BD), CD11b eFluor450 (Thermofisher Scientific), CD11c BV786 (BD), CD24 BUV496 (BD), Ly6C-Biotin and BV805-Streptavidin (BD), Ly6G PE-CF594 (BD), CD64 PE-Cy7 (Biolegend), Siglec F BV510 (BD), MHCII (IA/IE) PE (Biolegend, CA, USA), CD86 Alexa647 (Biolegend); (ii) pDC and T cell subsets: CD45 BUV395 (BD), CD11c APC (BD), Siglec H PE (ThermoFisher Scientific), Thy1.2 PB (Biolegend), CD4 BUV805 (BD), CD8a AlexaFluor488 (Biolegend), CD44 BUV737 (BD), CD62L BV605 (BD), CD45Ra BV786 (BD). Immune cell populations were defined according to the gating strategy shown in **Figure S4**.

For *in vitro* experiments, the antibodies used were as follows: (i) BMMO: CD11b eFluor450, F4/80 PerCP-Cy5.5, CD80 APC, CD86 PE, CD54 FITC, Live/Dead eFluor780 and (ii) BMDC: CD11c FITC, MHCII PB, CD86 PE, CD40 APC, CCR7 PE-Cy7, Live/Dead eFluor780. Cells were defined as follows: BMMO ($CD11b^+$, $F4/80^+$) and BMDC ($CD11c^+$ MHCII intermediate to high).

Stained cells were washed twice with FACS buffer before overnight fixation with 2% PFA. Flow cytometry was run using LSRFortessa X-20 analyzer (BD Biosciences) using UltraComp beads (Invitrogen) for single color controls. All flow cytometry analyses were conducted using FlowJo (v.10.5).

Syngeneic Mixed Lymphocyte Reaction (MLR)

M. bovis BCG-infected BMDC (3×10^4 cells) were pulsed with 10 ug/mL of MHC-I restricted OVA peptide 257–264 or MHC-II restricted OVA peptide 323–339, and co-treated with either BG (MOI 1 or 5) or a normalized dose of LPS (22.5 or 112.5 EU/mL) for 24 h. Splenic T cells (Tc) from C57BL/6 OTI or OTII transgenic mice were isolated using Pan T cell Isolation Kit (Miltenyi Biotec, Germany) and labeled with 5 uM CellTrace Violet (ThermoFisher Scientific). Labeled T cells were incubated with BMDC at a BMDC:Tc ratio of 1:10 for 96 h. Cells were stained with the following antibody panel for T cells: Thy1.2 APC, CD4 PE, CD8 AlexaFluor488, CD62L BV605, CD44 BUV737, and Live/Dead eFluor780, before overnight fixation. T cells were defined as follows: CD4 T cells ($Thy1.2^+$, $CD4^+$) and CD8 T cells ($Thy1.2^+$, $CD8^+$). Flow cytometry was ran using LSRFortessa X-20 analyzer (BD Biosciences) using UltraComp beads (eBioscience) for single color controls. Division and proliferation indices were derived using FlowJo's proliferation modeling tool. Division index represents the average number of cell divisions undergone by the whole cell population and includes undivided cells; it is calculated as follows:

$$\textit{Division index} = \frac{\textit{Total number of divisions}}{\textit{Initial number of cells}}.$$

Proliferation index is the total number of divisions divided by the number of dividing cells and excludes the undivided population:

$$\textit{Proliferation index} = \frac{\textit{Total number of divisions}}{\textit{Number of dividing cells}}.$$

Quantification of Cytokine Levels

BCG-infected or uninfected BMMO or BMDC (10^5 cells) were incubated with BG at MOI 40 and 5, respectively or a normalized dose of LPS (300 and 37.5 EU/mL, respectively) for 24 h. ELISA was conducted on cell culture supernatants to determine the levels of TNFα, IFNγ, IL-6, IL-10, IL-12p40, and IL-12p70 using mouse ELISA kits (Invitrogen), according to the manufacturer's instructions.

Nitric Oxide Determination

Nitrite oxide (NO) production in cell culture supernatants was quantified using Measure-iT high-sensitivity nitrite assay kit (ThermoFisher Scientific). Fluorescence readings were recorded at $\lambda_{ex/em}$ 365/450 nm.

RNA Sequencing and Functional Analyses

BMDC were treated with BG at MOI 5 or with a normalized dose of LPS (188 EU/mL) for 2 h, or left untreated before RNA extraction was conducted using QIAGEN RNeasy mini kit (Qiagen, Singapore). RNA integrity was checked using Agilent 4200 TapeStation System, and all samples had RNA integrity numbers ≥ 8.9. Libraries for RNASeq were made with TruSeq Stranded mRNA Library Prep Kit (Illumina) using 1–1.5 μg of RNA as input. Libraries were multiplexed and ran across two lanes on HiSeq 4000 Sequencing Systems (Illumina) to yield 2 × 151 bp paired-end reads with an average yield of ∼55 million reads/sample. All raw sequences have been deposited in NCBI Sequence Read Archive (SRA) under BioProject number PRJNA544586.

FASTQ files (paired end; 2 × 151) were mapped using STAR aligner against the Genome Reference Consortium Mouse Build 38 (GRCm38). The mapped paired-end reads were counted using HTSeq (46) and unambiguously mapped read pairs were binned per gene. Gene-based read counts were further processed using Bioconductor package EdgeR (47). Briefly, gene counts were transformed into counts per million (CPM) reads and only genes with CPM value ≥1 across all samples were used in downstream analysis. Gene counts were then adjusted for library size and normalized using trimmed mean of m-values (TMM) method. Differential gene expression was calculated using the Fisher's exact test and genes were considered significantly differentially

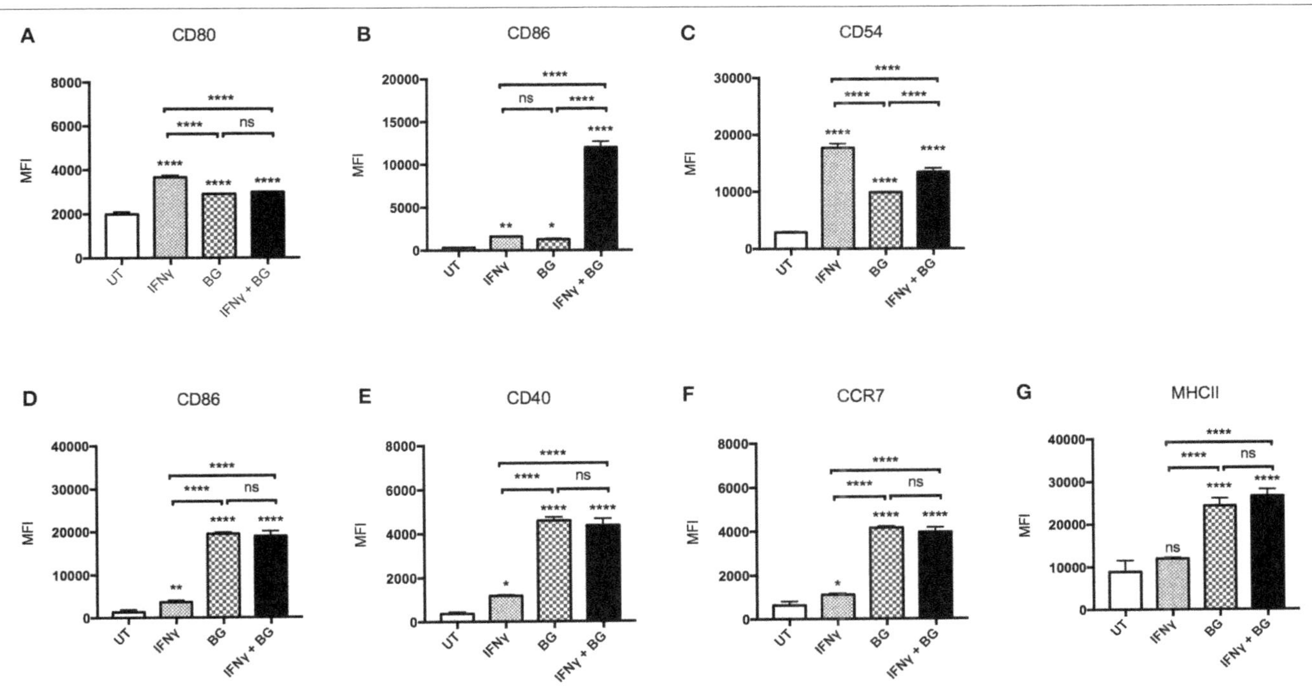

FIGURE 1 | Activation status of BMMO and BMDC upon IFNγ and BG treatment. BMMO and BMDC were left untreated (UT), or were incubated with recombinant murine IFNγ at 20 and 10 μg/ml, respectively, or with BG at MOI 40 and 5, respectively, or with a combination of both for 24 h. Expression of surface activation markers CD80, CD86, CD54 on BMMO **(A–C)** and CD86, CD40, CCR7, and MHCII on BMDC **(D–G)** was determined by flow cytometry. Results are expressed as mean ± SD of technical triplicates and are representative of two independent experiments. Significance values were derived using 1-way ANOVA with Holm-Sidak's multiple comparisons test (ns: not significant, *$p < 0.05$, **$p < 0.01$, ****$p < 0.0001$); asterisks above bars indicates significance with respect to UT control.

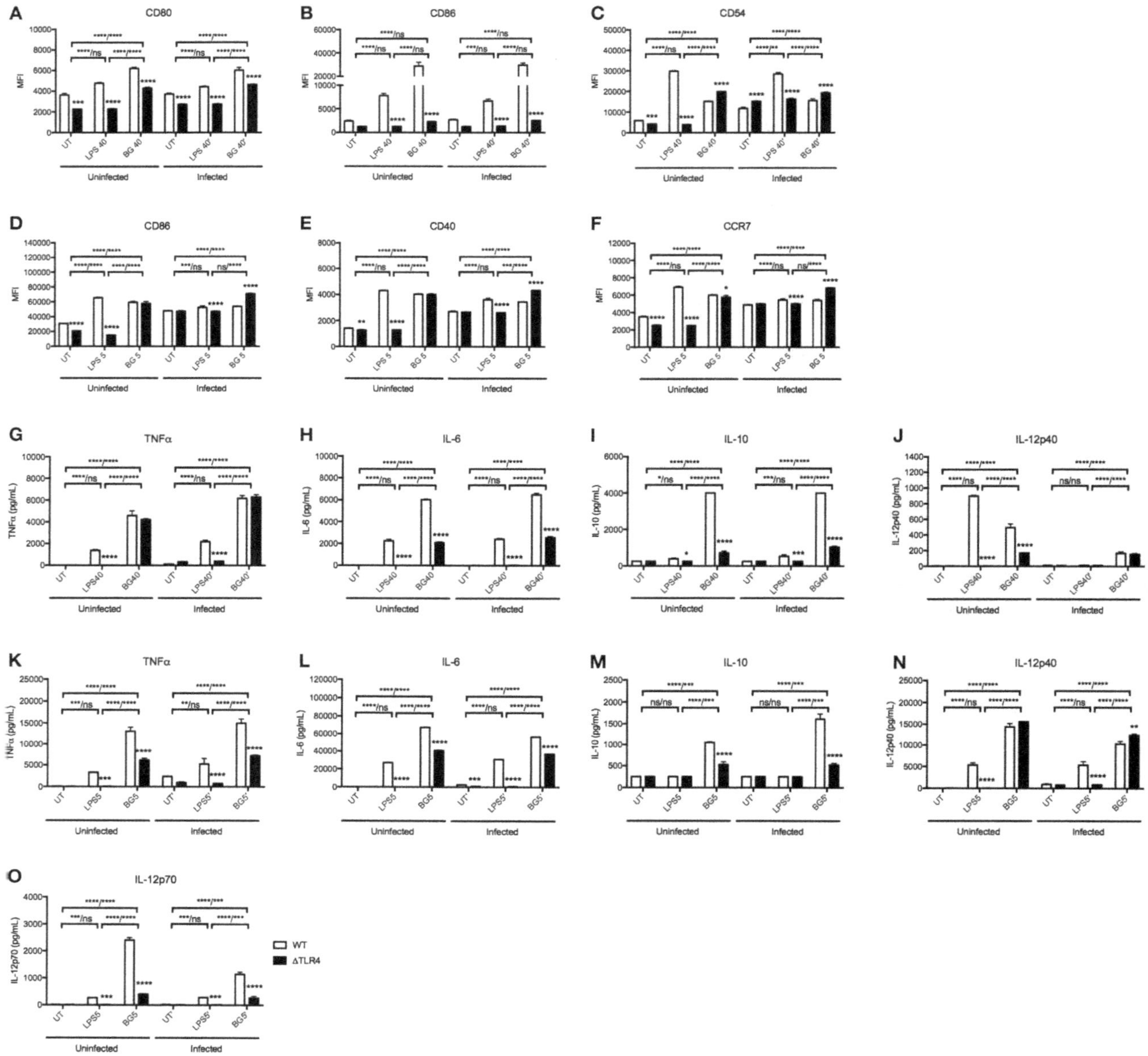

FIGURE 2 | Activation status and cytokine production of WT vs. ΔTLR4 BMMO and BMDC upon BG and LPS treatment. Uninfected and *M. bovis* BCG-infected BMMO and BMDC were treated with BG at MOI 40 and 5, respectively, or with a normalized amount of LPS (1,500 and 188 EU/mL, respectively) or left untreated (UT) for 24 h before analysis of surface activation markers by flow cytometry. Expression levels of CD80, CD86, CD54 for BMMO **(A–C)** and CD86, CD40, and CCR7 for BMDC **(D–F)** are shown for WT (open bar) and ΔTLR4 (black bar) cells. Cell culture supernatants were collected to quantify the levels of TNFα, IL-6, IL-10, IL12p40, and IL-12p70 produced by ELISA. Cytokine production was measured in WT and ΔTLR4 BMMO **(G–J)** and BMDC **(K–O)**. Results are expressed as mean ± SD of technical triplicates **(A–F)** or duplicates **(G–O)** and are representative of two independent experiments. Significance values were derived using 2-way ANOVA with Holm-Sidak's multiple comparisons test (ns: not significant, $^{*}p < 0.05$, $^{**}p < 0.01$, $^{***}p < 0.001$, $^{****}p < 0.0001$). Asterisks separated by a dash denote significance values between treatment groups within WT and KO samples, respectively (WT/KO), while those above bars indicate significance with respect to WT control. Dotted lines denote limit of detection.

expressed if they met the cut off criteria, i.e., false discovery rate (FDR) ≤ 0.05 and log2 fold change ≥ 1. Differential gene expression data was visualized as heatmap using R Bioconductor package heatmap3 (https://cran.r-project.org/package=heatmap3).

Functional annotation was performed using DAVID (version 6.8) (48, 49) and the gene term enrichment for the significantly enriched annotation terms were extracted from the functional annotation chart. Annotation terms were considered significant if they had a fold enrichment ≥ 1.5 and -$\log_{10}$ FDR ≥ 1.

Statistical Analyses

Statistical analyses were generated from Prism 7.0 (GraphPad, USA) and tests used are indicated in the figure legends. One-way and two-way ANOVA were conducted on experiments comparing across treatment groups under single and multiple conditions, respectively, with Holm-Sidak's correction as *post-hoc* test. Results with *p*-values <0.05 were defined as statistically significant.

RESULTS

Immunomodulatory Properties of BG on Macrophages and Dendritic Cells

The ability of BG to activate macrophages and dendritic cells was first examined. BMMO and BMDC were treated with BG at MOI 40 and 5, respectively, which corresponds to the maximum dose that did not lead to more than 20% cell death (data not shown). BG treatment resulted in a significant upregulation of all the activation markers tested (CD80, CD86, CD54, CD40, CCR7, MHCII) on bone marrow-derived macrophages (BMMO) (**Figures 1A–C**) and bone marrow-derived dendritic cells (BMDC) (**Figures 1D–G**) compared to untreated cells. However, the increased surface expression of CD80 and CD54 was significantly lower than that measured on BMMO treated with IFNγ alone (**Figures 1A–C**). In contrast, BG treatment led to significantly greater expression of all the activation markers on BMDC compared to treatment with IFNγ alone (**Figures 1D–G**). Notably, increased surface CCR7 expression on BG-treated BMDC suggested that BG might increase the migratory ability of DC (**Figure 1F**). When BMMO were co-incubated with both IFNγ and BG, significantly higher levels of CD86 and CD54 were measured compared to stimulation with BG alone, suggesting that IFNγ and BG may act synergistically to activate macrophages (**Figures 1B,C**). However, such synergy was not observed with BMDC (**Figures 1D–G**).

BG Has Distinct Immunomodulatory Properties From LPS

Since LPS is a major component of *E. coli* bacterial cell wall, we questioned whether LPS alone could recapitulate the immunostimulatory properties of BG. We thus compared the activation level of BMMO and BMDC treated with BG or with an amount of LPS equivalent to that present in the BG dose (see Methods), referred to as "normalized amount of

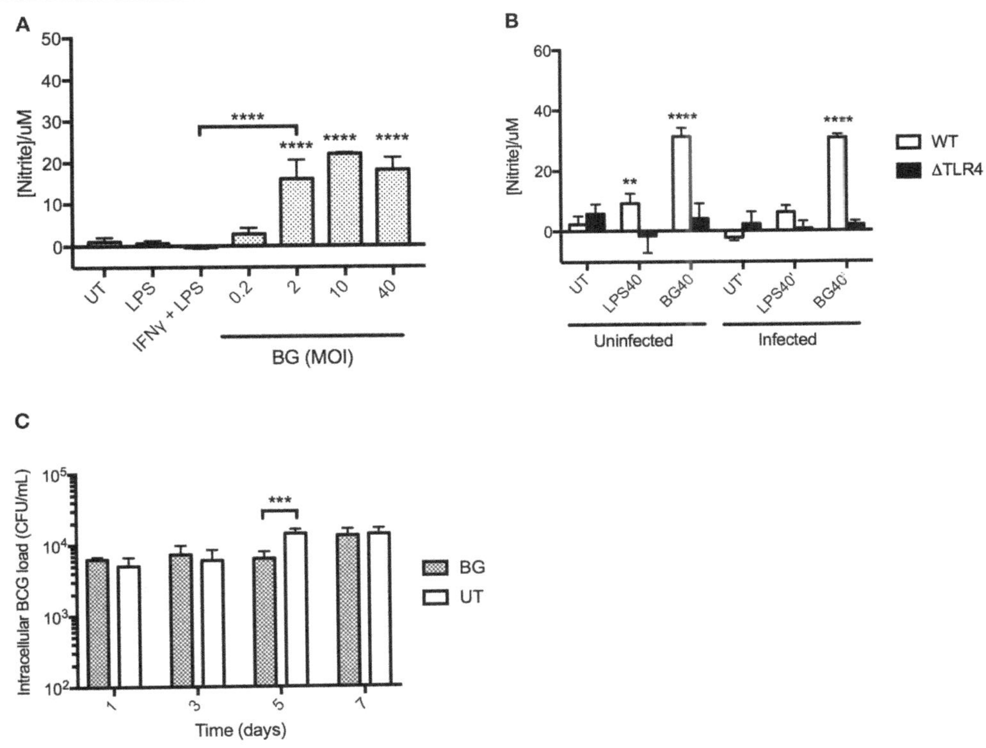

FIGURE 3 | NO production in BMMO upon BG and LPS treatment and killing efficacy. **(A)** BMMO were left untreated (UT), or treated with 10 ng/mL LPS, or with a combination of (20 ng/mL IFNγ +10 ng/mL LPS), or with a range of BG MOIs for 24 h before nitrite determination. **(B)** Uninfected or *M. bovis* BCG-infected WT and ΔTLR4 BMMO were treated with BG at MOI 40 (BG40) or with a normalized amount of LPS (LPS40, corresponding to 1,500 EU/mL) or left untreated (UT) for 24 h before nitrite quantification. **(C)** *M. bovis* BCG-infected BMMO were treated with BG (MOI 40) or left untreated (UT). Intracellular bacterial loads were determined at 1, 3, 5, and 7 days post-infection. Results are expressed as mean ± SD of technical triplicates and are representative of two independent experiments. Significance values were derived using 1-way ANOVA for **(A)** and 2-way ANOVA for **(B,C)** with Holm-Sidak's multiple comparisons test (**$p < 0.01$, ***$p < 0.001$, ****$p < 0.0001$); asterisks above bars indicates significance with respect to UT **(A,C)** and WT **(B)** control.

LPS" thereafter. Furthermore, since LPS immunostimulatory properties signal mainly through TLR4 (50), we examined the ability of BG to activate TLR4-deficient BMMO and BMDC. The results indicated that BG activated BMMO and BMDC to a greater extent than a normalized amount of LPS, as evidenced by higher expression of most activation markers in both *M. bovis* BCG-infected and uninfected contexts (**Figures 2A–F**). BG- and LPS-mediated activation were found to be partially dependent on TLR4: ΔTLR4 BMMO displayed lower surface expression of CD80 and CD86 compared to WT BMMO (**Figures 2A,B**). In contrast, the reduced expression of CD54 in ΔTLR4 BMMO was seen only upon LPS treatment, implying that BG-induced upregulation of CD54 expression is TLR4-independent (**Figure 2C**). In BMDC, BG-mediated upregulation of CD86, CD40, and CCR7 was largely independent of TLR4, unlike LPS treatment (**Figures 2D–F**).

Cytokine production in culture supernatant was also measured in BG- and LPS-treated WT vs. ΔTLR4 BMMO and BMDC (**Figures 2G–O**). BG treatment generally induced higher levels of TNFα, IL-6, and IL-10 compared to LPS treatment in both uninfected and *M. bovis* BCG-infected BMMO (**Figures 2G–J**); similar results were obtained with BMDC, including IL-12p70, an important Th1 cytokine (**Figures 2K–O**). Interestingly, production of IL-12p40 in uninfected BMMO was greater upon LPS stimulation compared to BG treatment (**Figure 2J**), while the converse was observed in BMDC (**Figure 2N**); this suggests that production of this cytokine subunit is mediated by different signaling pathways in both cell types. Production of IL-12p70 instead was found TLR4-dependent upon stimulation with both LPS and BG (**Figure 2O**). Furthermore, LPS-induced production of all tested cytokines was undetectable in ΔTLR4 BMMO and BMDC, whereas BG treatment resulted in no or partial decrease of these cytokine levels in the absence of TLR4.

Overall, the data demonstrates that BG treatment of BMMO and BMDC results in activation patterns and cytokine production profiles that differ from those observed upon LPS treatment. Moreover, unlike LPS, BG-mediated cytokine production in BMMO and BMDC is partially TLR4-dependent, supporting BGs' ability to trigger alternative signaling pathways in these innate immune cells.

BG-Induced NO Production Correlates With Enhanced Bacterial Killing in Macrophages

BGs' ability to activate macrophages suggested their propensity to produce NO, an important mycobactericidal element. To test this hypothesis, BMMO were treated with a range of BG MOIs or with positive controls including (i) 10 ng/mL LPS and (ii) a combination of (20 ng/mL IFNγ + 10 ng/mL LPS). A significantly greater production of NO was measured in BMMO treated with BG at MOI 2 and above, compared to untreated BMMO, and BMMO treated with LPS or (IFNγ + LPS) (**Figure 3A**). In comparison to a normalized amount of LPS, BG exhibited a superior ability to trigger NO production in both *M. bovis* BCG-infected and uninfected contexts (**Figure 3B**). Furthermore, BG treatment of ΔTLR4 BMMO resulted in NO levels that were close to the detection limit (**Figure 3B**), indicating that BG-induced NO production is largely TLR4-dependent. Importantly, BG-mediated NO production in BMMO correlated with a transient but significant decrease in the intracellular bacterial load at day 5 post-infection (p.i.) (**Figure 3C**). This indicates that NO-dependent mechanisms may contribute to improved killing in BG-treated macrophages.

Gene Expression Profile in BG-Treated and LPS-Treated Dendritic Cells

To compare the overall impact of BG vs. LPS treatment on BMDC, a transcriptomics (RNAseq) approach was carried out. The number of genes that were differentially modulated by BG treatment compared to untreated BMDC was significantly greater than upon LPS treatment (616 vs. 369 genes, respectively) (**Figure 4A**). Most of the genes induced by LPS were found in common with BG treatment, leaving 56 genes unique to LPS treatment (**Figure 4A**, **Tables S1**, **S2**), whereas 303 genes were uniquely induced by BG treatment (**Figure 4A**, **Table S3**). Heat map analysis showed that BG treatment modulated gene expression differently from LPS (**Figure 4B**). Functional annotation analysis revealed that immune system processes involving both the innate and adaptive immune responses were commonly modulated upon both LPS and BG treatment (**Figures 4C,D**): these genes include *Bcl10*, *CD86*, *IL-4*, *Icam1* (CD54), *IL-27*, *CCL22*, and *CD14*, which facilitates TLR4-mediated responses (**Tables S4**, **S5**). Unlike treatment with a normalized amount of LPS, BG treatment significantly modulated *Nfkb1* gene expression, which supports the superior immune activation potential of BG. BG treatment was also found to influence a greater variety of pathways and corresponding gene counts than LPS (**Figures 4C,D**). Interestingly, only LPS treatment modulated the pathway GO:0032496 (response to lipopolysaccharide); BG may contain other components that dampen the LPS pathway response in favor of others (**Figures 4C,D**). Additionally, BG-induced modulation of *Lyst*, a lysosomal trafficking regulator, supports DC internalization and processing of BG (**Tables S4**, **S5**). Overall, the RNAseq data confirm the superior and broader modulatory ability of BG in comparison to a normalized amount of LPS.

BG Modulates T Cell Proliferation and Differentiation *in vitro*

The ability of BG to increase the surface expression of co-stimulatory molecules CD80 and CD86 on BMDC, essential for T cell receptor binding, led us to investigate whether BG could promote T cell differentiation and proliferation. A syngeneic mixed lymphocyte reaction (MLR) assay was set up whereby uninfected or *M. bovis* BCG-infected BMDC were stimulated with OTI or OTII OVA peptide in the presence of BG or a normalized amount of LPS or in the absence of both,

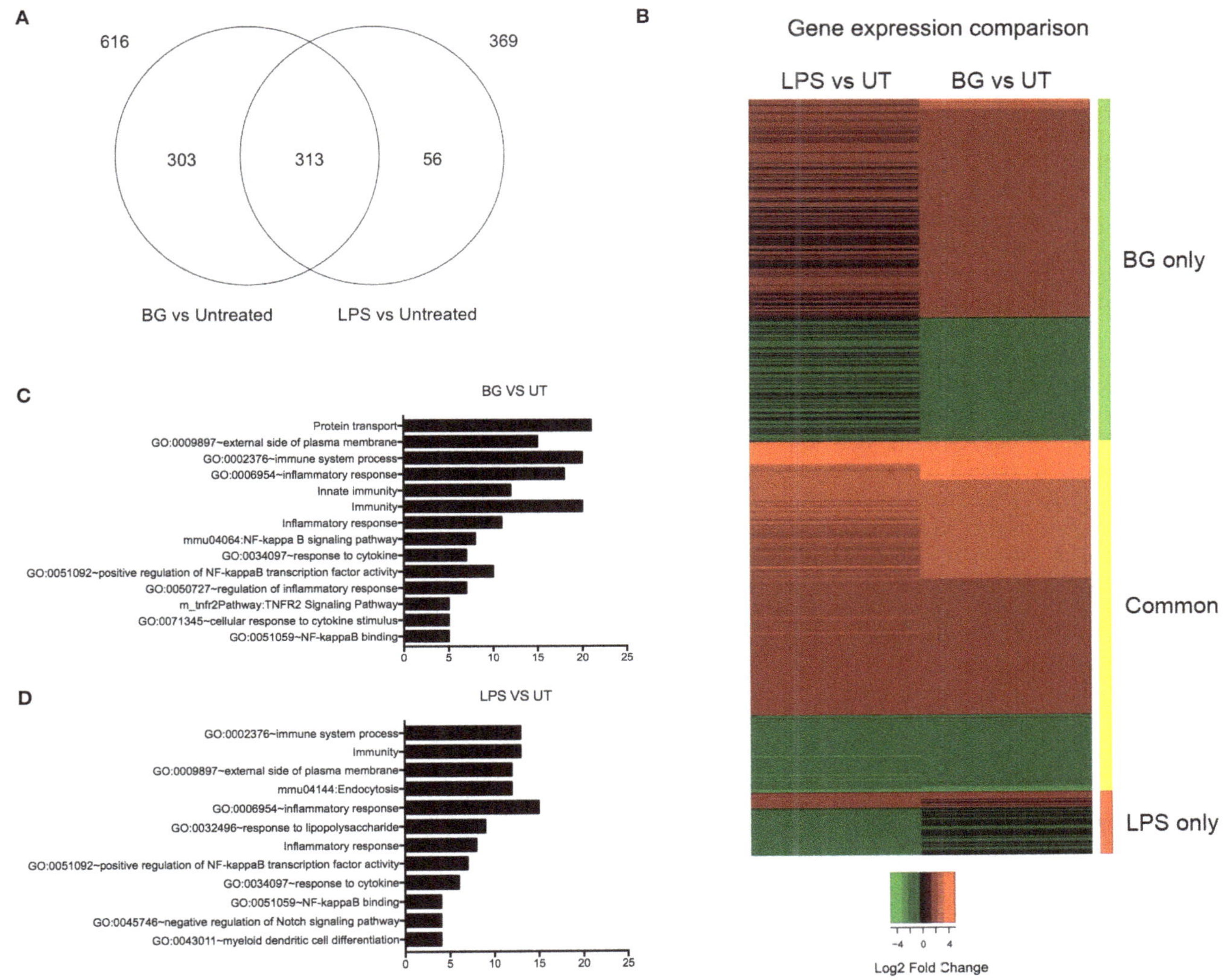

FIGURE 4 | Comparison of differential gene expression profiles of BG- and LPS-treated BMDC. BMDC were treated with BG MOI 5 or a normalized amount of LPS (188 EU/mL) for 2 h before total RNA was extracted and processed for RNA sequencing. **(A)** Venn diagram shows the differentially expressed gene counts between BG and LPS treatment relative to untreated (UT) controls 2 h post-treatment. 369 and 616 genes were found differentially modulated from untreated (UT) controls in consensus between two independent experiments upon BG and LPS treatment, respectively. 313 genes were found commonly modulated between both treatments, while 56 and 303 genes were BG- and LPS-specific, respectively. **(B)** Heat map representation of differentially expressed genes for the conditions: BG and LPS relative to UT controls. Color panel above the heat map indicate the three sides of the comparison, i.e., green: significant in BG only, yellow: common in both, and red: significant in LPS only. Legend indicates log2 fold change, where green indicates down-regulation and red, up-regulation relative to UT. **(C,D)** Bar charts showing total number of genes within manually curated subsets containing immunologically relevant, significant gene terms (fold enrichment ≥ 1.5 and $-\log_{10}$ FDR ≥ 1.0) derived from functional annotation of differentially expressed genes upon BG **(C)** and LPS **(D)** treatment relative to UT.

before being co-cultured with corresponding transgenic OTI and OTII T cells. T cell differentiation and proliferation, as well as cytokine production in the culture supernatants, were then measured.

Division and proliferation indices indicated that in the OTI system, comparable CD8 T cell proliferation was observed with BG-treated, LPS-treated and untreated BMDC, suggesting that BG treatment did not significantly impact on CD8 T cell proliferation (**Figures S1A,B**). However, BG treatment of BMDC resulted in a greater proportion of activated CD8 T cells compared to untreated and LPS-treated controls (**Figure S1D**). Interestingly, compared to untreated control, LPS or BG treatment of BMDC resulted in significantly lower proportion of naive (**Figure S1C**) as well as CD62L CD44 double positive CD8 T cells (**Figure S1E**), representative of central memory T cells (also $CCR7^{+}$). As for cytokine production, OTI T cells co-cultured with BG-treated BMDC produced significantly greater levels of IFNγ and similar levels of IL-12p40 compared to untreated and LPS-treated conditions (**Figures S1F,H**). Expectedly, IL-4, which is mainly produced by CD4 T cells, was lowly/not detected in all the groups (**Figure S1G**).

In the OTII system, the division index indicated that BG-treated BMDC induced a greater proportion of proliferating CD4 T cells in both the uninfected and infected contexts compared to untreated controls (**Figure 5A**). Moreover, BG treatment of infected BMDC resulted in a significantly higher proportion of CD4 T cells to undergo cell division compared to LPS treatment. The extent of proliferation was generally comparable or lower between BG-treated BMDC and the other groups (**Figure 5B**). Interestingly, BG treatment resulted in reduced proportion of activated CD4 T cells and a greater proportion of CD62L CD44 double positive CD4 T cells compared to untreated controls (**Figures 5C–E**). In term of cytokine production, similar levels of IL-12p40 were measured in BG-treated and LPS-treated groups (**Figure 5H**). Furthermore, slightly elevated levels of IFNγ and very low levels of IL-4 were obtained with BG-treated BMDC compared to untreated controls (**Figures 5F,G**), suggesting that BG treatment of BMDC promotes T cell differentiation into CD4 Th1 lineage.

Overall, the data obtained from these MLR experiments demonstrated that BG treatment of BMDC significantly influences the proliferation and/or differentiation of naïve T cells. BG-treated BMDC generally led to greater IFNγ production by both CD4 and CD8 T cells, which suggests that BG treatment may help to control mycobacterial replication more effectively.

BG Treatment Influences the Composition of Lung Immune Cell Populations and Cytokine Production in *M. bovis* BCG-Infected Mice

The immunostimulatory properties of BG were next examined *in vivo*. The impact of BG and a normalized dose of LPS on pulmonary cell populations was examined in an established *M. bovis* BCG infection mouse model in C57BL/6 mice. Starting at day 7 p.i., BG and LPS were administered intratracheally to *M. bovis* BCG-infected mice once weekly for 4 consecutive weeks. Pulmonary innate immune cell populations were analyzed at 1 day (day 29 p.i.) or 1 week (day 35 p.i.) after the last BG or LPS treatment dose. The number of neutrophils and interstitial macrophages (IM) was significantly higher at both time points in the BG-treated group compared to the other groups, which may suggest that both innate immune cell populations may play a significant role in mycobacteria killing. In contrast, increased levels of Ly6C^{+} monocytes were seen only at day 29 p.i. (**Figures 6A,B,F**). Elevated levels of CD11b^{+} DC, which are typically responsible for T cell activation (51) were also measured 1 day post-BG treatment (**Figure 6C**). Lung resident CD103^{+} DC, which acquire apoptotic cells and traffic to the draining lymph nodes (51), also displayed increased levels in BG-treated animals at day 35 p.i. (**Figure 6D**), which may reflect a greater antigen presentation activity in the lungs of these mice. Levels of resident alveolar macrophages (AM) were also raised at day 35 p.i. upon BG treatment (**Figure 6E**); this is in line with their role in protection of lung tissue from destruction by inflammatory mediators or damaging oxidative burst and in recruitment of monocyte-derived macrophages (52, 53). Interestingly, treatment with a normalized dose of LPS did not lead to any significant changes in the number of all these innate immune cell populations compared to untreated or vehicle-treated infected mice (**Figures 6A–F**).

We also analyzed the CD4 and CD8 T cell populations present in the lungs from BG- and LPS-treated *M. bovis* BCG-infected mice 1 day (day 29 p.i.) or 1 week (day 35 p.i.) after the last treatment dose. The total CD4 T cell count was significantly increased in BG-treated mice 1 week after the last treatment dose, compared to the other treatment groups (**Figure 6G**). This correlated with an increased number of activated CD4 T cells (**Figure 6I**), and effector and effector memory CD4 T cells (**Figures 6J,K**) compared to the other groups. These observations thus showed that BG treatment augmented the number of both short-lived CD4 effectors and transitional CD4 effector memory cells that possess rapid effector functions, including production of IFNγ and IL-4 (54). On the other hand, and consistent with our *in vitro* observations, BG treatment impacted minimally on the CD8 T cell populations, as evidenced by comparable levels of CD8 T cell subsets across all the infected groups (**Figures S2A–E**). A mild but significant increase in the number of CD8 effectors was nevertheless observed 1 day after the last BG dose, although this was not sustained after 1 week (**Figure S2D**). Again, LPS treatment did not significantly affect the CD4 and CD8 T cell populations, underscoring the superior immunostimulatory properties of BG over LPS.

Finally, the levels of key cytokines in the lung homogenates of BG-treated vs. LPS-treated mice were quantified. One day after the last treatment dose (day 29 p.i.), BG-treated animals displayed significantly higher levels of TNFα, IFNγ, IL-6, and IL-12p70 compared to those measured in vehicle-treated and untreated infected mice (**Figures 6L–O**), supporting the pro-inflammatory effect of BG. In contrast, LPS-treated infected mice did not display enhanced levels of pro-inflammatory cytokines compared to controls. No significant difference was found among the treatment groups for all cytokines tested 1 week after the last treatment dose (day 35 p.i.).

BG Treatment Reduces Lung Bacterial Loads in *M. bovis* BCG- and Mtb-Infected Mice

We next questioned whether the greater recruitment of immune cells observed in the lungs of BG-treated infected mice correlated with enhanced bacteria killing efficacy. Strikingly, BG-treated mice but not LPS-treated mice displayed significantly lower pulmonary bacterial loads at day 36 post-infection (1 week after the last treatment dose) compared to vehicle and untreated groups (**Figure 7A**). Both treatments were well-tolerated across all groups, with both BG- and LPS-treated groups displaying a body weight change profile similar to vehicle-treated and untreated groups (**Figure S3A**). Histological analysis of lung

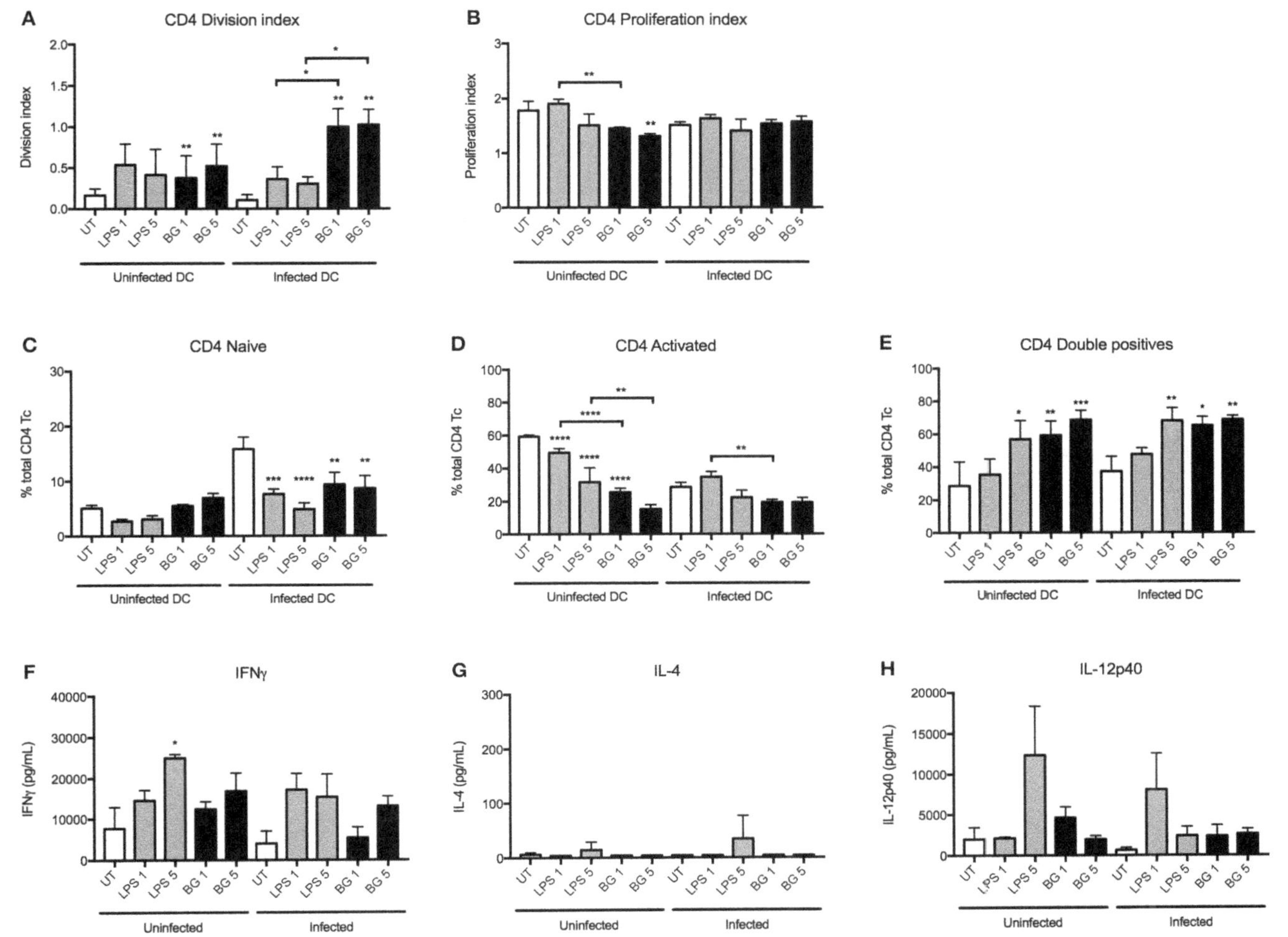

FIGURE 5 | CD4 T cell proliferation and cytokine production induced by LPS- and BG-treated DC in a mixed lymphocyte reaction. *M. bovis* BCG-infected or uninfected BMDC were left untreated (UT) (open bars), stimulated with BG (MOI 1 and 5) (black bars) or stimulated with a normalized amount of LPS (23 or 113 EU/mL, respectively) (gray bars) in the presence of OTII OVA peptide for 24 h, before co-culture with transgenic T cells for 96 h Division and proliferation indices of CD4 **(A,B)** T cells were derived. Proportion of naïve ($CD62L^+$ $CD44^-$), activated ($CD62L^-$ $CD44^+$) and double positive T cells were displayed as percentages of total CD4 T cells **(C–E)**. The levels of IFNγ, IL-4, and IL-12p40 produced after 96 h incubation were measured **(F–H)**. Results are expressed as mean ± SD of technical triplicates and are representative of two independent experiments. Significance values were derived using 1-way ANOVA with Holm-Sidak's multiple comparisons test ($^*p < 0.05$, $^{**}p < 0.01$, $^{***}p < 0.001$, $^{****}p < 0.0001$); asterisks above bars indicate significance with respect to UT control. Dotted lines denote limit of quantification.

sections examined at day 36 p.i. indicated no significant difference in BG- and LPS-treated animals compared to vehicle and untreated controls, implying that both treatments did not cause overt inflammation, nor did they adversely affect lung architecture (**Figure S3B**). To further characterize the BG-mediated effects, the bacterial loads were determined at day 14, 21, 28, and 35 p.i. A significant reduction in bacterial loads was observed at day 28 and 35 p.i. in the lungs from BG-treated mice compared to vehicle-treated controls (**Figure 7B**). Importantly, similar observations were made in Mtb-infected mice whereby a significant reduction in pulmonary bacterial loads was observed at day 28 and 35 p.i. in BG-treated mice (**Figure 7C**). It is worthy to note that reduction in bacterial burden started to be seen at day 28 p.i., which coincides with the activation of adaptive immunity. This suggests that the effector mechanisms responsible for improved mycobacterial killing involve the adaptive immunity. Interestingly, BG treatment significantly diminished the bacterial load in lymph nodes at day 35 p.i., 1 week after the last BG dose was administered in Mtb-infected mice (**Figure 7D**), but not in *M. bovis* BCG-infected ones (data not shown). This observation may suggest that BG immune stimulatory effects are greater in the context of infection with more virulent pathogens that may sensitize the host immunity to additional stimuli. Although the decrease in lung bacterial loads was sustained up to 1 week after the last BG dose (**Figures 7B,C**), it did not extend beyond 3, 4, and 5 weeks after the last BG dose—day 42, 49, and 56 p.i., respectively (**Figure S3C**). This latter observation indicates that weekly BG administration is necessary to sustain reduced pulmonary bacterial loads. Additionally, single dose BG treatment administered at day 7 p.i., or at day 21 or 28

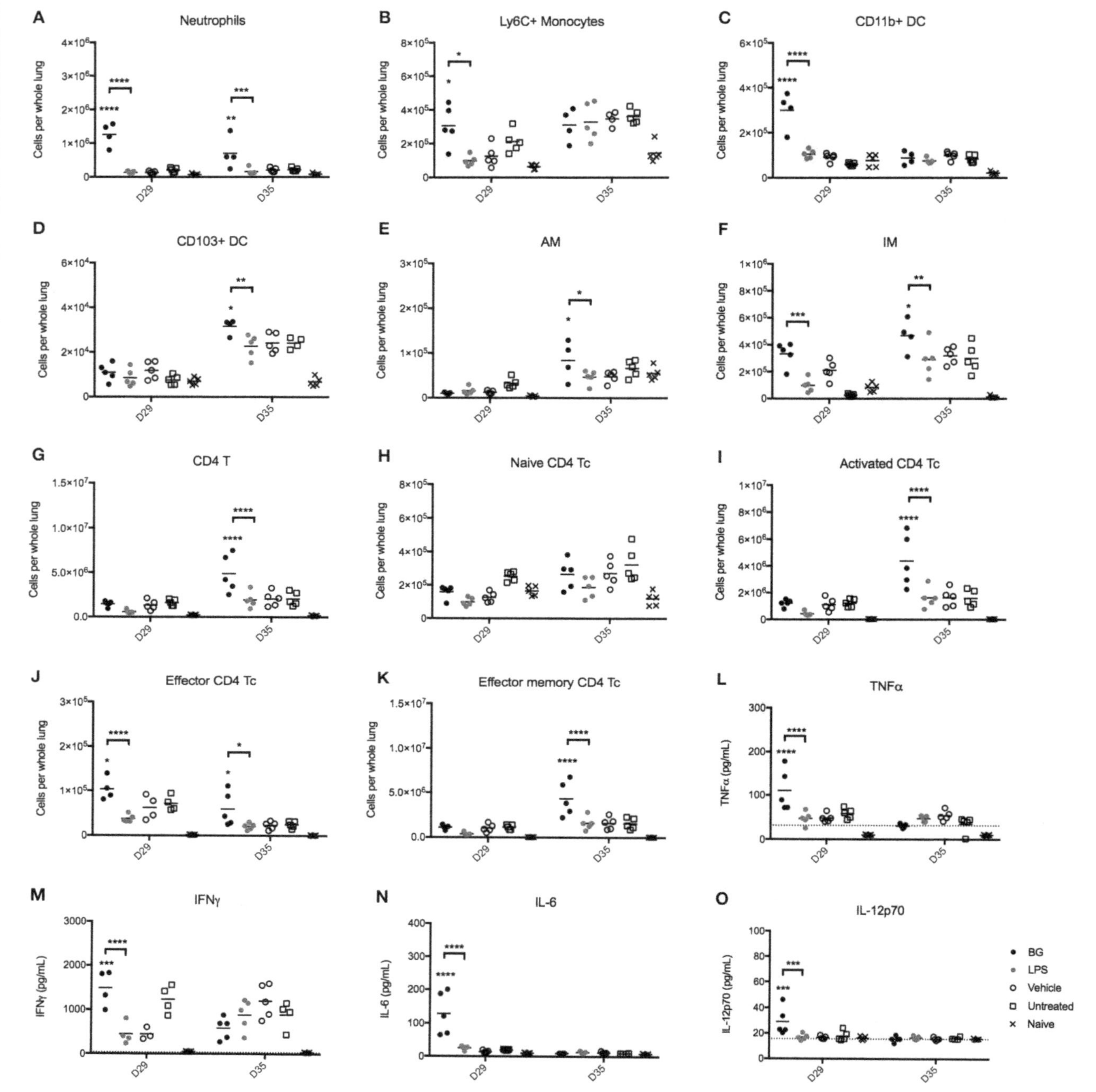

FIGURE 6 | Immune cell populations and cytokine production in lungs from BG-treated vs. LPS-treated *M. bovis* BCG-infected mice. Adult female C57BL/6 mice were infected intratracheally (IT) with 10^6 CFU of *M. bovis* BCG. Starting from day 7 post-infection, mice were administered IT weekly and for 4 consecutive weeks with 10^6 BG, a normalized amount of LPS (75 EU), vehicle or were left untreated (UT). Lungs were harvested 1 day (day 29 p.i.) or 1 week (day 35 p.i.) after the last dose administered and the myeloid **(A–F)** and CD4 T cell **(G–K)** populations were analyzed by flow cytometry. Levels of TNFα, IFNγ, IL-6, IL-10, IL12p40, and IL-12p70 in the lung homogenates **(L–O)** were determined by ELISA. Results are representative of two independent experiments and data points are shown for each mouse ($n = 4$–5 mice/group). Significance values were derived using 2-way ANOVA with Holm-Sidak's multiple comparisons test (*$p < 0.05$, **$p < 0.01$, ***$p < 0.001$, ****$p < 0.0001$); asterisks above bars indicate significance with respect to vehicle control. Dotted lines denote limit of quantification. pDC, plasmacytoid DC; AM, alveolar macrophages; IM, interstitial macrophages.

p.i. (when adaptive immunity has been activated) did not lead to significantly lower pulmonary bacterial loads at day 35 p.i. (**Figure S3D**). Neither did 2 weekly BG doses administered at day 21 and 28 p.i. (**Figure S3D**). These observations thus suggest that a regimen of at least 4 BG weekly doses is necessary to achieve significant reduction in bacterial load.

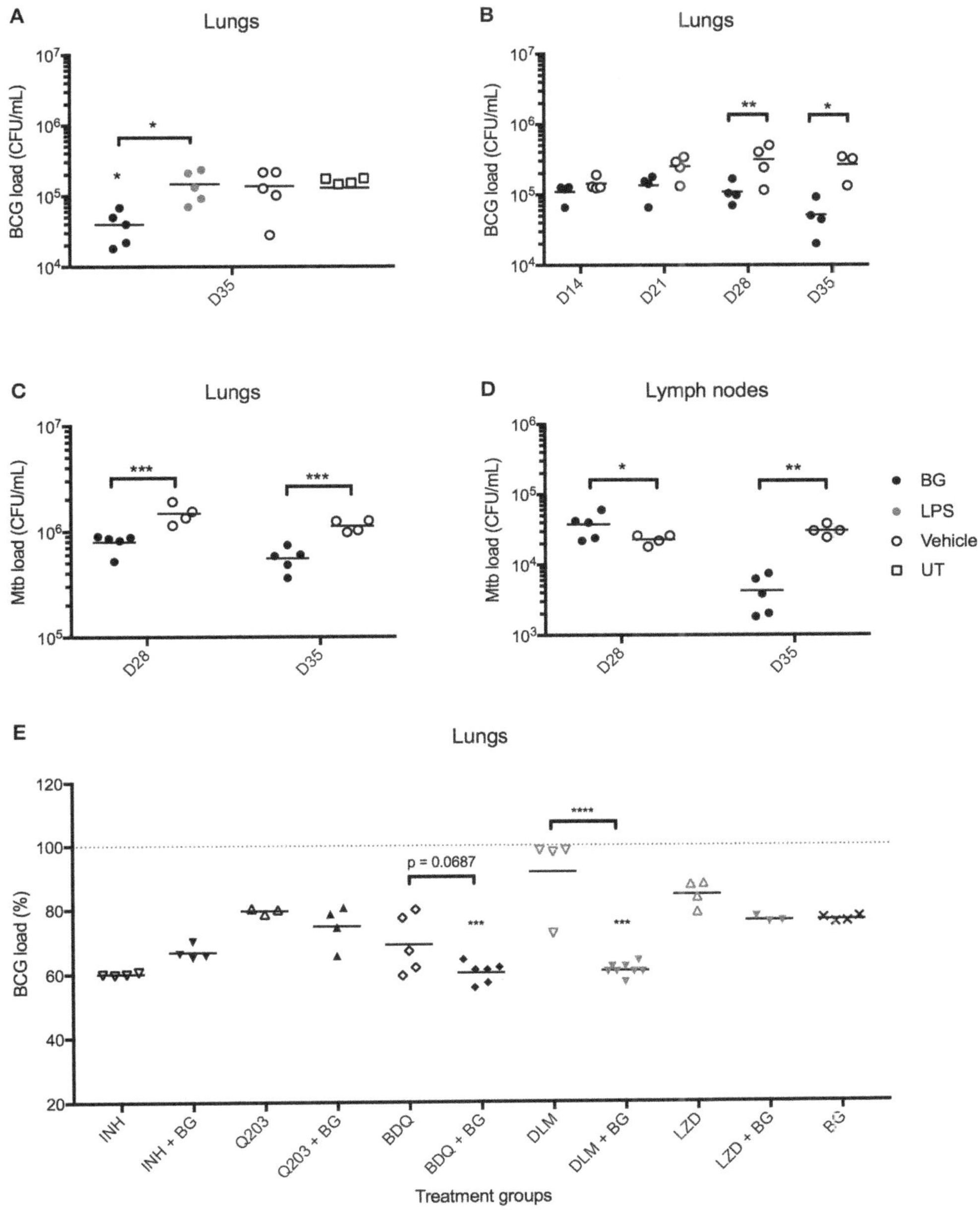

FIGURE 7 | Effect of BG treatment on lung bacterial loads in *M. bovis* BCG- and Mtb-infected mice. Adult female C57BL/6 mice were infected intratracheally (IT) with 10^6 CFU of *M. bovis* BCG **(A,B,E)** or 10^3 CFU Mtb H37Rv **(C,D)**. Treatment was administered as described in the legend of **Figure 6**. For BG adjunct therapy, infected mice were treated daily with INH (0.05 mg/mL) or thrice weekly with Q203 (10 mg/kg) BDQ (15 mg/kg), DLM (10 mg/kg) or LZD (50 mg/kg) via the oral route, in combination with IT administration of BG as described in the legend of **Figure 6**. Organs were harvested at day 35 p.i., unless otherwise indicated, and homogenates were plated for CFU enumeration. Data points are shown for each mouse (n = 3–8 mice/group) and *M. bovis* BCG load **(E)** is expressed as a percentage of vehicle control. Significance values were derived using 1-way **(E)** or 2-way **(A–D)** ANOVA with Holm-Sidak's multiple comparisons test (*$p < 0.05$, **$p < 0.01$, ***$p < 0.001$, ****$p < 0.0001$); asterisks above data points indicate significance with respect to vehicle control. Dotted lines denote percentage of *M. bovis* BCG load of vehicle control.

BG Treatment Synergizes With Second-Line TB Drugs

Given its potential in reducing mycobacterial load, BG treatment was evaluated in combination with selected anti-TB compounds. Since second-line drugs possess comparatively lower cidal potential and higher toxicity than their first-line counterparts, the potential synergistic killing effect between BG and various second-line agents bedaquiline (BDQ), delamanid (DLM) and linezolid (LZD) was examined *in vivo*. First-line drug isoniazid (INH), and phase II clinical drug candidate Q203 were also included. Oral dosing regimens were adapted from established drug regimens for each drug (55–57) to achieve a sub-optimal killing in order to observe any synergistic cidal effect when co-treated with BG. The results indicated that lower pulmonary bacterial loads were observed with BDQ + BG and DLM + BG groups compared to drug only-treated groups (**Figure 7E**). In contrast, BG treatment did not enhance killing efficacy in INH-, Q203-, and LZD-treated mice. Together, the data showed that BG synergizes with at least two second-line TB drugs DLM and BDQ.

DISCUSSION

Our work describes the immunostimulatory properties of BG in the context of mycobacterial infection, and demonstrates that pulmonary delivery of BG helps reduce lung mycobacterial loads. The significant reduction in bacterial loads in the lungs from BG-treated *M. bovis* BCG- and Mtb-infected mice correlated with increased numbers of key innate (neutrophils, macrophages, dendritic cells) and adaptive (CD4 effector cells) immune cell populations and elevated levels of key Th1 cytokines (TNFα, IFNγ, IL-12p70). Hence, BG treatment has the potential to improve the killing activity of innate immune cells and tip the Th1/Th2 balance toward the more protective Th1 response.

These *in vivo* observations were consistent with our *in vitro* data showing that BG effectively activated both macrophages and DC, as evidenced by the increased expression of surface activation markers—CD80/86, CD54, and MHCII—and increased production of TNFα, IL-6, IL-10, and IL-12p40. This finding is in agreement with previous BG stimulation studies conducted on murine BMDC (58), bovine monocyte-derived DC (59), and THP-1 macrophages (60). We also propose that BG may increase the migratory potential of DC through upregulation of CCR7, essential for activation of naïve T cells in the draining lymph nodes. Furthermore, in line with previous studies (45, 59, 61) our MLR experiments showed that BG-treated DC resulted in enhanced CD4 T cell proliferation and differentiation. Unlike previous studies however (38, 41, 45), we failed to observe a significant impact of BG treatment on CD8 T cell proliferation both *in vitro* and *in vivo*. Nevertheless, an increased proportion of activated CD8 T cells supports that BG treatment does potentiate CD8 T cells in their effector functions.

Consistent with a previous report (43), BG-activated macrophages were proficient in producing NO, the importance of which has been well-documented in controlling TB infection. iNOS knockout mice were found to be more susceptible to Mtb infection (62). Moreover, in TB patients, RNIs are capable of inactivating essential pathogenic components that limit mycobacterial persistence within the host (63, 64). The strong induction of NO production upon BG treatment may thus help counteract the limited amount of RNI produced during Mtb infection. However, only a moderate and transient reduction in intracellular bacterial loads was seen in *M. bovis* BCG-infected BMMO treated with BG. Thus, the main mechanism by which BG treatment leads to reduced mycobacterial loads in murine lungs may not predominantly rely on increased NO production. This hypothesis is further supported by the delayed effect of BG treatment on the pulmonary mycobacterial loads *in vivo*, that was observed only at day 28 and 35 p.i., but not at earlier time points, despite BG treatment commencing at day 7 p.i. Our data thus suggest that BG treatment impacts the adaptive immunity (in particular CD4 T cells) through potentiating innate immune cells (DC and macrophages mainly). The fact that several weekly BG doses were required to observe a significant reduction in the bacterial loads points at trained innate immunity, although this is purely speculative at this stage. Furthermore, the effect was not sustained beyond 1 week after the last BG dose, implying that continued BG dosing is necessary to maintain stimulation of both the innate and adaptive immunity.

Importantly, our work clearly demonstrates that treatment with an equivalent amount of purified LPS that is present in the BG dose could not recapitulate the effects seen with BG treatment. This was especially apparent *in vivo*, where LPS treatment of *M. bovis* BCG-infected mice did not influence the lung immune cell populations, cytokine levels and bacterial burden compared to infected controls. Consistently, we demonstrated that BG-induced innate immune activation is only partially TLR4-dependent (with the exception of NO production, which was fully mediated by TLR4), and involved a broader and stronger intracellular signaling response compared to LPS, although the latter observation was not verified at the protein level. The presence of a variety of TLR ligands on BG likely explains the greater immunostimulatory potential of BG over LPS, without overt inflammation.

Additionally, BG treatment enhanced the *in vivo* bactericidal efficacy of second-line drugs—DLM and BDQ. Such synergistic killing was not observed for INH + BG. A previous study reported that host cell activation by nitrosative stress induces tolerance to first-line drugs, including INH, in Mtb (65). Since BG treatment induces NO production in murine macrophages, it is thus possible that BG-mediated activation of macrophages could compromise the killing efficacy of INH. The lack of improved killing in mice treated with Q203 + BG or LZD + BG may be attributed to the immunomodulatory abilities of these drugs that could hinder and/or counteract those of BG. While this latter hypothesis remains to be experimentally explored, our data indicate that BG treatment is not universally compatible with all anti-TB agents/compounds, but can improve the efficacy of certain second-line agents.

This work paves the way toward the possible use of BG as an adjunct TB immunotherapy, although much work remains to be done. Specifically, it will be very important to confirm our observations in TB models. In addition, the cellular and molecular mechanisms involved in BG-mediated therapeutic effects should be deciphered. Furthermore, as BG production is limited to Gram-negative bacteria (to allow formation of the transmembrane tunnel), it is not possible to produce BG from mycobacteria. However, *E. coli* BG may be further engineered with mycobacterial antigens expressed on their surface in order to trigger a TB-specific immune response and further enhance the therapeutic potential of BG treatment.

ETHICS STATEMENT

The animal study was reviewed and approved by the Institutional Animal Care and Use Committee of National University of Singapore (NUS) under protocol R15-1030. All the animal experiments were performed in the AALAAC-accredited animal facilities.

AUTHOR CONTRIBUTIONS

JL, GP, and SA designed the experiments. JL, VK, SC, MV, BP, and DC performed the experiments. JL, VK, BP, PD, and SA analyzed the data. PK and WL provided the reagents. JL and SA wrote the manuscript.

ACKNOWLEDGMENTS

We thank Dr. Paul Hutchinson and team from the Flow Cytometry Core Facility at LSI for their assistance. We are also grateful to Prof. Laurent Renia [Singapore Immunology Network (SIgN), A*STAR, Singapore] for his gift of TLR4 KO mice, and Prof. Nicholas Gascoigne (Department of Microbiology & Immunology, NUS), and Dr. Amit Singhal (SIgN) for their gift of transgenic OTI and OTII mice, respectively.

REFERENCES

1. World Health Organization (WHO). *Global Tuberculosis Report 2017*. Geneva: World Health Organization (2018).
2. Glaziou P, Sismanidis C, Floyd K, Raviglione M. Global epidemiology of tuberculosis. *Cold Spring Harb Perspect Med.* (2015) 5:a017798. doi: 10.1101/cshperspect.a017798
3. World Health Organization (WHO). *The End TB Strategy* (2018). Available online at: http://www.who.int/tb/post2015_TBstrategy.pdf?ua=1
4. Schrager LK, Harris RC, Vekemans J. Research and development of new tuberculosis vaccines: a review. *F1000Res.* (2018) 7:1732. doi: 10.12688/f1000research.16521.1
5. Li Y, Sun F, Zhang W. Bedaquiline and delamanid in the treatment of multidrug-resistant tuberculosis: promising but challenging. *Drug Dev Res.* (2019) 80:98–105. doi: 10.1002/ddr.21498
6. Rohde K, Yates RM, Purdy GE, Russell DG. Mycobacterium tuberculosis and the environment within the phagosome. *Immunol Rev.* (2007) 219:37–54. doi: 10.1111/j.1600-065X.2007.00547.x
7. Noss EH, Harding CV, Boom WH. Mycobacterium tuberculosis inhibits MHC class II antigen processing in murine bone marrow macrophages. *Cell Immunol.* (2000) 201:63–74. doi: 10.1006/cimm.2000.1633
8. Hmama Z, Peña-Díaz S, Joseph S, Av-Gay Y. Immunoevasion and immunosuppression of the macrophage by *Mycobacterium tuberculosis*. *Immunol Rev.* (2015) 264:220–32. doi: 10.1111/imr.12268
9. Urdahl KB, Shafiani S, Ernst JD. Initiation and regulation of T-cell responses in tuberculosis. *Mucos Immunol.* (2011) 4:288–93. doi: 10.1038/mi.2011.10
10. Andersson J, Samarina A, Fink J, Rahman S, Grundstrom S. Impaired expression of perforin and granulysin in $CD8^+$ T cells at the site of infection in human chronic pulmonary tuberculosis. *Infect Immun.* (2007) 75:5210–22. doi: 10.1128/IAI.00624-07
11. Day CL, Moshi ND, Abrahams DA, van Rooyen M, O'rie T, de Kock M, et al. Patients with tuberculosis disease have *Mycobacterium tuberculosis*-specific CD8 T cells with a pro-apoptotic phenotype and impaired proliferative capacity, which is not restored following treatment. *PLoS ONE.* (2014) 9:e94949. doi: 10.1371/journal.pone.0094949
12. da Silva MV, Tiburcio MGS, Machado JR, Silva DAA, Rodrigues DBR, Rodrigues V, et al. Complexity and controversies over the cytokine profiles of T helper cell subpopulations in tuberculosis. *J Immunol Res.* (2015) 2015:639107. doi: 10.1155/2015/639107
13. Prezzemolo T, Guggino G, La Manna MP, Di Liberto D, Dieli F, Caccamo N. Functional signatures of human CD4 and CD8 T cell responses to *Mycobacterium tuberculosis*. *Front Immunol.* (2014) 5:180. doi: 10.3389/fimmu.2014.00180
14. Frank DJ, Horne DJ, Dutta NK, Shaku MT, Madensein R, Hawn TR, et al. Remembering the host in tuberculosis drug development. *J Infect Dis.* (2018) 219:1518–24. doi: 10.1093/infdis/jiy712
15. Kaufmann SHE, Lange C, Rao M, Balaji KN, Lotze M, Schito M, et al. Progress in tuberculosis vaccine development and host-directed therapies–a state of the art review. *Lancet Respir Med.* (2014) 2:301–20. doi: 10.1016/S2213-2600(14)70033-5
16. Brinkmann V, Geiger T, Alkan S, Heusser CH. Interferon alpha increases the frequency of interferon gamma-producing human $CD4^+$ T cells. *J Exp Med.* (1993) 178:1655–63. doi: 10.1084/jem.178.5.1655
17. Gao X-F, Yang Z-W, Li J. Adjunctive therapy with interferon-gamma for the treatment of pulmonary tuberculosis: a systematic review. *Int J Infect Dis.* (2011) 15:e594–e600. doi: 10.1016/j.ijid.2011.05.002
18. Giosuè S, Casarini M, Alemanno L, Galluccio G, Mattia P, Pedicelli G, et al. Effects of aerosolized interferon-α in patients with pulmonary tuberculosis. *Am J Respir Crit Care Med.* (1998) 158:1156–62. doi: 10.1164/ajrccm.158.4.9803065
19. Olivares N, Rodriguez Y, Zatarain-Barron ZL, Marquina B, Mata-Espinosa D, Barrios-Payán J, et al. A significant therapeutic effect of immunoglobulins administered alone, or in combination with conventional chemotherapy, in experimental pulmonary tuberculosis caused by drug-sensitive or drug-resistant strains. *Pathog Dis.* (2017) 75:ftx118. doi: 10.1093/femspd/ftx118
20. Roy E, Stavropoulos E, Brennan J, Coade S, Grigorieva E, Walker B, et al. Therapeutic efficacy of high-dose intravenous immunoglobulin in *Mycobacterium tuberculosis* infection in mice. *Infect Immun.* (2005) 73:6101–9. doi: 10.1128/IAI.73.9.6101-6109.2005
21. Roy E, Brennan J, Jolles S, Lowrie DB. Beneficial effect of anti-interleukin-4 antibody when administered in a murine model of tuberculosis infection. *Tuberculosis (Edinb).* (2008) 88:197–202. doi: 10.1016/j.tube.2007.11.005
22. Cheng CY, Gutierrez NM, Marzuki MB, Lu X, Foreman TW, Paleja B, et al. Host sirtuin 1 regulates mycobacterial immunopathogenesis and represents a therapeutic target against tuberculosis. *Sci Immunol.* (2017) 2:eaaj1789. doi: 10.1126/sciimmunol.aaj1789
23. Singhal A, Jie L, Kumar P, Hong GS, Leow MK-S, Paleja B, et al. Metformin as adjunct antituberculosis therapy. *Sci Transl Med.* (2014) 6:263ra159. doi: 10.1126/scitranslmed.3009885
24. Dlugovitzky D, Notario R, Martinel-Lamas D, Fiorenza G, Farroni M, Bogue C, et al. Immunotherapy with oral, heat-killed, Mycobacterium vaccae in patients with moderate to advanced pulmonary tuberculosis. *Immunotherapy.* (2010) 2:159–69. doi: 10.2217/imt.09.90
25. Vilaplana C, Montané E, Pinto S, Barriocanal AM, Domenech G, Torres F, et al. Double-blind, randomized, placebo-controlled phase I clinical trial of the therapeutical antituberculous vaccine RUTI®. *Vaccine.* (2010) 28:1106–16. doi: 10.1016/j.vaccine.2009.09.134

26 Vilaplana C, Gil O, Cáceres N, Pinto S, Díaz J, Cardona P-J. Prophylactic effect of a therapeutic vaccine against TB based on fragments of *Mycobacterium tuberculosis*. *PLoS ONE.* (2011) 6:e20404. doi: 10.1371/journal.pone.0020404
27 Paukner S, Stiedl T, Kudela P, Bizik J, Al Laham F, Lubitz W. Bacterial ghosts as a novel advanced targeting system for drug and DNA delivery. *Expert Opin Drug Deliv.* (2006) 3:11–22. doi: 10.1517/17425247.3.1.11
28 Witte A, Lubitz W, Bakker EP. Proton-motive-force-dependent step in the pathway of lysis of Escherichia coli induced by bacteriophage PhiX174 gene E product. *J Bacteriol.* (1987) 169:1750–2. doi: 10.1128/jb.169.4.1750-1752.1987
29. Witte A, Wanner G, Blasi U, Halfmann G, Szostak M, Lubitz W. Endogenous transmembrane tunnel formation mediated by phi X174 lysis protein E. *J Bacteriol.* (1990) 172:4109–14. doi: 10.1128/jb.172.7.4109-4114.1990
30. Haidinger W, Mayr UB, Szostak MP, Resch S, Lubitz W. *Escherichia coli* ghost production by expression of lysis gene E and staphylococcal nuclease. *Appl Environ Microbiol.* (2003) 69:6106–13. doi: 10.1128/AEM.69.10.6106-6113.2003
31. Mayr UB, Haller C, Haidinger W, Atrasheuskaya A, Bukin E, Lubitz W, et al. Bacterial ghosts as an oral vaccine: a single dose of *Escherichia coli* O157:H7 bacterial ghosts protects mice against lethal challenge. *Infect Immun.* (2005) 73:4810–7. doi: 10.1128/IAI.73.8.4810-4817.2005
32. Panthel K, Jechlinger W, Matis A, Rohde M, Szostak M, Lubitz W, et al. Generation of *Helicobacter pylori* ghosts by PhiX protein E-mediated inactivation and their evaluation as vaccine candidates. *Infect Immun.* (2003) 71:109–16. doi: 10.1128/IAI.71.1.109-116.2003
33. Vinod N, Noh HB, Oh S, Ji S, Park HJ, Lee K-S, et al. A *Salmonella typhimurium* ghost vaccine induces cytokine expression *in vitro* and immune responses *in vivo* and protects rats against homologous and heterologous challenges. *PLoS ONE.* (2017) 12:e0185488. doi: 10.1371/journal.pone.0185488
34. Jawale CV, Lee JH. Development of a biosafety enhanced and immunogenic *Salmonella enteritidis* ghost using an antibiotic resistance gene free plasmid carrying a bacteriophage lysis system. *PLoS ONE.* (2013) 8:e78193. doi: 10.1371/journal.pone.0078193
35. Eko FO, Lubitz W, McMillan L, Ramey K, Moore TT, Ananaba GA, et al. Recombinant *Vibrio cholerae* ghosts as a delivery vehicle for vaccinating against *Chlamydia trachomatis*. *Vaccine.* (2003) 21:1694–703. doi: 10.1016/S0264-410X(02)00677-1
36. Huter V, Szostak MP, Gampfer J, Prethaler S, Wanner G, Gabor F, et al. Bacterial ghosts as drug carrier and targeting vehicles. *J Control Release.* (1999) 61:51–63. doi: 10.1016/S0168-3659(99)00099-1
37. Hajam IA, Dar PA, Won G, Lee JH. Bacterial ghosts as adjuvants: mechanisms and potential. *Vet Res.* (2017) 48:37. doi: 10.1186/s13567-017-0442-5
38. Katinger A, Lubitz W, Szostak MP, Stadler M, Klein R, Indra A, et al. Pigs aerogenously immunized with genetically inactivated (ghosts) or irradiated *Actinobacillus pleuropneumoniae* are protected against a homologous aerosol challenge despite differing in pulmonary cellular and antibody responses. *J Biotechnol.* (1999) 73:251–60. doi: 10.1016/S0168-1656(99)00143-1
39. Kim CS, Hur J, Eo SK, Park S-Y, Lee JH. Generation of salmonella ghost cells expressing fimbrial antigens of enterotoxigenic *Escherichia coli* and evaluation of their antigenicity in a murine model. *Can J Vet Res.* (2016) 80:40–8.
40. Wen J, Yang Y, Zhao G, Tong S, Yu H, Jin X, et al. Salmonella typhi Ty21a bacterial ghost vector augments HIV-1 gp140 DNA vaccine-induced peripheral and mucosal antibody responses via TLR4 pathway. *Vaccine.* (2012) 30:5733–9. doi: 10.1016/j.vaccine.2012.07.008
41. Won G, Chaudhari AA, Lee JH. Protective efficacy and immune responses by homologous prime-booster immunizations of a novel inactivated *Salmonella gallinarum* vaccine candidate. *Clin Exp Vaccine Res.* (2016) 5:148–58. doi: 10.7774/cevr.2016.5.2.148
42. Eko FO, Mania-Pramanik J, Pais R, Pan Q, Okenu DMN, Johnson A, et al. *Vibrio cholerae* ghosts (VCG) exert immunomodulatory effect on dendritic cells for enhanced antigen presentation and induction of protective immunity. *BMC Immunol.* (2014) 15:584. doi: 10.1186/s12865-014-0056-x
43. Koller VJ, Dirsch VM, Beres H, Donath O, Reznicek G, Lubitz W, et al. Modulation of bacterial ghosts–induced nitric oxide production in macrophages by bacterial ghost-delivered resveratrol. *FEBS J.* (2013) 280:1214–25. doi: 10.1111/febs.12112
44. Dobrovolskiene N, Pašukoniene V, Darinskas A, Kraśko JA, Žilionyte K, Mlynska A, et al. Tumor lysate-loaded bacterial ghosts as a tool for optimized production of therapeutic dendritic cell-based cancer vaccines. *Vaccine.* (2018) 36:4171–80. doi: 10.1016/j.vaccine.2018.06.016
45. Michalek J, Hezova R, Turanek-Knötigova P, Gabkova J, Strioga M, Lubitz W, et al. Oncolysate-loaded *Escherichia coli* bacterial ghosts enhance the stimulatory capacity of human dendritic cells. *Cancer Immunol Immunother.* (2017) 66:149–59. doi: 10.1007/s00262-016-1932-4
46. Anders S, Pyl PT, Huber W. HTSeq—a Python framework to work with high-throughput sequencing data. *Bioinformatics.* (2015) 31:166–9. doi: 10.1093/bioinformatics/btu638
47. Robinson MD, McCarthy DJ, Smyth GK. edgeR: a bioconductor package for differential expression analysis of digital gene expression data. *Bioinformatics.* (2010) 26:139–40. doi: 10.1093/bioinformatics/btp616
48. Huang DW, Sherman BT, Lempicki RA. Systematic and integrative analysis of large gene lists using DAVID bioinformatics resources. *Nat Protoc.* (2009) 4:44–57. doi: 10.1038/nprot.2008.211
49. Huang DW, Sherman BT, Lempicki RA. Bioinformatics enrichment tools: paths toward the comprehensive functional analysis of large gene lists. *Nucleic Acids Res.* (2009) 37:1–13. doi: 10.1093/nar/gkn923
50. Dunzendorfer S, Lee H-K, Soldau K, Tobias PS. TLR4 is the signaling but not the lipopolysaccharide uptake receptor. *J Immunol.* (2004) 173:1166–70. doi: 10.4049/jimmunol.173.2.1166
51. Desch AN, Henson PM, Jakubzick CV. Pulmonary dendritic cell development and antigen acquisition. *Immunol Res.* (2013) 55:178–86. doi: 10.1007/s12026-012-8359-6
52. Guirado E, Schlesinger L. Modeling the *Mycobacterium tuberculosis* granuloma–the critical battlefield in host immunity and disease. *Front Immunol.* (2013) 4:98. doi: 10.3389/fimmu.2013.00098
53. Janssen WJ, Barthel L, Muldrow A, Oberley-Deegan RE, Kearns MT, Jakubzick C, et al. Fas determines differential fates of resident and recruited macrophages during resolution of acute lung injury. *Am J Respir Crit Care Med.* (2011) 184:547–60. doi: 10.1164/rccm.201011-1891OC
54. Vasconcelos JR, Dominguez MR, Araújo A, Ersching J, Tararam CA, Bruna-Romero O, et al. Relevance of long-lived $CD8^+$ T effector memory cells for protective immunity elicited by heterologous prime-boost vaccination. *Front Immunol.* (2012) 3:58. doi: 10.3389/fimmu.2012.00358
55. Rouan M-C, Lounis N, Gevers T, Dillen L, Gilissen R, Raoof A, et al. Pharmacokinetics and pharmacodynamics of TMC207 and its N-desmethyl metabolite in a murine model of tuberculosis. *Antimicrob Agents Chemother.* (2012) 56:1444–51. doi: 10.1128/AAC.00720-11
56. Swanson RV, Adamson J, Moodley C, Ngcobo B, Ammerman NC, Dorasamy A, et al. Pharmacokinetics and pharmacodynamics of clofazimine in a mouse model of tuberculosis. *Antimicrob Agents Chemother.* (2015) 59:3042–51. doi: 10.1128/AAC.00260-15
57. Tasneen R, Betoudji F, Tyagi S, Li S-Y, Williams K, Converse PJ, et al. Contribution of oxazolidinones to the efficacy of novel regimens containing bedaquiline and pretomanid in a mouse model of tuberculosis. *Antimicrob Agents Chemother.* (2016) 60:270–7. doi: 10.1128/AAC.01691-15
58. Ebensen T, Paukner S, Link C, Kudela P, de Domenico C, Lubitz W, et al. Bacterial ghosts are an efficient delivery system for DNA vaccines. *J Immunol.* (2004) 172:6858–65. doi: 10.4049/jimmunol.172.11.6858
59. Hajam IA, Dar PA, Appavoo E, Kishore S, Bhanuprakash V, Ganesh K. Bacterial ghosts of *Escherichia coli* drive efficient maturation of bovine monocyte-derived dendritic cells. *PLoS ONE.* (2015) 10:e0144397. doi: 10.1371/journal.pone.0144397
60. Haslberger AG, Kohl G, Felnerova D, Mayr UB, Fürst-Ladani S, Lubitz W. Activation, stimulation and uptake of bacterial ghosts in antigen presenting cells. *J Biotechnol.* (2000) 83:57–66. doi: 10.1016/S0168-1656(00)00298-4
61. Felnerova D, Kudela P, Bizik J, Haslberger A, Hensel A, Saalmuller A, et al. T cell-specific immune response induced by bacterial ghosts. *Med Sci Monit.* (2004) 10:BR362–370.
62. MacMicking JD, North RJ, LaCourse R, Mudgett JS, Shah SK, Nathan CF. Identification of nitric oxide synthase as a protective locus

against tuberculosis. *Proc Natl Acad Sci USA.* (1997) 94:5243–8. doi: 10.1073/pnas.94.10.5243

63. Chakraborty U, Goswami A, Saha S, Mukherjee T, Dey SK, Majumdar S, et al. Tumour necrosis factor-alpha and nitric oxide response in different categories of tuberculosis patients. *Int J Tuberc Lung Dis.* (2013) 17:505–10. doi: 10.5588/ijtld.12.0196
64. Nicholson S, Bonecini-Almeida MdG, Silva JRL, Nathan C, Xie QW, Mumford R, et al. Inducible nitric oxide synthase in pulmonary alveolar macrophages from patients with tuberculosis. *J Exp Med.* (1996) 183:2293–302. doi: 10.1084/jem.183.5.2293
65. Liu Y, Tan S, Huang L, Abramovitch RB, Rohde KH, Zimmerman MD, et al. Immune activation of the host cell induces drug tolerance in *Mycobacterium tuberculosis* both *in vitro* and *in vivo*. *J Exp Med.* (2016) 213:809–25. doi: 10.1084/jem.20151248

6

Clinical Relevance and Molecular Pathogenesis of the Emerging Serotypes 22F and 33F of *Streptococcus pneumoniae* in Spain

Julio Sempere[1], Sara de Miguel[2], Fernando González-Camacho[1], José Yuste[1,3]* and Mirian Domenech[1]*

[1] Centro Nacional de Microbiología, Instituto de Salud Carlos III, Madrid, Spain, [2] Servicio de Epidemiología de la Comunidad de Madrid, Dirección General de Salud Pública, Madrid, Spain, [3] Centro de Investigación Biomédica en Red de Enfermedades Respiratorias (CIBERES), Madrid, Spain

***Correspondence:**
José Yuste
jyuste@isciii.es
Mirian Domenech
mdomenech@isciii.es

Streptococcus pneumoniae is the main bacterial cause of respiratory infections in children and the elderly worldwide. Serotype replacement is a frequent phenomenon after the introduction of conjugated vaccines, with emerging serotypes 22F and 33F as frequent non-PCV13 serotypes in children and adults in North America and other countries. Characterization of mechanisms involved in evasion of the host immune response by these serotypes is of great importance in public health because they are included in the future conjugated vaccines PCV15 and PCV20. One of the main strategies of *S. pneumoniae* to persistently colonize and causes infection is biofilm formation. In this study, we have evaluated the influence of capsule polysaccharide in biofilm formation and immune evasion by using clinical isolates from different sources and isogenic strains with capsules from prevalent serotypes. Since the introduction of PCV13 in Spain in the year 2010, isolates of serotypes 22F and 33F are rising among risk populations. The predominant circulating genotypes are $ST433^{22F}$ and $ST717^{33F}$, being CC433 in 22F and CC717 in 33F the main clonal complexes in Spain. The use of clinical isolates of different origin, demonstrated that pediatric isolates of serotypes 22F and 33F formed better biofilms than adult isolates and this was statistically significant. This phenotype was greater in clinical isolates from blood origin compared to those from cerebrospinal fluid, pleural fluid and otitis. Opsonophagocytosis assays showed that serotype 22F and 33F were recognized by the PSGL-1 receptor on leukocytes, although serotype 22F, was more resistant than serotype 33F to phagocytosis killing and more lethal in a mouse sepsis model. Overall, the emergence of additional PCV15 serotypes, especially 22F, could be associated to an enhanced ability to divert the host immune response that markedly increased in a biofilm state. Our findings demonstrate that pediatric isolates of 22F and 33F, that form better biofilm than isolates from adults, could have an advantage to colonize the nasopharynx of children and therefore, be important in carriage and subsequent dissemination to the elderly. The increased ability of serotype 22F to avoid the host immune response, might explain the emergence of this serotype in the last years.

Keywords: *Streptococcus pneumoniae*, PCV-pneumococcal conjugate vaccine, biofilms, serotype 22F, serotype 33F, PSGL-1

INTRODUCTION

Streptococcus pneumoniae, also termed pneumococcus, colonizes asymptomatically the human nasopharynx although the bacterium has the capacity to reach the lower respiratory tract (LRT) producing pneumonia and disseminate producing invasive pneumococcal disease (IPD) (Bogaert et al., 2004). The burden of disease caused by this microorganism is of great relevance because is the major etiologic agent of community acquired pneumonia, non-epidemic meningitis and a frequent cause of bacterial sepsis (Bogaert et al., 2004). As a result, this devastating pathogen is responsible for high morbidity and mortality rates worldwide affecting mainly the children under the age of 5 years and adults older than 65 years. Indeed, nearly 2.38 million deaths are caused by LRT infections, being *S. pneumoniae* the major etiologic agent of these alarming rates (GBD 2016 Lower Respiratory Infections Collaborators, 2018). As a consequence, LRT infections are the sixth mortality cause for all ages and the first cause of death among children under 5 years old (GBD 2016 Lower Respiratory Infections Collaborators, 2018). While the use of available antibiotics is the best option to treat pneumococcal infections once they are established, the emergence of multidrug resistant strains can jeopardize the outcome of the infection in many cases (Aguinagalde et al., 2015; Azarian et al., 2018).

Prophylactic measures based on the administration of pneumococcal vaccines in children and adults, seems to be the best strategy to control the development of IPD and pneumonia and reduce the impact of antimicrobial resistance (Moore et al., 2015; Atkins et al., 2018; Wahl et al., 2018). In children under 2 years old, there are currently two vaccines available, a 10-valent conjugate vaccine (PCV10) and a 13-valent conjugate vaccine (PCV13). The use of PCV10 has decreased the burden of disease caused by serotypes covered in the vaccine but several countries using this vaccine have reported the emergence of non-PCV10 serotypes such as 19A after its introduction (Savulescu et al., 2017; Cassiolato et al., 2018; Rinta-Kokko et al., 2018). PCV13 has shown to be effective in children who were the main target for this vaccine but also has shown herd effects for the elderly population (Mackenzie et al., 2016). In adults, the 23-valent polysaccharide vaccine (PPV23) can be used to prevent IPD although its effectiveness against pneumonia is controversial (Huss et al., 2009; Andrews et al., 2012; Russell et al., 2015; Tin Tin Htar et al., 2017). The use of PCV13 has been shown to be effective avoiding IPD and pneumonia in the elderly population (Bonten et al., 2015; McLaughlin et al., 2018). The main limitation of these vaccines is that serotype replacement is a frequent phenomenon that occurs after the massive use of these vaccines based on capsular polysaccharides due to the wide antigenic variability of this bacterium with up to 99 serotypes described so far and emergence of virulent clones with vaccine-escape capsule (Brueggemann et al., 2007; Domenech et al., 2018). To target the emergence of non-vaccine types producing pneumococcal infection, a 15-valent conjugate vaccine (PCV15) including serotypes covered by PCV13 plus serotypes 22F and 33F is in clinical phase III with the advantage of inducing a higher title of antibodies against serotype 3 (Greenberg et al., 2018; Stacey et al., 2019). In addition, a 20-valent conjugate vaccine (PPV20) that contains serotypes in PCV15 plus serotypes 8, 10A, 12F, 11A, and 15B is also in clinical trials studies (Thompson et al., 2019).

The emergence of many of these serotypes in certain countries after the use of current PCVs is one of the main reasons for including these additional serotypes in newer conjugate vaccines. In United States, serotypes 22F and 33F were the main cause of IPD among non-PCV13 in children under 5 years old and adults ≥65 years (Moore et al., 2015). In Europe, several countries have shown the rise of non-PCV13 serotypes in children and adults including serotypes covered by PCV15 and PCV20 (Aguinagalde et al., 2015; Savulescu et al., 2017; Ladhani et al., 2018). Nevertheless, one aspect that is poorly investigated before the introduction of new conjugate vaccines is the pathogenic capacity of these additional serotypes.

It is been known that biofilm formation in *S. pneumoniae* provides the bacterium an advantage in terms of virulence because it increases the resistance to antimicrobial drugs and enhances the ability to avoid the host immune response (Donlan and Costerton, 2002; Domenech et al., 2013). For instance, serotypes 11A and 35B, which are serotypes frequently associated to multidrug resistance, are good biofilm formers (Domenech et al., 2015). Biofilm formation is a critical aspect from the pathogenesis perspective because *S. pneumoniae* has been reported to form biofilms in the upper respiratory tract (Wu et al., 2017; Iverson et al., 2019; Silva and Sillankorva, 2019) and nasopharyngeal colonization is the initial step in this process and the prerequisite for developing IPD (Bogaert et al., 2004). Interestingly, active infection is also associated to pneumococcal biofilms in meningitis by binding to brain microvascular endothelial cells and in persistent respiratory infection affecting patients with cystic fibrosis or chronic obstructive pulmonary disease (COPD) (Orihuela et al., 2009; Vidal et al., 2013; Vandevelde et al., 2014; Dennis et al., 2018). In the biofilm state, pneumococcal cells express the PspC protein in a higher extent, and this protein is the bacterial ligand associated to the recruitment of factor H and therefore to the cleavage of the C3 complement system protein deposited on the bacterial surface (Domenech et al., 2013). This is interesting in terms of virulence because when pneumococcal cells are released from the biofilm producing dissemination to the LRT, the bloodstream or crossing the blood brain barrier producing meningitis, these colonies express higher levels of the virulence factor PspC increasing the potential for IPD (Yuste et al., 2010).

In contrast to *Neisseria meningitidis*, bactericidal activity by the membrane attack complex of the complement system plays a minor role against *S. pneumoniae* and killing by professional phagocytes in the presence or not of specific antibodies, is the most efficacy mechanism to fight the pneumococcal infection (Standish and Weiser, 2009). For this reason opsonophagocytosis killing assays (OPKA) are the best parameter to measure the functional opsonic activity of antibodies to *S. pneumoniae* when a new vaccine is tested (Greenberg et al., 2018; Stacey et al., 2019; Thompson et al., 2019). Hence, investigating these aspects will contribute to increase the knowledge about the potential of non-vaccine serotypes to produce infection in the host. Differences in the recognition of pneumococcal serotypes by specific components of the host immune response may explain the prevalence of certain serotypes causing IPD (Hyams et al., 2011). In this sense, the human P-selectin glycoprotein ligand 1 is a novel receptor for *S. pneumoniae* that contributes to protection against IPD by controlling the severity of the infection (Ramos-Sevillano et al., 2016). This receptor is present on leukocytes that recognizes the pneumococcal capsular polysaccharide and the main autolytic enzyme of the bacterium (the amidase LytA) increasing the phagocytosis process (Ramos-Sevillano et al., 2016). Differences in the interaction of different pneumococcal capsules with PSGL-1 might explain the higher burden of disease caused by certain serotypes of *S. pneumoniae* (Ramos-Sevillano et al., 2016).

In this study, we have evaluated the impact of current vaccine strategies in the epidemiology of serotypes 22F and 33F during the period 2009–2018 including the circulating genotypes that cause IPD among these serotypes. In addition, we have characterized the ability of serotypes 22F and 33F to form biofilms and their capacity to avoid the phagocytosis process and produce infection because they are important aspects that are missing for these additional serotypes covered in the new PCV15. For comparison purposes, we also included pneumococcal serotypes that are prevalent in IPD and/or because they are associated to multidrug resistance.

MATERIALS AND METHODS

Strains, Media and Genetic Transformation

The pneumococcal strains of the different serotypes used in this study are listed in **Table 1**. The Spanish Pneumococcal Reference Lab (SPRL) receives the IPD cases from hospitals located at all the Spanish regions through a passive surveillance system with minimal required information accompanying isolates (hospital and city, sample, age of the patient and date of isolation). The SPRL notifies annually to the European Center for Disease Control (ECDC) all the IPD cases received following a passive surveillance system that cover 80% of the national level according to estimates by the National Center for Epidemiology reported to ECDC (ECDC, 2018). Unfortunately, vaccine coverage data is not available and that is the reason that effectiveness of the different vaccines cannot be included in this study. Initially, PCV7 coverage based on vaccine sales was low, but its use increased from 2002 onward with reported vaccine coverage below 50% before 2006 and missing data on PCV coverage at national level in further years (Fenoll et al., 2015).

All pneumococcal strains were grown in C medium supplemented (C+Y medium) or in Mueller Hinton agar supplemented with 5% defibrinated sheep blood (Becton Dickinson GmbH; Heidelberg, Germany). Bacterial growth was monitored by measuring the absorbance at 550 nm (A_{550}). *S. pneumoniae* was transformed with chromosomal DNA by treating pre-competent cells with 100 ng/ml of synthetic competence-stimulating pheromone 1 at 37°C for 10 min to induce competence, followed by incubation at 30°C during DNA uptake. Encapsulated transformants of strain M11 were enriched by successive transfers of the transformed culture to C medium containing 0.08% bovine serum albumin, and supplemented with 0.5 μl/ml of anti-R antiserum before plating (Mollerach et al., 1998; Domenech et al., 2015). Anti-R (antisomatic) antiserum contains group-specific agglutinins, which, at the proper dilution, agglutinate only non-encapsulated pneumococci. In this study, we have used isogenic mutants in CPS in order to reduce the influence of genetic variability within the strains. To confirm the absence of mutations in other parts of the genome, we used two independent transformants of each serotype with not differences in the phenotype. Based on this, only one transformed strain of each serotype was further studied for the rest of the experiments. The selection of pneumococcal isolates for immune response characterization and biofilm formation was randomly chosen. We selected five clinical isolates from each source (20 clinical isolates of serotype 22F and another 20 clinical isolates of serotype 33F) from different geographical locations in Spain (**Table 1**). Moreover, we did biofilm formation trials in parallel with clinical strains of the serotypes studied as control.

S. pneumoniae Typification

In addition to strains showed in **Table 1**, we included the clinical isolates of serotypes 22F and 33F received at the Spanish Pneumococcal Reference Laboratory (SPRL) since 2009 to analyze the evolution of IPD caused by both serotypes in Spain. We considered IPD clinical isolates those isolated from sterile sites. Serotyping was performed by Quellung reaction, dot blot assay (Fenoll et al., 2015) using specific antisera from the Statens Serum Institut (Copenhagen, Denmark) and/or by molecular capsular sequence typing methodology (Elberse et al., 2011).

Multilocus sequence typing (MLST) was determined with the tools provided by the MLST website[1]. Data were analyzed using Lasergene® SeqMan Pro (DNAStar, Madison,WI, United States). Sequence types (STs) were identified based on the allelic profiles of seven housekeeping genes (*aroE, ddl, gdh, gki, recP, spi*, and *xpt*). We used the eBURST tool to determine the clonal complex (CC) (Feil et al., 2004). STs were considered from the same CC if they demonstrated ≥5 MLST allele numbers in common.

Biofilm Formation Assay

Biofilm formation assays were performed following the methodology previously described (Domenech et al., 2015) and it was determined by the ability of cells to adhere to the walls and base of 96-well, flat-bottomed polystyrene microtiter dishes (Falcon 353072, Corning Incorporated, New York, NY, United States). Unless stated otherwise, cells were grown in C+Y medium to an A_{550} of ≈0.5–0.6, sedimented by centrifugation, resuspended in an equal volume of the indicated pre-warmed medium, diluted 1/100, and then dispensed 200 μl per well. After 5 h of incubation at 34°C, the A_{595} was determined using Tecan Infinite F200 (Tecan Group Ltd., Switzerland). The biofilm formed was stained with 0.2% crystal violet (Sigma-Aldrich) and rinsed three times with distilled water to remove non-adherent bacteria. Biofilm formation was quantified solubilizing

[1]http://pubmlst.org/spneumoniae

TABLE 1 | Strains of *S. pneumoniae* used in this study[a].

Strain	Description/serotype (source)b ST/CCc	References/sourced
M11	Non-encapsulated strain derived from R6 (Hex$^-$, lytA$^+$)	Domenech et al., 2014
YNM2	M11 transformant with DNA from strain 1734/19; serotype 8	This study
1734/19	8(blood)	SPRL
YNM3	M11 transformant with DNA from strain 1732/19; serotype 11A	This study
1732/19	11A(blood)	SPRL
YNM4	M11 transformant with DNA from strain 1228/19; serotype 19A	This study
1228/19	19A(blood)	SPRL
P007	M11 transformant with DNA from strain 406; serotype 3	Domenech et al., 2009
P224	M11 transformant with DNA from strain 3017/13; serotype 24F	Domenech et al., 2014
P244	M11 transformant with DNA from strain 3014/13; serotype 22F	Domenech et al., 2015
1407/18	22F(blood/pediatric) ST3134/CC1439	SPRL
1000/18	22F(blood/adult) ST13692/CC698	SPRL
1155/18	22F(CSF/pediatric) ST433/CC433	SPRL
523/18	22F(CSF/adult) ST13692/CC698	SPRL
223/11	22F(PF/pediatric) ST433/CC433	SPRL
1285/18	22F(PF/adult) ST698/CC698	SPRL
2780/17	22F(Otic/adult) ST13692/CC698	SPRL
100/08	22F(Otic/pediatric) ST433/CC433	SPRL
1766/18	22F(blood/pediatric) ST3134/CC1439	SPRL
2597/17	22F(blood/pediatric) ST433/CC433	SPRL
194/17	22F(blood/pediatric) ST433/CC433	SPRL
2153/17	22F(blood/pediatric) ST433/CC433	SPRL
212/18	22F(blood/adult) ST698/CC698	SPRL
250/18	22F(blood/adult) ST433/CC433	SPRL
306/18	22F(blood/adult) ST433/CC433	SPRL
613/18	22F(blood/adult) ST7314/CC433	SPRL
P017	M11 transformant with DNA from strain SSISP33F/1; serotype 33F	Domenech et al., 2015
1833/18	33F(blood/pediatric) ST717/CC717	SPRL
1950/18	33F(blood/adult) ST13320/CC717	SPRL
1088/16	33F(CSF/pediatric) ST717/CC717	SPRL
934/19	33F(CSF/adult) ST717/CC717	SPRL
800/18	33F(PF/pediatric) ST717/CC717	SPRL
363/18	33F(PF/adult) ST717/CC717	SPRL
782/15	33F(Otic/pediatric) ST1012/CC1012	SPRL
1945/15	33F(Otic/pediatric) ST717/CC717	SPRL
644/18	33F(blood/pediatric) ST717/CC717	SPRL
1018/18	33F(blood/pediatric) ST717/CC717	SPRL
1992/18	33F(blood/pediatric) ST4668/CC717	SPRL
2316/17	33F(blood/pediatric) ST13320/CC717	SPRL
1897/18	33F(blood/adult) ST717/CC717	SPRL
2027/18	33F(blood/adult) ST717/CC717	SPRL
627/18	33F(blood/adult) ST717/CC717	SPRL
840/18	33F(blood/adult) ST717/CC717	SPRL

[a]*Strains are organized by serotype.* [b]*CSF, cerebrospinal fluid; PF, pleural fluid.* [c]*ST, sequence type; CC, clonal complex.* [d]*SPRL, Spanish Pneumococcal Reference Laboratory.*

the biofilm in 95% ethanol (200 μl per well) and measuring the A_{595}.

Phagocytosis of *S. pneumoniae* Biofilms and Planktonic Cultures

Experiments investigating human neutrophil phagocytosis were performed by OPKA using HL-60 cells (CCL-240; ATCC) differentiated to granulocytes (Domenech et al., 2013). The presence of complement receptors on HL-60 granulocytes has been previously documented and therefore expression of CD11b (iC3b receptor and CR3 α-chain), a marker of granulocytic differentiation, was measured prior to phagocytic assays to confirm the presence of the receptor (Ramos-Sevillano et al., 2016). After the incubation process at 34°C (previously described in biofilm formation), bacterial cultures growing as biofilms in microtiter plates or the planktonic cultures in tubes were washed with fresh C medium and resuspended in Hank's buffered salt solution (HBSS) in the presence of calcium and magnesium ions. Biofilm disaggregation was performed by gently pipetting and slow vortexing before the opsonization process to avoid possible bias by morphological differences between the two growing stages. The number of biofilm-forming CFU was determined by viable counts of bacteria and a similar number of planktonic cells were used in each phagocytosis assay. OPKA were performed using 10^5 HL-60 cells and 2.5 × 10^2 CFU of *S. pneumoniae* strains (MOI of 400 HL-60:1 *S. pneumoniae*) that were previously opsonized for 1 h with 1/20 of rabbit serum in the case of planktonic cultures, and 20 min with 1/5 of rabbit serum in the case of biofilm cultures. First, the corresponding bacterial suspensions (10 µl) were added to microtiter round bottom polystyrene plates (Nunclon Delta Surface; Themo Fisher Scientific) containing 10 µl of rabbit serum diluted 1/20 or 1/5 in phosphate-buffered saline (PBS, pH 7.0) previously described (Domenech et al., 2013). After incubation at 37°C with shaking (150 rpm) to allow opsonization by the different serum components, HL-60 cells were added and the plate was incubated at 37°C with shaking (150 rpm) for 45 min. The mixture was plated on blood agar plates for bacterial counts determination and results were expressed as bacterial killing. Blood agar plates were incubated at 37°C with 5% CO2 during 24 h for determinate viable cells.

Phagocytosis Mediated by PSGL-1 Receptor

To analyze the function of the PSGL-1 receptor in recognizing the CPS of the new emerging serotypes 22F and 33F, and isogenic strains expressing different CPS, we followed the methodology previously described (Ramos-Sevillano et al., 2016). To block PSGL-1, HL-60 cells were incubated for 1 h at 37°C with 25 µg/ml of the KPL-1 antibody (mouse antihuman PSGL-1; MBL) or IgG isotype control (mouse anti-human IgG; Novus Biologicals). The phagocytosis killing assays were performed in the absence of rabbit serum using a proportion of 10^5 HL-60 cells with the PSGL-1 receptor either active or blocked and 2.5 × 10^2 CFU of *S. pneumoniae*. Then, as mentioned above, we plated on blood agar plates serial dilutions of culture for bacterial counts determination. Results were expressed normalizing CFU/ml to percentage of phagocytosis using the IgG isotype control as the 100%.

Mouse Model of *S. pneumoniae* Sepsis

Experimental procedures involving mice were performed at Instituto de Salud Carlos III (ISCIII) conforming to the Spanish government legislation (RD 53/2013, ECC/566/2015) and European Community regulations (2010/63/EU). C57BL/6 male mice (8–12 weeks old) weighing about 20 g were bred by the ISCIII animal facility. Animal procedures followed the guidelines of the Bioethical and Animal Welfare Committee of ISCIII that reviewed and approved protocols (CBA PA 52-2011-v2 and PROEX 218/15). Studies investigating pneumococcal sepsis were performed using groups of five mice and infected as previously described (Ramos-Sevillano et al., 2016). Briefly, for sepsis, mice were challenged with 2 × 10^7 CFU/mouse for P244, P017, 1407/18, 1000/18, 1833/18, and 1950/18 strains (**Table 1**) (in a volume of 200 µl) by the intraperitoneal route. Bacterial levels in blood, from the tail vein, were determined from every infected mouse at 24 h. The lower limit of detection was 10^2 CFU/ml. Results were expressed as Log_{10} CFU/ml of bacteria recovered from the blood and survival curves were determined after 7 days of follow up.

Statistical Analysis

Data represent results obtained from repeated independent experiments, each one conducted as a triplicate, representing at least three replicates. Statistical analysis was performed by using two-tailed Student's *t*-test. The log-rank (Mantel-Cox) test was used for survival curves. Incidence rates were calculated considering the number of cases divided by the population using data provided by the Spanish National Institute of Statistics. Serotype trends were obtained by comparing the rates of the current situation (2017–2018) vs. the rates of different periods by calculating relative risks (IRR) with 95% confidence intervals through Poisson regression models. We included the pre-PCV13 period (2009), the early PCV13 effect (2010–2012) and the middle PCV13 period (2013–2016) when this vaccine was included in the pediatric calendar at national level at the end of 2016. Statistical analyses for epidemiological data were analyzed using Stata v.14. GraphPad InStat version 8.0 (GraphPad Software, San Diego, CA) was used for the rest of analysis. Differences were considered statistically significant with $^*P < 0.05$ and highly significant with $^{**}P < 0.01$ and $^{***}P < 0.001$.

RESULTS

Evolution of Invasive Pneumococcal Disease by Serotypes 22F and 33F in Spain

The epidemiological situation of IPD cases by clinical isolates of serotypes 22F and 33F was investigated during the last 10 years including 2009 which is the pre-PCV13 year and 2018 which is the last year when epidemiological data is fully registered in Spain.

The data contain cases, proportion among all IPD cases and incidences by these two serotypes. Incidences were calculated considering the number of cases divided by the population using data provided by the Spanish National Institute of Statistics. Incidence rate ratios with 95% confidence intervals were estimated to compare the current situation (2017–2018) vs. different periods including the pre-PCV13 period (2009), the early PCV13 effect (2010–2012) and the middle PCV13 period (2013–2016) when this vaccine was included in the pediatric calendar at national level at the end of 2016.

In children, IPD cases by serotype 22F showed a similar trend until 2016 (6 cases in 2009 vs. 8 cases in 2016) which is the year when PCV13 was introduced at the national pediatric vaccination calendar (**Figure 1A**). However, since 2016 we observed a

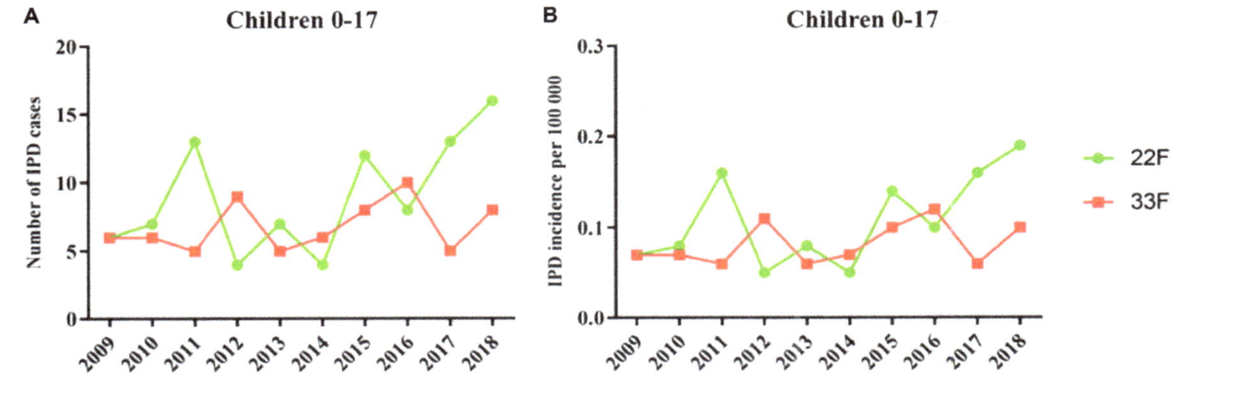

FIGURE 1 | Trends in IPD incidence due to serotypes 22F and 33F producing IPD episodes in the pediatric population during the period 2009–2018 in Spain. **(A)** Number of IPD cases. **(B)** Incidence of IPD cases. Green line with dots is the evolution of serotype 22F whereas red line with squares is the evolution of serotype 33F.

continuous rise with 13 cases in 2017 and 16 cases in 2018 or 29 cases in the last epidemiological period 2017–2018 showing the emerging of this serotype in children (**Figure 1**). The proportion of IPD cases by serotype 22F was 1.08% in 2009 and 6.23% in 2018 confirming that this serotype is rising and increasing its proportion over total serotypes in the pediatric population. IPD cases by serotype 33F in children show a moderate rise during the last 10 years when comparing 2009 vs. 2018 increasing from 6 cases in 2009 to 8 cases in 2018 and 13 cases for the last 2 years (**Figure 1**). Incidence rate ratios (IRR) for serotype 22F demonstrate an increasing trend (IRR 2.38; 95% CI 0.99–5.74 for the period 2017–2018 vs. 2009, IRR 1.82; 95% CI 1.06–3.12 for 2017–2018 vs. 2010–2012, and IRR 1.88; 95% CI 1.13–3.11 for 2017–2018 vs. 2013–2016 (**Table 2**). However, for serotype 33F the situation is relatively stable in the last 10 years (IRR 1.07; 95% CI 0.41–2.81 for the period 2017–2018 vs. 2009, IRR 0.98; 95% CI 0.49–1.97 for 2017–2018 vs. 2010–2012, IRR 0.90; 95% CI 0.47–1.73 for 2017–2018 vs. 2013–2016 (**Table 2**). Overall, our results suggest that serotype 22F is more prevalent in Spanish children than serotype 33F with a more pronounced effect in the last 2 years concurring with the introduction of PCV13 in the national immunization pediatric calendar.

In adults of all ages, serotypes 22F and 33F show an increase of 52% (64 cases vs. 132 cases) and 48% (26 cases vs. 50 cases), respectively, when the pre-PCV13 period (year 2009) is compared to the last year 2018 (**Figure 2**). Hence, incidence by serotype 22F increased from 0.17 cases per 100000 in 2009 to 0.24 cases per 100000 in 2013–2016 and 0.32 cases per 100000 in 2017–2018. Incidence rate ratios show that serotype 22F rapidly increase after PCV13 was introduced in Spain with a constant increasing trend until 2018 (IRR 1.95; 95% CI 1.48–2.56 for 2017–2018 vs. 2009, IRR 1.39; 95% CI 1.17–1.65 for 2017–2018 vs. 2010–2012 and IRR 1.37; 95% CI 1.16–1.61 for 2017–2018 vs. 2013–2016) (**Table 2**). For serotype 33F, a similar pattern was observed after the introduction of PCV13 (IRR 1.70; 95% CI 1.10–2.64 for 2017–2018 vs. 2009, IRR 1.86; 95% CI 1.36–2.54 for 2017–2018 vs. 2010–2012 and IRR 1.41; 95% CI 1.15–1.74 for 2017–2018 vs. 2013–2016) (**Table 2**). In adults 18–64 years old, only serotype 22F increased since the introduction of PCV13 from 0.09 cases per 100000 in 2009 to 0.16 cases per 100000 in 2017–2018 (IRR 1.82; 95% CI 1.18–2.78). For adults ≥65 years, an increased in the incidence of both serotypes has been observed comparing 2009 and 2017–2018 (IRR 1.83; 95% CI 1.28–2.62 for serotype 22F and IRR 2.00; 95% CI 1.1–3.64 for serotype 33F). Hence, these data demonstrate that both serotypes 22F and 33F are emerging in adults being serotype 22F one of the most prevalent in 2018 for Spanish adults ≥65 years (3rd cause of IPD) whereas serotype 33F is the 16th cause of IPD in this age group (unpublished data from our laboratory).

Genetic Analysis of Circulating Clones Among Clinical Isolates of Serotypes 22F and 33F

Genetic diversity of clinical isolates of serotypes 22F and 33F producing IPD in Spain was assessed by MLST. We chose the year 2018 to know the circulating genotypes of 22F and 33F because is an early time-point after the introduction of PCV13 in the pediatric calendar by the end of 2016 and even in the adult calendar of certain Spanish regions. In Spain, PCV7 was mainly used in private market and low selection pressure is expected.

Isolates of serotype 22F contained five different sequence types being ST433 the most frequent with up to 58% of the isolates belonging to this sequence type (**Table 3**). These genotypes were grouped into three different clonal complexes although CC433 was associated to 71% of the isolates of serotype 22F (**Table 3**). Isolates of serotype 33F also had five different genotypes being ST717 the most popular containing 71% of the strains, followed by ST 13320 with 18% of the isolates (**Table 3**). In contrast to serotype 22F, isolates of serotype 33F showed a less variable diversity in terms of clonal complexes with CC717 being the most frequent with up to 93% of the strains (**Table 3**). Overall, clinical isolates of serotypes 22F and 33F that are producing the majority of the IPD cases in the Spanish population seem to be very conserved with ST433 and ST717 being the most frequent genotypes among 22F and 33F, respectively (**Table 3**).

TABLE 2 | Number of cases and incidence of IPD in 2017–2018 compared to 2009 (pre-vaccine period), 2010–2012 (early effect after private use of PCV13 in Spanish children), and 2013–2016 (middle effect after PCV13 introduction).

		2009 Pre-vaccine		2010–2012 Early vaccine effect (private market)		2013–2016 Middle vaccine effect		2017–2018		2017–18 vs. 2009		2017–18 vs. 2010–12		2017–18 vs. 2013–16	
		Cases	Incidence (per 100000)	Cases	Incidence (per 100000)	Cases	Incidence (per 100000)	Cases	Incidence (per 100000)	IRR	95% CI	IRR	95% CI	IRR	95% CI
<18 years	22F	6	0.07	24	0.10	31	0.09	29	0.17	2.38	0.99–5.74	1.82	1.06–3.12	1.88	1.13–3.11
	33F	6	0.07	20	0.08	29	0.09	13	0.08	1.07	0.41–2.81	0.98	0.49–1.97	0.90	0.47–1.73
All adults	22F	64	0.17	271	0.23	364	0.24	248	0.32	1.95	1.48–2.56	1.39	1.17–1.65	1.37	1.16–1.61
	33F	26	0.07	72	0.06	125	0.08	88	0.11	1.70	1.10–2.64	1.86	1.36–2.54	1.41	1.15–1.74
18–64 years	22F	27	0.09	103	0.11	134	0.11	94	0.16	1.82	1.18–2.78	1.43	1.08–1.89	1.42	1.16–1.74
	33F	13	0.04	33	0.4	52	0.04	29	0.05	1.16	0.6–2.24	1.37	0.83–2.26	1.13	0.79–1.63
≥65 years	22F	37	0.48	168	0.69	230	0.68	154	0.87	1.83	1.28–2.62	1.26	1.01–1.57	1.29	1.1–1.51
	33F	13	0.17	39	0.16	73	0.21	59	0.33	2.00	1.1–3.64	2.08	1.39–3.11	1.56	1.21–2.01
Total IPD by all serotypes		3099	6.63	7009	4.95	8096	4.32	5243	5.62	0.85	0.81–0.89	1.13	1.09–1.18	1.30	1.25–1.34

IRR = incidence rate ratio. CI = confidence interval.

Pneumococcal Biofilms of Serotypes 22F y 33F From Different Sources

Figure 3 shows the biofilm formation capacity of clinical isolates of serotypes 22F (**Figure 3A**) and 33F (**Figure 3B**) from four different sources: blood, cerebrospinal fluid (CSF), pleural fluid (PF) and otic (**Table 1**). We also wanted to detect if there were differences in biofilm formation when the clinical isolate was either pediatric or adult (except for an adult clinical isolate of serotype 33F from otitis, which could not be tested). As biofilm formation controls, we used the non-encapsulated *S. pneumoniae* M11 strain, and isogenic mutants containing the genetic background of strain M11 and the capsules of serotypes 22F (P244) or 33F (P017). One clinical isolate of each serotype and origin were analyzed in detail. Although pneumococci of every serotype tested produced less biofilm than the non-encapsulated strain M11, significant differences were noted in the biofilm formation capacity of several pairs of clinical strains of the same serotype. The pediatric isolates formed greater biofilm than adult isolates, this difference being statistically significant in the case of clinical isolates from blood and otitis of serotype 22F (**Figure 3A**) and from blood and CSF of serotype 33F (**Figure 3B**). We also observed that there are clinical isolates of serotypes 22F or 33F that formed more or less biofilm than the isogenic transformant P244 or P017 (**Figure 3**). These results confirm previous observations indicating that the genetic background, and not only the CPS, modulates pneumococcal attachment to the artificial substrate (Moscoso et al., 2006; Domenech et al., 2014, 2015).

Comparing globally all the results of biofilm formation of pediatric isolates with those from adults (**Figure 4A**), biofilm formation was greater in clinical isolates of pediatric origin being statistically significant ($^{***}P < 0.001$). In **Figure 3**, we observed that, clinical pediatric isolates from blood were the best biofilm formers than isolates from the others sources (CSF, PF, otic) regardless of the serotype analyzed. In addition, if we compare a higher number of pediatric isolates from blood with adult isolates of each serotype (**Figure 4B**), we observed again, that pediatric blood isolates formed better biofilms than adult isolates and this phenotype was serotype-independent.

Comparison of ST and clonal complexes with biofilm formation based on the clinical origin of the isolates does not allow establishing a possible relationship between the genotype of the strain (**Table 1** and **Figures 3, 4**), biofilm formation capacity and the origin of the sample.

Opsonophagocytosis of Different Serotypes With the Same Genetic Background Growing as Planktonic or Biofilms Cultures

To explore the potential of different serotypes to avoid the opsonophagocytosis process by human neutrophils which could explain differences in the burden of disease at the epidemiological level, isogenic transformants of M11 strain were used (**Figure 5**). For this study, PCV13 serotypes such as 3 and 19A and non-PCV13/PCV15 serotypes such as 8, 11A and 24F were

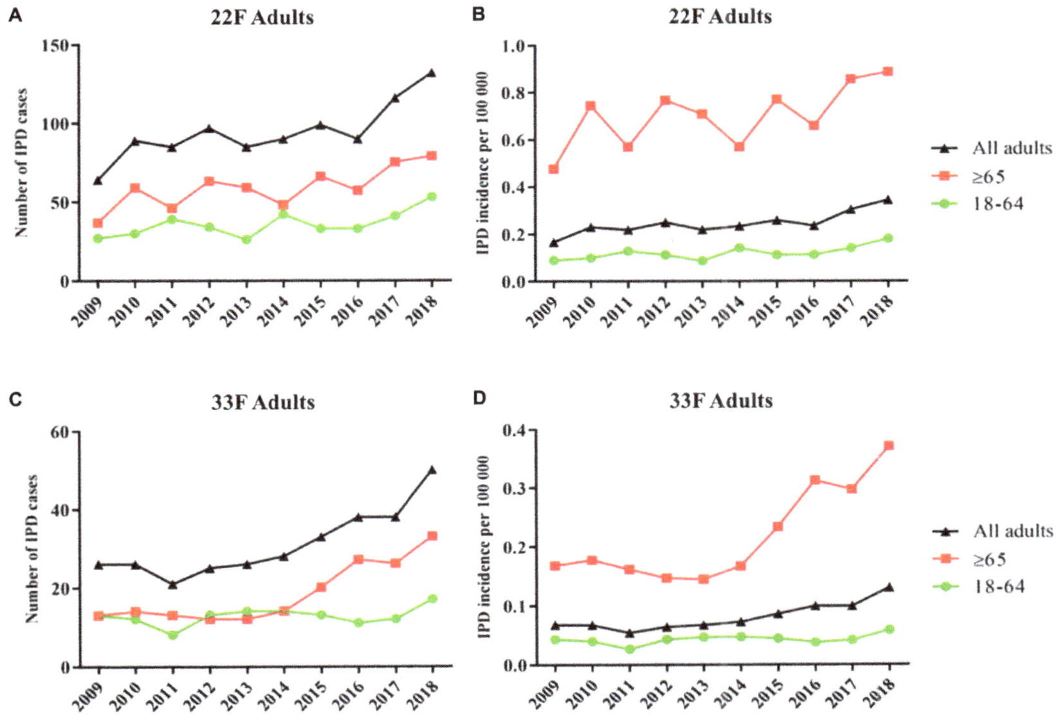

FIGURE 2 | Trends in IPD incidence due to serotypes 22F and 33F producing IPD episodes in adults during the period 2009–2018 in Spain. **(A)** Number of IPD cases of serotype 22F. **(B)** Incidence of IPD cases of serotype 22F. **(C)** Number of IPD cases of serotype 33F. **(D)** Incidence of IPD cases of serotype 33F. Black line with triangles is the evolution in adults of all ages. Green line with dots is the evolution in adults 18–64 years. Red line with squares is the evolution in adults ≥65 years.

TABLE 3 | Genotype and clonal complex distribution of *S. pneumoniae* 22F and 33F clinical isolates from the year 2018.

Serotype/Clonal complex (CC)	Number of isolates	Percentage of total (%)
Serotype 22F	24	
CC433	17	70,83
ST433	14	58,33
ST7314	3	12,5
CC698	5	20,83
ST698	2	8,33
ST13692	3	12,5
CC1439	2	8,33
ST3134	2	8,33
Serotype 33F	28	
CC717	26	92,86
ST717	20	71,43
ST13320	5	17,86
ST4668	1	3,57
CC1012	1	3,57
ST1012	1	3,57
CC433	1	3,57
ST7314	1	3,57

included based in their high prevalence rates of these serotypes causing IPD in Europe (Fenoll et al., 2015). Serotype 11A is an emerging multidrug resistant phenotype and a good biofilm former (Aguinagalde et al., 2015; Domenech et al., 2015), whereas serotypes 22F and 33F contained in PCV15 were included for comparison purposes.

The use of the M11 strain for constructing all the isogenic transformants, being the CPS as the only difference among the strains, is the best strategy to assess variations in the phagocytosis process mediated by the CPS and not by differences related to the genetic background of the strains. OPKA was measured using bacteria growing as planktonic culture or biofilms.

In planktonic cultures, the analysis of the two most frequent PCV13 serotypes, confirmed that isolate with CPS of type 3 was more resistant to the phagocytosis than the isolate expressing serotype 19A proving than the CPS of serotype 3 conferred more resistance to the phagocytosis than the capsule of type 19A (****P* < 0.001) (**Figure 5A**). The two new additional serotypes included in PCV15 showed a different pattern of recognition by the phagocytic cells. The capsule 22F was more resistant to the phagocytosis process than the capsule 33F (****P* < 0.001) (**Figure 5A**). These results may explain why serotype 22F is more frequent causing IPD in children and adults than serotype 33F (**Figures 1**, **2**). Strains expressing the CPS of types 8 and 11A had the most resistant phenotype whereas the strain with the CPS of type 24F was phagocytosed as the same level than the CPS of 19A (**Figure 5A**).

In biofilm cultures, the strain expressing serotype 3 was more resistant to the phagocytosis process than serotype 19A upholding the marked resistant level of serotype 3 to the

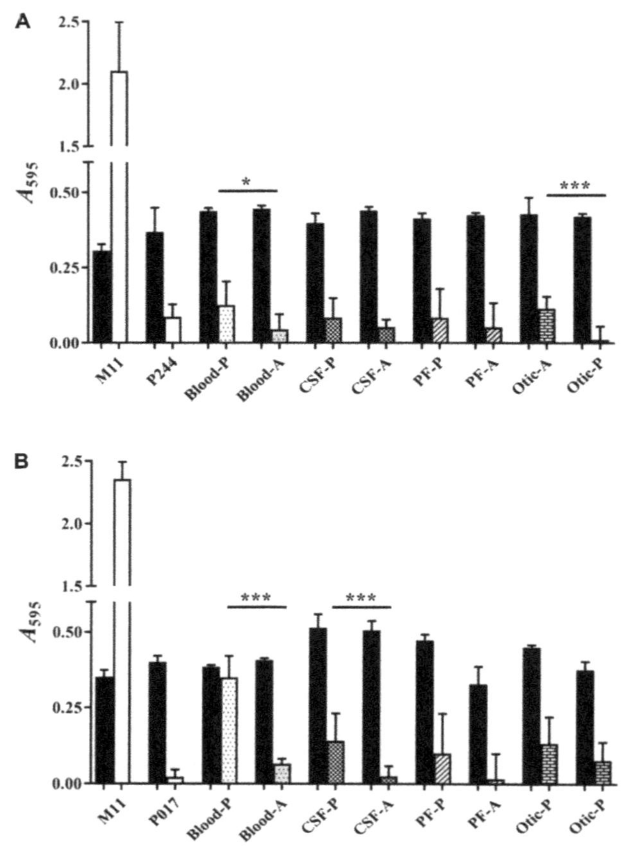

FIGURE 3 | Biofilm formation of pediatric and adult clinical isolates from four different origins. **(A)** Represents clinical isolates of serotype 22F **(B).** Represents clinical isolates of serotypes 33F. M11, non-encapsulated strain; P244, 22F isogenic transformant; P017, 33F isogenic transformant; P, pediatric isolates; A, adult isolates; CSF, cerebrospinal fluid; PF, pleural fluid. Black bars represent growth and pattern or pattern-less bars represent biofilm formation. All data were normalized to the A_{595} CV blanks. Error bars represent standard deviations, and asterisks mark results that are statistically significant (two-tailed Student's *t*-test: $^{*}P < 0.05$; $^{**}P < 0.01$; $^{***}P < 0.001$).

phagocytosis (**Figure 5B**, $^{***}P < 0.001$). Among the two additional serotypes included in PCV15, the strain expressing the CPS of serotype 22F was more resistant to phagocytosis than the strain of serotype 33F suggesting that serotype 22F may have an enhanced ability to colonize and produce persistent infection associated to biofilms than serotype 33F (**Figure 5B**). The strain with the CPS of type 8 had a similar pattern of phagocytosis evasion than the strain expressing the serotype 19A (**Figure 5B**). Finally, serotypes 11A and 24F avoided very efficiently the phagocytosis in comparison to the control strain (**Figure 5B**).

Evasion of Phagocytosis by Clinical Isolates of Serotypes 22F and 33F From Children and Adults

In this study, we analyzed the recognition of pneumococcal serotypes 22F and 33F by phagocytic cells using clinical isolates from blood obtained from children and adults with IPD and grown as planktonic or biofilms (**Figure 6**). For serotype 22F, no differences were found between pediatric or adult isolates suggesting that this serotype may affect both target populations at a similar level and therefore, it may be useful to vaccinate children and adults against serotype 22F (**Figure 6**). In the case of serotype 33F, a higher resistance level to phagocytosis was observed in the pediatric isolate grown as planktonic culture (**Figure 6A**) whereas no differences were observed between isolates as biofilms (**Figure 6B**), suggesting that children may be more susceptible to IPD by this serotype.

Role of PSGL-1 Receptor in the Phagocytosis of Prevalent Pneumococcal Serotypes Included or Not in Conjugate Vaccines

The interaction of pneumococcal serotypes with the PSGL-1 receptor was studied in the absence of serum to avoid any effect on phagocytosis by serum-mediated receptors such as complement receptors. In the absence of pneumococcal capsule (control strain M11), we did not observe any difference on phagocytosis independently of the functionality of the PSGL-1 receptor, confirming that the capsule is necessary for the PSGL-1 mediated phagocytosis (**Figure 7**). For serotypes 3 and 19A, blocking of PSGL-1 by treatment with KPL1 antibody, increased the viability of bacterial cells, confirming that PSGL-1 recognizes pneumococcal CPS of types 3 and 19A inducing phagocytosis (**Figure 7**). Similar results were obtained for the additional serotypes included in PCV15 and for serotype 8 as inhibition of PSGL-1 receptor on human neutrophils by KPL1 allowed greater levels of viable bacteria of these serotypes, demonstrating that this receptor is important for the phagocytosis of serotypes 22F, 33F and 8 (**Figure 7**). However, uptake of serotypes 11A and 24F remained similar in the presence or absence of PSGL-1 (**Figure 7**) suggesting that these two serotypes are not recognized by this receptor which may explain the emergence of these two serotypes causing IPD cases in the last years.

Virulence of Isolates of Serotypes 22Fand 33F in a Mouse Sepsis Model of Infection

Infection assays using the isogenic transformants of M11 strain expressing the CPS of type 22F (P244) or 33F (P017) confirmed that the CPS of serotype 22F confers a higher invasive capacity than the CPS of serotype 33F as in these two strains the genetic background is the same and the only difference is the CPS expressed (**Figure 8**). The M11 strain expressing 22F had a higher ability to replicate in blood (**Figure 8A**) and lethality was increased compared to M11 with CPS of type 33F (**Figure 8B**). This finding is consistent with the epidemiological results mentioned above showing that serotype 22F is more prevalent than serotype 33F in IPD in Spain. When clinical isolates of both serotypes were analyzed, we found that serotype 22F is very lethal regardless of the origin of the strain, killing all the mice within the first 30 h (**Figure 8**). However, in serotype 33F, the replication in blood of the pediatric isolate was markedly higher compared to the adult isolate (**Figure 8A**) showing a marked

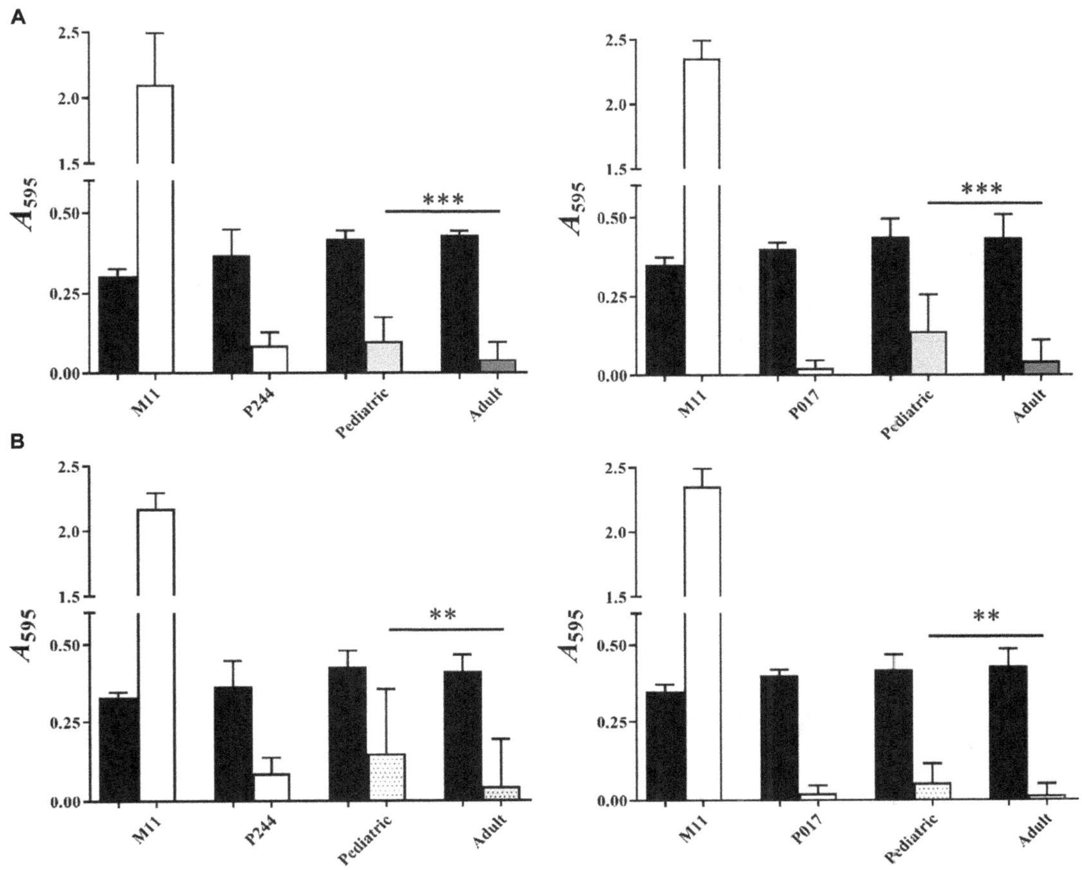

FIGURE 4 | Analysis of biofilm formation of pediatric and adult clinical isolates. **(A)** Represents the comparison between adult and pediatric clinical isolates from four different origins: 22F (left) and 33F (right). **(B)** Represents the comparison between 8 additional adult and pediatric clinical isolates from blood: 22F (left) and 33F (right). M11, non-encapsulated strain; P244, 22F isogenic transformant; P017, 33F isogenic transformant. Black bars represent growth and white or color bars represent biofilm formation. All data were normalized to the A_{595} CV blanks. Error bars represent standard deviations, and asterisks mark results that are statistically significant (two-tailed Student's *t*-test: $^{*}P < 0.05$; $^{**}P < 0.01$; $^{***}P < 0.001$).

lethality (**Figure 8C**) which explains the higher resistance to the phagocytosis of this strain in the planktonic cultures (**Figure 6A**).

DISCUSSION

The effectiveness of current pneumococcal conjugate vaccines against targeted serotypes has been very successful decreasing the burden of disease caused by these serotypes, although unfortunately some countries have reported an increase of IPD cases by certain non-vaccine types in recent years (Feikin et al., 2013; Savulescu et al., 2017; Ladhani et al., 2018; Lewnard and Hanage, 2019). This is the case for serotypes 22F and 33F with different countries reporting increased rates in children and adults after PCV13 (Kaplan et al., 2013; Pichon et al., 2013; Moore et al., 2015; Golden et al., 2016; Balsells et al., 2017; Cui et al., 2017). Serotypes 22F and 33F are also important in terms of quality adjusted life years (QALY) as they caused the highest QALY loss among non-PCV13 serotypes in children (van Hoek et al., 2012). In Spain, our data show an increase of IPD cases for serotype 22F in children and adults and a moderate increase for serotype 33F mainly in adults which is consistent with the situation of other countries worldwide described above. Interestingly, serotype 22F significantly increased not only in adults up to 64 years old but also in adults ≥65 years old between 2009 and the 2017–2018 period (IRR 1.82; 95% CI 1.18–2.78 and IRR 1.83; 95% CI 1.28–2.62, respectively), whereas serotype 33F only increased significantly in the population ≥65 years (IRR 2.00; 95% CI 1.1–3.64). The higher trend to infect adults regardless the age in the case of serotype 22F may explain why this serotype is increasing at a higher proportion than serotype 33F in other countries (Golden et al., 2016; Ladhani et al., 2018). The clonal spread of pneumococcal population allows the dissemination of hypervirulent clones and multidrug resistant genotypes that may contribute to the expansion of certain serotypes and genotypes (Brueggemann and Spratt, 2003; Ardanuy et al., 2014; Aguinagalde et al., 2015; Azarian et al., 2018). Our data demonstrate that genotype ST433 is the most frequent cause of IPD among clinical isolates of serotype 22F in Spain. This is consistent with results from other countries

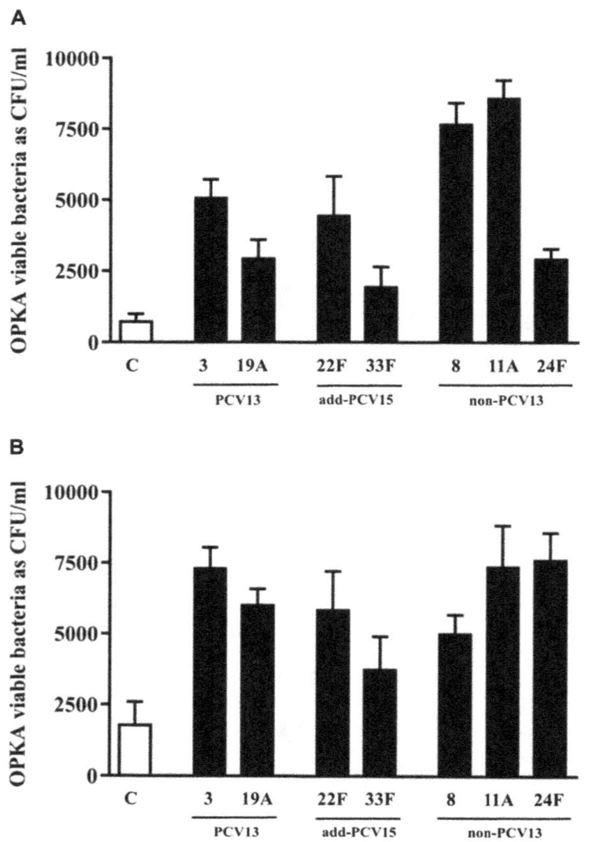

FIGURE 5 | Influence of different CPS in the evasion of opsonophagocytosis. **(A)** Bacterial survival of control strain M11 expressing different CPS and grown as a planktonic culture. **(B)** Bacterial survival of control strain M11 expressing different CPS and grown as a biofilm. Error bars represent standard deviations, and asterisks mark results that are statistically significant (two-tailed Student's *t*-test: $^{*}P < 0.05$; $^{**}P < 0.01$; $^{***}P < 0.001$).

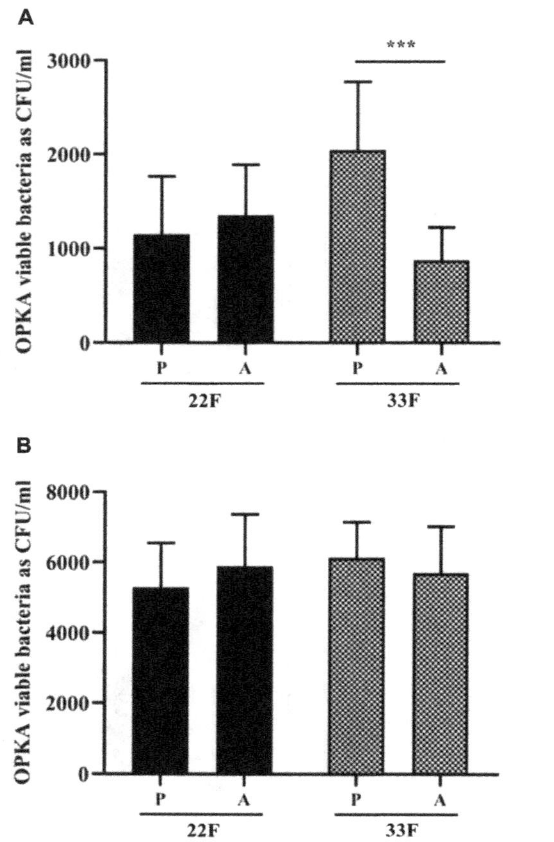

FIGURE 6 | Evasion of opsonophagocytosis of 22F and 33F clinical isolates. **(A)** Bacterial survival of clinical strains from pediatric (P) and adult (A) patients and grown as a planktonic culture. **(B)** Bacterial survival of clinical strains from pediatric (P) and adult (A) patients and grown as a biofilm. Error bars represent standard deviations, and asterisks mark results that are statistically significant (two-tailed Student's *t*-test: $^{***}P < 0.001$).

for this serotype causing IPD (Golden et al., 2016) although it also has been found associated to nasopharyngeal carriage (Sa-Leao et al., 2011). For serotype 33F, our results show up to five different genotypes whereas isolates of this serotype from other countries show a more clonal diversity with up to eight different genotypes (Golden et al., 2018). In addition, the majority of the clinical isolates of serotype 33F that are circulating in Spain, belonged to the genotype ST717, which is different to the situation in other countries such as Canada where ST100 is the most frequent cause of IPD for serotype 33F (Golden et al., 2016).

The use of isogenic transformants to make comparisons of biofilm formation is very useful to avoid differences of each clinical isolate (Domenech et al., 2014, 2015), since biofilm formation is a multifactorial process (Domenech et al., 2013). Hence, to analyze the influence of the CPS, the most reasonable thing would be to use bacterial lines with the same genetic background. Biofilm formation is a tool that can help to predict the clinical impact and emergence of new serotypes that colonize the nasopharynx after the introduction of new vaccines (Domenech et al., 2014). These authors observed that serotype 19A was an excellent biofilm former with a marked capacity of nasopharyngeal colonization (Domenech et al., 2014). This ability to form thick biofilms can contribute to the pathogenesis process of serotype 19A, explaining why is one of the most predominant PCV13 serotypes in IPD (Domenech et al., 2014; Fenoll et al., 2015; Ladhani et al., 2018). A similar approach can be useful to explain the emergence of serotype 11A because is also a good biofilm former and is associated to multidrug resistance (Aguinagalde et al., 2015; Domenech et al., 2015). Serotypes 8 and 3, despite forming little biofilm, remain two of the most important serotypes in IPD, with serotype 8 being the most predominant in Europe and the second in Spain, which shows that biofilm formation is not the only factor to take into account when determining the clinical impact of serotypes and their future impact on the incidence of the disease. *S. pneumoniae* isolates of serotypes 22F and 33F, which were found both in carriage and causing IPD, and which are potentially highly invasive (Yildirim et al., 2010), failed to produce substantial amounts of biofilms *in vitro*. We observed the formation of

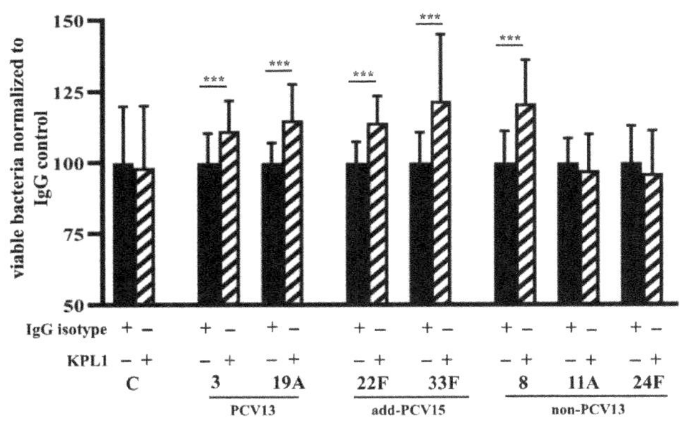

FIGURE 7 | Phagocytosis mediated by PSGL-1 receptor. Results represent bacterial survival of control strain M11 expressing different CPS and grown as a planktonic culture. Phagocytic cells were incubated with an IgG isotype negative control that does not block PSGL-1 (black bars), whereas cells exposed to the KPL-1 antibody had the PSGL-1 blocked (hatched bars). Error bars represent standard deviations, and asterisks mark results that are statistically significant (two-tailed Student's *t*-test: ***$P < 0.001$).

pneumococcal biofilm for clinical strains expressing capsules of types 22F or 33F although in the majority of the cases it was weak in agreement with previous observations using isogenic transformants with CPS 22F and 33F (Domenech et al., 2015). The biofilm levels of the control strain M11 in our study are lower than those found in the study by Domenech et al., mentioned above, but this aspect does not affect the findings of the manuscript as we used the same M11 strain to construct the isogenic mutants. The use of different brands of multiwell plates, cristal violet, and a different multiplate reader may have contributed to the variations of absorbance values. In our study, the formation of biofilm does not explain the increase in IPD by serotypes 22F and 33F, since being bad biofilm formers, an expected phenotype that was already described in previous work (Domenech et al., 2015), they should not be very frequent in IPD. However, considering that colonization of the nasopharynx is a multifactorial process and that although the capsule is a prerequisite for the virulence of the microorganism, there are numerous virulence factors that also contribute to the pathogenesis of IPD and for serotypes 22F and 33F may be playing a predominant role (Geno et al., 2015). The CPS, determines the pneumococcal surface charge, and this aspect influences colonization, because negatively charged surfaces are associated with increased colonization (Weinberger et al., 2009). Most pneumococcal capsules are anionic and most pneumococcal clinical isolates have negative charge (Geno et al., 2015; Morais et al., 2018). This anionic charge helps preventing clearance by the mucus and helps repelling phagocytosis. There are many examples of capsule-negative strains that colonize the nasopharynx and also cause disease, such as serotype 19A, which is a good biofilm former *in vitro* (Domenech et al., 2014), colonizes efficiently the human nasopharynx (Adler et al., 2019) and is one of the main PCV13 serotypes causing IPD. In addition, anionic charge of the capsule does not seem to be an impediment to colonize the upper respiratory tract and produce IPD, but there are capsule-negative serotypes that are good biofilm formers such as 35B and capsule-negative serotypes that are bad biofilm formers such as 24F (Domenech et al., 2015). This phenomenon would explain that serotype 22F is more prevalent in the population, since due to the structure of its CPS its net charge is negative whereas the CPS of 33F is neutral (Geno et al., 2015). These differences in the CPS charge on 22F could contribute to a better colonizing phenotype, and could explain why there is a greater burden of disease due to serotype 22F compared to 33F.

The heterogeneity in biofilm formation using clinical isolates of this study is not surprising, since it confirms evidence published before, where the genetic background and not only the CPS modulate the adhesion of the pneumococcus and formation of a biofilm on an artificial substrate (Moscoso et al., 2006; Domenech et al., 2009, 2014). The novelty of this work, resides in the differences found between pediatric biofilms and adult biofilms, more precisely, the tendency of pediatric isolates to form greater biofilms. These results are compatible with the fact that the pediatric population is the largest carrier of pneumococcus with up to 20–40% of asymptomatic colonization in healthy children (Chaguza et al., 2019) suggesting that pneumococcal isolates can modulate its ability to interact with the nasopharyngeal epithelium by a mechanism related to increased activation of intrinsic factors associated with biofilm formation. The source of the strain (pediatric or adult) is certainly not the only difference between the phenotype of the strains and although the genotype did not contribute to our results, other unrelated factors may be affecting.

Resolution of IPD is finely regulated by the efficient recognition and clearance of *S. pneumoniae* by professional phagocytes (Standish and Weiser, 2009; van der Poll and Opal, 2009). The pneumococcal CPS that surrounds the bacterium and it is used to determine the serotype, is the most well-established virulence factor, although the genetic background also contributes significantly to the pathogenesis process (Hyams et al., 2011; McAllister et al., 2011). Our study using strains with the same genetic background but expressing different CPS, demonstrates that the strain with capsule of type 3 was more resistant to the phagocytosis process that the strain expressing the capsule 19A. This is interesting because serotype 3 remains as one of the most frequent causes of IPD in adults worldwide (Moore et al., 2015; Ladhani et al., 2018). The higher resistant phenotype conferred by the capsule of type 3 may be due to the higher size and even abundance of the CPS expressed on these strains (Choi et al., 2015). Among the two additional serotypes covered by PCV15, the strain expressing the CPS of type 22F was more resistant to the phagocytosis and much more virulent in a mouse sepsis model than the strain of serotype 33F. This is consistent with the epidemiological data presented in our study showing a higher burden of disease caused by serotype 22F and may explain why in other countries, serotype 22F is also more prevalent than serotype 33F (Moore et al., 2015; Golden et al., 2016; Ladhani et al., 2018). In bacteria growing as biofilms, strains expressing the CPS of type 3, 11A and 24F were among the most resistant strains to be phagocytosed. This is interesting as serotype 3 remains as major cause of pneumonia in adults (Menéndez et al., 2017) and

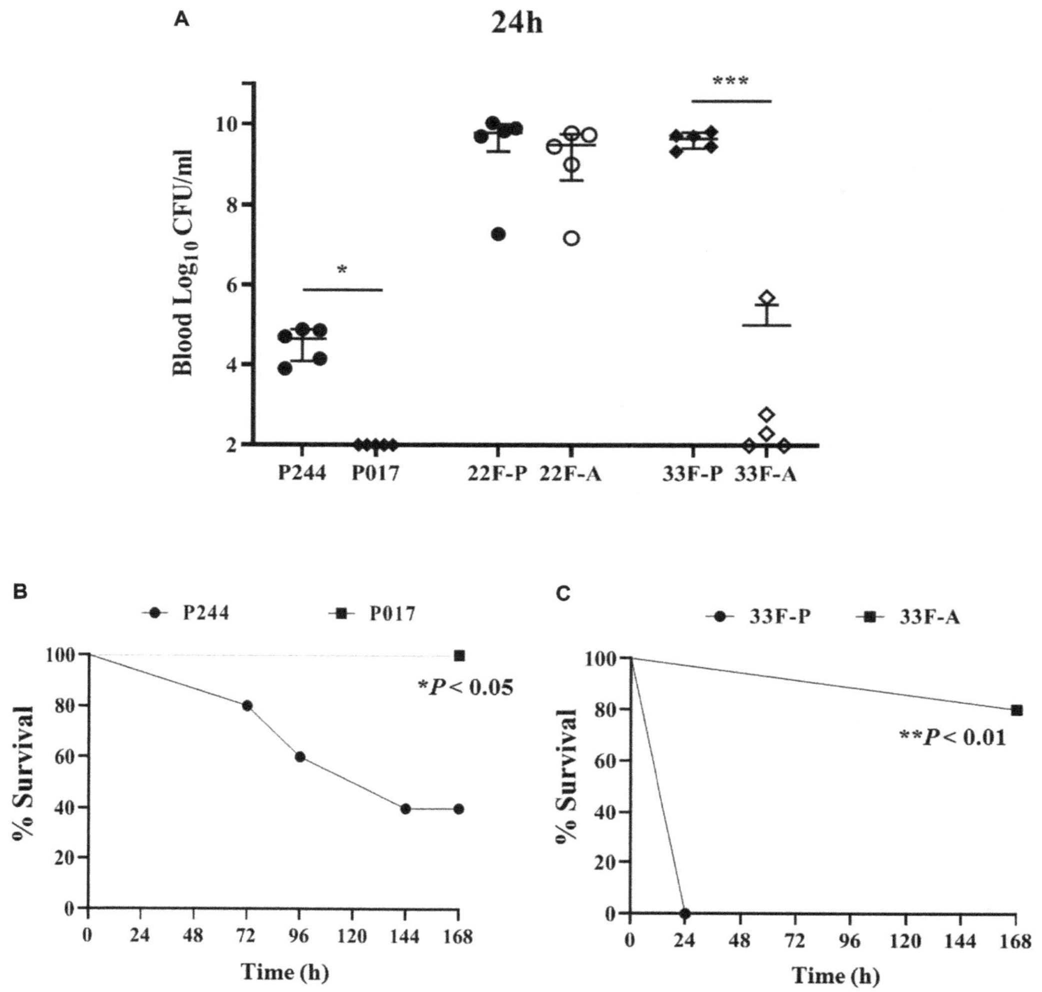

FIGURE 8 | Virulence of isolates of serotypes 22F and 33F in a sepsis model of infection. **(A)** Colony counts expressed as Log_{10} CFU/ml from the blood of mice infected with M11 strain expressing serotype 22F (P244) or serotype 33F (P017) or with clinical isolates of serotypes 22F or 33F from pediatric origin (P) or adult origin (A). **(B)** Survival curves of P244 vs. P017 strains. **(C)** Survival curves of clinical isolates of serotype 33F from pediatric origin (P) or adult (A). Error bars represent standard deviations, and asterisks mark results that are statistically significant (two-tailed Student's *t*-test: $^*P < 0.05$; $^{***}P < 0.001$ for bacterial counts; and Log-rank test $^*P < 0.05$; $^{**}P < 0.01$ for survival curves).

in patients with COPD, serotypes 3 and 11A are among the most prevalent (Shoji et al., 2018). In addition, serotype 24F is more prone to cause meningitis, showing an increase in clinical severity (Balsells et al., 2018) which could be associated to the increase resistant pattern to phagocytosis when replicating as a biofilm.

The repertoire of cellular receptors involved in the phagocytosis of invading pathogens is critical for the outcome of the infection. PSGL-1 on leukocytes plays a critical role in host defense against pneumococcal infection. As a consequence of pathogen-recognition by PSGL-1, pneumococcal strains are efficiently phagocytosed and killed intracellularly, reducing bacterial replication and dissemination in the host, contributing therefore, to control the severity of the IPD process (Ramos-Sevillano et al., 2016). Our results show that PSGL-1 receptor is important for the phagocytosis of different serotypes including the additional serotypes covered by PCV15. However, for serotypes 11A and 24F, cells expressing PSGL-1 did not kill efficiently these particular serotypes suggesting that strains expressing these two CPS, may have an increased ability to produce IPD. This is consistent with the emergence of amoxicillin-resistant variants of serotype 11A with genotype ST6521 that avoid efficiently the phagocytosis process and are good biofilm formers (Aguinagalde et al., 2015) and with the increased severity of infection by isolates of serotype 24F (Balsells et al., 2018).

Overall, the results of this study may be of relevance to understand critical aspects of the pathogenesis process such as biofilm formation and interaction with phagocytes by prevalent serotypes including the additional serotypes covered by the new PCV15. Surveillance studies and characterization of emergent pneumococcal strains remains necessary in order to explain what features lead to the success of individual serotypes and genotypes.

ETHICS STATEMENT

Animal procedures followed the guidelines of the Bioethical and Animal Welfare Committee of ISCIII that reviewed and approved protocols (CBA PA 52-2011-v2 and PROEX 218/15) and were performed conforming to the Spanish Government legislation (RD 53/2013, ECC/566/2015) and European Community regulations (2010/63/EU).

AUTHOR CONTRIBUTIONS

JS, MD, and JY conceived and designed the experiments and wrote the manuscript. SM carried out the epidemiology analyses. JS and MD performed the experiments. FG-C helped with the interpretation of the data. SM and FG-C reviewed the results and contributed to the final version of the manuscript.

ACKNOWLEDGMENTS

The authors thank D. Vicioso, I. del Rio, and B. López for skillful technical assistance.

REFERENCES

1. Adler, H., Nikolaou, E., Gould, K., Hinds, J., Collins, A. M., Connor, V., et al. (2019). Pneumococcal colonization in healthy adult research participants in the conjugate vaccine era, United Kingdom, 2010-2017. *J. Infect. Dis.* 219, 1989–1993. doi: 10.1093/infdis/jiz034
2. Aguinagalde, L., Corsini, B., Domenech, A., Domenech, M., Camara, J., Ardanuy, C., et al. (2015). Emergence of amoxicillin-resistant variants of Spain9V-ST156 pneumococci expressing serotype 11A correlates with their ability to evade the host immune response. *PLoS One* 10:e0137565. doi: 10.1371/journal.pone. 0137565
3. Andrews, N. J., Waight, P. A., George, R. C., Slack, M. P., and Miller, E. (2012). Impact and effectiveness of 23-valent pneumococcal polysaccharide vaccine against invasive pneumococcal disease in the elderly in England and Wales. *Vaccine* 30, 6802–6808. doi: 10.1016/j.vaccine.2012.09.019
4. Ardanuy, C., de la Campa, A. G., Garcia, E., Fenoll, A., Calatayud, L., and Cercenado, E. (2014). Spread of *Streptococcus pneumoniae* serotype 8- ST63 multidrug-resistant recombinant Clone, Spain. *Emerg. Infect. Dis.* 20, 1848–1856. doi: 10.3201/eid2011.131215
5. Atkins, K. E., Lafferty, E. I., Deeny, S. R., Davies, N. G., Robotham, J. V., and Jit, M. (2018). Use of mathematical modelling to assess the impact of vaccines on antibiotic resistance. *Lancet Infect. Dis.* 18, e204–e213. doi: 10.1016/S1473- 3099(17)30478-4
6. Azarian, T., Mitchell, P. K., Georgieva, M., Thompson, C. M., Ghouila, A., Pollard, A. J., et al. (2018). Global emergence and population dynamics of divergent serotype 3 CC180 pneumococci. *PLoS Pathog.* 14:e1007438. doi: 10.1371/ journal.ppat.1007438
7. Balsells, E., Dagan, R., Yildirim, I., Gounder, P. P., Steens, A., Munoz-Almagro, C., et al. (2018). The relative invasive disease potential of *Streptococcus pneumoniae* among children after PCV introduction: a systematic review and meta-analysis. *J. Infect.* 77, 368–378. doi: 10.1016/j.jinf.2018.06.004
8. Balsells, E., Guillot, L., Nair, H., and Kyaw, M. H. (2017). Serotype distribution of *Streptococcus pneumoniae* causing invasive disease in children in the post- PCV era: a systematic review and meta-analysis. *PLoS One* 12:e0177113. doi: 10.1371/journal.pone.0177113
9. Bogaert, D., De Groot, R., and Hermans, P. W. (2004). *Streptococcus pneumoniae* colonisation: the key to pneumococcal disease. *Lancet Infect. Dis.* 4, 144–154. doi: 10.1016/S1473-3099(04)00938-7
10. Bonten, M. J., Huijts, S. M., Bolkenbaas, M., Webber, C., Patterson, S., Gault, S., et al. (2015). Polysaccharide conjugate vaccine against pneumococcal pneumonia in adults. *N. Engl. J. Med.* 372, 1114–1125. doi: 10.1056/ NEJMoa1408544
11. Brueggemann, A. B., Pai, R., Crook, D. W., and Beall, B. (2007). Vaccine escape recombinants emerge after pneumococcal vaccination in the United States. *PLoS Pathog.* 3:e168. doi: 10.1371/journal.ppat.0030168
12. Brueggemann, A. B., and Spratt, B. G. (2003). Geographic distribution and clonal diversity of *Streptococcus pneumoniae* serotype 1 isolates. *J. Clin. Microbiol.* 41, 4966–4970. doi: 10.1128/jcm.41.11.4966-4970.2003
13. Cassiolato, A. P., Almeida, S. C. G., Andrade, A. L., Minamisava, R., and Brandileone, M. C. C. (2018). Expansion of the multidrug-resistant clonal complex 320 among invasive *Streptococcus pneumoniae* serotype 19A after the introduction of a ten-valent pneumococcal conjugate vaccine in Brazil. *PLoS One* 13:e0208211. doi: 10.1371/journal.pone.0208211
14. Chaguza, C., Heinsbroek, E., Gladstone, R. A., Tafatatha, T., Alaerts, M., Peno, C., et al. (2019). Early signals of vaccine driven perturbation seen in pneumococcal carriage population genomic data. *Clin. Infect. Dis.* ciz404. doi: 10.1093/cid/ciz404
15. Choi, E. H., Zhang, F., Lu, Y. J., and Malley, R. (2015). Capsular polysaccharide release by serotype 3 pneumococcal strains reduces the protective effect of anti- type 3 capsular antibodies. *Clin. Vaccine Immunol.* 23, 162–167. doi: 10.1128/ CVI.00591-15
16. Cui, Y. A., Patel, H., O'Neil, W. M., Li, S., and Saddier, P. (2017). Pneumococcal serotype distribution: a snapshot of recent data in pediatric and adult populations around the world. *Hum. Vaccin Immunother.* 13, 1–13. doi: 10. 1080/21645515.2016.1277300
17. Dennis, E. A., Coats, M. T., Griffin, S., Pang, B., Briles, D. E., and Crain, M. J. (2018). Hyperencapsulated mucoid pneumococcal isolates from patients with cystic fibrosis have increased biofilm density and persistence in vivo. *Pathog. Dis.* 76:fty073. doi: 10.1093/femspd/fty073
18. Domenech, M., Araujo-Bazan, L., García, E., and Moscoso, M. (2014). *In vitro* biofilm formation by *Streptococcus pneumoniae* as a predictor of post- vaccination emerging serotypes colonizing the human nasopharynx. *Environ. Microbiol.* 16, 1193–1201. doi: 10.1111/1462-2920.12370
19. Domenech, M., Damian, D., Ardanuy, C., Linares, J., Fenoll, A., and Garcia, E. (2015). Emerging, non-PCV13 serotypes 11A and 35B of *Streptococcus pneumoniae* show high potential for biofilm formation *in vitro*. *PLoS One* 10:e0125636. doi: 10.1371/journal.pone.0125636
20. Domenech, M., García, E., and Moscoso, M. (2009). Versatility of the capsular genes during biofilm formation by *Streptococcus pneumoniae*. *Environ. Microbiol.* 11, 2542–2555 doi: 10.1111/j.1462-2920.2009.01979.x
21. Domenech, M., Ramos-Sevillano, E., García, E., Moscoso, M., and Yuste, J. (2013). Biofilm formation avoids complement immunity and phagocytosis of *Streptococcus pneumoniae*. *Infect. Immun.* 81, 2606–2615. doi: 10.1128/IAI. 00491-13
22. Domenech, M., Sempere, J., de Miguel, S., and Yuste, J. (2018). Combination of antibodies and antibiotics as a promising strategy against multidrug-resistant pathogens of the respiratory tract. *Front. Immunol.* 9:2700. doi: 10.3389/fimmu. 2018.02700
23. Donlan, R. M., and Costerton, J. W. (2002). Biofilms: survival mechanisms of clinically relevant microorganisms. *Clin. Microbiol. Rev.* 15, 167–193. doi: 10. 1128/cmr.15.2.167-193.2002
24. ECDC (2018). *Invasive Pneumococcal Disease-Annual Epidemiological Report for 2016*. Stockholm: ECDC.
25. Elberse, K. E., van de Pol, I., Witteveen, S., van der Heide, H. G., Schot, C. S., van Dijk, A., et al. (2011). Population structure of invasive *Streptococcus pneumoniae* in the Netherlands in the pre-vaccination era assessed by MLVA and capsular sequence typing. *PLoS One* 6:e20390. doi: 10.1371/journal.pone. 0020390
26. Feikin, D. R., Kagucia, E. W., Loo, J. D., Link-Gelles, R., Puhan, M. A., Cherian, T., et al. (2013). Serotype-specific changes in invasive pneumococcal disease after pneumococcal conjugate vaccine introduction: a pooled analysis of multiple surveillance sites. *PLoS Med.* 10:e1001517. doi: 10.1371/journal.pmed.1001517
27. Feil, E. J., Li, B. C., Aanensen, D. M., Hanage, W. P., and Spratt, B. G.

(2004). eBURST: inferring patterns of evolutionary descent among clusters of related bacterial genotypes from multilocus sequence typing data. *J. Bacteriol.* 186, 1518–1530. doi: 10.1128/jb.186.5.1518-1530.2004
28. Fenoll, A., Granizo, J. J., Giménez, M. J., Yuste, J., and Aguilar, L. (2015). Secular trends (1990-2013) in serotypes and associated non-susceptibility of S. pneumoniae isolates causing invasive disease in the pre-/post-era of pneumococcal conjugate vaccines in Spanish regions without universal paediatric pneumococcal vaccination. *Vaccine* 33, 5691–5699. doi: 10.1016/j. vaccine.2015.08.009
29. GBD 2016 Lower Respiratory Infections Collaborators (2018). Estimates of the global, regional, and national morbidity, mortality, and aetiologies of lower respiratory infections in 195 countries, 1990-2016: a systematic analysis for the global burden of disease study 2016. *Lancet Infect. Dis.* 18, 1191–1210. doi: 10.1016/S1473-3099(18)30310-4
30. Geno, K. A., Gilbert, G. L., Song, J. Y., Skovsted, I. C., Klugman, K. P., Jones, C., et al. (2015). Pneumococcal capsules and their types: past, present, and future. *Clin. Microbiol. Rev.* 28, 871–899. doi: 10.1128/CMR.00024-15
31. Golden, A. R., Adam, H. J., Karlowsky, J. A., Baxter, M., Nichol, K. A., and Martin, I. (2018). Molecular characterization of predominant *Streptococcus pneumoniae* serotypes causing invasive infections in Canada: the SAVE study, 2011-15. *J. Antimicrob. Chemother.* 73(Suppl. 7), vii20–vii31. doi: 10.1093/jac/dky157
32. Golden, A. R., Adam, H. J., Zhanel, G. G., and Canadian Antimicrobial Resistance Alliance (2016). Invasive *Streptococcus pneumoniae* in Canada, 2011-2014: characterization of new candidate 15-valent pneumococcal conjugate vaccine serotypes 22F and 33F. *Vaccine* 34, 2527–2530. doi: 10.1016/j.vaccine.2016.03.058
33. Greenberg, D., Hoover, P. A., Vesikari, T., Peltier, C., Hurley, D. C., McFetridge, R. D., et al. (2018). Safety and immunogenicity of 15-valent pneumococcal conjugate vaccine (PCV15) in healthy infants. *Vaccine* 36, 6883–6891. doi: 10.1016/j.vaccine.2018.02.113
34. Huss, A., Scott, P., Stuck, A. E., Trotter, C., and Egger, M. (2009). Efficacy of pneumococcal vaccination in adults: a meta-analysis. *CMAJ* 180, 48–58. doi: 10.1503/cmaj.080734
35. Hyams, C., Opel, S., Hanage, W., Yuste, J., Bax, K., Henriques-Normark, B., et al. (2011). Effects of *Streptococcus pneumoniae* strain background on complement resistance. *PLoS One* 6:e24581. doi: 10.1371/journal.pone.0024581
36. Iverson, A., Meyer, C. J., Vogel, P., Waidyarachchi, S., Das, N., and Bruhn, D. F. (2019). Efficacy of aminomethyl spectinomycins against complex upper respiratory tract bacterial infections. *Antimicrob. Agents Chemother.* 63:e02096- 18. doi: 10.1128/AAC.02096-18
37. Kaplan, S. L., Barson, W. J., Lin, P. L., Romero, J. R., Bradley, J. S., Tan, T. Q., et al. (2013). Early trends for invasive pneumococcal infections in children after the introduction of the 13-valent pneumococcal conjugate vaccine. *Pediatr. Infect. Dis. J.* 32, 203–207. doi: 10.1097/INF.0b013e318275614b
38. Ladhani, S. N., Collins, S., Djennad, A., Sheppard, C. L., Borrow, R., Fry, N. K., et al. (2018). Rapid increase in non-vaccine serotypes causing invasive pneumococcal disease in England and Wales, 2000-17: a prospective national observational cohort study. *Lancet Infect. Dis.* 18, 441–451. doi: 10.1016/S1473-3099(18) 30052-5
39. Lewnard, J. A., and Hanage, W. P. (2019). Making sense of differences in pneumococcal serotype replacement. *Lancet Infect. Dis.* 19, e213–e220. doi: 10.1016/S1473-3099(18)30660-1
40. Mackenzie, G. A., Hill, P. C., Jeffries, D. J., Hossain, I., Uchendu, U., Ameh, D., et al. (2016). Effect of the introduction of pneumococcal conjugate vaccination on invasive pneumococcal disease in The Gambia: a population-based surveillance study. *Lancet Infect. Dis.* 16, 703–711. doi: 10.1016/S1473-3099(16)00054-2
41. McAllister, L. J., Ogunniyi, A. D., Stroeher, U. H., Leach, A. J., and Paton, J. C. (2011). Contribution of serotype and genetic background to virulence of serotype 3 and serogroup 11 pneumococcal isolates. *Infect. Immun.* 79, 4839–4849. doi: 10.1128/IAI.05663-11
42. McLaughlin, J. M., Jiang, Q., Isturiz, R. E., Sings, H. L., Swerdlow, D. L., Gessner, B. D., et al. (2018). Effectiveness of 13-valent pneumococcal conjugate vaccine against hospitalization for community-acquired pneumonia in older us adults: a test-negative design. *Clin. Infect. Dis.* 67, 1498–1506. doi: 10.1093/cid/ciy312
43. Menéndez, R., Espana, P. P., Pérez-Trallero, E., Uranga, A., Méndez, R., Cilloniz, C., et al. (2017). The burden of PCV13 serotypes in hospitalized pneumococcal pneumonia in Spain using a novel urinary antigen detection test. CAPA study. *Vaccine* 35, 5264–5270. doi: 10.1016/j.vaccine.2017.08.007
44. Mollerach, M., López, R., and García, E. (1998). Characterization of the *galU* gene of *Streptococcus pneumoniae* encoding a uridine diphosphoglucose pyrophosphorylase: a gene essential for capsular polysaccharide biosynthesis. *J. Exp. Med.* 188, 2047–2056. doi: 10.1084/jem.188.11.2047
45. Moore, M. R., Link-Gelles, R., Schaffner, W., Lynfield, R., Lexau, C., Bennett, N. M., et al. (2015). Effect of use of 13-valent pneumococcal conjugate vaccine in children on invasive pneumococcal disease in children and adults in the USA: analysis of multisite, population-based surveillance. *Lancet Infect. Dis.* 15, 301–309. doi: 10.1016/s1473-3099(14)71081-3
46. Morais, V., Dee, V., and Suarez, N. (2018). Purification of capsular polysaccharides of *Streptococcus pneumoniae*: traditional and new methods. *Front. Bioeng. Biotechnol.* 6:145. doi: 10.3389/fbioe.2018.00145
47. Moscoso, M., García, E., and López, R. (2006). Biofilm formation by *Streptococcus pneumoniae*: role of choline, extracellular DNA, and capsular polysaccharide in microbial accretion. *J. Bacteriol.* 188, 7785–7795. doi: 10.1128/JB.00673-06
48. Orihuela, C. J., Mahdavi, J., Thornton, J., Mann, B., Wooldridge, K. G., Abouseada, N., et al. (2009). Laminin receptor initiates bacterial contact with the blood brain barrier in experimental meningitis models. *J. Clin. Invest.* 119, 1638–1646. doi: 10.1172/JCI36759
49. Pichon, B., Ladhani, S. N., Slack, M. P., Segonds-Pichon, A., Andrews, N. J., Waight, P. A., et al. (2013). Changes in molecular epidemiology of *Streptococcus pneumoniae* causing meningitis following introduction of pneumococcal conjugate vaccination in England and Wales. *J. Clin. Microbiol.* 51, 820–827. doi: 10.1128/JCM.01917-12
50. Ramos-Sevillano, E., Urzainqui, A., de Andres, B., González-Tajuelo, R., Domenech, M., González-Camacho, F., et al. (2016). PSGL-1 on leukocytes is a critical component of the host immune response against invasive pneumococcal disease. *PLoS Pathog.* 12:e1005500. doi: 10.1371/journal.ppat.1005500
51. Rinta-Kokko, H., Palmu, A. A., Auranen, K., Nuorti, J. P., Toropainen, M., Siira, L., et al. (2018). Long-term impact of 10-valent pneumococcal conjugate vaccination on invasive pneumococcal disease among children in Finland. *Vaccine* 36, 1934–1940. doi: 10.1016/j.vaccine.2018.03.001
52. Russell, K. L., Baker, C. I., Hansen, C., Poland, G. A., Ryan, M. A., Merrill, M. M., et al. (2015). Lack of effectiveness of the 23-valent polysaccharide pneumococcal vaccine in reducing all-cause pneumonias among healthy young military recruits: a randomized, double-blind, placebo-controlled trial. *Vaccine* 33, 1182–1187. doi: 10.1016/j.vaccine.2014.12.058
53. Sa-Leao, R., Pinto, F., Aguiar, S., Nunes, S., Carrico, J. A., Frazao, N., et al. (2011). Analysis of invasiveness of pneumococcal serotypes and clones circulating in Portugal before widespread use of conjugate vaccines reveals heterogeneous behavior of clones expressing the same serotype. *J. Clin. Microbiol.* 49, 1369–1375. doi: 10.1128/JCM.01763-10
54. Savulescu, C., Krizova, P., Lepoutre, A., Mereckiene, J., Vestrheim, D. F., Ciruela, P., et al. (2017). Effect of high-valency pneumococcal conjugate vaccines on invasive pneumococcal disease in children in SpIDnet countries: an observational multicentre study. *Lancet Respir. Med.* 5, 648–656. doi: 10.1016/ S2213-2600(17)30110-8
55. Shoji, H., Vázquez-Sánchez, D. A., González-Díaz, A., Cubero, M., Tubau, F., Santos, S., et al. (2018). Overview of pneumococcal serotypes and genotypes causing diseases in patients with chronic obstructive pulmonary disease in a Spanish hospital between 2013 and 2016. *Infect. Drug Resist.* 11, 1387–1400. doi: 10.2147/IDR.S165093
56. Silva, M. D., and Sillankorva, S. (2019). Otitis media pathogens – A life entrapped in biofilm communities. *Crit. Rev. Microbiol.* 45, 595–612. doi: 10.1080/1040841X. 2019.1660616
57. Stacey, H. L., Rosen, J., Peterson, J. T., Williams-Diaz, A., Gakhar, V., Sterling, T. M., et al. (2019). Safety and immunogenicity of 15-valent pneumococcal conjugate vaccine (PCV-15) compared to PCV-13 in healthy older adults. *Hum. Vaccin Immunother.* 15, 530–539. doi: 10.1080/21645515.2018.1532249
58. Standish, A. J., and Weiser, J. N. (2009). Human neutrophils kill *Streptococcus pneumoniae* via serine proteases. *J. Immunol.* 183, 2602–2609. doi: 10.4049/ jimmunol.0900688
59. Thompson, A., Lamberth, E., Severs, J., Scully, I., Tarabar, S., Ginis, J., et al. (2019). Phase 1 trial of a 20-valent pneumococcal conjugate vaccine in healthy adults. *Vaccine* 37, 6201–6207. doi: 10.1016/j.vaccine.2019.08.048
60. Tin Tin Htar, M., Stuurman, A. L., Ferreira, G., Alicino, C., Bollaerts, K., Paganino, C., et al. (2017). Effectiveness of pneumococcal vaccines in preventing pneumonia in adults, a systematic review and meta-analyses of observational studies. *PLoS One* 12:e0177985. doi: 10.1371/journal.pone.0177985
61. van der Poll, T., and Opal, S. M. (2009). Pathogenesis, treatment, and prevention of pneumococcal pneumonia. *Lancet* 374, 1543–1556. doi: 10.1016/S0140- 6736(09)61114-4
62. van Hoek, A. J., Andrews, N., Waight, P. A., George, R., and Miller, E. (2012). Effect of serotype on focus and mortality of invasive pneumococcal disease: coverage of different vaccines and insight into non-vaccine serotypes. *PLoS One* 7:e39150. doi: 10.1371/journal.pone.0039150
63. Vandevelde, N. M., Tulkens, P. M., Diaz Iglesias, Y., Verhaegen, J., Rodriguez-Villalobos, H., Philippart, I., et al. (2014). Characterisation of a collection of *Streptococcus pneumoniae* isolates from patients suffering from acute

exacerbations of chronic bronchitis: in vitro susceptibility to antibiotics and biofilm formation in relation to antibiotic efflux and serotypes/serogroups. *Int. J. Antimicrob. Agents* 44, 209–217. doi: 10.1016/j.ijantimicag.2014.05.016

64. Vidal, J. E., Howery, K. E., Ludewick, H. P., Nava, P., and Klugman, K. P. (2013). Quorum-sensing systems LuxS/autoinducer 2 and Com regulate *Streptococcus pneumoniae* biofilms in a bioreactor with living cultures of human respiratory cells. *Infect. Immun.* 81, 1341–1353. doi: 10.1128/IAI.01096-12
65. Wahl, B., O'Brien, K. L., Greenbaum, A., Majumder, A., Liu, L., Chu, Y., et al. (2018). Burden of *Streptococcus pneumoniae* and *Haemophilus influenzae* type b disease in children in the era of conjugate vaccines: global, regional, and national estimates for 2000-15. *Lancet Glob. Health* 6, e744–e757. doi: 10.1016/ S2214-109X(18)30247-X
66. Weinberger, D. M., Trzcinski, K., Lu, Y. J., Bogaert, D., Brandes, A., Galagan, J., et al. (2009). Pneumococcal capsular polysaccharide structure predicts serotype prevalence. *PLoS Pathog.* 5:e1000476. doi: 10.1371/journal.ppat.10 00476
67. Wu, X., Jacobs, N. T., Bozio, C., Palm, P., Lattar, S. M., and Hanke, C. R. (2017). Competitive dominance within biofilm consortia regulates the relative distribution of pneumococcal nasopharyngeal density. *Appl. Environ. Microbiol.* 83:e00953-17. doi: 10.1128/AEM.009 53-17
68. Yildirim, I., Hanage, W. P., Lipsitch, M., Shea, K. M., Stevenson, A., Finkelstein, J., et al. (2010). Serotype specific invasive capacity and persistent reduction in invasive pneumococcal disease. *Vaccine* 29, 283–288. doi: 10.1016/j.vaccine. 2010.10.032
69. Yuste, J., Khandavilli, S., Ansari, N., Muttardi, K., Ismail, L., Hyams, C., et al. (2010). The effects of PspC on complement-mediated immunity to *Streptococcus pneumoniae* vary with strain background and capsular serotype. *Infect. Immun.* 78, 283–292. doi: 10.1128/IAI.00541-09

7

Unique Roles for *Streptococcus pneumoniae* Phosphodiesterase 2 in Cyclic di-AMP Catabolism and Macrophage Responses

*Alicia K. Wooten[1,2], Anukul T. Shenoy[1], Emad I. Arafa[1,2], Hisashi Akiyama[3], Ian M. C. Martin[1], Matthew R. Jones[1,2], Lee J. Quinton[1,2,3,4], Suryaram Gummuluru[3], Guangchun Bai[5] and Joseph P. Mizgerd[1,2,3,6]**

[1] Pulmonary Center, Boston University School of Medicine, Boston, MA, United States, [2] Department of Medicine, Boston University School of Medicine, Boston, MA, United States, [3] Department of Microbiology, Boston University School of Medicine, Boston, MA, United States, [4] Department of Pathology and Laboratory Medicine, Boston University School of Medicine, Boston, MA, United States, [5] Department of Immunology and Microbial Disease, Albany Medical College, Albany, NY, United States, [6] Department of Biochemistry, Boston University School of Medicine, Boston, MA, United States

***Correspondence:**
Joseph P. Mizgerd
jmizgerd@bu.edu

Cyclic di-AMP (c-di-AMP) is an important signaling molecule for pneumococci, and as a uniquely prokaryotic product it can be recognized by mammalian cells as a danger signal that triggers innate immunity. Roles of c-di-AMP in directing host responses during pneumococcal infection are only beginning to be defined. We hypothesized that pneumococci with defective c-di-AMP catabolism due to phosphodiesterase deletions could illuminate roles of c-di-AMP in mediating host responses to pneumococcal infection. Pneumococci deficient in phosphodiesterase 2 (Pde2) stimulated a rapid induction of interferon β (IFNβ) expression that was exaggerated in comparison to that induced by wild type (WT) bacteria or bacteria deficient in phosphodiesterase 1. This IFNβ burst was elicited in mouse and human macrophage-like cell lines as well as in primary alveolar macrophages collected from mice with pneumococcal pneumonia. Macrophage hyperactivation by Pde2-deficient pneumococci led to rapid cell death. STING and cGAS were essential for the excessive IFNβ induction, which also required phagocytosis of bacteria and triggered the phosphorylation of IRF3 and IRF7 transcription factors. The select effects of Pde2 deletion were products of a unique role of this enzyme in c-di-AMP catabolism when pneumococci were grown on solid substrate conditions designed to enhance virulence. Because pneumococci with elevated c-di-AMP drive aberrant innate immune responses from macrophages involving hyperactivation of STING, excessive IFNβ expression, and rapid cytotoxicity, we surmise that c-di-AMP is pivotal for directing innate immunity and host-pathogen interactions during pneumococcal pneumonia.

Keywords: cyclic di-AMP, innate immunity, interferon-β, macrophages, pneumococcus, pneumonia, STING

INTRODUCTION

Pneumonia is a leading cause of morbidity and mortality worldwide (1). Children under 5 and adults over 60 years of age have the greatest risk of developing pneumonia (2). The most common bacterial cause of community acquired pneumonia is the gram-positive extracellular bacterium, *Streptococcus pneumoniae* (pneumococcus). Pneumococcus can colonize the nasopharynx asymptomatically, or it can cause diseases such as otitis media, bacteremia, or meningitis, in addition to pneumonia (3). Despite advances with pneumococcal vaccines, infections with non-vaccine serotypes remain important (4). A better understanding of the pathogen and the host immune response may help develop novel prophylactics and therapeutics to lower the disease burden caused by *S. pneumoniae*.

In the lungs, alveolar macrophages are among the first lines of immune defense (5). Multiple receptors on the surface of macrophages recognize bacteria, leading to phagocytosis and the expression of cytokines and chemokines. During pneumococcal pneumonia, NF-κB activation in macrophages is required to rapidly ramp up cytokine expression andneutrophil recruitment (6). Cytokines such as TNFα, IL-1, CXCL2, and IFNβ are produced by macrophages to elicit lung immunity (5). TNFα, IL-1, and CXCL2 all contribute to neutrophil-mediated killing of pneumococcus in the lungs (7, 8). IFNβ and its receptor IFNAR1 help mediate resistance against pneumococcal infection by decreasing nasal colonization (9), enhancing compartmentalization of bacteria within the infected respiratory tract (10), and increasing lung epithelial cell resilience against the infectious and inflammatory challenges of pneumonia (11). However, excessive or inappropriate type I interferon signaling compromises immune defense and predisposes the host to pneumococcal pneumonia (12–14). The induction of IFNβ by pneumococcus is mediated via a pathway in which the endoplasmic reticulum transmembrane protein STimulator of Interferon Genes (STING) triggers the TANK Binding Kinase 1 (TBK1) to activate the transcription factor interferon regulatory factor 3 (IRF3) (9, 15). STING is an adaptor molecule and receptor for cyclic dinucleotides in the cytosol including the bacterial metabolites cyclic di-GMP and cyclic di-AMP (c-di-AMP), as well as the mammalian-derived cyclic GMP-AMP (cGAMP) produced by the cyclic GMP-AMP synthase (cGAS) enzyme (16–18). Induction of IFNβ by pneumococcus requires both STING and cGAS (19), which was interpreted as evidence that pneumococcal DNA but not pneumococcal c-di-AMP triggers STING-dependent IFNβ induction (19). However, a cGAS-STING complex is essential to IFNβ induction by purified c-di-AMP (20), which could contribute to the requirement for cGAS in pneumococcus-induced signaling. Specific effects of pneumococcal c-di-AMP on macrophage responses remain to be demonstrated.

The roles of c-di-AMP in bacteria are diverse and include potassium transport, resistance to cell wall stress, peptidoglycan homeostasis, biofilm formation, and modulating the cellular size of the bacteria (21–25). Pneumococcus generates c-di-AMP using a diadenylate cyclase, CdaA (26). c-di-AMP is degraded in pneumococcus by two phosphodiesterase enzymes, Phosphodiesterase 1 (Pdel) and Pde2 (26). Pdel converts c-di-AMP to 5′-phosphoadenylyl-adenosine (pApA), while Pde2 is capable of catabolizing both c-di-AMP and pApA, in each case resulting in AMP as a product. Deletion of one or both of the phosphodiesterase enzymes impairs c-di-AMP catabolism, increasing its concentrations in the mutant pneumococci (26). The effects of pneumococcal c-di-AMP metabolism on host-pathogen interactions are largely unclear. We hypothesized that pneumococci deficient in the phosphodiesterase enzymes degrading c-di-AMP could illuminate macrophage pathways involved in innate immune responses to bacterial cyclic dinucleotides during infection.

RESULTS

Elevated Macrophage NF-κB Responses to Phosphodiesterase-Mutant Pneumococci

Macrophage NF-κB is important to pneumococcal infection of the lung. During pneumococcal pneumonia, NF-κB RelA in macrophages is crucial for early cytokine expression, neutrophil recruitment, and lung defense (6). Macrophage activation of NF-κB is heterogeneous across clinical isolates, and lower NF-κB activators cause more severe lung infection in mouse models and associate with more severe pneumonia in human patients (27). To determine whether variations in c-di-AMP levels may influence the magnitude of macrophage NF-κB activation, we compared macrophage responses to 4 pneumococcal strains: a wild type (WT) strain and strains in which one (Δ*pdel* or Δ*pde2*) or both (Δ*pdel*Δ*pde2*) c-di-AMP-catabolizing enzymes were deleted, all in the isogenic D39 genetic background (26). Macrophage NF-κB activity was quantified using a mouse macrophage-like RAW264.7 cell line that was stably transduced to express firefly luciferase driven by tandem NF-κB binding sites (27, 28). All three pneumococcal phosphodiesterase mutants significantly increased NF-κB activity compared to the WT strain (**Figure 1A**). The different mutant strains had similar effects on macrophage NF-κB activation (**Figure 1A**). To determine if this influenced cytokine expression, we quantified TNFα and IL-1β induction. TNFα mRNA levels were significantly elevated after infection with the phosphodiesterase-deficient pneumococci, with comparable effects noted for all the mutant bacteria (**Figure 1B**). At the protein level, TNFα was elevated in cell culture supernatants which included bacteria, with those containing Δ*pde2* or Δ*pdel*Δ*pde2* pneumococci reaching statistical significance (mean ± SEM concentrations of 1790 ± 264, 2390 ± 157, 2370 ± 173, 2580 ± 108, and 2620 ± 37 in cultures containing no, WT, Δ*pdel*, Δ*pde2*, or Δ*pdel*Δ*pde2* pneumococci, respectively, from $N = 3$ independent experiments; P values compared to the no pneumococci group of 0.11, 0.12, 0.03, and 0.02, respectively, using one-way ANOVA and the Sidak *post hoc* test). IL-1β mRNA induction showed a similar trend but had more variability and did not reach statistical significance (**Figure 1C**). IL-1β protein was not detectable by ELISA in any culture supernatants at this 2-h time-point. Altogether, these

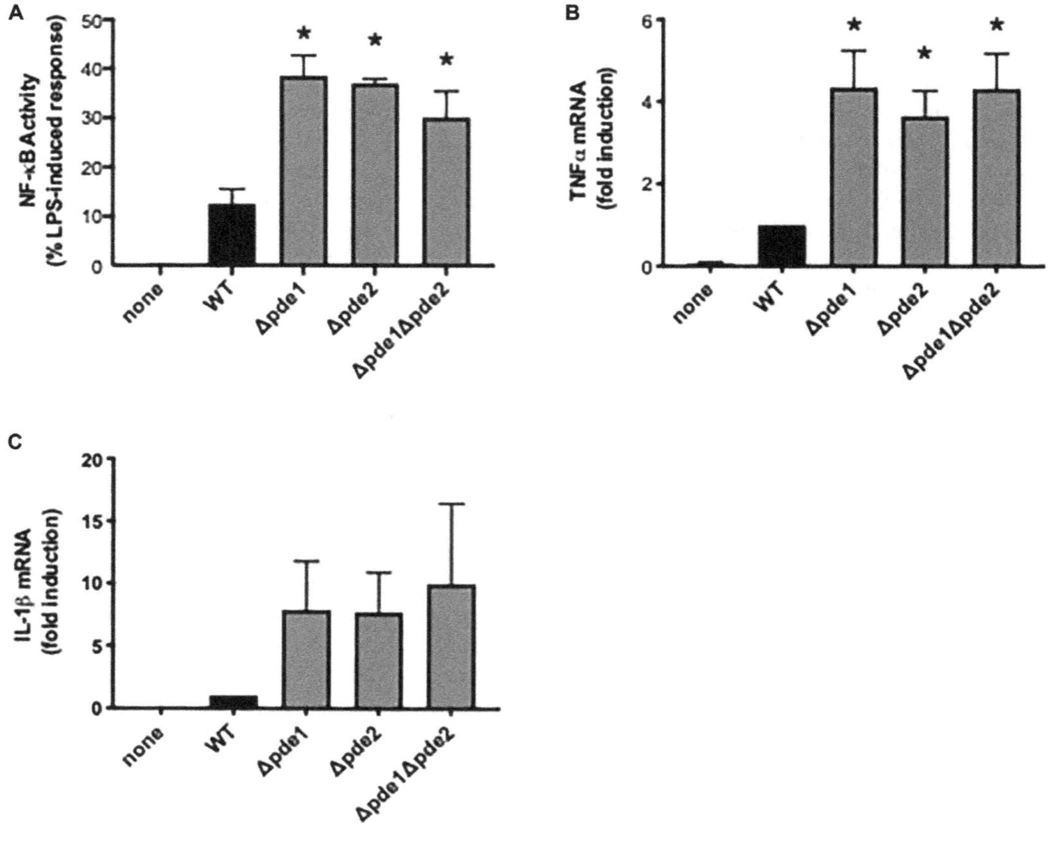

FIGURE 1 | Phosphodiesterase mutations increase pneumococcus-induced NF-κB activity. **(A)** Relative NF-κB-mediated gene expression was measured using a mouse macrophage-like RAW264.7 cell line which had been stably transduced with a firefly luciferase transgene responsive to NF-κB. Cultures were infected 2 h with the indicated bacteria, and luciferase values were quantified using a luminometer and expressed relative to LPS positive control wells run in parallel ($N = 9$ experiments). **(B)** Relative induction of TNFα mRNA was measured in RAW264.7 cell cultures infected 2 h with the indicated bacteria. TNFα mRNA was measured and normalized to 18S rRNA using qPCR, and expressed relative to the cells infected by WT bacteria ($N = 3$ experiments). **(C)** Relative induction of IL-1β mRNA was measured in RAW264.7 cell cultures infected 2 h with the indicated bacteria. IL-1β mRNA was measured and normalized to 18S rRNA using qPCR, and expressed relative to the cells infected by WT bacteria ($N = 3$ experiments). Throughout panels, asterisk (*) indicates $P < 0.05$ compared to WT.

data reveal that phosphodiesterase enzymes are determinants of macrophage innate immune responses to pneumococcus, and loss of the pneumococcal enzymes that catabolize c-di-AMP increases NF-κ B activity.

Mixed Macrophage IFNβ Responses to the Phosphodiesterase Mutants

The innate immune response most directly responsive to c-di-AMP is type I IFN induction (29). To investigate if pneumococcal c-di-AMP could be a modulator of type I interferon responses, RAW264.7 macrophage-like cells were infected with the phosphodiesterase mutants and mRNA was collected so that IFNβ expression could be measured. We expected one of three outcomes: consistently elevated IFNβ responses across the mutant pneumococci, matching the observations with NF-κB activity (**Figure 1**); a ramping up of IFNβ responses with peak levels after infection by the double mutant Δ*pde1*Δ*pde2* strain, based on how c-di-AMP content in pneumococci increase due to phosphodiesterase mutations (26); or no effect of phosphodiesterase mutation, based on the postulate that pneumococcal DNA but not c-di-AMP drives IFNβ responses (19). Surprisingly, macrophage IFNβ responses matched none of these expectations. Instead, only macrophages infected with the Δ*pde2* mutant bacteria displayed enhanced levels of IFNβ after 2 h of infection (**Figure 2A**). In contrast to Δ*pde2* pneumococci, neither Δ*pde1* nor Δ*pde1*Δ*pde2* pneumococci stimulated this burst of type I IFN expression. To determine whether this was a peculiarity of IFNβ alone, we measured another gene in this activation pathway. CXCL10 is also transcribed by the IRF3 transcription factor which STING activates (30, 31). Like IFNβ, CXCL10 expression was only elevated by phosphodiesterase mutation when *pde2* alone was targeted, not after infection with the Δ*pde1* or Δ*pde1*Δ*pde2* pneumococci (**Figure 2B**). These results suggest, for the first time to our knowledge, that the two phosphodiesterase enzymes in *S. pneumoniae* have distinct and non-overlapping roles relating to infection and immunity.

In order to determine whether these results were robust and generalizable, we tested for macrophage IFNβ induction

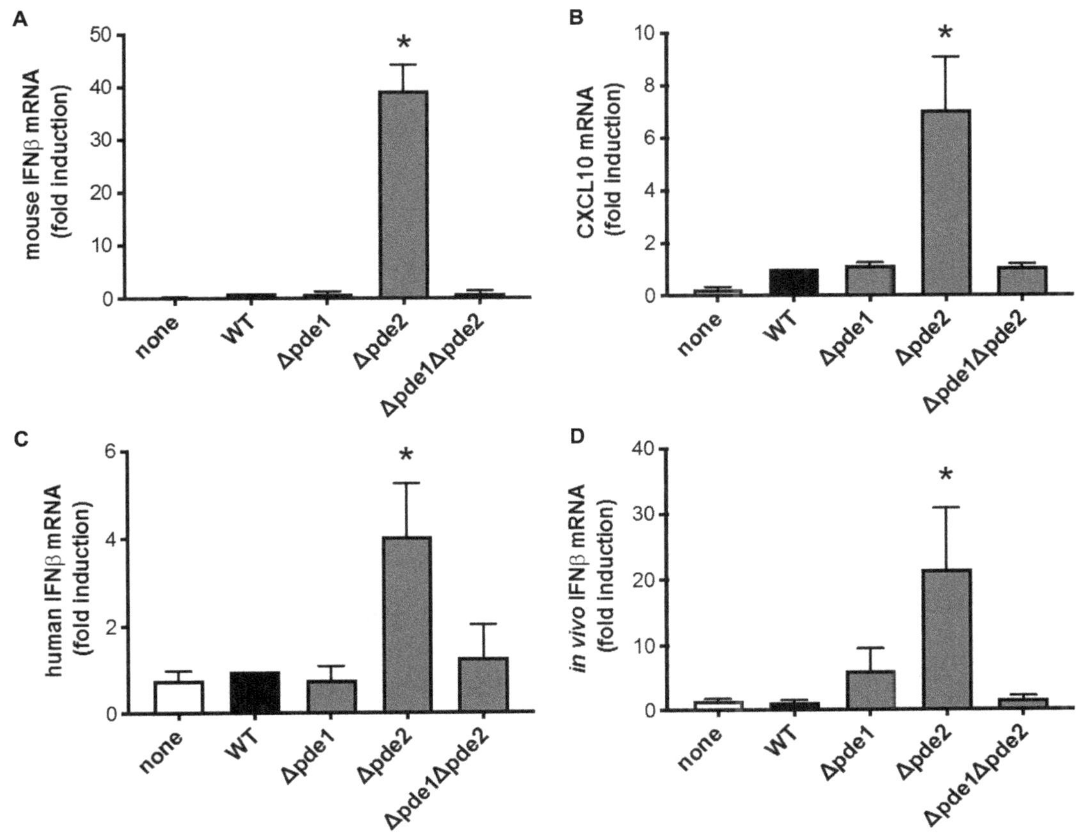

FIGURE 2 | Phosphodiesterase 2 mutation in pneumococcus elicits a distinctive burst of IFNβ expression from macrophages **(A)** Relative induction of IFNβ mRNA was measured in mouse macrophage-like RAW264.7 cell cultures infected 2 h with the indicated bacteria. Mouse IFNβ mRNA was measured and normalized to 18S rRNA using qPCR, and expressed relative to the cells infected by WT bacteria ($N = 3$ experiments). **(B)** Relative induction of mouse CXCL10 mRNA was measured and normalized to 18S rRNA using qPCR, and expressed relative to the cells infected by WT bacteria ($N = 3$ experiments). **(C)** Relative induction of IFNβ mRNA was measured in human THP-1 cell cultures that were matured to macrophage-like phenotypes using PMA before being infected 2 h with the indicated bacteria. Human IFNβ mRNA was measured and normalized to 18S rRNA using qPCR, and expressed relative to the cells infected by WT bacteria ($N = 6$ experiments). **(D)** Relative induction of IFNβ mRNA was measured in mouse alveolar macrophages collected by bronchoalveolar lavage 3 h after *in vivo* infection of mice by intratracheal instillation with the indicated bacteria. Mouse IFNβ mRNA in these cells collected from infected lungs was measured and normalized to 18S rRNA using qPCR, and expressed relative to the cells collected from mice infected by WT bacteria ($N = 11$–16 mice per group, over 4 experiments). Throughout panels, asterisk (*) indicates $P < 0.05$ compared to WT.

using a cell line from a different species (human instead of mouse) and using primary cells during an *in vivo* infection (alveolar macrophages collected from pneumonic lungs, instead of the RAW264.7 cell line in culture). Although the magnitude of response from human THP-1 cells was modest compared to mouse RAW264.7 cells, the relative effects of the different bacterial strains were similar across the different cell lines and species, showing increased IFNβ induction in response to Δ*pde2* bacteria compared to any and all other bacterial strains examined (**Figure 2C**). Thus, human and mouse cells share this distinctive response to Δ*pde2* mutant pneumococci. Mice were infected with pneumococci in their lungs, and bronchoalveolar lavage cells were collected after 3 h of *in vivo* infection (before neutrophil recruitment into the air spaces). IFNβ expression was measured in these cells using qRT-PCR, and the Δ*pde2* mutants showed significantly greater IFNβ induction than any of the other strains, which all behaved similar to each other (**Figure 2D**). Thus, the selective effects of mutation in phosphodiesterase 2 extend beyond *in vitro* cell lines and apply to primary alveolar macrophages from pneumonia experiments *in vivo*.

Outcome of Infection With the Phosphodiesterase Mutants

We measured IFNβ protein in supernatants from infected RAW264.7 cells, expecting to see increased cytokine accumulation in cultures of the Δ*pde2* mutant infections compared to other bacteria. Cultures included living bacteria for 2 h, after which antibiotics were provided to restore sterility to the cell cultures. All the bacteria stimulated IFNβ production, but over time the Δ*pde2* mutant infections stimulated significantly less IFNβ compared to the WT pneumococci (**Figure 3A**). This protein result after 12 or more hours of infection was the opposite

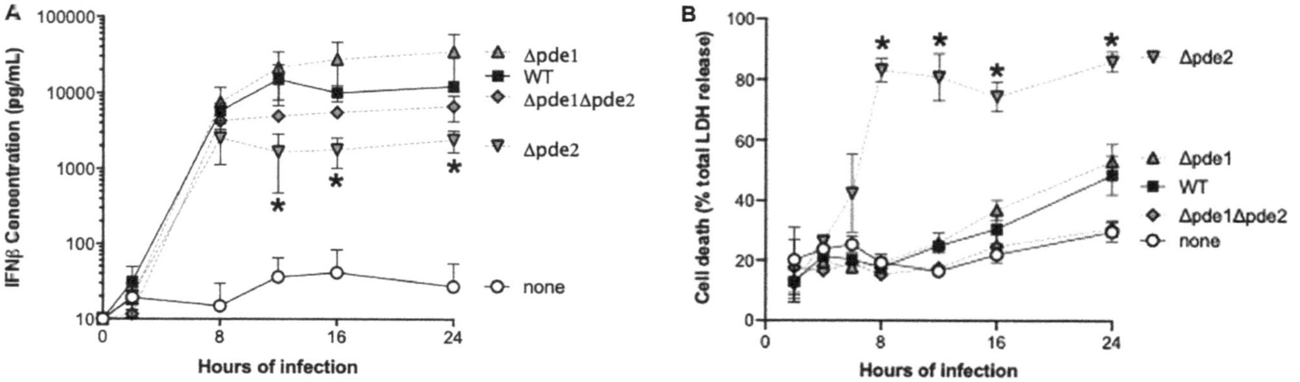

FIGURE 3 | Outcome of infection is dictated by pneumococcal phosphodiesterase 2. **(A)** Time-course of IFNβ protein accumulation in the supernatant was measured in mouse macrophage-like RAW264.7 cell cultures infected with the indicated bacteria. Mouse IFNβ concentration was measured using ELISA (*N* = 3 experiments). **(B)** Time-course of cell death was measured in mouse macrophage-like RAW264.7 cell cultures infected with the indicated bacteria. Concentration of the cytosolic enzyme lactate dehydrogenase (LDH) was measured using a commercially available cytotoxicity assay kit, and expressed relative to concentrations measured after cells were completely lysed by detergent (*N* = 3 experiments). Throughout panels, asterisk (*) indicates $P < 0.05$ compared to WT.

of the early mRNA induction measured after 2–3 h of infection (**Figure 2**). This led us to question whether macrophage cultures infected with the Δ*pde2* mutant bacteria might deteriorate over time. We assessed macrophage viability after stimulation with the different strains of pneumococci using an LDH assay for cellular necrosis (**Figure 3B**). Again, there was a unique phenotype in macrophages infected with phosphodiesterase 2 mutant bacteria. By 8 h, more than 80% of the cultured cells were already dead when infected with the Δ*pde2* bacteria, whereas other strains exhibited only limited cytotoxicity at this time-point. Thus, the unique phenotypic responses of macrophages to Δ*pde2* mutant pneumococci includes rapid cytotoxicity. We therefore focused attention on early responses to infection with these mutants.

Signaling Requirements for Exaggerated IFN Responses From the Phosphodiesterase Mutants

We endeavored to elucidate the pathway by which Δ*pde2* mutant bacteria led to an elevated IFNβ burst. To determine if phagocytic uptake is involved, RAW264.7 cells were pretreated with the actin polymerization inhibitor cytochalasin D before infection with pneumococcus. Inhibition of actin polymerization prevented the burst of IFNβ expression after 2 h of infection by the Δ*pde2* mutant bacteria (**Figure 4A**). All strains, particularly the Δ*pde2* mutant, had diminished IFNβ expression, suggesting that phagocytosis is essential for the rapid and strong IFNβ induction by *pde2*-deficient bacteria. To determine roles of phagolysosomal

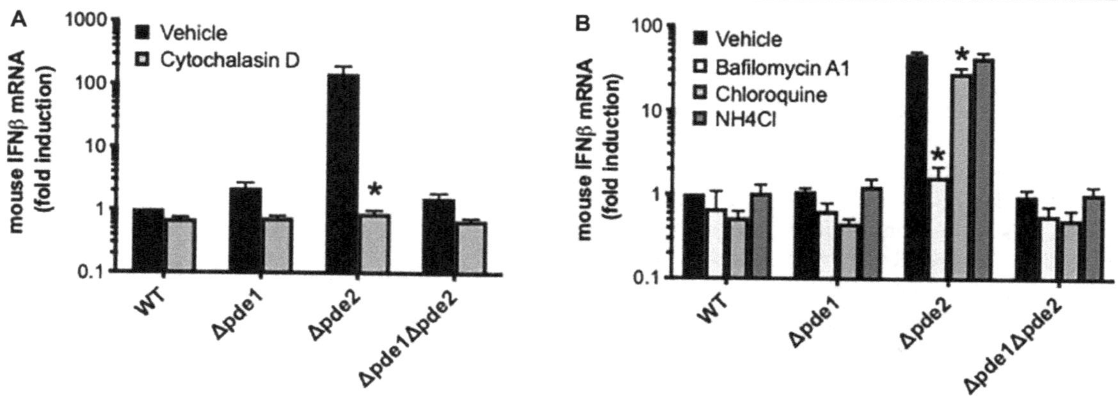

FIGURE 4 | The induction of IFNβ by phosphodiesterase 2 mutant pneumococci requires phagocytosis. **(A)** Relative induction of IFNβ mRNA was measured in mouse macrophage-like RAW264.7 cell cultures infected 2 h with the indicated bacteria in the presence or absence of cytochalasin D as a means of inhibiting actin polymerization (*N* = 3 experiments). **(B)** Relative induction of IFNβ mRNA was measured in mouse macrophage-like RAW264.7 cell cultures infected 2 h with the indicated bacteria in the presence or absence of the indicated inhibitors pf phagosomal processing (*N* = 3 experiments). For both panels, mouse IFNβ mRNA was measured and normalized to 18S rRNA using qPCR, and expressed relative to the cells infected by WT bacteria. For both panels, asterisk (*) indicates $P < 0.05$ compared to vehicle.

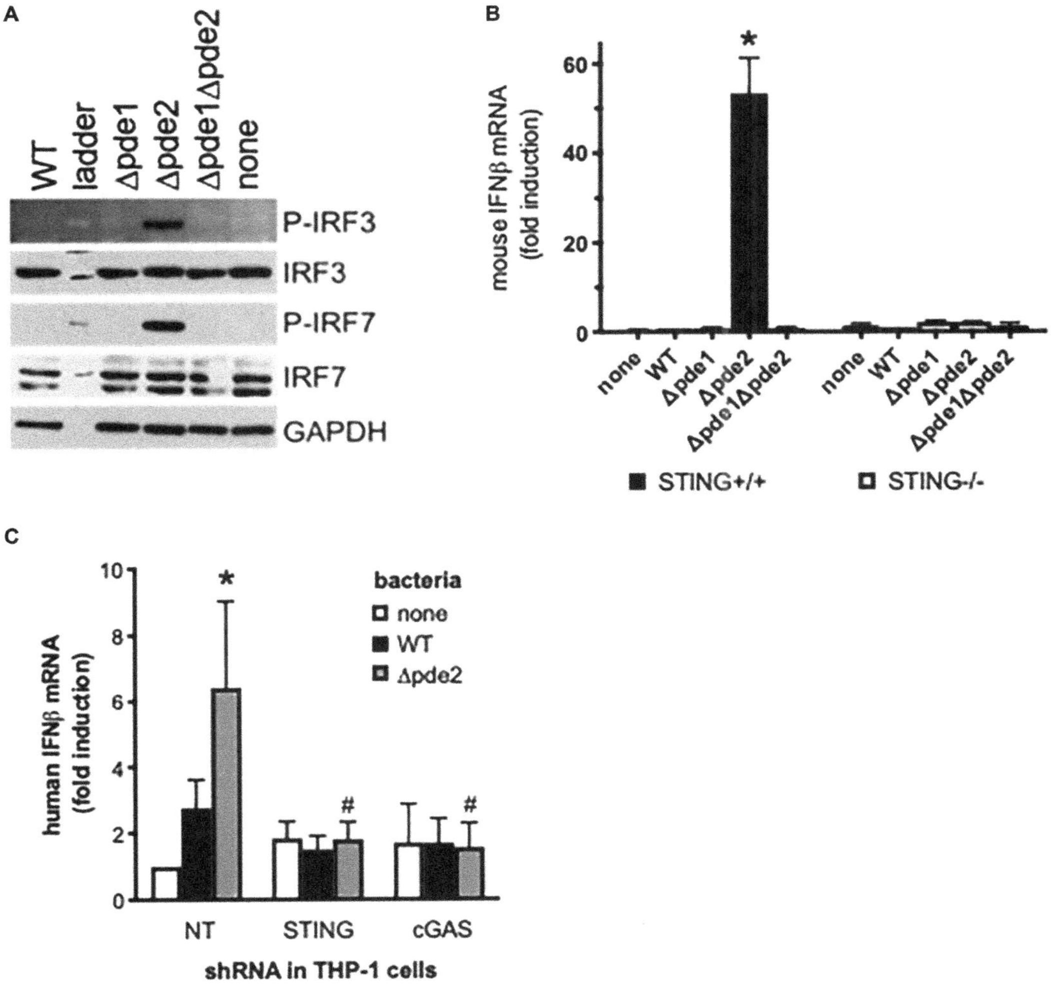

FIGURE 5 | IFNβ expression elicited by phosphodiesterase 2 mutant pneumococci is mediated by the STING-cGAS-IRF3-IRF7 signaling pathway. **(A)** Relative contents of phosphorylated IRF3 and phosphorylated IRF7 protein were measured using immunoblot in cell lysates from mouse macrophage-like RAW264.7 cell cultures infected 2 h with the indicated bacteria. Relative contents of total IRF3 and IRF7 were measured for comparison, as well as GAPDH for loading control (image shown was from one experiment, representative of 2 independent experiments). **(B)** Relative induction of IFNβ mRNA was measured in parallel cultures of mouse macrophage-like RAW264.7 cells, one of which was deficient in STING due to gene targeting. Cultures were infected for 2 h with the indicated bacteria. Mouse IFNβ mRNA was measured and normalized to 18S rRNA using qPCR, and expressed relative to the cells infected by WT bacteria ($N = 3$ experiments). Asterisk (*) indicates $P < 0.05$ compared to WT. **(C)** Relative induction of IFNβ mRNA was measured in parallel cultures of human THP-1 cell cultures that were stably transduced with lentiviruses encoding shRNA that was non-targeting (NT) or which targeted STING or cGAS. THP-1 cells were matured to macrophage-like phenotypes using PMA before being infected 2 h with the indicated bacteria. Human IFNβ mRNA was measured and normalized to 18S rRNA using qPCR, and expressed relative to the uninfected cells transduced with NT shRNA ($N = 5$ experiments). Asterisk (*) indicates $P < 0.05$ compared to WT bacteria in cells transduced by the same shRNA, and hashtag (#) indicates $P < 0.05$ compared to NT shRNA-transduced cells infected by same bacteria.

fusion and acidification, we pretreated RAW264.7 cells with phagolysosome inhibitors. Bafilomycin A1, which inhibits vacuolar H^+-ATPases and disrupts phagolysosome acidification and fusion, completely prevented IFNβ induction by the Δ*pde2* mutant bacteria (**Figure 4B**). Chloroquine and ammonium chloride (NH_4Cl), lysosomotropic agents that can raise vacuolar pH without affecting fusion events, had more modest effects (**Figure 4B**). The profound effects of cytochalasin D and bafilomycin A1 on IFNβ induction suggest that Δ*pde2* mutant pneumococci stimulate macrophages after their phagocytosis and phagosomal processing.

The canonical pathway by which pneumococcus and c-di-AMP stimulate IFNβ expression is via STING-mediated activation of IRF3 and IRF7 (29). The early phosphorylation of IRF3 and IRF7 was particularly triggered by infection with the *pde2* mutant (**Figure 5A**), implicating this pathway in the select responses of macrophages to these Δ*pde2* bacteria. To determine if STING was required for IFNβ induction by Pde2-deficient pneumococci, responses were compared between control RAW264.7 cells and STING-deficient RAW264.7 cells. The strong induction of IFNβ by Δ*pde2* mutants was abrogated by the absence of STING (**Figure 5B**).

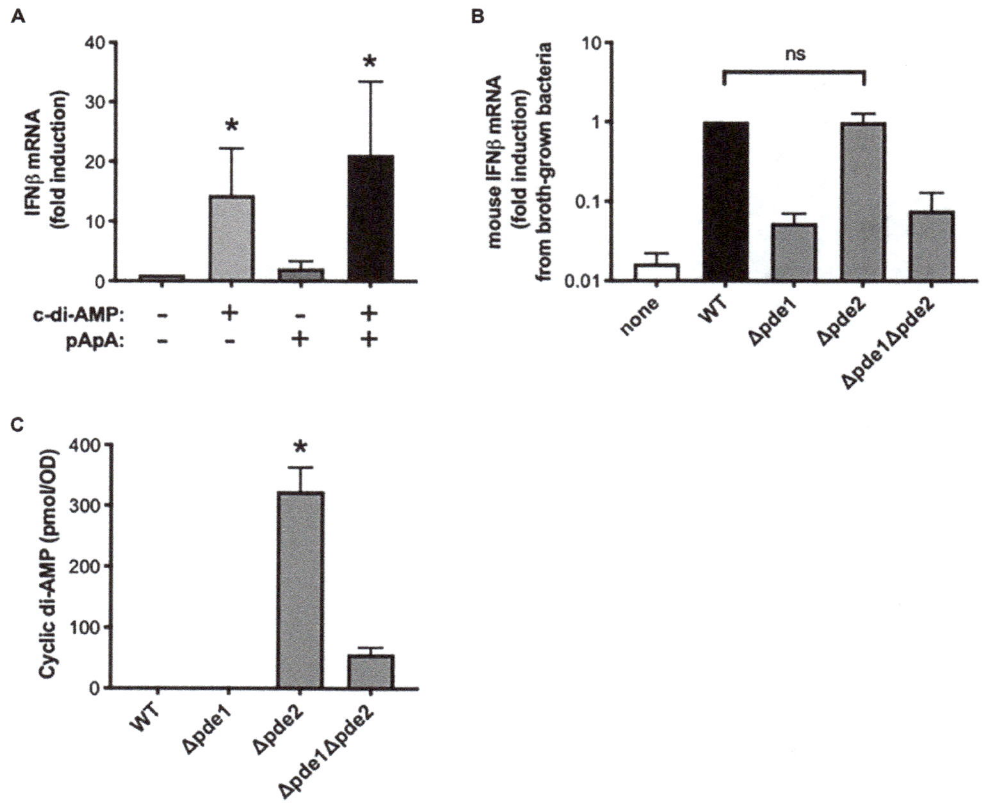

FIGURE 6 | Dinucleotides involved in the distinctive effects of phosphodiesterase 2 mutant pneumococci. **(A)** Relative induction of IFNβ mRNA was measured in human THP-1 cell cultures that were matured to macrophage-like phenotypes using PMA before being stimulated 2 h with the indicated dinucleotides at a final concentration of 30 μg/ml. Human IFNβ mRNA was measured and normalized to 18S rRNA using qPCR, and expressed relative to the unstimulated cells ($N = 3$ experiments). Asterisk (*) indicates $P < 0.05$ compared to unstimulated cells. **(B)** Relative induction of IFNβ mRNA was measured in mouse macrophage-like RAW264.7 cell cultures infected 2 h with the indicated bacteria that were cllected after growth in roth culture instead of on blood agar plates. Mouse IFNβ mRNA was measured and normalized to 18S rRNA using qPCR, and expressed relative to the cells infected by WT bacteria ($N = 3$ experiments). **(C)** Relative c-di-AMP content was measured in pneumococcal cultures that were grown as used throughout experiments (except for in **B**), on inverted tryptic soy agar plates containing 5% sheep's blood and in a 5% CO_2 environment. Cyclic di-AMP was measured using a competitive ELISA ($N = 4$ experiments) and normalized to the bacterial density at a given optical density (OD). Asterisk (*) indicates $P < 0.05$ compared to other bacterial strains. "ns" indicates not significant ($P > 0.05$).

In contrast to IFNβ induction, cell death induced by pde2-deficient bacteria was not abrogated by STING deficiency ($P = 0.15$ from unpaired Student *t*-test on 3 independent experiments; 57 ± 6 and 51 ± 3 percent LDH after 24 h in STING-deficient and control RAW264.7 cells, respectively), dissociating these outcomes and suggesting that this bacteria-induced cell death may not require excessive IFNβ expression. The STING-dependent IFNβ induction was corroborated with independent experiments in which STING expression was knocked down by shRNA in human THP-1 cells. STING knock down inhibited IFNβ induction by the Δ*pde2* mutant pneumococci (**Figure 5C**). The STING-mediated induction of IFNβ stimulated by c-di-AMP requires cGAS (20). In parallel studies of human THP-1 macrophages in which cGAS was targeted by shRNA, induction of IFNβ mRNA by Δ*pde2* mutant pneumococci was reduced by cGAS knock down as effectively as the knock down of STING (**Figure 5C**). Altogether, these results implicate the cGAS-STING and IRF3/IRF7 pathways that mediate IFNβ induction by purified c-di-AMP (20) as underlying mechanisms of the distinctive responses of macrophages to Δ*pde2* mutant pneumococci.

Dinucleotides Connecting the Phosphodiesterase Mutants to IFNβ Induction

Although the pathways activated in macrophages by *pde2*-deficient pneumococci matched those induced by c-di-AMP, the Δ*pde2* mutant pneumococci were not expected to have higher levels of c-di-AMP than the other mutant strains, based on prior analyses (26). We considered whether Pde2 could have unique roles in bacteria that lead to different types of metabolites accumulating. Based on the different substrate specificities of the pneumococcal phosphodiesterases (26), the *pde2* deletion could result in the buildup of pApA in ways that the Δ*pde1* or Δ*pde1*Δ*pde2* mutants would not. To investigate whether excessive pApA could be a contributing factor to the burst of IFNβ expression in macrophages, we tested whether the pApA dinucleotide metabolite could stimulate macrophage IFNβ expression either alone or in combination with c-di-AMP. The pApA metabolite did not stimulate IFNβ expression at doses sufficient for c-di-AMP to do so (**Figure 6A**). Furthermore, no synergistic effects were seen when pApA was added to c-di-AMP (**Figure 6A**). These results do not support a role for pApA in either stimulating or exacerbating macrophage IFNβ expression.

Next, we considered whether the distinct responses of Δ*pde2* mutants could be due to unanticipated effects of phosphodiesterase mutations on c-di-AMP content in these bacteria. Previous studies of these pneumococcal strains reveal increased c-di-AMP in the Δ*pde1* and Δ*pde2* strains, with the greatest increase in the Δ*pde1*Δ*pde2* double mutants (26). We assumed those effects of phosphodiesterase mutations would apply to bacteria in the present studies. However, the present studies involved bacteria grown on blood agar plates in humidified 5% CO_2 environments, designed to enrich for virulence, whereas the prior studies were of bacteria grown in liquid broth and room air. Bacterial growth conditions can influence gene expression and metabolism (32, 33). Unlike with plate-grown bacteria, broth-grown Δ*pde2* mutants did not elicit a stronger induction of IFNβ mRNA compared to WT bacteria (**Figure 6B**), suggesting that mode of growth influences the phenotypes of bacteria and their interactions with macrophages. To investigate effects of the phosphodiesterase mutations on c-di-AMP content in bacteria as grown throughout the current studies (**Figures 1–5**), we measured relative c-di-AMP levels using an ELISA (34) in pneumococci that were grown on blood agar plates. Under these conditions, WT pneumococci did not have detectable c-di-AMP (**Figure 6C**). Similarly, the Δ*pde1* mutant grew with c-di-AMP levels remaining beneath the detection limit (**Figure 6C**). However, the Δ*pde2* and Δ*pde1*Δ*pde2* double mutants accumulated c-di-AMP, with by far the greatest amounts in the Δ*pde2* single mutant bacteria (**Figure 6C**). These data suggest that growth conditions may have substantial effects on c-di-AMP metabolism, and that pneumococcal Pde2 has especially important roles in limiting c-di-AMP during the more biofilm-like and virulence-enhancing growth conditions used here. In conjunction with the prior data revealing distinct IFNβ responses from the Δ*pde2* mutant bacteria, these data strongly support the interpretation that macrophage responses are directly influenced by c-di-AMP levels in pneumococcus during infection.

DISCUSSION

This study suggests that the pneumococcal phosphodiesterase 2 enzyme has distinct and prominent roles in dictating bacterial c-di-AMP content and macrophage innate immunity. Deletion of the phosphodiesterase 2 gene resulted in multiple phenotypes that were not seen with other phosphodiesterase mutants, including pronounced c-di-AMP accumulation. In macrophages, the *pde2*-mutant pneumococci induced a rapid and strong induction of IFNβ and cytotoxicity, neither of which was observed after macrophage interactions with other pneumococci. These results were robust, observed *in vitro* with mouse and human cell lines as well as *in vivo* with primary murine alveolar macrophages. These data highlight a previously unappreciated complexity in how pneumococcal phosphodiesterase enzymes regulate c-di-AMP metabolism in bacteria and immunity in mammals.

It was unexpected that the *pde2*-mutant but not the *pde1*-mutant bacteria would substantially increase c-di-AMP levels in pneumococci grown as cultured here. These data suggest that when cultured on blood agar plates in a 5% CO_2 environment, *pde2* is especially important for catabolizing c-di-AMP. It was further curious that the compound deletion of *pde2* with *pde1* had less pronounced effects, suggesting that other c-di-AMP regulatory mechanisms (24, 25) may compensate to diminish c-di-AMP levels when both of these 2 phosphodiesterase enzymes are absent from pneumococci. The present results with pneumococcus grown on solid media (a more biofilm-like condition) contrast with prior studies of these bacteria grown in a strictly planktonic liquid broth culture (26), suggesting that c-di-AMP metabolism varies across types of bacterial growth. This is plausible given the many roles c-di-AMP plays in bacterial physiology, including evidence that c-di-AMP itself helps determine planktonic vs. biofilm organization in streptococci (22, 35–38). Some virulence factors, like pneumolysin which can induce macrophage cytotoxicity as observed here, are more strongly expressed in biofilm-like growth states of pneumococci (32, 33). During infection, pneumococci transition between biofilm and planktonic phenotypes, and genetically identical pneumococci exhibit markedly different behaviors and transcriptomes in different anatomical sites involving planktonic or biofilm growth (33). In addition, there are different selection pressures on the pneumococcal phosphodiesterase enzymes that catabolize c-di-AMP across infected sites within a host, leading to the emergence of pneumococci with different phosphodiesterase gene mutations in different anatomic sites within infected individuals (39). Altogether, these data suggest strikingly dynamic roles of pneumococcal phosphodiesterases with impacts on c-di-AMP metabolism, pneumococcal phenotype, and infection that are highly context-dependent.

Macrophage signaling in response to c-di-AMP in the context of bacterial infection is incompletely understood. The steps involved in macrophage responses to extracellular cyclic dinucleotides (including c-di-AMP) are different from the pathways by which macrophages respond to cyclic dinucleotides delivered directly into the cytoplasm (20). Notably, extracellular cyclic dinucleotides require phagocytosis and phagosomal acidification before they can gain access to the cytosol (20). The membrane folate antiporter SLC19A1 mediates the transport of c-di-AMP across the membrane from phagosome lumen into cytosol (40). In the cytosol, c-di-AMP is recognized by a cGAS-STING complex which forms a signaling platform that leads to phosphorylation of IRF transcription factors (41). Our studies suggest similar pathways for c-di-AMP signaling during live bacterial infections. The triggering of IFNβ expression by *pde2*-mutant bacteria was prevented by an inhibitor of phagocytosis or of phagosome acidification, by cGAS knockdown, and by STING deficiency or knockdown. These results are consistent with a model in which macrophages ingest bacteria and bacteria-derived c-di-AMP into acidic phagosomes where the bacteria are degraded and c-di-AMP is released into the phagosomal lumen. Transport of c-di-AMP across the membrane into the cytosol then allows signaling via STING and cGAS to activate IRF3- and IRF7-mediated transcription of the gene for IFNβ .

The effects of *pde2* deletion on c-di-AMP metabolism in an *in vivo* infection would be multifactorial. Most importantly, the dysregulation of c-di-AMP metabolism due to phosphodiesterase deletion(s) can be disastrous for pneumococcal physiology, rendering them much more sensitive to diverse stresses including heat, osmotic shock, or UV radiation (26). They grow more slowly, exhibit altered morphology, and display reduced virulence (26, 42). Thus, such bacteria may be less fit or even incapable of effectively establishing infection. However, altered macrophage responses can also impact infection. Increased type I interferons can have complex effects during pneumococcal pneumonia. For example, type I IFN in pneumococcus infected lungs can induce *Sectm1* in lung epithelial cells to recruit neutrophils (43), which augments host defense but increases lung injury risk. Type I IFN signaling to the respiratory epithelium also helps to maintain a vigorous and resilient mucosal barrier against invasive pneumococcal disease (9–11). In contrast to this epithelial resilience, excessive IFNβ induced by *Salmonella* or inflammatory stimuli can kill macrophages by necroptosis (44, 45). In the present studies, the early IFNβ burst but not the later cell death triggered by Pde2-deficient pneumococci required STING, suggesting that excessive IFNβ might not be necessary for the cell death due to this strain of bacteria. Although the Pde2-deficient and c-di-AMP-rich pneumococci rapidly caused macrophage necrosis, the mode of cell death was not defined. Macrophage death can be detrimental during pneumonia in many ways (5). Across pneumococcal strains, those that more rapidly induce necroptosis tend to be more virulent in the lung (27), suggesting this mode of cell death to be a maladaptive pathway during pneumococcal pneumonia. In contrast, macrophage cell death by apoptosis appears to be a healthy response to pneumococcal infection, since specifically preventing macrophage apoptosis results in more severe lung infections (46). Pneumococcus-induced macrophage death is a complicated but important contributor to pneumonia outcomes. More research is needed to understand the natural variations in phosphodiesterase enzymes and c-di-AMP metabolism among pneumococci in the community and how these variations may influence cell death pathways including necroptosis, apoptosis, and more.

Finally, it was curious that all deletions of phosphodiesterase enzymes (*pde1*, *pde2*, or both) caused similar changes in macrophage NF-κB activity, including downstream cytokines like TNFα. Unlike the macrophage IRF phosphorylation, IFNβ induction, and cytotoxicity, macrophage NF-κB activity, and TNFα induction appear to dissociate from the bacterial c-di-AMP content. This could possibly result from non-canonical STING-dependent pathways through which DNA triggers NF-κB (47). These data suggest that some effects of phosphodiesterase enzymes in pneumococcus may be independent from their role in modulating c-di-AMP, implying novel substrates of pneumococcal phosphodiesterases yet to be identified.

The Pde2 enzyme appears to have distinct roles in c-di-AMP metabolism in pneumococci, which vary across growth conditions and perhaps infection settings. Loss of pneumococcal Pde2 function can profoundly elevate c-di-AMP and skew macrophage responses, including a dysregulated burst of IFNβ expression followed quickly by cell death. These results suggest that c-di-AMP in pneumococci is a pivotal factor driving innate immune responses in infection. Pneumococcal c-di-AMP may influence pneumonia and invasive pneumococcal disease. Additional studies should elucidate further the roles of phosphodiesterase 2 in bacterial physiology and host immune responses to pneumococcus.

MATERIALS AND METHODS

Bacteria Strains and Growth Conditions

The strains of *S. pneumoniae* used here have been described in detail (23, 26). Unless otherwise specified, bacteria were grown for 10–15 h at 37°C in a 5% CO_2 environment on inverted tryptic soy agar plates containing 5% sheep blood before being suspended in serum-free and antibiotic-free media to the desired optical density as a means of estimating concentration. For broth-grown bacteria, pneumococci were grown for 8 h in Todd Hewitt Broth with 0.5% Yeast extract (THY) as preculture, and preculture aliquots were used to seed planktonic cultures grown in THY for 6 h to ensure log-phase growth of all bacteria. Bacterial concentrations were initially estimated using optical density and then confirmed *post hoc* using serial dilution CFU assays.

Cell Culture and Infection

For growth and maintenance, RAW264.7 cells (ATCC) were cultured at 37°C with 5% CO_2 in Dulbecco's Modified Eagle's Medium (DMEM, Gibco) supplemented with 10% heat inactivated fetal bovine serum (Gibco), 100 IU of penicillin/mL, and 100 μg/mL of streptomycin. STING-deficient RAW264.7 cells (RAW-Lucia ISG-KO-STING cells; Invivogen) were maintained in the same media with Zeocin supplementation at 200 ug/mL. THP-1 Scrambled, STING knockdown, and cGAS knockdown cells were generated by transducing THP-1 cells with lentiviral vectors expressing shRNA targeting a scrambled sequence (48), STING (48), or cGAS (Sigma, TRCN0000149984), and maintained in RPMI 1640 (Gibco) supplemented with 10% heat inactivated fetal bovine serum (Gibco), 100 IU of penicillin/mL, 100 μg/mL of streptomycin, and 2ug/mL of puromycin, and incubated at 37°C with 5% CO_2. For differentiation of THP-1 cells into a macrophage state, cells were resuspended in culture medium containing 100 nM phorbol myristate acetate (PMA, Sigma) for 24 h. Macrophages were lifted using Versene (Gibco) and replated for infection. For dinucleotide stimulation, pApA and c-di-AMP were purchased (InvivoGen) and added to PMA-matured THP-1 cells to a final concentration of 30 μg/ml. In infection experiments, cells were cultured in antibiotic-free media and *S. pneumoniae* were added at a dose of 10^7 colony forming units (CFU) per well for 2 h at 37°C with 5% CO_2. Indicated experiments included a 30-min preincubation with 2 μM cytochalasin D (Life Technologies), 200 nM bafilomycin A1 (Sigma), 50 μM chloroquine (Sigma), or 5 mM ammonium chloride (Sigma). None of the bacterial strains increased CFU/ml over 2 h in cell culture; while there was a possible trend for living Δ*pde2* and Δ*pde1*Δ*pde2* mutants to decrease more than WT (suggesting poor stress responses), this did not reach statistical significance ($P = 0.10$ across groups in one-way ANOVA). For cell culture infection experiments lasting longer than 2 h, the antibiotic-free media was replaced with antibiotic-containing media after 2 h of culture with live bacteria. Studies with the NFκB-luciferase reporter RA264.7 cell line were performed as previously reported (27, 28).

RNA Preparation and qRT-PCR

Total RNA was isolated with TRIzol reagent (Invitrogen) and Direct-zol RNA Kit (Zymo). qRT-PCR was performed using the RNA-to-Ct kit (Life Technologies) with the following primers and probes – mouse IFNβ: forward 5′-ACAGCCCTCTCCATCAACTATAA-3′, reverse 5′-CATCTT CTCCGTCATCTCCAT-3′, probe 5′-FAM-AGCTCCAGC/ZEN/ TCCAAGAA-3′; mouse TNFα: forward 5′-TCATACCAG GAGAAAGTCAACCTC-3′, reverse 5′-TGGAAGACTCCT CCCAGGTATATG-3′, probe 5′-FAM-TGCCGTCAA/ZEN/ GAGCCCCTG-3′; mouse IL-1β: forward 5′-GCCACCTTTTGA CAGTGATGA-3′, reverse 5′-GATGTGCTGCTGCCGAGA TT-3′, probe 5′-FAM-CTGCTTCCA/ZEN/AACCTTTGA-3′; mouse CXCL10: forward 5′-GGCCATAGGGAAGCTTGAA AT-3′, reverse 5′-GACATCTCTGCTCATCATTCTTT-3′, probe 5′-FAM-ATCGTGGCA/ZEN/ATGATCTCA-3′; mouse 18S ribosomal RNA: forward 5′-ATTCGAACGTCTGCCCTAT CA-3′, reverse 5′-GTCACCCGTGGTCACCATG-3′, probe 5′-FAM-TCGATGGTA/ZEN/GTCGCCGTG-3′. TaqMan Gene Expression Assays for human IFNβ were purchased from Applied Biosystems.

Murine Model of Pneumococcal Pneumonia

C57BL/6 mice were purchased from Jackson Laboratory and housed in a pathogen free environment with access to food and water *ad libitum*. Mice were anesthetized using intraperitoneal injection of ketamine (50 mg/kg) and xylazine (5 mg/kg) and the trachea was surgically exposed. A 50 μL volume containing 10^7 CFU of *S. pneumoniae* of specified strains (or saline vehicle as negative control) was intratracheally instilled via angiocatheter into the left lobe. Three hours after infection, mice were euthanized and the lungs were lavaged with 10 mL of phosphate buffered saline (PBS). Bronchoalveolar lavage cells were isolated by centrifugation and used as sources for RNA purification.

Enzyme Linked Immunosorbent Assay (ELISA)

Cytokine levels of IFNβ were measured in a sandwich ELISA using rat anti-mouse IFNβ mAb (ab24324; Abcam) for capture, rabbit anti-mouse IFNβ polyclonal Ab (32400-1; PBL Biomedical Laboratories) for detection, HRP-conjugated donkey anti-rabbit IgG (711-036-152; Jackson ImmunoResearch Laboratories), and recombinant mouse IFNβ standard (12400-1; PBL Biomedical Laboratories). The detection limit of the IFNβ ELISA was 130 pg/ml. Cytokine levels of TNFα and IL-1β were determined using ELISA kits from R&D systems.

Cell Death Assays

Cell death was measured by supernatant lactate dehydrogenase (LDH) using the Cytotox 96 Non-Radioactive Cytotoxicity Assay (Promega).

Measurement of c-di-AMP

Bacterial strains were grown overnight on tryptic soy agar plates with 5% sheep blood at 37°C with 5% CO_2. *S. pneumoniae* were suspended in DMEM to an OD_{620} of 0.4. After centrifugation of 6-ml aliquots, the bacterial pellets were resuspended in 500 μL 50 mM Tris–HCl pH 8.0 and lysed by sonication, followed by heating for 10 min at 95°C. Quantities of c-di-AMP were measured in the lysates using a competitive ELISA, as described (34). The amount of c-di-AMP was normalized to the bacterial density recorded at OD_{620}.

Statistics

Statistical analyses were performed using GraphPad Prism 8 (GraphPad Software). Data were presented as mean and standard error of the mean (SEM). All data were analyzed by one-way or two-way analysis of variance (ANOVA) with Sidak or Dunnett tests to correct for multiple comparisons. Values were log-transformed prior to analyses if they did not pass the F test for equal variance. Differences with $p < 0.05$ were considered statistically significant.

ETHICS STATEMENT

The animal study was reviewed and approved by the Boston University Institutional Care and Use Committee.

AUTHOR CONTRIBUTIONS

AW, GB, and JM contributed to the conception and overall design of the study. GB generated mutant bacteria and performed c-di-AMP analyses. AW, AS, EA, and IM helped with designing, performing, and interpreting the individual experiments. HA and SG provided tools and insights relevant to STING and cGAS in human cells. AW performed statistical analyses. MJ, LQ, SG, GB, and JM helped with data analyses and interpretations. AW and JM wrote the first draft of the manuscript. JM managed the project. All authors provided help with the written manuscript including revisions and edits, and approved the submitted version.

REFERENCES

1. Walker CLF, Rudan I, Liu L, Nair H, Theodoratou E, Bhutta ZA, et al. Global burden of childhood pneumonia and diarrhoea. *Lancet.* (2013) 381:1405–16. doi: 10.1016/S0140-6736(13)60222-6
2. Quinton LJ, Mizgerd JP. Dynamics of lung defense in pneumonia: resistance, resilience, and remodeling. *Annu Rev Physiol.* (2015) 77:407–30. doi: 10.1146/annurev-physiol-021014-071937
3. Drijkoningen JJ, Rohde GG. Pneumococcal infection in adults: burden of disease. *Clin Microbiol Infect.* (2014) 20(Suppl. 5):45–51. doi: 10.1111/1469-0691.12461
4. Weinberger DM, Malley R, Lipsitch M. Serotype replacement in disease after pneumococcal vaccination. *Lancet (London, England).* (2011) 378:1962–73.
5. Quinton LJ, Walkey AJ, Mizgerd JP. Integrative physiology of pneumonia. *Physiol Rev.* (2018) 98:1417–64. doi: 10.1152/physrev.00032.2017
6. Pittet LA, Quinton LJ, Yamamoto K, Robson BE, Ferrari JD, Algul H, et al. Earliest innate immune responses require macrophage RelA during pneumococcal pneumonia. *Am J Respir Cell Mol Biol.* (2011) 45:573–81. doi: 10.1165/rcmb.2010-0210OC
7. Jones MR, Simms BT, Lupa MM, Kogan MS, Mizgerd JP. Lung NF-kappaB activation and neutrophil recruitment require IL-1 and TNF receptor signaling during pneumococcal pneumonia. *J Immunol.* (2005) 175:7530–5.
8. Gauthier JF, Fortin A, Bergeron Y, Dumas MC, Champagne ME, Bergeron MG. Differential contribution of bacterial N-formyl-methionyl-leucyl-phenylalanine and host-derived CXC chemokines to neutrophil infiltration into pulmonary alveoli during murine pneumococcal pneumonia. *Infect Immun.* (2007) 75:5361–7.
9. Parker D, Martin FJ, Soong G, Harfenist BS, Aguilar JL, Ratner AJ, et al. *Streptococcus pneumoniae* DNA initiates type I interferon signaling in the respiratory tract. *mBio.* (2011) 2:e00016-11. doi: 10.1128/mBio.00016-11
10. LeMessurier KS, Hacker H, Chi L, Tuomanen E, Redecke V. Type I interferon protects against pneumococcal invasive disease by inhibiting bacterial transmigration across the lung. *PLoS Pathog.* (2013) 9:e1003727. doi: 10.1371/journal.ppat.1003727
11. Maier BB, Hladik A, Lakovits K, Korosec A, Martins R, Kral JB, et al. Type I interferon promotes alveolar epithelial type II cell survival during pulmonary *Streptococcus pneumoniae* infection and sterile lung injury in mice. *Eur J Immunol.* (2016) 46:2175–86. doi: 10.1002/eji.201546201
12. Li W, Moltedo B, Moran TM. Type I interferon induction during influenza virus infection increases susceptibility to secondary *Streptococcus pneumoniae* infection by negative regulation of gammadelta T cells. *J Virol.* (2012) 86:12304–12. doi: 10.1128/JVI.01269-12
13. Shahangian A, Chow EK, Tian X, Kang JR, Ghaffari A, Liu SY, et al. Type I IFNs mediate development of postinfluenza bacterial pneumonia in mice. *J Clin Invest.* (2009) 119:1910–20. doi: 10.1172/JCI35412
14. Tian X, Xu F, Lung WY, Meyerson C, Ghaffari AA, Cheng G, et al. Poly I:C enhances susceptibility to secondary pulmonary infections by gram-positive bacteria. *PLoS One.* (2012) 7:e41879. doi: 10.1371/journal.pone.0041879
15. Koppe U, Hogner K, Doehn JM, Muller HC, Witzenrath M, Gutbier B, et al. *Streptococcus pneumoniae* stimulates a STING- and IFN regulatory factor 3-dependent type I IFN production in macrophages, which regulates RANTES production in macrophages, cocultured alveolar epithelial cells, and mouse lungs. *J Immunol.* (2012) 188:811–7. doi: 10.4049/jimmunol.1004143
16. McWhirter SM, Barbalat R, Monroe KM, Fontana MF, Hyodo M, Joncker NT, et al. A host type I interferon response is induced by cytosolic sensing of the bacterial second messenger cyclic-di-GMP. *J Exp Med.* (2009) 206:1899–911. doi: 10.1084/jem.20082874
17. Woodward JJ, Iavarone AT, Portnoy DA. c-di-AMP secreted by intracellular *Listeria monocytogenes* activates a host type I interferon response. *Science.* (2010) 328:1703–5. doi: 10.1126/science.1189801
18. Burdette DL, Monroe KM, Sotelo-Troha K, Iwig JS, Eckert B, Hyodo M, et al. STING is a direct innate immune sensor of cyclic di-GMP. *Nature.* (2011) 478:515–8. doi: 10.1038/nature10429
19. Ruiz-Moreno JS, Hamann L, Jin L, Sander LE, Puzianowska-Kuznicka M, Cambier J, et al. The cGAS/STING pathway detects *Streptococcus pneumoniae* but appears dispensable for antipneumococcal defense in mice and humans. *Infect Immun* (2018) 86:e00849-17. doi: 10.1128/IAI.00849-17
20. Liu H, Moura-Alves P, Pei G, Mollenkopf HJ, Hurwitz R, Wu X, et al. cGAS facilitates sensing of extracellular cyclic dinucleotides to activate innate immunity. *EMBO Rep* (2019) 20:e46293. doi: 10.15252/embr.201846293
21. Corrigan RM, Abbott JC, Burhenne H, Kaever V, Grundling A. c-di-AMP is a new second messenger in *Staphylococcus aureus* with a role in controlling cell size and envelope stress. *PLoS Pathog.* (2011) 7:e1002217. doi: 10.1371/journal.ppat.1002217
22. Fahmi T, Faozia S, Port G, Cho KH. The second messenger c-di-AMP regulates diverse cellular pathways involved in stress response, biofilm formation, cell wall homeostasis, SpeB expression and virulence in *Streptococcus pyogenes. Infect Immun* (2019) 8:e00147-19. doi: 10.1128/IAI.00147-19
23. Bai Y, Yang J, Zarrella TM, Zhang Y, Metzger DW, Bai G. Cyclic di-AMP impairs potassium uptake mediated by a cyclic di-AMP binding protein in *Streptococcus pneumoniae. J Bacteriol.* (2014) 196:614–23. doi: 10.1128/JB.01041-13
24. Commichau FM, Heidemann JL, Ficner R, Stulke J. Making and breaking of an essential poison: the cyclases and phosphodiesterases that produce and degrade the essential second messenger cyclic di-AMP in bacteria. *J Bacteriol* (2019) 201:e00462-18. doi: 10.1128/JB.00462-18
25. Huynh TN, Woodward JJ. Too much of a good thing: regulated depletion of c-di-AMP in the bacterial cytoplasm. *Curr Opin Microbiol.* (2016) 30:22–9. doi: 10.1016/j.mib.2015.12.007
26. Bai Y, Yang J, Eisele LE, Underwood AJ, Koestler BJ, Waters CM, et al. Two DHH subfamily 1 proteins in *Streptococcus pneumoniae* possess cyclic di-AMP phosphodiesterase activity and affect bacterial growth and virulence. *J Bacteriol.* (2013) 195:5123–32. doi: 10.1128/JB.00769-13
27. Coleman FT, Blahna MT, Kamata H, Yamamoto K, Zabinski MC, Kramnik I, et al. Capacity of pneumococci to activate macrophage nuclear factor kappaB: influence on necroptosis and pneumonia severity. *J Infect Dis.* (2017) 216:425–35. doi: 10.1093/infdis/jix159
28. Wilson AA, Kwok LW, Porter EL, Payne JG, McElroy GS, Ohle SJ, et al. Lentiviral delivery of RNAi for in vivo lineage-specific modulation of gene expression in mouse lung macrophages. *Mol Ther.* (2013) 21:825–33. doi: 10.1038/mt.2013.19
29. Devaux L, Kaminski PA, Trieu-Cuot P, Firon A. Cyclic di-AMP in host-pathogen interactions. *Curr Opin Microbiol.* (2018) 41:21–8. doi: 10.1016/j.mib.2017.11.007
30. Ashley CL, Abendroth A, McSharry BP, Slobedman B. Interferon-independent upregulation of interferon-stimulated genes during human cytomegalovirus infection is dependent on IRF3 expression. *Viruses* (2019) 11:246. doi: 10.3390/v11030246
31. Sung PS, Hong SH, Lee J, Park SH, Yoon SK, Chung WJ, et al. CXCL10 is produced in hepatitis a virus-infected cells in an IRF3-dependent but IFN-independent manner. *Sci Rep.* (2017) 7:6387. doi: 10.1038/s41598-017-06784-x
32. Hakansson AP, Orihuela CJ, Bogaert D. Bacterial-host interactions: physiology and pathophysiology of respiratory infection. *Physiol Rev.* (2018) 98:781–811. doi: 10.1152/physrev.00040.2016
33. Shenoy AT, Brissac T, Gilley RP, Kumar N, Wang Y, Gonzalez-Juarbe N, et al. *Streptococcus pneumoniae* in the heart subvert the host response through biofilm-mediated resident macrophage killing. *PLoS Pathog.* (2017) 13:e1006582. doi: 10.1371/journal.ppat.1006582
34. Underwood AJ, Zhang Y, Metzger DW, Bai G. Detection of cyclic di-AMP using a competitive ELISA with a unique pneumococcal cyclic di-AMP binding protein. *J Microbiol Methods.* (2014) 107:58–62. doi: 10.1016/j.mimet.2014.08.026
35. Peng X, Zhang Y, Bai G, Zhou X, Wu H. Cyclic di-AMP mediates biofilm formation. *Mol Microbiol.* (2016) 99:945–59. doi: 10.1111/mmi.13277
36. Du B, Ji W, An H, Shi Y, Huang Q, Cheng Y, et al. Functional analysis of c-di-AMP phosphodiesterase, GdpP, in *Streptococcus suis* serotype 2. *Microbiol Res* (2014) 169:749–58. doi: 10.1016/j.micres.2014.01.002
37. Konno H, Yoshida Y, Nagano K, Takebe J, Hasegawa Y. Biological and biochemical roles of two distinct cyclic dimeric adenosine 3′, 5′-monophosphate- associated phosphodiesterases in *Streptococcus mutans Front Microbiol.* (2018) 9:2347. doi: 10.3389/fmicb.2018.02347
38. Teh WK, Dramsi S, Tolker-Nielsen T, Yang L, Givskov M. Increased intracellular cyclic di-AMP levels sensitize *Streptococcus gallolyticus* subsp.

gallolyticus to osmotic stress and reduce biofilm formation and adherence on intestinal cells. *J Bacteriol.* (2019) 201:e00597-18. doi: 10.1128/JB.00597-18

39. Lees JA, Brouwer M, van der Ende A, Parkhill J, van de Beek D, Bentley SD. Within-host sampling of a natural population shows signs of selection on Pde1 during bacterial meningitis. *Infect Immun.* (2017) 85:e01061-16.
40. Luteijn RD, Zaver SA, Gowen BG, Wyman SK, Garelis NE, Onia L, et al. SLC19A1 transports immunoreactive cyclic dinucleotides. *Nature.* (2019) 573:434–8. doi: 10.1038/s41586-019-1553-0
41. Ablasser A, Goldeck M, Cavlar T, Deimling T, Witte G, Röhl I, et al. cGAS produces a 2'-5'-linked cyclic dinucleotide second messenger that activates STING. *Nature.* (2013) 498:380–384. doi: 10.1038/nature12306
42. Cron LE, Stol K, Burghout P, van Selm S, Simonetti ER, Bootsma HJ, et al. Two DHH subfamily 1 proteins contribute to pneumococcal virulence and confer protection against pneumococcal disease. *Infect Immun.* (2011) 79:3697–710. doi: 10.1128/IAI.01383-10
43. Kamata H, Yamamoto K, Wasserman GA, Zabinski MC, Yuen CK, Lung WY, et al. Epithelial cell-derived secreted and transmembrane 1a signals to activated neutrophils during pneumococcal pneumonia. *Am J Respir Cell Mol Biol.* (2016) 55:407–18. doi: 10.1165/rcmb.2015-0261OC
44. Robinson N, McComb S, Mulligan R, Dudani R, Krishnan L, Sad S. Type I interferon induces necroptosis in macrophages during infection with *Salmonella enterica* serovar Typhimurium. *Nat Immunol.* (2012) 13:954–62. doi: 10.1038/ni.2397
45. McComb S, Cessford E, Alturki NA, Joseph J, Shutinoski B, Startek JB, et al. Type-I interferon signaling through ISGF3 complex is required for sustained Rip3 activation and necroptosis in macrophages. *Proc Natl Acad Sci USA.* (2014) 111:E3206–13. doi: 10.1073/pnas.1407068111
46. Preston JA, Bewley MA, Marriott HM, McGarry Houghton A, Mohasin M, Jubrail J, et al. Alveolar macrophage apoptosis-associated bacterial killing helps prevent murine pneumonia. *Am J Respir Crit Care Med.* (2019) 200:84–97. doi: 10.1164/rccm.201804-0646OC
47. Dunphy G, Flannery SM, Almine JF, Connolly DJ, Paulus C, Jonsson KL, et al. Non-canonical activation of the DNA sensing adaptor STING by ATM and IFI16 mediates NF-kappaB signaling after nuclear DNA damage. *Mol Cell* (2018) 71:745–60.e5. doi: 10.1016/j.molcel.2018.07.034
48. Akiyama H, Miller CM, Ettinger CR, Belkina AC, Snyder-Cappione JE, Gummuluru S. HIV-1 intron-containing RNA expression induces innate immune activation and T cell dysfunction. *Nat Commun.* (2018) 9:3450.

8

Out-Smarting the Host: Bacteria Maneuvering the Immune Response to Favor their Survival

***Nastaran Mues*† *and Hong Wei Chu**†**

Department of Medicine, National Jewish Health, Denver, CO, United States

****Correspondence:***
Hong Wei Chu
ChuH@NJHealth.org

† These authors have contributed equally to this work

Bacteria adapt themselves to various environmental conditions in nature, which can lead to bacterial adaptation and persistence in the host as commensals or pathogens. In healthy individuals, host defense mechanisms prevent the opportunistic bacteria/commensals from becoming a pathological infection. However, certain pathological conditions can impair normal defense barriers leading to bacterial survival and persistence. Under pathological conditions such as chronic lung inflammation, bacteria employ various mechanisms from structural changes to protease secretion to manipulate and evade the host immune response and create a niche permitting commensal bacteria to thrive into infections. Therefore, understanding the mechanisms by which pathogenic bacteria survive in the host tissues and organs may offer new strategies to overcome persistent bacterial infections. In this review, we will discuss and highlight the complex interactions between airway pathogenic bacteria and immune responses in several major chronic inflammatory diseases such as asthma and chronic obstructive pulmonary disease (COPD).

Keywords: toll like receptors, bacterial infection, immune response, airways, inflammation

INTRODUCTION

Human lungs are in constant interaction with different bacteria and bacterial particles and are exposed to a variety of environmental threats. The healthy human lungs used to be considered sterile, but recent studies have reshaped this belief. In fact, human lungs are colonized with diverse bacteria including the genera *Prevotella, Streptococcus, Klebsiella, Veillonella, Neisseria, Haemophilus, pseudomonas, and Fusobacterium* (1, 2). These bacterial species can particularly persist in the lungs and often give rise to super infections particularly followed by viral infections. Microbes maintain a lower density in a healthy lung (about 10^3–10^5 CFU per gram of the tissue) as compared to the gut with a load of 10^{11} CFU per gram of the tissue. It has been shown that in airway chronic inflammatory diseases such as asthma, there is a shift in the lung microbiota toward a greater diversity in species richness (3).

Normal human lung resident cells such as macrophages and epithelial cells employ a complex defense mechanism to cope with the pathogenic infection vs. commensal bacteria and their products. The innate immune response is the first line of defense that protects the lungs from pathogenic microbes and their secreted products. The lung epithelium cells act as a barrier with goblet cells secreting mucus and ciliated cells transporting mucus containing microbes and microbial particles away from the distal lung. In chronic respiratory diseases, such as cystic fibrosis (CF), COPD, and asthma, mucus hypersecretion and dysfunctional ciliated cells can disturb this barrier leading to less to no clearance of the bacteria from the lungs (3–5). Alveolar macrophages act as the primary phagocytes of the innate immunity in the lung. Airway epithelial cells and macrophages also secrete inflammatory cytokines in response to pathogens and their particles (6). Immune system utilizes several pathways such as toll like receptors (TLRs), NOD like receptors (NLRs), and inflammasome to recognize microbial particles and induce the production of antimicrobial proteins and peptides like lyzozymes, defensins and cathelicidines that effectively stop microbial infection (7–9). Some of these antimicrobial peptides like defensins and cathelicidines have chemotactic properties and recruit immune cells like macrophages and neutrophils to the site of infection (10, 11).

Although inflammation is a pivotal response to microbial infections, it may damage the host cells or tissues and create an environment that allows pathogenic bacteria to employ evading mechanisms to outsmart the host for their survival and persistence. The major goal of this review is to present some unique survival mechanisms exploited by several strains of bacteria commonly seen in lung infectious and inflammatory processes related to the utilization of the host TLR signaling pathways. In addition, our review is mainly focused on the evasion of bacterial infection in chronic inflammatory lung diseases, and there is no doubt that these examples only scratch the surface of this forthcoming research area. We foresee that current research is moving toward investigating bacterial infections in specific niche environments of the host, and that these insights discussed here can enhance our perspective in which the pathogen evade the immune system.

TLRS SIGNALING: A TWO-EDGE SWORD IN BACTERIAL INFECTION OF ASTHMATIC OR ALLERGIC AIRWAYS

Toll like receptors are a family of highly conserved and pattern recognition receptors (PRRs) that bind to microbial pathogen associated molecular patterns (PAMPs) also called microbial associated molecular patterns (MAMPs). TLRs also bind to endogenous molecules released from the host dying cells known as danger associated molecular pattern (DAMPs). Different TLRs are expressed on different cell types including immune cells and airway epithelial cells and bind to different ligands, which upon activation in healthy individuals can promote an appropriate inflammatory response. TLR ligands consists of, but not limited to, bacterial cell wall components like lipopolysaccharides (LPS) in Gram-negative bacteria and teichoic acid in Gram-positive bacteria, viral double stranded RNA, single stranded or double stranded DNA, flagellin, etc (5, 12). TLRs are transmembrane receptors that contain a leucine rich extracellular domain and a highly conserved Toll interleukin-1 receptor (TIR) domain. So far, there have been 10 human and 12 murine TLRs identified, and each recognizes a specific set of molecular pattern. In humans, TLR1, 2, 4, 5, and 6 reside on the cell membrane, while TLR3, 7, 8, and 9 are located in endosomes, lysosomes, or endoplasmic reticulum (ER). Upon binding to their ligand, TLRs initiate the inflammatory response by activating their target downstream signaling pathways, including the recruitment of adaptor proteins such as myeloid differentiation factor 88 (MyD88) to the TIR domain. MyD88 activates downstream signaling targets including IRAK family kinases and results in activation of transcription factors of nuclear factor-κB (NF-κB), mitogen-activated protein kinases (MAPK), and activator protein-1 (AP-1). These transcription factors facilitate up-regulation of pro-inflammatory cytokines and type I interferons transcription (13).

Toll like receptors-mediated proper inflammatory response in healthy individuals leads to inflammation induction and bacterial clearance from the lungs. In the field of experimental asthma and allergic airways, the pre-existing type 2 inflammation environment reduces normal TLR function to allow the bacteria to survive and hide from the immune response in part by inhibiting the production of antimicrobial substances (**Figure 1**). The persistence of bacteria in turn attempts to suppress the type 2 inflammatory response, but it may fail to do so, leading to asthma exacerbations. One of the mechanisms is that bacterial products can hijack the immune system for their benefit by recruiting regulatory T cells (14, 15). Efforts of reducing inflammation can be at the cost of higher risk of opportunistic/commensal bacteria persistence in the lungs as an appropriate pro-inflammatory response is critical to recruit leukocytes such as neutrophils to eliminate pathogens. Collectively, insufficient TLR signaling activation by bacteria in allergic airways and asthma may lead to bacterial survival and persistence.

EVADING MECHANISMS OF BACTERIA IN LUNG DISEASES

Patients with chronic airway inflammatory diseases are generally susceptible to opportunistic bacterial infections that can persist from months or even years. Notably, about more than 50% of COPD infective exacerbations are due to bacterial infections (16). These infections can cause disease exacerbations and promote disease progression. Here, we will discuss how several common bacterial species utilize their tactics to evade the host effective defending mechanisms.

NON-TYPEABLE *HAEMOPHILUS INFLUENZAE*, AN UNWANTED GUEST IN SMALL AIRWAYS

Non-typeable *Haemophilus influenzae* (NTHi) is a non-capsulated Gram-negative bacterium, which resides in human nasopharynx as a common commensal. Interestingly, NTHi is a common opportunistic and human exclusive pathogen bacterium of lower respiratory tract and small airways causing chronic and repetitive infections and structural damages especially in COPD patients (17). It has consistently been shown that NTHi can survive in the lungs by attaching and or entering human airway epithelial cells (18–20). NTHi invasion and entry into airway epithelial cells can be through microvilli and lamellipodia extensions of epithelial cells that form a vesicle

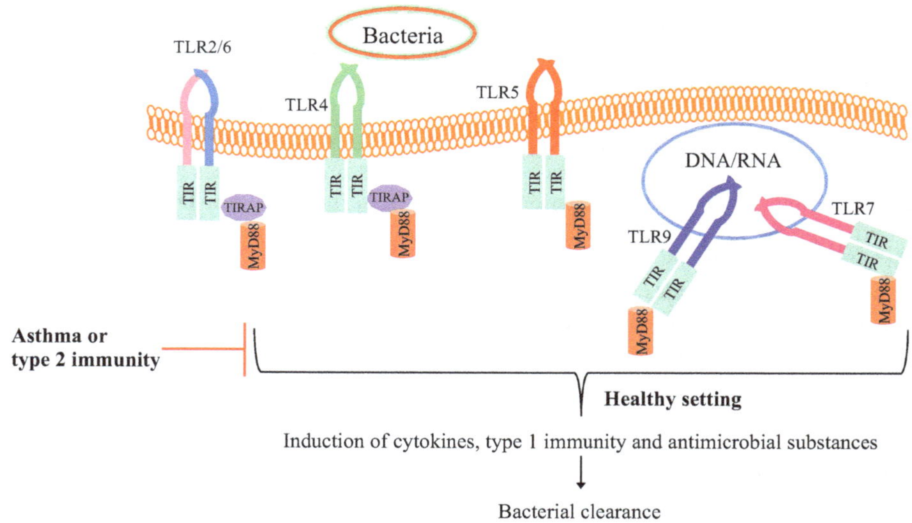

FIGURE 1 | TLR signaling in healthy individuals and asthmatics. Bacteria and their components bind to TLRs on the cell membrane (TLR2/6, TLR4, or TLR5) or enter the cell cytoplasm and bind to endosomal TLRs (TLR 7 or TLR9). Upon binding the bacterial particle to its receptor, TLR recruit MyD88 and subsequently induce host defense cytokines and antimicrobial mediators as well as the type 1 immune response, enhancing bacterial clearance from the tissue (e.g., lung). However, in allergic asthma or type 2 inflammation environment, TLR activity is dampened, which allows the bacteria to survive and hide from the normal defense mechanisms.

around the live bacteria and facilitate NTHi entrance into these cells (21). Additionally, the role of actin and tubulin cytoskeletons was confirmed in NTHi internalization since inhibiting actin and tubulin construction with Cytochalasin D and colchicine, constrained NTHi invasion into epithelial cells (18, 20, 22). Another mechanism for NTHi cell entry is endocytosis mediated by lipid rafts since lipid raft inhibitors were able to hinder NTHi invasion (23). Lipid rafts are cholesterol enriched areas on the epithelial cells plasma membrane that play pivotal roles in trafficking and signal transduction (24). Receptor mediated endocytosis or Clathrin mediated endocytosis was suggested as a possible way for the NTHi bacteria to invade airway epithelial cells and alveolar macrophages and evade the immune system by hiding in these cells (21, 25). NTHi infection has been shown to reduce E-cadherin, a protein required for tight junction formation and airway epithelial integrity (26). The mechanism in which NTHi reduces E-cadherin in airway epithelial cells is currently unknown. Nonetheless, NTHi-mediated reduction of E-cadherin in airway epithelial cells can lead to bacterial colonization at the basal lamina and result in perturbations of the airway epithelial cell barrier (27).

Recent studies have emphasized on the important role of NTHi-derived human IgA-protease B1 and B2 in cleaving human lysosomal-associated membrane protein 1 (LAMP1) that mediates NTHi survival inside the airway epithelial cells (17, 28) The mechanism by which LAMP1 cleavage results in NTHi survival within the airway epithelial cells needs to be further studied. Additionally, NTHi secreted IgA protease cleaves the human IgA_1. IgA attaches to the bacteria and this attachment prevents binding of NTHi to the epithelial cells and inactivates the bacterial toxins (29). Remarkably, the secreted IgA levels in COPD and asthma patients are reduced compared to healthy individuals (30). By cleaving the remaining IgA in airways, NTHi can escape the immune surveillance of IgA to facilitate their survival within the cells.

By hiding in airway epithelial cells and undergo structural changes, secreting proteases and reducing host defense mediators, NTHi can cause repetitive and chronic infections of the lower respiratory tract.

EVADING MECHANISMS BY *KLEBSIELLA PNEUMONIAE*

Klebsiella pneumoniae (Kp) is a Gram-negative bacterium most commonly known as a pulmonary pathogen (31). Kp infection has gained more attention due to its immunomodulatory effects and antibiotic resistance features. Interestingly, it has been shown in asthma and allergic inflammation environments, the lung Kp burden increases (32).

Klebsiella pneumoniae can overcome the human immune system and cause persistent infections in the lung. One mechanism employed by Kp to survive within the airways is to reduce airway neutrophil production of α-defensin, an antimicrobial peptide. Thijs et al. demonstrated that the nasal levels of α-defensins are significantly lower in asthma patients who are more susceptible to Kp infections (33). Furthermore, Kp hijacks airway cells by employing deubiquitinase cylindromatosis (CYLD) that is involved in NF-κB signaling inactivation (34, 35). Additionally, Kp can inhibit the production of inflammatory mediators and α-defensins from airway epithelial cells through inhibiting MAPK signaling pathway by upregulating MAPK phosphatase-1 (MKP-1) and activating nucleotide-binding oligomerization domain-containing protein 1 (NOD1). NOD1 is an intracellular PRR that responds to bacterial particles. MKP-1 and CYLD can synergistically inhibit production of neutrophil chemoattractant IL-8 from airway epithelial cells (36–38). Manipulating the immune system with these mechanisms can contribute to persistence of Kp infections in the lung. It has been shown that Kp-specific Outer membrane protein A (OmpA) favors an anti-inflammatory response in early stages of pneumonia (39). Fagundes et al. demonstrated that Kp infection in germfree mice was able to induce IL-10 production in the lung and inhibit the inflammatory response development by restricting production of pro-inflammatory mediators (40). Furthermore, Kp exploits the IL-10 production to attenuate the innate immune response through activation of its downstream target signal transducer and activator of transcription 3 (STAT3) (41). Interestingly, Greenberger et al. showed that neutralizing and inhibiting IL-10 was able to enhance the Kp clearance from the lung (42). To further support role of IL-10 in Kp infection, Dolgachey et al. showed that overexpression of IL-10 in the lung of Kp infected mice significantly increased bacterial survival and mouse mortalities (43).

In summary, Kp exploits several mechanisms to evade host immune system in order to persist in the lungs, which include inhibition of anti-inflammatory peptides, host defense inflammatory cytokines and chemokines, and promotion of anti-inflammatory cytokines.

PSEUDOMONAS AERUGINOSA IMPAIRS HUMAN AIRWAY INNATE IMMUNITY

Pseudomonas aeruginosa (Pa), is a Gram-negative opportunistic bacterium that causes acute infections in patients with CF, COPD, ventilator-associated pneumonia, and bronchiectasis (44). This facultative anaerobe bacterium is capable of adhering to human airway epithelial cells via their flagellum, pili, and other cell membrane components (45). Pa secretes several virulence factors that potentially sabotage innate immunity (45, 46).

In CF airway chronic Pa infection, the bacterium changes from an active moving form to a passive form by down-regulating its flagellin expression (47). Pa flagellin is one of the best known PAMPs that activate TLR5 signaling pathway through MyD88 and induce multiple pro-inflammatory cytokines (IL-8, IL-1ß) from airway epithelial cells and macrophages to recruit neutrophils and other inflammatory cells into the airways (48–50). Pa uses different strategies to escape the protective role of flagellin-mediated host immune response. Notably, Pa can secrete alkaline protease AprA and elastase LasB, which cleave the exogenous flagellin as a mechanism to evade flagellin mediated immune responses (47). Interestingly, degradation of flagellin monomers by AprA and LasB can reduce TLR5 activation induced inflammatory responses (47). In addition, Pa secretes other proteases including LasA and protease IV. These proteases interact with a wide range of molecules including the host and the bacteria as mentioned above, resulting in structural component and inflammatory mediator degradation and dampening the immune responses. Pa proteases have been shown to degrade a variety of host defense mediators and components including but not limited to IL-8, CXCL1, CXCL5, IFN-γ, IL-6, immunoglobulins, and antimicrobial peptides (51–54).

The effects of elastase LasB in modulating the immune response during Pa infections have been well studied. Pa exploits LasB to inhibit alveolar macrophages oxidative burst and down-regulate reactive oxygen species (ROS) generation during phagocytosis (55). LasB is also involved in degradation of surfactant protein SP-A resulting in phagocytosis resistance of the bacteria (56, 57). Another LasB dependent immune modulating function is lysis of the thrombin protein resulting in formation of the FYT21 peptide that inhibits the activation of transcription factors NF-κB and AP-1 (58). Remarkably, asthma patients have about 20% more thrombin concentration compared to healthy individuals (59).

An additional strategy developed by Pa in chronic infections is that it is capable of halting the expression of the type III secretion system (T3SS) (60). T3SS is a needle like secretion machinery complex in Gram-negative bacteria that injects bacterial effectors into the host cells (61). This machinery complex has been implicated in pathogenesis of acute Pa infections by causing tissue damage and bacterial spreading (62, 63). By inhibiting T3SS expression, bacteria escape T3SS mediated inflammasome activation by chronic Pa infection in CF patients (64).

Notably, Pa can form biofilms, a specific bacteria self-aggregates via their extracellular matrix to form a multicellular matrix (65). The host response to Pa biofilm is rather intricate since it can both incite or inhibit the immune response. It has been shown that during the biofilm stage, Pa down-regulates flagellin and T3SS resulting in lower complement system activation (66–68). On the other hand, biofilms can conceal the surface bacterial factors from the host and helping Pa to evade the immune system. In contrast, Pa biofilms can stimulate the neutrophilic response and furthermore cause necrotic killing of neutrophils leading to a further robust inflammation and tissue damage (69, 70).

Mucoid Pa, the most common in CF chronic infections, produces excess amount of extracellular polysaccharide alginate called mucoidy (71). It has been shown that over-production of alginate can impair the immune response and allow for persistence of the bacteria with different strategies. Alginate interferes with opsonic phagocytosis and compliment system activation and disrupts ROS production during phagocytosis (65, 72). Alginate is also responsible for bacterial resistance to antimicrobial peptides like LL-37 (73). Furthermore, it has been shown that due to co-regulation of alginate and flagellin, mucoidy can inhibit synthesis of flagellin and thus reduce TLR5 activation (74, 75).

Another adaptive mechanism in which Pa escapes the host immune system is synthetic and structural changes to LPS in chronic infections. LPS structure is recognized by TLR4 and is composed of three components: lipid A, core oligosaccharide, and the O antigen. The O antigen is the main component which shows high variability in immunogenic oligosaccharides and interacts with extracellular surroundings (76). During Pa chronic infection, the bacterial LPS undergoes adaptive structural and synthetic changes which results in lipid A modification/acetylation, loss of O antigen polysaccharide, and downregulation of LPS synthesis (76). These adaptive changes are considered to be possible mechanisms that Pa exploits to escape the immune system perhaps through being unrecognizable to TLR4 (77). Moreover, lipid A undergoes acetylation, which prevents binding of host antimicrobial peptides to the bacteria (78). It seems that Pa causing the chronic infection has more tendency to undergo genetic mutations resulting in significant lower expression to no expression of the O antigen involved in lower clearance of the bacteria from the lungs of CF patients (79–81).

Together, Pa uses various mechanisms to sustain lung chronic infections, such as reducing the recognition of flagellin by TLR5 and LPS by TLR4 through cleaving the TLR ligands, degrading host immune mediators or their transcription factors via secreting proteases, undergoing structural changes like forming biofilm, and producing excess amount of mucoid to evade host defense mechanisms and persist in the lungs.

CRAFTY *STAPHYLOCOCCUS AUREUS* MANIPULATES HOST IMMUNE RESPONSES

Staphylococcus aureus (Sa) is a Gram-positive bacterium contributing to a range of diseases. Sa is a commensal of the human nose without showing any symptoms, but it can cause life-threatening diseases like pneumonia, endocarditis and septicemia (82). Sa is not an intracellular pathogen, but it can bind the epithelial and macrophage cell surface type F scavenger receptor SREC-I through the bacterial glycol-polymer cell wall teichoic acid (83). Furthermore, clumping factor B (ClfB) and iron-regulated surface determinant A (IsdA) are also involved in adherence of Sa to epithelial cells (84).

One of the mechanisms by which Sa can evade the immune system of the lung is to produce peptides that disturb accumulation of the complement system on the surface of the bacteria. Staphylococcal immunoglobulin binding protein (Sbi) depletes complement factor 3 (C3) (85). Moreover, the chemotaxis inhibitory protein of Sa (CHIPS) hinders the function of complement factor C5a. CHIPS also impedes the function of formylated peptide receptors on neutrophils that are required for neutrophil chemotaxis and recruitment to the site of infection (86).

There are multiple Sa proteases that can play a pivotal role in dampening the innate immune system. One of these proteases is Staphopain A, a serine protease, cleaves the N terminal domain of CXCR2, which inhibits the binding of CXCR2 to its ligand IL-8 and subsequently neutrophil chemotaxis and activation (87) Meanwhile, Staphopain B can cleave CD31, a member of immunoglobulin superfamily, expressed on neutrophils, and lead to reduced functionality of neutrophils (88). Besides, the Zn dependent metalloprotease, Aureolysin, can cleave and deactivate LL-37, an antimicrobial peptide (89). Another mechanism employed by Sa to dampen the immune system is by expressing a sortase anchored protein to dephosphorylate and activate adenosine (90). Adenosine is an effective mediator of the immune response and it binds to different G proteins coupled receptors. Upon binding adenosine to its receptor, the anti-inflammatory signaling pathways activate and result in inhibition of neutrophils degranulation and superoxide burst, platelet aggregation, and secretion of anti-inflammatory cytokine IL-10 from the innate immune cells (91).

Coagulation is the conversion of the fibrinogen to fibrin by activated thrombin and forming fibrin clots. Coagulation is one of the innate immunity defense mechanisms involved in immobilization of the bacteria and recruiting/activating the immune cells to the lungs to clear the bacteria by phagocytosis. Sa secretes coagulase (Coa) and von Willebrand Factor-binding protein (vWbp) which activate a prothrombin named staphylothrombin that only cleaves fibrinogen A and B peptides and creates fibrils of fibrin (92). Staphylothrombin avoids clotting activation and inflammation by only cleaving fibrinogen A and B but not other thrombin substrates (93, 94).

In summary, Sa utilizes a variety of elaborated mechanisms to evade the immune response including adhering to the epithelial cells and other airway innate immune cells, disrupting and depleting the complement system and neutrophil macrophages, cleaving and deactivating antimicrobial peptides, and activating adenosine mediated anti-inflammatory signaling pathways. These mechanisms may contribute to antibiotic resistance of Sa, and thus need to be further investigated for developing alternative therapies.

NON-TUBERCULOUS MYCOBACTERIA VEIL FROM THE HOST IMMUNE SYSTEM

Non-tuberculous mycobacterium (NTM) has emerged as a significant cause of infection in the lungs of immunocompromized patients or patients with CF, COPD, and bronchiectasis. Different from *Mycobacterium tuberculosis*, NTMs are opportunistic bacteria that can cause airways infection in altered lung environment specifically in chronic inflammatory lung diseases (95, 96). Interestingly, patients under corticosteroid therapies are more susceptible to NTM infections. The underlying mechanism of this susceptibility is unknown.

Non-tuberculous mycobacterium bacteria are composed of more than 170 species with various virulence potencies. Among these species, *Mycobacterium avium* and *Mycobacterium abscessus* are the most frequent causes of NTM related pulmonary diseases (95–100).

Wide spectrum antibiotic resistances of NTMs are well studied but these bacteria also benefit from a variety of mechanisms that they can exploit and evade the immune system.

Non-tuberculous mycobacterium can grow inside and outside of cells. *M. avium* and *M. abscessus* can reside within macrophages and hide from the immune system and anti-microbial mediators. *M. avium* can be discharged from macrophages and infect other macrophages and spread (101). In contrast, *M. abscessus* is able to deter phagocytosis by restricting

intra-phagosomal acidification and as a result persist within macrophages (102, 103).

Defective cilia functionality and excess mucus in the lungs of patients with chronic inflammatory lung diseases allow persistence of the bacteria. It has been shown that *M. abscessus* can enter a slow growth phase and persist better in the mucus of CF patients (104, 105).

Another mechanism in which *M. avium* and *M. abscessus* escape the immune response is to form biofilms. NTMs can develop biofilms within thickened alveolar airways in CF patients or within the lung cavities of COPD patients (106, 107). The biofilm can create a shield to prevent antimicrobial mediators penetration and allow persistence of the bacteria in the lungs (108–111).

Interestingly, the smooth variant of *M. abscessus* expresses glycopeptidolipid (GPL), which has been shown to mask the bioactive, immunostimulatory cell wall lipids of the bacteria. This coverage results in becoming unrecognizable from the TLRs and inhibition of production of inflammatory mediators and antimicrobial peptides and the innate immune response (112).

Therefore, NTMs continue to pose a huge health concern especially in patients with compromised immunity as they undergo physiological adaptations and mechanisms in the lung, such as persisting within macrophages or deterring phagocytosis, entering a slow growth phase, and masking immunostimulatory cell wall components via GPL expression or biofilm formation.

CONCLUSION AND PERSPECTIVES

One of the pivotal responsibilities of the immune system is to induce an appropriate inflammatory response to colonizing pathogens. However, many of these pathogens exploit diseased environments and impaired defense mechanisms in the host to develop various strategies and genetic polymorphisms to either stimulate tolerance, escape the immune response, or manipulate the immune system to survive in the body. As mentioned above, in allergic airways, pathogenic bacteria either inactivate the TLRs to modulate the immune system to their benefit or become unrecognizable to the TLRs. One example is Pa in CF airways reducing its flagellin expression and evades the consequences of being recognized by TLR5 to induce inflammation. Reducing anti-microbial peptides and inflammatory mediators, increasing anti-inflammatory mediators, secreting proteases, hiding within the host cells, and structural changes are other mechanisms employed by bacteria in chronic inflammatory airway diseases resulting in reduced clearance of the pathogens and persistence of the bacterial infection in the lungs of these patients. Current studies are exploring the immune response evasion mechanisms of pathogenic bacteria in disease environments. Under the circumstances that host diseased environment can affect the pathogenicity and persistence of the bacteria in the lungs is a significant area of ongoing research.

In the future, the mechanisms behind differential regulation and functions of TLRs in healthy individuals vs. patients in various host environments should be considered for further investigation aimed to unravel this complex system. Moreover, the host and pathogen factors that help pathogens evolve very sophisticated strategies to evade the immune system and inflammation should be further determined. For example, how therapies like corticosteroids commonly used in chronic inflammatory diseases such as COPD and asthma affect bacterial evading mechanisms remain unclear, and could be carefully evaluated. Given significant growth of antibiotic resistant bacterial strains, new therapies targeting the host rather than the bacteria can be developed to allow the host to outsmart the pathogens.

AUTHOR CONTRIBUTIONS

Both authors listed have made a substantial, direct and intellectual contribution to the work, and approved it for publication.

ACKNOWLEDGMENTS

We would like to thank the investigators working in this field and apologize to ones whose work was not cited in this review article.

REFERENCES

1. Hilty M, Burke C, Pedro H, Cardenas P, Bush A, Bossley C, et al. Disordered microbial communities in asthmatic airways. *PLoS One.* (2010) 5:e8578. doi: 10.1371/journal.pone.0008578
2. O'Dwyer DN, Dickson RP, Moore BB. The lung microbiome, immunity, and the pathogenesis of chronic lung disease. *J Immunol.* (2016) 196:4839–47. doi: 10.4049/jimmunol.1600279
3. Mathieu E, Escribano-Vazquez U, Descamps D, Cherbuy C, Langella P, Riffault S, et al. Paradigms of lung microbiota functions in health and disease, particularly, in asthma. *Front Physiol.* (2018) 9:1168. doi: 10.3389/fphys.2018.01168
4. Cohen TS, Prince A. Cystic fibrosis: a mucosal immunodeficiency syndrome. *Nat Med.* (2012) 18:509–19. doi: 10.1038/nm.2715
5. Su Y-C, Jalalvand F, Thegerström J, Riesbeck K. The interplay between immune response and bacterial infection in COPD: focus upon non-typeable *Haemophilus influenzae. Front Immunol.* (2018) 9:2530. doi: 10.3389/fimmu.2018.02530
6. Lafferty EI, Qureshi ST, Schnare M. The role of toll-like receptors in acute and chronic lung inflammation. *J Inflamm.* (2010) 7:57–57. doi: 10.1186/1476-9255-7-57
7. Ganz T. Defensins: antimicrobial peptides of innate immunity. *Nat Rev Immunol.* (2003) 3:710–20. doi: 10.1136/ard.62.suppl_2.ii17
8. Vladimer GI, Marty-Roix R, Ghosh S, Weng D, Lien E. Inflammasomes and host defenses against bacterial infections. *Curr Opin Microbiol.* (2013) 16:23–31. doi: 10.1016/j.mib.2012.11.008
9. Askarian F, Van Sorge NM, Sangvik M, Beasley FC, Henriksen JR, Sollid JUE, et al. A *Staphylococcus aureus* TIR domain protein virulence factor

blocks TLR2-mediated NF-κB signaling. *J Innate Immun.* (2014) 6:485–98. doi: 10.1159/000357618

10. De Y, Chen Q, Schmidt AP, Anderson GM, Wang JM, Wooters J, et al. LL-37, the neutrophil granule- and epithelial cell-derived cathelicidin, utilizes formyl peptide receptor-like 1 (FPRL1) as a receptor to chemoattract human peripheral blood neutrophils, monocytes, and T cells. *J Exp Med.* (2000) 192:1069–74. doi: 10.1084/jem.192.7.1069
11. Cole AM, Ganz T, Liese AM, Burdick MD, Liu L, Strieter RM. Cutting edge: IFN-inducible ELR CXC chemokines display defensin-like antimicrobial activity. *J Immunol.* (2001) 167:623. doi: 10.4049/jimmunol.167.2.623
12. Zakeri A, Russo M. Dual role of toll-like receptors in human and experimental asthma models. *Front Immunol.* (2018) 9:1027. doi: 10.3389/fimmu.2018.01027
13. Gu J, Liu Y, Xie B, Ye P, Huang J, Lu Z. Roles of toll-like receptors: from inflammation to lung cancer progression. *Biomed Rep.* (2018) 8:126–32. doi: 10.3892/br.2017.1034
14. Navarro S, Cossalter G, Chiavaroli C, Kanda A, Fleury S, Lazzari A, et al. The oral administration of bacterial extracts prevents asthma via the recruitment of regulatory T cells to the airways. *Mucosal Immunol.* (2011) 4:53–65. doi: 10.1038/mi.2010.51
15. Kearney SC, Dziekiewicz M, Feleszko W. Immunoregulatory and immunostimulatory responses of bacterial lysates in respiratory infections and asthma. *Ann Allergy Asthma Immunol.* (2015) 114:364–9. doi: 10.1016/j.anai.2015.02.008
16. Ko FW, Chan KP, Hui DS, Goddard JR, Shaw JG, Reid DW, et al. Acute exacerbation of COPD. *Respirology.* (2016) 21:1152–65. doi: 10.1111/resp.12780
17. Clementi CF, Håkansson AP, Murphy TF. Internalization and trafficking of nontypeable *Haemophilus influenzae* in human respiratory epithelial cells and roles of IgA1 proteases for optimal invasion and persistence. *Infect Immun.* (2014) 82:433–44. doi: 10.1128/IAI.00864-13
18. St Geme JW III, Falkow S. *Haemophilus influenzae* adheres to and enters cultured human epithelial cells. *Infect Immun.* (1990) 58:4036–44.
19. van Schilfgaarde M, Eijk P, Regelink A, Van Ulsen P, Everts V, Dankert J, et al. *Haemophilus influenzae*localized in epithelial cell layers is shielded from antibiotics and antibody-mediated bactericidal activity. *Microb Pathog.* (1999) 26:249–62. doi: 10.1006/mpat.1998.0269
20. Ahrén IL, Williams DL, Rice PJ, Forsgren A, Riesbeck K. The importance of a β-glucan receptor in the nonopsonic entry of nontypeable *Haemophilus influenzae* into human monocytic and epithelial cells. *J Infect Dis.* (2001) 184:150–8. doi: 10.1086/322016
21. Swords WE, Ketterer MR, Shao J, Campbell CA, Weiser JN, Apicella MA. Binding of the non-typeable *Haemophilus influenzae* lipooligosaccharide to the PAF receptor initiates host cell signalling. *Cell Microbiol.* (2001) 3:525–36. doi: 10.1046/j.1462-5822.2001.00132.x
22. Holmes KA, Bakaletz LO. Adherence of non-typeable*Haemophilus influenzae*promotes reorganization of the actin cytoskeleton in human or chinchilla epithelial cellsin vitro. *Microb Pathog.* (1997) 23:157–66. doi: 10.1006/mpat.1997.0145
23. Morey P, Cano V, Martí-Lliteras P, López-Gómez A, Regueiro V, Saus C, et al. Evidence for a non-replicative intracellular stage of nontypable *Haemophilus influenzae* in epithelial cells. *Microbiology.* (2011) 157:234–50. doi: 10.1099/mic.0.040451-0
24. Donaldson JG, Porat-Shliom N, Cohen LA. Clathrin-independent endocytosis: a unique platform for cell signaling and PM remodeling. *Cell Signal.* (2009) 21:1–6. doi: 10.1016/j.cellsig.2008.06.020
25. Swords WE, Buscher BA, Ver Steeg Ii K, Preston A, Nichols WA, Weiser JN, et al. Non-typeable *Haemophilus influenzae* adhere to and invade human bronchial epithelial cells via an interaction of lipooligosaccharide with the PAF receptor. *Mol Microbiol.* (2000) 37:13–27. doi: 10.1046/j.1365-2958.2000.01952.x
26. Kaufhold I, Osbahr S, Shima K, Marwitz S, Rohmann K, Drömann D, et al. Nontypeable *Haemophilus influenzae* (NTHi) directly interfere with the regulation of E-cadherin in lung epithelial cells. *Microb Infect.* (2017) 19:560–6. doi: 10.1016/j.micinf.2017.07.002
27. Singh B, Fleury C, Jalalvand F, Riesbeck K. Human pathogens utilize host extracellular matrix proteins laminin and collagen for adhesion and invasion of the host. *FEMS Microbiol Rev.* (2012) 36:1122–80. doi: 10.1111/j.1574-6976.2012.00340.x
28. Murphy TF, Kirkham C, Gallo MC, Yang Y, Wilding GE, Pettigrew MM. Immunoglobulin a protease variants facilitate intracellular survival in epithelial cells by nontypeable *Haemophilus influenzae* that persist in the human respiratory tract in chronic obstructive pulmonary disease. *J Infect Dis.* (2017) 216:1295–302. doi: 10.1093/infdis/jix471
29. Murphy TF, Kirkham C, Jones MM, Sethi S, Kong Y, Pettigrew MM. Expression of IgA proteases by *Haemophilus influenzae* in the respiratory tract of adults with chronic obstructive pulmonary disease. *J Infect Dis.* (2015) 212:1798–805. doi: 10.1093/infdis/jiv299
30. Pilette C, Durham SR, Vaerman J-P, Sibille Y. Mucosal immunity in asthma and chronic obstructive pulmonary disease. *Proc Am Thorac Soc.* (2004) 1:125–35. doi: 10.1513/pats.2306032
31. Ko W-C, Paterson DL, Sagnimeni AJ, Hansen DS, Von Gottberg A, Mohapatra S, et al. Community-acquired *Klebsiella pneumoniae* bacteremia: global differences in clinical patterns. *Emerg Infect Dis.* (2002) 8:160–6. doi: 10.3201/eid0802.010025
32. Dulek DE, Newcomb DC, Goleniewska K, Cephus J, Zhou W, Reiss S, et al. Allergic airway inflammation decreases lung bacterial burden following acute *Klebsiella pneumoniae* infection in a neutrophil- and CCL8-dependent manner. *Infect Immun.* (2014) 82:3723–39. doi: 10.1128/IAI.00035-14
33. Thijs W, Janssen K, Van Schadewijk AM, Papapoulos SE, Le Cessie S, Middeldorp S, et al. Nasal levels of antimicrobial peptides in allergic asthma patients and healthy controls: differences and effect of a short 1,25(OH)2 Vitamin D3 treatment. *PLoS One.* (2015) 10:e0140986. doi: 10.1371/journal.pone.0140986
34. Sun S-C. Deubiquitylation and regulation of the immune response. *Nat Rev Immunol.* (2008) 8:501–11. doi: 10.1038/nri2337
35. Frank CG, Reguerio V, Rother M, Moranta D, Maeurer AP, Garmendia J, et al. *Klebsiella pneumoniae* targets an EGF receptor-dependent pathway to subvert inflammation. *Cell Microbiol.* (2013) 15:1212–33. doi: 10.1111/cmi.12110
36. Wu JH, Hong L-C, Tsai Y-Y, Chen H-W, Chen W-X, Wu TS. Mitogen-activated protein kinase (MAPK) signalling pathways in HepG2 cells infected with a virulent strain of *Klebsiella pneumoniae. Cell Microbiol.* (2006) 8:1467–74. doi: 10.1111/j.1462-5822.2006.00725.x
37. Moranta D, Regueiro V, March C, Llobet E, Margareto J, Larrarte E, et al. *Klebsiella pneumoniae* capsule polysaccharide impedes the expression of beta-defensins by airway epithelial cells. *Infect Immun.* (2010) 78:1135–46. doi: 10.1128/IAI.00940-09
38. Regueiro V, Moranta D, Frank CG, Larrarte E, Margareto J, March C, et al. *Klebsiella pneumoniae* subverts the activation of inflammatory responses in a NOD1-dependent manner. *Cell Microbiol.* (2011) 13:135–53. doi: 10.1111/j.1462-5822.2010.01526.x
39. March C, Moranta D, Regueiro V, Llobet E, Tomás A, Garmendia J, et al. *Klebsiella pneumoniae* outer membrane protein A is required to prevent the activation of airway epithelial cells. *J Biol Chem.* (2011) 286:9956–67. doi: 10.1074/jbc.M110.181008
40. Fagundes CT, Amaral FA, Vieira AT, Soares AC, Pinho V, Nicoli JR, et al. Transient TLR activation restores inflammatory response and ability to control pulmonary bacterial infection in germfree mice. *J Immunol.* (2012) 188:1411. doi: 10.4049/jimmunol.1101682
41. Gabryšová L, Howes A, Saraiva M, O'garra A. The regulation of IL-10 expression. *Curr Top Microbiol Immunol.* (2014) 380:157–90. doi: 10.1007/978-3-662-43492-5_8
42. Greenberger MJ, Strieter RM, Kunkel SL, Danforth JM, Goodman RE, Standiford TJ. Neutralization of IL-10 increases survival in a murine model of Klebsiella pneumonia. *J Immunol.* (1995) 155:722.
43. Dolgachev VA, Yu B, Sun L, Shanley TP, Raghavendran K, Hemmila MR. Interleukin 10 overexpression alters survival in the setting of gram-negative pneumonia following lung contusion. *Shock.* (2014) 41:301–10. doi: 10.1097/SHK.0000000000000123
44. Lin CK, Kazmierczak BI. Inflammation: a double-edged sword in the response to *Pseudomonas aeruginosa* infection. *J Innate Immun.* (2017) 9:250–61. doi: 10.1159/000455857
45. Saint-Criq V, Villeret B, Bastaert F, Kheir S, Hatton A, Cazes A, et al. *Pseudomonas aeruginosa* LasB protease impairs innate immunity in mice and humans by targeting a lung epithelial cystic fibrosis transmembrane

regulator–IL-6–antimicrobial–repair pathway. *Thorax.* (2018) 73:49–61. doi: 10.1136/thoraxjnl-2017-210298

46. Curran CS, Bolig T, Torabi-Parizi P. Mechanisms and targeted therapies for *Pseudomonas aeruginosa* lung infection. *Am J Respir Crit Care Med.* (2018) 197:708–27. doi: 10.1164/rccm.201705-1043SO
47. Casilag F, Lorenz A, Krueger J, Klawonn F, Weiss S, Häussler S. The LasB elastase of *Pseudomonas aeruginosa* acts in concert with alkaline protease AprA to prevent flagellin-mediated immune recognition. *Infect Immun.* (2015) 84:162–71. doi: 10.1128/IAI.00939-15
48. Hayashi F, Smith KD, Ozinsky A, Hawn TR, Yi EC, Goodlett DR, et al. The innate immune response to bacterial flagellin is mediated by Toll-like receptor 5. *Nature.* (2001) 410:1099–103. doi: 10.1038/35074106
49. Descamps D, Le Gars M, Balloy V, Barbier D, Maschalidi S, Tohme M, et al. Toll-like receptor 5 (TLR5), IL-1β secretion, and asparagine endopeptidase are critical factors for alveolar macrophage phagocytosis and bacterial killing. *Proc Natl Acad Sci USA.* (2012) 109:1619–24. doi: 10.1073/pnas.1108464109
50. Beaudoin T, Lafayette S, Roussel L, Bérubé J, Desrosiers M, Nguyen D, et al. The level of p38α mitogen-activated protein kinase activation in airway epithelial cells determines the onset of innate immune responses to planktonic and biofilm *Pseudomonas aeruginosa. J Infect Dis.* (2013) 207:1544–55. doi: 10.1093/infdis/jit059
51. Heck LW, Alarcon PG, Kulhavy RM, Morihara K, Russell MW, Mestecky JF. Degradation of IgA proteins by *Pseudomonas aeruginosa* elastase. *J Immunol.* (1990) 144:2253.
52. Parmely M, Gale A, Clabaugh M, Horvat R, Zhou WW. Proteolytic inactivation of cytokines by *Pseudomonas aeruginosa. Infect Immun.* (1990) 58:3009–14.
53. Schmidtchen A, Frick I-M, Andersson E, Tapper H, Björck L. Proteinases of common pathogenic bacteria degrade and inactivate the antibacterial peptide LL-37. *Mol Microbiol.* (2002) 46:157–68. doi: 10.1046/j.1365-2958.2002.03146.x
54. Matheson Nancy R, Potempa J, Travis J. Interaction of a novel form of *Pseudomonas aeruginosa* alkaline protease (aeruginolysin) with interleukin-6 and interleukin-8. *Biol Chem.* (2006) 387:911–5. doi: 10.1515/BC.2006.115
55. Bastaert F, Kheir S, Saint-Criq V, Villeret B, Dang PM-C, El-Benna J, et al. *Pseudomonas aeruginosa* LasB subverts alveolar macrophage activity by interfering with bacterial killing through downregulation of innate immune defense, reactive oxygen species generation, and complement activation. *Front Immunol.* (2018) 9:1675. doi: 10.3389/fimmu.2018.01675
56. Mun JJ, Tam C, Kowbel D, Hawgood S, Barnett MJ, Evans DJ, et al. Clearance of *Pseudomonas aeruginosa* from a healthy ocular surface involves surfactant protein D and is compromised by bacterial elastase in a murine null-infection model. *Infect Immun.* (2009) 77:2392–8. doi: 10.1128/IAI.00173-09
57. Kuang Z, Hao Y, Hwang S, Zhang S, Kim E, Akinbi HT, et al. The *Pseudomonas aeruginosa* flagellum confers resistance to pulmonary surfactant protein-A by impacting the production of exoproteases through quorum-sensing. *Mol Microbiol.* (2011) 79:1220–35. doi: 10.1111/j.1365-2958.2010.07516.x
58. van der Plas MJA, Bhongir RKV, Kjellström S, Siller H, Kasetty G, Mörgelin M, et al. *Pseudomonas aeruginosa* elastase cleaves a C-terminal peptide from human thrombin that inhibits host inflammatory responses. *Nat Commun.* (2016) 7:11567–11567. doi: 10.1038/ncomms11567
59. Bazan-Socha S, Mastalerz L, Cybulska A, Zareba L, Kremers R, Zabczyk M, et al. Asthma is associated with enhanced thrombin formation and impaired fibrinolysis. *Clin Exp Allergy.* (2016) 46:932–44. doi: 10.1111/cea.12734
60. Moss J, Ehrmantraut ME, Banwart BD, Frank DW, Barbieri JT. Sera from adult patients with cystic fibrosis contain antibodies to *Pseudomonas aeruginosa* type III apparatus. *Infect Immun.* (2001) 69:1185–8. doi: 10.1128/IAI.69.2.1185-1188.2001
61. Hauser AR. The type III secretion system of *Pseudomonas aeruginosa*: infection by injection. *Nat Rev Microbiol.* (2009) 7:654–65. doi: 10.1038/nrmicro2199
62. Shaver CM, Hauser AR. Relative contributions of *Pseudomonas aeruginosa* ExoU, ExoS, and ExoT to virulence in the lung. *Infect Immun.* (2004) 72:6969–77. doi: 10.1128/IAI.72.12.6969-6977.2004
63. Rangel SM, Diaz MH, Knoten CA, Zhang A, Hauser AR. The role of ExoS in dissemination of *Pseudomonas aeruginosa* during pneumonia. *PLoS Pathog.* (2015) 11:e1004945. doi: 10.1371/journal.ppat.1004945
64. Huus KE, Joseph J, Zhang L, Wong A, Aaron SD, Mah T-F, et al. Clinical isolates of *Pseudomonas aeruginosa* from chronically infected cystic fibrosis patients fail to activate the inflammasome during both stable infection and pulmonary exacerbation. *J Immunol.* (2016) 196:3097. doi: 10.4049/jimmunol.1501642
65. Mann EE, Wozniak DJ. *Pseudomonas* biofilm matrix composition and niche biology. *FEMS Microbiol Rev.* (2012) 36:893–916. doi: 10.1111/j.1574-6976.2011.00322.x
66. Jensen ET, Kharazmi A, Garred P, Kronborg G, Fomsgaard A, Mollnes TE, et al. Complement activation by *Pseudomonas aeruginosa* biofilms. *Microb Pathog.* (1993) 15:377–88. doi: 10.1006/mpat.1993.1087
67. Whiteley M, Bangera MG, Bumgarner RE, Parsek MR, Teitzel GM, Lory S, et al. Gene expression in *Pseudomonas aeruginosa* biofilms. *Nature.* (2001) 413:860–4.
68. Sauer K, Camper AK, Ehrlich GD, Costerton JW, Davies DG. *Pseudomonas aeruginosa* displays multiple phenotypes during development as a biofilm. *J Bacteriol.* (2002) 184:1140–54. doi: 10.1128/jb.184.4.1140-1154.2002
69. Jesaitis AJ, Franklin MJ, Berglund D, Sasaki M, Lord CI, Bleazard JB, et al. Compromised host defense on *Pseudomonas aeruginosa* biofilms: characterization of neutrophil and biofilm interactions. *J Immunol.* (2003) 171:4329. doi: 10.4049/jimmunol.171.8.4329
70. Jensen PØ, Bjarnsholt T, Phipps R, Rasmussen TB, Calum H, Christoffersen L, et al. Rapid necrotic killing of polymorphonuclear leukocytes is caused by quorum-sensing-controlled production of rhamnolipid by *Pseudomonas aeruginosa. Microbiology.* (2007) 153:1329–38. doi: 10.1099/mic.0.2006/003863-0
71. Ryall B, Carrara M, Zlosnik JEA, Behrends V, Lee X, Wong Z, et al. The mucoid switch in *Pseudomonas aeruginosa* represses quorum sensing systems and leads to complex changes to stationary phase virulence factor regulation. *PLoS One.* (2014) 9:e96166. doi: 10.1371/journal.pone.0096166
72. Leid JG, Willson CJ, Shirtliff ME, Hassett DJ, Parsek MR, Jeffers AK. The exopolysaccharide alginate protects *Pseudomonas aeruginosa* biofilm bacteria from IFN-γ-mediated macrophage killing. *J Immunol.* (2005) 175:7512. doi: 10.4049/jimmunol.175.11.7512
73. Malhotra S, Limoli DH, English AE, Parsek MR, Wozniak DJ. Mixed communities of mucoid and nonmucoid *Pseudomonas aeruginosa* exhibit enhanced resistance to host antimicrobials. *mBio.* (2018) 9:e00275-18. doi: 10.1128/mBio.00275-18
74. Firoved AM, Ornatowski W, Deretic V. Microarray analysis reveals induction of lipoprotein genes in mucoid *Pseudomonas aeruginosa*: implications for inflammation in cystic fibrosis. *Infect Immun.* (2004) 72:5012–8. doi: 10.1128/IAI.72.9.5012-5018.2004
75. Tart AH, Blanks MJ, Wozniak DJ. The AlgT-dependent transcriptional regulator AmrZ (AlgZ) inhibits flagellum biosynthesis in mucoid, nonmotile *Pseudomonas aeruginosa* cystic fibrosis isolates. *J Bacteriol.* (2006) 188:6483–9. doi: 10.1128/JB.00636-06
76. Pier GB. *Pseudomonas aeruginosa* lipopolysaccharide: a major virulence factor, initiator of inflammation and target for effective immunity. *Int J Med Microbiol.* (2007) 297:277–95. doi: 10.1016/j.ijmm.2007.03.012
77. Di Lorenzo F, Silipo A, Bianconi I, Lore NI, Scamporrino A, Sturiale L, et al. Persistent cystic fibrosis isolate *Pseudomonas aeruginosa* strain RP73 exhibits an under-acylated LPS structure responsible of its low inflammatory activity. *Mol Immunol.* (2015) 63:166–75. doi: 10.1016/j.molimm.2014.04.004
78. Ernst RK, Adams KN, Moskowitz SM, Kraig GM, Kawasaki K, Stead CM, et al. The *Pseudomonas aeruginosa* lipid A deacylase: selection for expression and loss within the cystic fibrosis airway. *J Bacteriol.* (2006) 188:191–201. doi: 10.1128/JB.188.1.191-201.2006
79. Cigana C, Curcurù L, Leone MR, Ieranò T, Lorè NI, Bianconi I, et al. *Pseudomonas aeruginosa* exploits lipid A and muropeptides modification as a strategy to lower innate immunity during cystic fibrosis lung infection. *PLoS One.* (2009) 4:e8439. doi: 10.1371/journal.pone.0008439
80. Cramer N, Klockgether J, Wrasman K, Schmidt M, Davenport CF, Tümmler B. Microevolution of the major common *Pseudomonas aeruginosa* clones C and PA14 in cystic fibrosis lungs. *Environ Microbiol.* (2011) 13:1690–704. doi: 10.1111/j.1462-2920.2011.02483.x
81. Dettman JR, Rodrigue N, Aaron SD, Kassen R. Evolutionary genomics of epidemic and nonepidemic strains of *Pseudomonas aeruginosa. Proc Natl Acad Sci USA.* (2013) 110:21065–70. doi: 10.1073/pnas.1307862110

82. Kluytmans J, Van Belkum A, Verbrugh H. Nasal carriage of *Staphylococcus aureus*: epidemiology, underlying mechanisms, and associated risks. *Clin Microbiol Rev.* (1997) 10:505–20.
83. Baur S, Rautenberg M, Faulstich M, Grau T, Severin Y, Unger C, et al. A nasal epithelial receptor for *Staphylococcus aureus* WTA governs adhesion to epithelial cells and modulates nasal colonization. *PLoS Pathog.* (2014) 10:e1004089. doi: 10.1371/journal.ppat.1004089
84. Lacey KA, Geoghegan JA, Mcloughlin RM. The role of *Staphylococcus aureus* virulence factors in skin infection and their potential as vaccine antigens. *Pathogens.* (2016) 5:22. doi: 10.3390/pathogens5010022
85. Burman JD, Leung E, Atkins KL, O'seaghdha MN, Lango L, Bernadó P, et al. Interaction of human complement with Sbi, a staphylococcal immunoglobulin-binding protein: indications of a novel mechanism of complement evasion by *Staphylococcus aureus*. *J Biol Chem.* (2008) 283:17579–93. doi: 10.1074/jbc.M800265200
86. Postma B, Poppelier MJ, Van Galen JC, Prossnitz ER, Van Strijp JAG, De Haas CJC, et al. Chemotaxis inhibitory protein of *Staphylococcus aureus* binds specifically to the C5a and formylated peptide receptor. *J Immunol.* (2004) 172:6994. doi: 10.4049/jimmunol.172.11.6994
87. Laarman AJ, Mijnheer G, Mootz JM, Van Rooijen WJM, Ruyken M, Malone CL, et al. *Staphylococcus aureus* Staphopain A inhibits CXCR2-dependent neutrophil activation and chemotaxis. *EMBO J.* (2012) 31:3607–19. doi: 10.1038/emboj.2012.212
88. Smagur J, Guzik K, Bzowska M, Kuzak M, Zarebski M, Kantyka T, et al. Staphylococcal cysteine protease staphopain B (SspB) induces rapid engulfment of human neutrophils and monocytes by macrophages. *Biol Chem.* (2009) 390:361–71. doi: 10.1515/BC.2009.042
89. Sieprawska-Lupa M, Mydel P, Krawczyk K, Wójcik K, Puklo M, Lupa B, et al. Degradation of human antimicrobial peptide LL-37 by *Staphylococcus aureus*-derived proteinases. *Antimicrob Agents Chemother.* (2004) 48:4673–9. doi: 10.1128/AAC.48.12.4673-4679.2004
90. Thammavongsa V, Kern JW, Missiakas DM, Schneewind O. *Staphylococcus aureus* synthesizes adenosine to escape host immune responses. *J Exp Med.* (2009) 206:2417–27. doi: 10.1084/jem.20090097
91. Csóka B, Németh ZH, Virág L, Gergely P, Leibovich SJ, Pacher P, et al. A2A adenosine receptors and C/EBPbeta are crucially required for IL-10 production by macrophages exposed to *Escherichia coli*. *Blood.* (2007) 110:2685–95. doi: 10.1182/blood-2007-01-065870
92. McCarthy AJ, Lindsay JA. Genetic variation in *Staphylococcus aureus* surface and immune evasion genes is lineage associated: implications for vaccine design and host-pathogen interactions. *BMC Microbiol.* (2010) 10:173. doi: 10.1186/1471-2180-10-173
93. Friedrich R, Panizzi P, Fuentes-Prior P, Richter K, Verhamme I, Anderson PJ, et al. Staphylocoagulase is a prototype for the mechanism of cofactor-induced zymogen activation. *Nature.* (2003) 425:535–9. doi: 10.1038/nature01962
94. Panizzi P, Friedrich R, Fuentes-Prior P, Richter K, Bock PE, Bode W. Fibrinogen substrate recognition by staphylocoagulase.(pro)thrombin complexes. *J Biol Chem.* (2006) 281:1179–87. doi: 10.1074/jbc.M507956200
95. Andréjak C, Nielsen R, Thomsen VØ, Duhaut P, Sørensen HT, Thomsen RW. Chronic respiratory disease, inhaled corticosteroids and risk of non-tuberculous mycobacteriosis. *Thorax.* (2013) 68:256. doi: 10.1136/thoraxjnl-2012-201772
96. Park IK, Olivier KN. Nontuberculous mycobacteria in cystic fibrosis and non-cystic fibrosis bronchiectasis. *Semin Respir Crit Care Med.* (2015) 36:217–24. doi: 10.1055/s-0035-1546751
97. Skolnik K, Kirkpatrick G, Quon BS. Nontuberculous mycobacteria in cystic fibrosis. *Curr Treat Options Infect Dis.* (2016) 8:259–74. doi: 10.1007/s40506-016-0092-6
98. van Ingen J, Wagner D, Gallagher J, Morimoto K, Lange C, Haworth CS, et al. Poor adherence to management guidelines in nontuberculous mycobacterial pulmonary diseases. *Eur Respir J.* (2017) 49:1601855. doi: 10.1183/13993003.01855-2016
99. Viviani L, Harrison MJ, Zolin A, Haworth CS, Floto RA. Epidemiology of nontuberculous mycobacteria (NTM) amongst individuals with cystic fibrosis (CF). *J Cyst Fibros.* (2016) 15:619–23. doi: 10.1016/j.jcf.2016.03.002
100. Martiniano SL, Nick JA, Daley CL. Nontuberculous mycobacterial infections in cystic fibrosis. *Thorac Surg Clin.* (2019) 29:95–108. doi: 10.1016/j.thorsurg.2018.09.008
101. Early J, Fischer K, Bermudez LE. *Mycobacterium avium* uses apoptotic macrophages as tools for spreading. *Microb Pathog.* (2011) 50:132–9. doi: 10.1016/j.micpath.2010.12.004
102. Roux A-L, Viljoen A, Bah A, Simeone R, Bernut A, Laencina L, et al. The distinct fate of smooth and rough *Mycobacterium abscessus* variants inside macrophages. *Open Biol.* (2016) 6:160185. doi: 10.1098/rsob.160185
103. Kim S-W, Subhadra B, Whang J, Back YW, Bae HS, Kim H-J, et al. Clinical *Mycobacterium abscessus* strain inhibits autophagy flux and promotes its growth in murine macrophages. *Pathog Dis.* (2017) 75:ftx107. doi: 10.1093/femspd/ftx107
104. Thomas SR, Ray A, Hodson ME, Pitt TL. Increased sputum amino acid concentrations and auxotrophy of *Pseudomonas aeruginosa* in severe cystic fibrosis lung disease. *Thorax.* (2000) 55:795. doi: 10.1136/thorax.55.9.795
105. Miranda-CasoLuengo AA, Staunton PM, Dinan AM, Lohan AJ, Loftus BJ. Functional characterization of the *Mycobacterium abscessus* genome coupled with condition specific transcriptomics reveals conserved molecular strategies for host adaptation and persistence. *BMC Genomics.* (2016) 17:553. doi: 10.1186/s12864-016-2868-y
106. Brodlie M, Aseeri A, Lordan JL, Robertson AGN, Mckean MC, Corris PA, et al. Bile acid aspiration in people with cystic fibrosis before and after lung transplantation. *Eur Respir J.* (2015) 46:1820. doi: 10.1183/13993003.00891-2015
107. Fennelly KP, Ojano-Dirain C, Yang Q, Liu L, Lu L, Progulske-Fox A, et al. Biofilm formation by *Mycobacterium abscessus* in a lung cavity. *Am J Respir Crit Care Med.* (2016) 193:692–3.
108. Teng R, Dick T. Isoniazid resistance of exponentially growing *Mycobacterium smegmatis* biofilm culture. *FEMS Microbiol Lett.* (2003) 227:171–4. doi: 10.1016/S0378-1097(03)00584-6
109. Falkinham JO. Growth in catheter biofilms and antibiotic resistance of *Mycobacterium avium*. *J Med Microbiol.* (2007) 56:250–4. doi: 10.1099/jmm.0.46935-0
110. Greendyke R, Byrd TF. Differential antibiotic susceptibility of *Mycobacterium abscessus* variants in biofilms and macrophages compared to that of planktonic bacteria. *Antimicrob Agents Chemother.* (2008) 52:2019. doi: 10.1128/AAC.00986-07
111. McNabe M, Tennant R, Danelishvili L, Young L, Bermudez LE. *Mycobacterium avium* ssp. hominissuis biofilm is composed of distinct phenotypes and influenced by the presence of antimicrobials. *Clin Microbiol Infect.* (2011) 17:697–703. doi: 10.1111/j.1469-0691.2010.03307.x
112. Davidson LB, Nessar R, Kempaiah P, Perkins DJ, Byrd TF. *Mycobacterium abscessus* glycopeptidolipid prevents respiratory epithelial TLR2 signaling as measured by HβD2 gene expression and IL-8 release. *PLoS One.* (2011) 6:e29148. doi: 10.1371/journal.pone.0029148

9

Caspase-11 Non-Canonical Inflammasomes in the Lung

*Changhoon Oh, Ambika Verma and Youssef Aachoui**

Department of Microbiology and Immunology, Center for Microbial Pathogenesis and Host Responses, University of Arkansas for Medical Sciences, Little Rock, AR, United States

Correspondence:
Youssef Aachoui
yaachoui@uams.edu

The airway epithelium and underlying innate immune cells comprise the first line of host defense in the lung. They recognize pathogen-associated molecular patterns (PAMPs) using membrane-bound receptors, as well as cytosolic receptors such as inflammasomes. Inflammasomes activate inflammatory caspases, which in turn process and release the inflammatory cytokines IL-1β and IL-18. Additionally, inflammasomes trigger a form of lytic cell death termed pyroptosis. One of the most important inflammasomes at the host-pathogen interface is the non-canonical caspase-11 inflammasome that responds to LPS in the cytosol. Caspase-11 is important in defense against Gram-negative pathogens, and can drive inflammatory diseases such as LPS-induced sepsis. However, pathogens can employ evasive strategies to minimize or evade host caspase-11 detection. In this review, we present a comprehensive overview of the function of the non-canonical caspase-11 inflammasome in sensing of cytosolic LPS, and its mechanism of action with particular emphasis in the role of caspase-11 in the lung. We also explore some of the strategies pathogens use to evade caspase-11.

Keywords: caspase-11, gasdermin D, inflammasomes, pore intracellular traps (PIT), *Burkholderia thailandensis* lung defense, Gbps, LPS

INTRODUCTION

Bacterial infections of the respiratory tract remain a leading cause of global morbidity and mortality (1). As the first line of defense against infection, the airway epithelium and innate immune cells play a critical role in limiting infection. As such, they are especially sensitive to pathogen associated molecular patterns (PAMPs), expressing an array of membrane-bound and cytosolic receptors that recognize specific structural motifs shared by classes of microbes (2). For example, Toll-like receptor 5 (TLR5) and NOD-like receptor 4 (NLRC4) detect and respond to bacterial flagellin. TLR5 detects extracellular flagellin (3), while NLRC4 detects its cytosolic presence (4, 5).

Many pathogens infect cells and exploit intracellular niches to facilitate their replication and spread (6). In turn, host cells have evolved mechanisms to detect and counteract these efforts. For example, intracellular sensors like inflammasomes are expressed in innate immune cells, lung epithelium, and endothelium to enable detection of pathogens and subsequent protective responses (6–8). Inflammasomes lead to the activation of inflammatory caspases, which in turn process and release the inflammatory cytokines IL-1β and IL-18. Additionally, inflammasomes trigger a form of lytic cell death termed pyroptosis that plays important role in clearance of offending pathogens (6).

Virulent intracellular bacteria usually evade intracellular sensors or suppress inflammasome activity by suppressing or modifying the structural features of their PAMPs (9). These strategies diminish the ability of inflammasomes to respond to these pathogens. For instance, *Salmonella enterica* serovar typhimurium utilizes two pathogenicity islands, SPI-1 and SPI-2, which encode distinct type three secretion systems (T3SSs). The T3SS apparatus encoded by SPI-1 functions primarily during epithelial cell invasion, is co-expressed with flagellin, and is readily detected by the inflammasome NLRC4. In contrast, the SPI-2 T3SS is expressed in the vacuolar compartment of both epithelial cells and macrophages, and is not detected by inflammasomes. *S. typhimurium* suppresses transcription of flagellin during SPI-2 inducing conditions, thereby avoiding detection by NLRC4 (10, 11). Here, we present a comprehensive overview of the function of the caspase-11 inflammasome in sensing of cytosolic LPS, and its mechanism of action with particular emphasis in the lung. We also explore some of the strategies pathogens use to evade caspase-11.

INFLAMMASOMES ACTIVATE INFLAMMATORY CASPASE-1 AND -11

Caspases are a family of aspartate-specific, cysteine proteases that are activated by homodimerization or cleavage to mediate several cellular events including cell death (12). Cell death is an essential process that maintains tissue homeostasis, and recently, it has emerged as an important defense mechanism against infection (13). Caspases are divided into inflammatory (in mouse these include caspase-1,-11, and -12) or apoptotic caspases (caspase-2,-3,-6,-7,-8, and -9). Apoptotic caspases are further subdivided into initiators (caspase-2,-8, and -9) or executioners (caspase-3,-6, and -7) (12). A discussion of the activation and role of apoptotic caspases during infection is important; however, it is beyond the scope of this review, and we refer the reader to previously published reviews (12).

Inflammatory caspases are able to distinguish virulent from avirulent bacteria, and to alert the immune system to a pathogenic infection. Like apoptotic initiator caspases, inflammatory caspases contain a death fold prodomain termed the caspase activation and recruitment domain (CARD) (12). The CARD domain is essential to the recruitment and activation of inflammatory caspases-1 and-11 within the inflammasomes. Inflammasomes are large, multiprotein complexes typically comprising a NOD-like receptor (NLR) or AIM2-like receptor (ALR) such as NLRP3, NLRC4, or AIM2, sometimes an adaptor protein called ASC, and an executioner caspase, which is typically caspase-1 (6). Several inflammasomes that activate caspase-1 in response to contamination of the cytosol or perturbation of cellular physiology have been characterized, and each one is named after its NLR or ALR protein scaffold. The NLRP3 inflammasome is activated in response to the widest array of stimuli, including particulates, crystals, ATP, K^+ efflux, lysosomal disruption, and oxidized mitochondrial DNA. However, the precise signal that NLRP3 detects remains controversial (14). In contrast to the diverse stimuli that activate NLRP3, other inflammasomes respond to a limited set of stimuli. For instance, The AIM2 detects cytosolic dsDNA (15–17), which may be encountered in the cytosol during pathogenic infection. The NLRC4 inflammasome responds to flagellin and the activity of type III secretion system (T3SS) and type IV secretion system (T4SS) (10, 18, 19). Unlike other inflammasomes, activation of NLRC4 involves members of the NAIP subfamily of NLRs, forming mixed NLRC4-NAIP oligomeric inflammasome platforms. The murine NAIP locus is highly polymorphic. C57BL/6 mice encode four NAIPs; NAIP1 binds the T3SS needle, NAIP2 binds the T3SS rod, and NAIP5 and NAIP6 bind flagellins. By contrast, humans have a single NAIP that detects the T3SS needle (18–21). Upon activation, NLRs forming inflammasomes recruit the ASC adaptor, composed of a CARD and a PYD, via homotypic interactions. Additional ASC molecules are incorporated via CARD-CARD and PYD-PYD interactions, until all ASC are collected into a single focus called a "speck." Attraction of caspase-1 into the ASC speck via CARD-CARD interaction results in caspase-1 dimerization and proximity-induced autoproteolytic processing into p10 and p20 subunits (6). Active caspase-1 processes pro-IL-1β and pro-IL-18 to their mature forms; it additionally triggers a lytic form of programmed cell death called pyroptosis by cleaving and activating the pore-forming protein gasdermin D (GSDMD; discussed in more detail below) (6, 22). Activation of inflammasomes can also promote the release of IL-1α. IL-1α is considered an endogenous danger signal that is widely and constitutively expressed, active in its uncleaved form, and passively released after pyrpotosis (23).

Caspase-1 was long thought to be the only inflammatory caspase activated within an inflammasome and the sole mediator of pyroptosis because caspase-1-deficient bone marrow macrophages (BMMs) were resistant to inflammasome activation-induced cell death. However, the Dixit lab showed that the process of backcrossing the caspase-1 knockout allele into the C57BL/6 background carried a passenger mutation in caspase-11 from the 129 background, effectively making *Casp1-Casp11*^{DKO} animals (24). Examination of the single *Casp11*$^{-/-}$ mice revealed that, caspase-11 drives pyroptosis upon *in vitro* activation like the closely related caspase-1, but it does not directly mediate IL-1β and IL-18 secretion. Instead, caspase-11 can activate an indirect NLRP3-ASC-caspase-1 pathway leading to IL-1β/IL-18 processing and release (24). The caspase-11 pathway was thus termed the "caspase-11 non-canonical inflammasome" to contrast it with the caspase-1-activating canonical inflammasomes (NLRP3, NLRC4, AIM2, etc.). These revelations ignited interest into the study of caspase-11.

CASPASE-11 DIRECTLY DETECTS THE CYTOSOLIC PRESENCE OF LPS

Caspase-11 was identified almost 23 years ago in a mouse cDNA library screen for homologs of caspase-1 (25). Back then, caspase-11 was found to be a key mediator in LPS-induced septic shock model since *Casp11*$^{-/-}$ mice are more resistant to lethal doses of LPS compared to wild-type mice (25, 26), though its mechanism of activation remained elusive. 15 years later, caspase-11 regained the center stage after Kayagaki et al. demonstrated that exposure to cholera toxin B (CTB) and certain Gram-negative bacteria, such as *Escherichia coli*, *Citrobacter rodentium*, and *Vibrio cholera*, activates caspase-11 to trigger pyroptosis, albeit after long exposure times (~16–24 h) (24). We

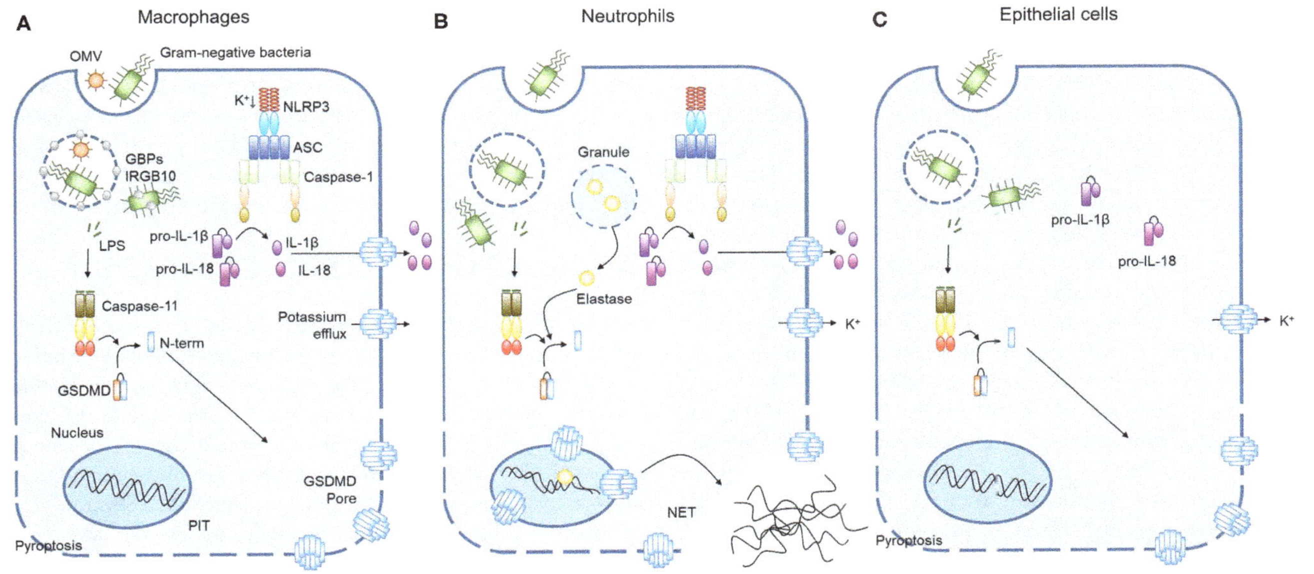

FIGURE 1 | Caspase-11 non-canonical inflammasome activation by intracellular LPS in different cells. **(A)** Cooperation of GBPchr3 with IRGB10 expose LPS from intracellular bacteria or OMVs in macrophages. Cytoplasmic LPS directly bind to the CARD motif of caspase-11 with their lipid A moiety, leading to oligomerization of caspase-11 to activate the non-canonical inflammasome. Active caspase-11 cleaves GSDMD to release its N-terminal domain, which is subsequently inserted into plasma membrane to form membrane pores. Potassium efflux through GSDMD pores additionally triggers NLRP3 inflammasome, inducing the processing and release of IL-1β and IL-18. Pyroptosis pores in the plasma membrane are large enough to permit soluble proteins to defuse to the extracellular milieu, but small enough to trap organelles and intracellular bacteria. This process is termed the pore-induced intracellular trap (PIT). **(B)** In neutrophils, both caspase-11 and elastase can cleave GSDMD to trigger neutrophil extracellular traps (NETs). Cleaved GSDMD targets the nucleus in addition to the plasma membrane and drives nuclear permeabilization, chromatin relaxation and plasma membrane rupture in elastase or caspase-11 dependent manner. These processes induce neutrophil to extrude NETs which restrict bacterial replication, dissemination, and enhance bacteria killing. **(C)** In contrast to the broadly expressed caspase-11 and GSDMD, caspase-1 inflammasome components are not detectable in lung epithelial cells. Therefore, the caspase-11 non-canonical inflammasome activation in lung epithelial cells only triggers pyroptosis without the processing and release of IL-1β and IL-18.

subsequently showed that caspase-11 specifically differentiates Gram-negative bacteria that invade the cytosol from bacteria that remain extracellular or confined to the vacuole, with the former activating caspase-11 rapidly (27) (**Figure 1**). However, like the experiments before, vacuolar and extracellular Gram-negative bacteria could still activate caspase-11 after sufficient time (28–31). These observations precipitated interest in the discovery of the identity of the common non-canonical activating agonist(s) and sensor(s). Two independent studies by the Miao and Dixit groups discovered that activation of caspase-11 is induced by LPS that has gained access to the host cytosol (32, 33). Of note, it was later determined that the activation of caspase-11 by CTB in LPS-primed macrophages was triggered by the aberrant delivery of LPS by CTB to the cytosol, rather than the direct action of CTB itself (32). The fact that LPS is the cytosolic ligand that activates caspase-11 also shed light on the role of caspase-11 in septic shock, and why septic shock could occur in the absence of TLR4, the cell-surface LPS receptor (32, 33). Therefore, LPS is detected by two receptors: extracellularly or within the recycling endosomes by TLR4 and in the cytosol via caspase-11. It is also important to note that LPS also co-localizes with intracellular TLR4 in the golgi apparatus or the endoplasmic reticulum (34, 35).

Shortly afterward, the Shao lab found that caspase-11 is the direct sensor of LPS. This was in clear contrast to the caspase-1 canonical inflammasome, where sensor and executioner functions were separated into two proteins, often bridged by the adapter ASC (36). Shi et al. demonstrated that the caspase-11 inflammasome is initiated by the CARD motif of caspase-11 directly binding to the lipid A moiety of LPS. The binding of LPS to the CARD of caspase-11 not only triggers its oligomerization but also its catalytic activation (36, 37).

In humans, caspase-11 is duplicated as caspase-4 and -5, both of which have been shown to detect directly cytosolic LPS (36). The reason for this duplication remains a mystery. One distinction is that caspase-4 expression is high in unstimulated macrophages (38–40), while murine caspase-11 and human caspase-5 are expressed at low and extremely low levels, respectively, without stimulation (39–41). Upon exposure to LPS or other toll agonists, however, macrophages rapidly induce transcription of caspase-11 and caspase- 5. Indeed, caspase-11 is non-responsive in the absence of priming through interferon-β (IFN-β) or interferon-γ (IFN-γ) (24, 27–30). Thus, as one hypothesis, caspase-11 duplication may enable a new priming-independent response through caspase-4.

CASPASE-11 CLEAVES GSDMD TO DRIVE PYROPTOSIS

Inflammatory caspases 11 and its human homologs caspase-4 and 5 cleave the pyroptosis effector protein, GSDMD, separating its N-terminal pore-forming domain from the C-terminal repressor domain (42–44). The N-terminal domain is inserted into the plasma membrane, and then oligomerizes to form large pores in the membrane that drive swelling and membrane rupture (22, 45–47). Additionally, pore formation leads to potassium efflux, which triggers the NLRP3/ASC/caspase-1 inflammasome and subsequent processing of pro-IL-1β and pro-IL-18 to their mature forms *in vitro* (48–51) (**Figure 1**); however, this pathway has not yet been confirmed *in vivo*. Additionally, GSDMD pores allow inflammasomes effectors such as IL-1α, IL-1β, IL-18, and inflammatory mediators such as eicosanoids to be released into the extracellular milieu (22, 52, 53). Although membrane pores release soluble cytosolic contents, they are small enough to retain organelles and entrap bacteria to prevent their dissemination, resulting in a structure called the pore-induced intracellular trap (PIT) (54). The PIT coordinates innate immune responses via complement and scavenger receptors to drive recruitment of and efferocytosis by neutrophils that ultimately kill the invading pathogen (54). GSDMD-dependent pores will ultimately lead to membrane rupture, but before that, cells can potentially repair membrane pores to negatively regulate pyroptosis and cytokines release. Rühl et al. showed that in macrophages, this process is coordinated by the endosomal sorting complexes required for transport (ESCRT). ESCRTs are recruited to damaged membrane in a Ca^{2+} influx-dependent manner and they remove pores from the plasma membrane (55).

In a conceptual analog to macrophage PITs, the Zychlinsky lab recently found that neutrophil GSDMD can also be cleaved by the serine protease elastase to drive formation of neutrophil extracellular traps (NETs) (56). In this situation, GSDMD cleavage releases the granular proteins including elastase that may enter the nucleus, triggering NETosis, while GSDMD forms pores in the plasma membrane to release these granules and form the NET (56) (**Figure 1**). Interestingly, the Schroder group showed that neutrophil exposure to cytosolic LPS drives caspase-11 activation and GSDMD cleavage, leading to the extruding of antimicrobial NETs independent of elastase (57). In this case, the combined actions of GSDMD and caspase-11 drive nuclear permeabilization, chromatin relaxation, and plasma membrane rupture prior to NETs release (57). NETs can restrict bacterial replication in the cells, entrap the bacteria to prevent their dissemination and enhance direct bacteria killing through the action of neutrophil granular contents. However, an excess of NETs has been reported for several pulmonary diseases, including asthma, cystic fibrosis (CF), influenza, bacterial pneumonia, and tuberculosis (58).

Caspase-11 and GSDMD are widely expressed in hematopoietic and non-hematopoietic cells, including macrophages, neutrophils, epithelial and endothelial cells. Lung epithelial and endothelial cells express caspase-11 and were found to be sensitive to stimulation with cytosolic LPS (7, 8). Interestingly, lung epithelial cells do not express the caspase-1 inflammasomes components NLRP3 or NLRC4 (7). Therefore, the activation of these cells through the caspase-11 non-canonical inflammasome triggers only pyroptosis without the processing of pro-IL-1β or pro-IL-18 (7) (**Figure 1**). Activation of caspase-11 can also induces the shedding of intestinal epithelial cells after detection of intracellular *S. typhimurium* during gut infection (59), and may perform a similar function in lung epithelial cells.

ACCESS TO THE CYTOSOL BY LPS

Access of LPS to the cytosol is a key factor during the activation of caspase-11. Cytosol -invasive pathogens such as *Burkholderia thailandensis* and its more virulent relative *Burkholderia pseudomallei* use T3SS to escape from the vacuole to the cytosol (60). This exit provides an explanation of how LPS can gain access to the cytosol. However, several Gram-negative bacteria also activate caspase-11 but are not cytosolic. Several studies showed that LPS cytosolic access can also be mediated by the activity of host factors, such as guanylate binding proteins (GBPs) (61, 62). GBPs are cytosolic GTPases that localize to the vacuole or endosome and contribute to cell-autonomous defense against cytosolic and non-cytosolic pathogens via several mechanisms including limiting intracellular bacterial survival and motility (63–66). GBPs are well conserved among vertebrates, and are found in both mice and humans (67). Genes encoding murine GBPs are clustered on chromosome 3 and are known collectively as GBPchr3 (GBP1, GBP2, GBP3, GBP5, and GBP7) or clustered on chromosome 5 (GBP4, GBP6, GBP8, GBP9, GBP10, and GBP11). In contrast, the family is reduced in humans to encode 7 GBPs genes (GBP1-GBP7) that are clustered on chromosome 1 (68–71). Intriguingly, like caspase-11, GBPs are interferon-stimulated genes, and require interferon signaling to be upregulated (62, 68). GBP-dependent effects in the activation of caspase-11 have been established in several intracellular pathogens including, *S. typhimurium*, *Legionella pneumophila*, *C. rodentium*, T3SS-negative *Pseudomonas aeruginosa*, *Vibrio cholerae*, *Chlamydia trachomatis*, and *Chlamydia muridarum* (61, 62, 72, 73). For instance, macrophages from mice that lack GBPs on Chromosome 3 exhibited less caspase-11-mediated pyroptosis in response to *S. typhimurium* and *L. pneumophila* relative to wild-type macrophages (61, 62, 74).

Whereas, the role of GBPs in general cytosolic sensing is well-established, the precise mechanism of GBPs function in LPS sensing is still the subject of ongoing research. Nonetheless, most studies suggest that GBPs are either recruited to the pathogen-containing vacuoles (PCVs), which might promote lysis of PCVs and consequent exposure of vacuolar LPS to caspase-11, or alternatively, GBPs are recruited to spontaneously ruptured bacteria-containing vacuoles or directly to cytosolic bacteria, where they act to extract or expose lipid A buried in bacterial membranes for recognition by caspase-11 (61, 62, 75, 76). In support of this latter hypothesis, human guanylate binding protein-1 (hGBP1) associates with the surface of intracellular Gram-negative bacterial pathogens after vacuolar escape (77, 78). Then, GBP1 polymerizes to coat the bacteria and initiate the recruitment of GBP2-4 to assemble a platform for caspase-4 activation (77–79). hGBP1 binds directly to LPS (77–79) and exerts a detergent-like effect of clustering LPS, which disrupts bacterial surfaces (79), thereby exposing the membrane-embedded lipid A for caspase-4 detection. In mice, GBPs can serve as a docking platform to recruit another interferon-inducible protein, IRGB10 that can co-localize to the intracellular bacteria to disrupt the bacterial cell membrane and to liberate bacterial ligands, including LPS and DNA, for innate immune recognition (80).

Virulence-associated secretion systems in Gram-negative pathogens can also drive LPS exposure in the cytosol. Gram-negative bacteria produce and release outer membrane vesicles (OMVs) during infection that are internalized by macrophages and function as vehicles that deliver LPS (and several other surface antigens) into the host cytosol (81). LPS on OMVs can trigger caspase-11 activation during *E. coli* infection. In addition, the OMVs from Gram-negative bacteria *S. typhimurium*, *L. pneumophila*, *P. aeruginosa*, and *Shigella flexneri* activate caspase-11 in a GBPchr3-dependent manner. In this case, GBPs may disrupt OMVs causing the release of LPS to cytosol where it engages caspase-11 (82).

CASPASE-11-MEDIATED DEFENSE AGAINST GRAM-NEGATIVE BACTERIA IN THE LUNG

Since caspase-11 is expressed broadly in the lung tissue, caspase-11-dependent LPS-sensing is poised to play an important role in defense against Gram-negative bacteria. As noted above, pyroptosis accomplishes the dual task of restricting intracellular bacterial growth by lysing infected cells, and releasing the cytokines IL-1β and IL-18 (6), which promote host defense via pleiotropic mechanisms. IL-1α can induce neutrophil recruitment to facilitate bacterial clearance and IL-1β is best known to promote local inflammation and to recruit neutrophils to the site of infection. In turn, IL-18 is best known to induce IFN-γ secretion by natural killer cells and cytotoxic T lymphocytes (83). During systemic infection, caspase-11 is essential for host defense against cytosol-invasive bacteria, including *B. thailandensis* and *B. pseudomallei* (27). Mice deficient in caspase-11 are extremely susceptible to even mild infection with *B. thailandensis*, while wild-type mice are completely resistant to higher doses of infection (27, 39). We showed that the NLRC4 inflammasome detects *B. thailandensis*, and activates caspase-1 to trigger pyroptosis and IL-18 secretion. Curiously, we found that *in vitro*, *B. thailandensis* efficiently triggers both caspase-1 and—11-dependent pyroptosis in macrophages. *In vivo*, however, caspase-1-dependent pyroptosis plays only a minor role and cannot substitute for caspase-11-dependent pyroptosis. On the other hand, caspase-1-driven IL-18 was needed only to clear early infection. IL-18 promotes a robust and rapid production of IFN-γ, which primes caspase-11. This coordinated response clears even high dose infections in 1 day (39). In the absence of IL-18 signaling, *B. thailandensis* continues to replicate *in vivo* for 3 days. This prolonged bacterial burden triggers weak IFN-γ production via another undefined pathway, which is nonetheless sufficient to prime caspase-11 during medium or low dose infection and rescue the mice from lethality In high dose infections, this pathway comes too little and too late and *Il18*$^{-/-}$ mice succumb to infection. Intriguingly, while endogenous type I interferons were insufficient to prime caspase-11 in the absence of IFN-γ, injection of poly (I:C), a known inducer of IFN-β, successfully bypassed the IFN-γ requirement and primed caspase-11 *in vivo* (39). It is important to note that there are no examples in the literature of any pathogen–be it bacterial, fungal, viral, or parasite–in which the magnitude of protection conferred by caspase-11 inflammasomes approaches what is seen with *B. thailandensis* (84).

Caspase-11 also provides host protection in the lung in response to infection by Gram-negative bacterial pathogens, including *B. thailandensis* (7, 85), *Acinetobacter baumannii* (86), *Klebsiella pneumoniae* (87), *L. pneumophila* (88), and *L. gratiana* (88). As mentioned above, we found that *B. thailandensis* is detected by both caspase-1 and-11 in macrophages. Additionally, Wang et al. found that caspase-1 is the most important in response to *B. thailandensis in vitro*, and he showed that the absence of caspase-1 completely ablates release of IL-1β and IL-18 as well as pyroptosis of *Burkholderia*-infected macrophages. In contrast, pyroptosis, IL-1β and IL-18 of macrophages were not affected by deficiency of caspase-11. Interestingly, during pulmonary infection, mice lacking either caspase-1, 11 or GSDMD were significantly more susceptible than wild type mice to intranasal infection with *B. thailandensis* (7, 85). To account for this phenotype, Wang et al. showed that unlike macrophages, lung epithelial cells do not express caspase-1 canonical inflammasome components and are thus incompetent for caspase-1-mediated pyroptosis (7). Therefore, macrophages are protected by both caspase-1 and—11. However, lung epithelial cells solely depended on caspase-11 to restrict intracellular *B. thailandensis* replication in these cells (7).

A. baumannii, a pathogenic bacterium that can cause severe pulmonary infection, can activate caspase-1 through the NLRP3 inflammasome, leading to increased IL-1β release by macrophages. However, IL-1β release is partially abrogated in caspase-11-deficient macrophages, indicating that *A. baumannii* can also activate the caspase-11 non-canonical inflammasomes (86). Furthermore, caspase-11 deficiency completely ablates IL-1α secretion and reduces the cytotoxicity of *A. baumannii* in macrophages (86). Therefore, these data suggest that caspase-11 deficiency may impair the innate immune response to *A. baumannii* infection. Indeed, caspase-11-deficient mice register higher bacterial burdens in the BALF and lung tissue during *A. baumannii* infection. Additionally, caspase-11 deficiency causes mice to exhibit exacerbated pulmonary pathology due to extensive neutrophil Infiltration (86). Similarly, pulmonary infection of *Casp11*$^{-/-}$ with *K. pneumoniae*, showed that lack of caspase-11-dependent release of IL-1α impeded neutrophil recruitment in the early stage of *K. pneumoniae* infection and was accompanied by impaired bacterial clearance as well as exaggerated pulmonary pathological changes (87). Therefore, caspase-11 functions in the lung by promoting pyroptosis to prevent the bacteria from establishing an intracellular niche in macrophages and the lung epithelial. Additionally, caspase-11 pyroptosis can drive IL-1α and IL-1β release to recruit neutrophils that eventually will efferocytose and eliminate the offending bacteria.

CASPASE-11 HYPER-ACTIVATION DRIVES INFLAMMATORY LUNG DISEASES

Caspase-11-dependent pyroptosis and cytokines are important for combating respiratory infections. However, their excessive activation may contribute to the development of severe diseases in the lung. Acute lung injury (ALI) is a leading cause of death in bacterial sepsis (8). ALI is characterized by massive destruction of the lung endothelial barrier which results in lung edema, influx of pro-inflammatory leukocytes and sever hypoxemia (8). During endotoxemia, high concentrations of LPS may persist and aberrantly localize to the cytoplasm, triggering the hyper-activation of caspase-11 and resulting in massive pyroptosis. The hyper-activation of caspase-11 drives endotoxin shock independently of TLR4 (32, 33). During an ALI model, Cheng et al. show that the activation of caspase-11 with LPS causes severe endothelial pyroptosis that results in ALI (8). Exposure to LPS has also been shown to play a major role in asthma development (89) and recently, caspase-11 response was implicated as a critical contributor to asthma (90). Using the ovalbumin model of allergic airway inflammation, Zaslona et al. found that expression of caspase-11 is elevated in the lung of wild type mice with allergic airway inflammation. Interestingly, they found that caspase-11-deficient mice are strongly resistant to this pathology (90). However, how caspase-11 is activated in this model isn't clear. Zaslona et al. suggest that the lung is a non-sterile environment, and LPS released from naturally occurring lung bacteria might activate caspase-11, leading to airway inflammation and asthma in susceptible individuals.

In patients with cystic fibrosis (CF), *P. aeruginosa* can cause chronic airway infection that is characterized by an exaggerated pro-inflammatory cytokine response and sustained, neutrophil-dominant inflammation (91). Previous studies have demonstrated a role of NLRP3 and NLRC4 inflammasome activation in response to *P. aeruginosa* infection in CF patients (73, 92). However, *P. aeruginosa* strains isolated from chronically infected CF patients have either defective T3SS or are non-motile, enabling them to evade NLRC4-caspase-1 inflammasome detection (93–95). Balakrishan et al. showed that caspase-11 can detect these T3SS-negative *P. aeruginosa* isolates (73). However, whether this detection takes place *in vivo* to drive inflammation and disease in CF has yet to be determined.

OUT-SMARTING THE CASPASE-11 NON-CANONICAL INFLAMMASOME

Caspase-11 protects against lethal infection mediated by cytosol-invasive pathogens (27), it is particularly important for protection against ubiquitous environmental bacteria that have not evolved to escape cytosolic detection, such as the aforementioned *B. thailandensis*. However, it is not surprising that a number of organisms have evolved specific strategies to avoid the activation of this innate immune signaling pathway. These strategies include limiting LPS access to the cytosol, modifying the structural features of LPS to avoid binding to caspase-11, or suppressing caspase-11 and/or GBPs activity.

As noted above, preventing access of LPS to the cytosol using vacuolar niches or by remaining extracellular are prominent ways to avoid caspase-11 activation. For instance, *S. typhimurium* and *L. pneumophila* use T3SS and T4SS, respectively, to translocate effector proteins that work in concert to establish and maintain an intracellular vacuolar growth niche. Loss of the *S. typhimurium SifA* or *L. pneumophila SdhA* effectors causes rupture of the vacuole and release of bacteria into the cytosol (96–98). As we might expect, these two bacteria are poorly detected by caspase-11, while their isogenic mutants for these proteins are readily detected by caspase-11, with half the attenuation of the *S. typhimurium* Δ*sifA* mutant in mice explained by caspase-11 activation alone (27).

Another strategy is to modify the chemical structure of LPS to avoid detection. Caspase-11 uses its CARD domain to bind penta- or hexa-acylated lipid A moieties on LPS (32, 33, 36). As such, several tetra-acyl lipid A structures from pathogens like *Francisella novicida*, *Yersinia pestis*, and *S. flexenri* have been shown to evade caspase-11/4 detection (33, 99). Indeed, during pulmonary infection, bacteria often appear to exploit these structural requirements in order to evade caspase-11. For example, *F. novicida*, a Gram-negative cytosolic bacterium, is not detected by caspase-11 (33). *F. novicida* initially synthesizes a penta-acylated lipid A structure with two phosphates, but then removes the 4' phosphate and 3′ acyl chain resulting in under-acylated LPS that does not activate caspase-11 (100, 101). A similar strategy is used by *Y. pestis*, which removes two acyl chains from its lipid A upon transition from growth at 25°C to 37°C (102). Caspase-11 detects hexa-acylated lipid A from *Y. pestis* grown at 25°C, but not tetra-acylated lipid A from bacteria grown at 37°C (33). Surprisingly, Lagrange et al. found that one of the human homologs of caspase-11, caspase-4, is able to respond to tetra-acylated LPS from *F. novicida* (103), suggesting that the caspase-11 duplication in human may have evolved to accommodate a broader LPS repertoire than that of mice.

Other strategies to evade caspase-11 detection may involve directly inhibiting the caspase-11 signaling pathway, as in the case of *S. flexneri*, which uses its OspC3 effector to specifically inhibit LPS detection by caspase-4 (104). Additionally, *Shigella* delivers an array of effector factors such as the ubiquitin ligase effector IpaH9.8 to target GBPs for proteasomal degradation (64, 65). Finally, host factors also can suppress the activity of caspase-11. For instance, L-adrenaline inhibits caspase-11 inflammasome activation through the ADRA2B receptor and the intracellular cAMP metabolism pathway in mouse macrophages or human monocytes (105). It is plausible that pathogens may manipulate this host metabolic pathway to their advantage.

CONCLUDING REMARKS

Lung tissue is a unique epithelial space constantly exposed to a variety of assaults from infectious and non-infectious stimuli. Innate immune detection of, and responses to, intracellular pathogens that invade host cells is paramount in defending against infections. The caspase-11 non-canonical inflammsome plays a key role in this response. It is widely expressed in both hematopoietic and non-hematopoietic cells of the lung, functioning as a general sensor of Gram-negative bacteria whose activation results in protective innate immune effectors including pyroptosis, NETosis, and inflammatory cytokines. Therefore, it is not surprising that bacterial pathogens have evolved several strategies to outsmart caspase-11-mediated sensing of LPS and subsequent activation. Indeed, the importance of this pathway is demonstrated by those species that have not evolved to evade caspase-11, such as *B. thailandensis*, which strongly triggers caspase-11-dependent effector mechanisms that quickly lead to sterilization of the infection. This remarkable protection highlights an important role of inflammasomes in defense against environmental pathogens. Similarly, pathogens that poorly activate the caspase-11 inflammasome can multiply to uncontrolled levels in the lung, resulting in higher levels of LPS that will eventually access the cell cytosol and hyper-activate caspase-11, leading to LPS induced lung injury and sepsis. Future studies uncovering the structural features of lipid A that activate caspase-11 and the cell-specific roles of the caspase-11 inflammasome in lung tissue could identify new therapeutic avenues to treat infection, sepsis, and immune-mediated pathologies within the lung.

AUTHOR CONTRIBUTIONS

CO, AV, and YA wrote the article. CO and YA contributed to designing the figure. All authors contributed to the article and approved the submitted version.

ACKNOWLEDGMENTS

We wish to thank Alan Tubbs and Stephen Kovacs for their suggestions and editing the manuscript. We also acknowledge the UAMS Center for Microbial Pathogenesis and Host Inflammatory Responses (CMPHIR) for continued support.

REFERENCES

1. GBD 2016 Lower Respiratory Infections Collaborators. Estimates of the global, regional, national morbidity. mortality, and aetiologies of lower respiratory infections in 195 countries, 1990-2016: a systematic analysis for the Global burden of disease study 2016. *Lancet Infect Dis.* (2018) 18:1191–210. doi: 10.1016/S1473-3099(18)30310-4
2. Akira S, Uematsu S, Takeuchi O. Pathogen recognition and innate immunity. *Cell.* (2006) 124:783–801. doi: 10.1016/j.cell.2006.02.015
3. Hayashi F, Smith KD, Ozinsky A, Hawn TR, Yi EC, Goodlett DR, et al. The innate immune response to bacterial flagellin is mediated by Toll-like receptor 5. *Nature.* (2001) 410:1099–103. doi: 10.1038/35074106
4. Miao EA, Alpuche-Aranda CM, Dors M, Clark AE, Bader MW, Miller SI, et al. Cytoplasmic flagellin activates caspase-1 and secretion of interleukin 1β via Ipaf. *Nat Immunol.* (2006) 7:569–75. doi: 10.1038/ni1344
5. Franchi L, Amer A, Body-Malapel M, Kanneganti T-D, Özören N, Jagirdar R, Inohara N, et al. Cytosolic flagellin requires Ipaf for activation of caspase-1 and interleukin 1β in salmonella-infected macrophages. *Nat Immunol.* (2006) 7:576–82. doi: 10.1038/ni1346
6. Aachoui Y, Sagulenko V, Miao EA, Stacey KJ. Inflammasome-mediated pyroptotic and apoptotic cell death, and defense against infection. *Curr Opin Microbiol.* (2013) 16:319–26. doi: 10.1016/j.mib.2013.04.004
7. Wang J, Sahoo M, Lantier L, Warawa J, Cordero H, Deobald K, et al. Caspase-11-dependent pyroptosis of lung epithelial cells protects from melioidosis while caspase-1 mediates macrophage pyroptosis and production of IL-18. *PLoS Pathog.* (2018) 14:e1007105. doi: 10.1371/journal.ppat.1007105
8. Cheng KT, Xiong S, Ye Z, Hong Z, Di A, Tsang KM, et al. Caspase-11-mediated endothelial pyroptosis underlies endotoxemia-induced lung injury. *J Clin Invest.* (2017) 127:4124–4135. doi: 10.1172/JCI94495
9. Ulland TK, Ferguson PJ, Sutterwala FS. Evasion of inflammasome activation by microbial pathogens. *J Clin Invest.* (2015) 125:469–77. doi: 10.1172/JCI75254
10. Miao EA, Mao DP, Yudkovsky N, Bonneau R, Lorang CG, Warren SE, et al. Innate immune detection of the type III secretion apparatus through the NLRC4 inflammasome. *Proc Natl Acad Sci USA.* (2010) 107:3076–80. doi: 10.1073/pnas.0913087107
11. Miao EA, Leaf IA, Treuting PM, Mao DP, Dors M, Sarkar A, et al. Caspase-1-induced pyroptosis is an innate immune effector mechanism against intracellular bacteria. *Nat Immunol.* (2010) 11:1136–42. doi: 10.1038/ni.1960
12. van Opdenbosch N, Lamkanfi M. Caspases in cell death, inflammation, and disease. *Immunity.* (2019) 50:1352–64. doi: 10.1016/j.immuni.2019.05.020
13. Jorgensen I, Rayamajhi M, Miao EA. Programmed cell death as a defence against infection. *Nat Rev Immunol.* (2017) 17:151–64. doi: 10.1038/nri.2016.147
14. Swanson KV, Deng M, Ting JPY. The NLRP3 inflammasome: molecular activation and regulation to therapeutics. *Nat Rev Immunol.* (2019) 19:477–89. doi: 10.1038/s41577-019-0165-0
15. Hornung V, Ablasser A, Charrel-Dennis M, Bauernfeind F, Horvath G, Caffrey DR, et al. AIM2 recognizes cytosolic dsDNA and forms a caspase-1-activating inflammasome with ASA. *Nature.* (2009) 458:514–8. doi: 10.1038/nature07725
16. Fernandes-Alnemri T, Yu JW, Datta P, Wu J, Alnemri ES. AIM2 activates the inflammasome and cell death in response to cytoplasmic DNA. *Nature.* (2009) 458:509–13. doi: 10.1038/nature07710
17. Roberts TL, Idris A, Dunn JA, Kelly GM, Burnton CM, Hodgson S, et al. HIN-200 proteins regulate caspase activation in response to foreign cytoplasmic DNA. *Science.* (2009) 323:1057–60. doi: 10.1126/science.1169841
18. Kofoed EM, Vance RE. Innate immune recognition of bacterial ligands by NAIPs determines inflammasome specificity. *Nature.* (2011) 477:592–5. doi: 10.1038/nature10394
19. Zhao Y, Yang J, Shi J, Gong Y-N, Lu Q, Xu H, et al. The NLRC4 inflammasome receptors for bacterial flagellin and type III secretion apparatus. *Nature.* (2011) 477:596–600. doi: 10.1038/nature10510
20. Rayamajhi M, Zak DE, Chavarria-Smith J, Vance RE, Miao EA. Cutting edge: mouse NAIP1 detects the type III secretion system needle protein. *J Immunol.* (2013) 191:3986–9. doi: 10.4049/jimmunol.1301549
21. Yang J, Zhao Y, Shi J, Shao F. Human NAIP and mouse NAIP1 recognize bacterial type III secretion needle protein for inflammasome activation. *Proc Natl Acad Sci USA.* (2013) 110:14408–13. doi: 10.1073/pnas.1306376110

22. Kovacs SB, Miao EA. Gasdermins: effectors of pyroptosis. *Trends Cell Biol.* (2017) 27:673–84. doi: 10.1016/j.tcb.2017.05.005
23. Di Paolo NC, Shayakhmetov DM. *Interleukin.* 1α and the inflammatory process. *Nat Immunol.* (2016) 17:906–13. doi: 10.1038/ni.3503
24. Kayagaki N, Warming S, Lamkanfi M, Walle LV, Louie S, Dong J, et al. Non-canonical inflammasome activation targets caspase-11. *Nature.* (2011) 479:117–21. doi: 10.1038/nature10558
25. Wang S, Miura M, Jung Y, Zhu H, Gagliardini V, Shi L, et al. Identification and characterization of Ich-3, a member of the interleukin-1beta converting enzyme (ICE)/Ced-3 family and an upstream regulator of ICE. *J Biol Chem.* (1996) 271:20580–7. doi: 10.1074/jbc.271.34.20580
26. Wang S, Miura M, Jung YK, Zhu H, Li E, Yuan J. Murine caspase-11, an ICE-interacting protease, is essential for the activation of ICE. *Cell.* (1998) 92:501–9. doi: 10.1016/S0092-8674(00)80943-5
27. Aachoui Y, Leaf IA, Hagar JA, Fontana MF, Campos CG, Zak DE, et al. Caspase-11 protects against bacteria that escape the vacuole. *Science.* (2013) 339:975–8. doi: 10.1126/science.1230751
28. Broz P, Ruby T, Belhocine K, Bouley DM, Kayagaki N, Dixit VM, et al. Caspase-11 increases susceptibility to Salmonella infection in the absence of caspase-1. *Nature.* (2012) 490:288–91. doi: 10.1038/nature11419
29. Gurung P, Malireddi RK, Anand PK, Demon D, Vande Walle L, Liu Z, et al. Toll or interleukin-1 receptor (TIR) domain-containing adaptor inducing interferon-beta (TRIF)-mediated caspase-11 protease production integrates Toll-like receptor 4 (TLR4) protein- and Nlrp3 inflammasome-mediated host defense against enteropathogens. *J Biol Chem.* (2012) 287:34474–83. doi: 10.1074/jbc.M112.401406
30. Rathinam VAK, Vanaja SK, Waggoner L, Sokolovska A, Becker C, Stuart LM, et al. Fitzgerald. TRIF licenses caspase-11-dependent NLRP3 inflammasome activation by gram-negative bacteria. *Cell.* (2012) 150:606–19. doi: 10.1016/j.cell.2012.07.007
31. Case CL, Kohler LJ, Lima JB, Strowig T, de Zoete MR, Flavell RA, et al. Caspase-11 stimulates rapid flagellin-independent pyroptosis in response to Legionella pneumophila. *Proc Natl Acad Sci USA.* (2013) 110:1851–6. doi: 10.1073/pnas.1211521110
32. Kayagaki N, Wong MT, Stowe IB, Ramani SR, Gonzalez LC, Akashi-Takamura S, et al. Noncanonical inflammasome activation by intracellular LPS independent of TLR4. *Science.* (2013) 341:1246–9. doi: 10.1126/science.1240248
33. Hagar JA, Powell DA, Aachoui Y, Ernst RK, Miao EA. Cytoplasmic LPS activates caspase-11: implications in TLR4-independent endotoxic shock. *Science.* (2013) 341:1250–3. doi: 10.1126/science.1240988
34. Hornef MW, Frisan T, vandewalle A, Normark S, Richter-Dahlfors A. Toll-like receptor 4 resides in the golgi apparatus and colocalizes with internalized lipopolysaccharide in intestinal epithelial cells. *J Exp Med.* (2002) 195:559–70. doi: 10.1084/jem.20011788
35. Hornef MW, Normark BH, Vandewalle A, Normark S. Intracellular recognition of lipopolysaccharide by toll-like receptor 4 in intestinal epithelial cells. *J Exp Med.* (2003) 198:1225–35. doi: 10.1084/jem.20022194
36. Shi J, Zhao Y, Wang Y, Gao W, Ding J, Li P, et al. Inflammatory caspases are innate immune receptors for intracellular LPS. *Nature.* (2014) 514:187–92. doi: 10.1038/nature13683
37. Lee BL, Stowe IB, Gupta A, Kornfeld OS, Roose-Girma M, Anderson K, et al. Caspase-11 auto-proteolysis is crucial for noncanonical inflammasome activation. *J Exp Med.* (2018) 215:2279–88. doi: 10.1084/jem.20180589
38. Kajiwara Y, Schiff T, Voloudakis G, Gama Sosa MA, Elder G, Bozdagi O, et al. A critical role for human caspase-4 in endotoxin sensitivity. *J Immunol.* (2014) 193:335–43. doi: 10.4049/jimmunol.1303424
39. Aachoui Y, Kajiwara Y, Leaf IA, Mao D, Ting J-PY, Coers J, et al. Canonical inflammasomes drive IFN-γ to prime caspase-11 in defense against a cytosol-invasive bacterium. *Cell Host Microbe.* (2015) 18:320–32 doi: 10.1016/j.chom.2015.07.016
40. Lin XY, Choi MS, Porter AG. Expression analysis of the human caspase-1 subfamily reveals specific regulation of the CASP5 gene by lipopolysaccharide and interferon-gamma. *J Biol Chem.* (2000) 275:39920–6. doi: 10.1074/jbc.M007255200
41. Schauvliege R, vanrobaeys J, Schotte P, Beyaert R. Caspase-11 gene expression in response to lipopolysaccharide and interferon-gamma requires nuclear factor-kappa B and signal transducer and activator of transcription (STAT) 1. *J Biol Chem.* (2002) 277:41624–30. doi: 10.1074/jbc.M207852200
42. He W-t, Wan H, Hu L, Chen P, Wang X, Huang Z, et al. Gasdermin D is an executor of pyroptosis and required for interleukin-1β secretion. *Cell Research.* (2015) 25:1285–98. doi: 10.1038/cr.2015.139
43. Kayagaki N, Stowe IB, Lee BL, O'Rourke K, Anderson K, Warming S, et al. Caspase-11 cleaves gasdermin D for non-canonical inflammasome signalling. *Nature.* (2015) 526:666–71. doi: 10.1038/nature15541
44. Shi J, Zhao Y, Wang K, Shi X, Wang Y, Huang H, et al. Cleavage of GSDMD by inflammatory caspases determines pyroptotic cell death. *Nature.* (2015) 526:660–5. doi: 10.1038/nature15514
45. Sborgi L, Rühl S, Mulvihill E, Pipercevic J, Heilig R, Stahlberg H, et al. GSDMD membrane pore formation constitutes the mechanism of pyroptotic cell death. *EMBO J.* (2016) 35:1766–78. doi: 10.15252/embj.201694696
46. Liu X, Zhang Z, Ruan J, Pan Y, Magupalli VG, Wu H, et al. Inflammasome-activated gasdermin D causes pyroptosis by forming membrane pores. *Nature.* (2016) 535:153–8. doi: 10.1038/nature18629
47. Ding J, Wang K, Liu W, She Y, Sun Q, Shi J, et al. Pore-forming activity and structural autoinhibition of the gasdermin family. *Nature.* (2016) 535:111–6. doi: 10.1038/nature18590
48. Muñoz-Planillo R, Kuffa P, Martínez-Colón G, Smith BL, Rajendiran TM, Núñez G. K+ efflux is the common trigger of NLRP3 inflammasome activation by bacterial toxins and particulate matter. *Immunity.* (2013) 38:1142–53. doi: 10.1016/j.immuni.2013.05.016
49. Kanneganti T-D, Lamkanfi M. K+ drops tilt the NLRP3 inflammasome. *Immunity.* (2013) 38:1085–8. doi: 10.1016/j.immuni.2013.06.001
50. Ruhl S, Broz P. Caspase-11 activates a canonical NLRP3 inflammasome by promoting K(+) efflux. *Eur J Immunol.* (2015) 45:2927–36. doi: 10.1002/eji.201545772
51. Baker PJ, Boucher D, Bierschenk D, Tebartz C, Whitney PG, D'Silva DB, et al. NLRP3 inflammasome activation downstream of cytoplasmic LPS recognition by both caspase-4 and caspase-5. *Eur J Immunol.* (2015) 45:2918–26. doi: 10.1002/eji.201545655
52. Evavold CL, Ruan J, Tan Y, Xia S, Wu H, Kagan JC. The pore-forming protein gasdermin d regulates interleukin-1 secretion from living macrophages. *Immunity.* (2018) 48:35–44.e6. doi: 10.1016/j.immuni.2017.11.013
53. Heilig R, Dick MS, Sborgi L, Meunier E, Hiller S, Broz P. The Gasdermin-D pore acts as a conduit for IL-1β secretion in mice. *Eur J Immunol.* (2018) 48:584–92. doi: 10.1002/eji.201747404
54. Jorgensen I, Zhang Y, Krantz BA, Miao EA. Pyroptosis triggers pore-induced intracellular traps (PITs) that capture bacteria and lead to their clearance by efferocytosis. *J Exp Med.* (2016) 213:2113–28. doi: 10.1084/jem.20151613
55. Rühl S, Shkarina K, Demarco B, Heilig R, Santos JC, Broz P. ESCRT-dependent membrane repair negatively regulates pyroptosis downstream of GSDMD activation. *Science.* (2018) 362:956–60. doi: 10.1126/science.aar7607
56. Sollberger G, Choidas A, Burn GL, Habenberger P, Di Lucrezia R, Kordes S, et al. Gasdermin D plays a vital role in the generation of neutrophil extracellular traps. *Sci Immunol.* (2018) 3:eaar6689. doi: 10.1126/sciimmunol.aar6689
57. Chen KW, Monteleone M, Boucher D, Sollberger G, Ramnath D, Condon ND, et al. Noncanonical inflammasome signaling elicits gasdermin D-dependent neutrophil extracellular traps. *Sci Immunol.* (2018) 3:eaar6676. doi: 10.1126/sciimmunol.aar6676
58. Porto BN, Stein RT. Neutrophil extracellular traps in pulmonary diseases: too much of a good thing? *Front Immunol.* (2016) 7:311. doi: 10.3389/fimmu.2016.00311
59. Knodler LA, Crowley SM, Sham HP, Yang H, Wrande M, Ma C, et al. Noncanonical inflammasome activation of caspase-4/caspase-11 mediates epithelial defenses against enteric bacterial pathogens. *Cell Host Microbe.* (2014) 16:249–56. doi: 10.1016/j.chom.2014.07.002
60. Wiersinga WJ, van der Poll T, White NJ, Day NP, Peacock SJ. Melioidosis: insights into the pathogenicity of Burkholderia pseudomallei. *Nat Rev Microbiol.* (2006) 4:272–82. doi: 10.1038/nrmicro1385
61. Pilla DM, Hagar JA, Haldar AK, Mason AK, Degrandi D, Pfeffer K, et al. Guanylate binding proteins promote caspase-11–dependent pyroptosis in response to cytoplasmic LPS. *Proc Natl Acad Sci.* (2014) 111:6046–51. doi: 10.1073/pnas.1321700111

62. Meunier E, Dick MS, Dreier RF, Schurmann N, Kenzelmann Broz D, Warming S, et al. Caspase-11 activation requires lysis of pathogen-containing vacuoles by IFN-induced GTPases. *Nature.* (2014) 509:366–70. doi: 10.1038/nature13157
63. Kravets E, Degrandi D, Ma Q, Peulen TO, Klumpers V, Felekyan S, et al. Guanylate binding proteins directly attack *Toxoplasma gondii* via supramolecular complexes. *Elife.* (2016) 5:e11479. doi: 10.7554/eLife.11479
64. Li P, Jiang W, Yu Q, Liu W, Zhou P, Li J, et al. Ubiquitination and degradation of GBPs by a Shigella effector to suppress host defence. *Nature.* (2017) 551:378–83. doi: 10.1038/nature24467
65. Wandel MP, Pathe C, Werner EI, Ellison CJ, Boyle KB, von der Malsburg A, et al. GBPs inhibit motility of shigella flexneri but are targeted for degradation by the bacterial ubiquitin ligase IpaH9.8. *Cell Host Microbe.* (2017) 22:507–18.e5. doi: 10.1016/j.chom.2017.09.007
66. Thurston TL, Matthews SA, Jennings E, Alix E, Shao F, Shenoy AR, et al. Growth inhibition of cytosolic Salmonella by caspase-1 and caspase-11 precedes host cell death. *Nat Commun.* (2016) 7:13292. doi: 10.1038/ncomms13292
67. Man SM, Place DE, Kuriakose T, Kanneganti TD. Interferon-inducible guanylate-binding proteins at the interface of cell-autonomous immunity and inflammasome activation. *J Leukoc Biol.* (2017) 101:143–50. doi: 10.1189/jlb.4MR0516-223R
68. Kim BH, Shenoy AR, Kumar P, Das R, Tiwari S, MacMicking JD. A family of IFN-gamma-inducible 65-kD GTPases protects against bacterial infection. *Science.* (2011) 332:717–21. doi: 10.1126/science.1201711
69. Olszewski MA, Gray J, Vestal DJ. In silico genomic analysis of the human and murine guanylate-binding protein (GBP) gene clusters. *J Interferon Cytokine Res.* (2006) 26:328–52. doi: 10.1089/jir.2006.26.328
70. Degrandi D, Konermann C, Beuter-Gunia C, Kresse A, Wurthner J, Kurig S, et al. Extensive characterization of IFN-induced GTPases mGBP1 to mGBP10 involved in host defense. *J Immunol.* (2007) 179:7729–40. doi: 10.4049/jimmunol.179.11.7729
71. Shenoy AR, Kim BH, Choi HP, Matsuzawa T, Tiwari S, MacMicking JD. Emerging themes in IFN-gamma-induced macrophage immunity by the p47 and p65 GTPase families. *Immunobiology.* (2007) 212:771–84. doi: 10.1016/j.imbio.2007.09.018
72. Finethy R, Jorgensen I, Haldar AK, de Zoete MR, Strowig T, Flavell RA, et al. Guanylate binding proteins enable rapid activation of canonical and noncanonical inflammasomes in Chlamydia-infected macrophages. *Infect Immun.* (2015) 83:4740–9. doi: 10.1128/IAI.00856-15
73. Balakrishnan A, Karki R, Berwin B, Yamamoto M, Kanneganti T-D. Guanylate binding proteins facilitate caspase-11-dependent pyroptosis in response to type 3 secretion system-negative Pseudomonas aeruginosa. *Cell Death Discov.* (2018) 4:66. doi: 10.1038/s41420-018-0068-z
74. Feeley EM, Pilla-Moffett DM, Zwack EE, Piro AS, Finethy R, Kolb JP, et al. Galectin-3 directs antimicrobial guanylate binding proteins to vacuoles furnished with bacterial secretion systems. *Proc Natl Acad Sci USA.* (2017) 114:E1698–706. doi: 10.1073/pnas.1615771114
75. Kim BH, Chee JD, Bradfield CJ, Park ES, Kumar P, MacMicking JD. Interferon-induced guanylate-binding proteins in inflammasome activation and host defense. *Nat Immunol.* (2016) 17:481–9. doi: 10.1038/ni.3440
76. Pilla-Moffett D, Barber MF, Taylor GA, Coers J. Interferon-inducible GTPases in host resistance, inflammation and disease. *J Mol Biol.* (2016) 428:3495–513. doi: 10.1016/j.jmb.2016.04.032
77. Santos JC, Boucher D, Schneider LK, Demarco B, Dilucca M, Shkarina K, et al. Human GBP1 binds LPS to initiate assembly of a caspase-4 activating platform on cytosolic bacteria. *Nat Commun.* (2020) 11:3276. doi: 10.1038/s41467-020-16889-z
78. Wandel MP, Kim BH, Park ES, Boyle KB, Nayak K, Lagrange B, et al. Guanylate-binding proteins convert cytosolic bacteria into caspase-4 signaling platforms. *Nat Immunol.* (2020) 21:880–91. doi: 10.1038/s41590-020-0697-2
79. Kutsch M, Sistemich L, Lesser CF, Goldberg MB, Herrmann C, Coers J. Direct binding of polymeric GBP1 to LPS disrupts bacterial cell envelope functions. *EMBO J.* (2020) 39:e104926. doi: 10.15252/embj.2020104926
80. Man SM, Karki R, Sasai M, Place DE, Kesavardhana S, Temirov J, et al. IRGB10 liberates bacterial ligands for sensing by the AIM2 and caspase-11-NLRP3 inflammasomes. *Cell.* (2016) 167:382–96.e17. doi: 10.1016/j.cell.2016.09.012
81. Vanaja SK, Russo AJ, Behl B, Banerjee I, Yankova M, Deshmukh SD, et al. Bacterial outer membrane vesicles mediate cytosolic localization of LPS and caspase-11 activation. *Cell.* (2016) 165:1106–19. doi: 10.1016/j.cell.2016.04.015
82. Santos JC, Dick MS, Lagrange B, Degrandi D, Pfeffer K, Yamamoto M, et al. LPS targets host guanylate-binding proteins to the bacterial outer membrane for non-canonical inflammasome activation. *EMBO J.* (2018) 37:e98089. doi: 10.15252/embj.201798089
83. Dinarello CA. IL-18: A TH1-inducing, proinflammatory cytokine and new member of the IL-1 family. *J Allergy Clin Immunol.* (1999) 103(1 Pt 1):11–24. doi: 10.1016/S0091-6749(99)70518-X
84. Maltez VI, Miao EA. Reassessing the evolutionary importance of inflammasomes. *J Immunol.* (2016) 196:956–62. doi: 10.4049/jimmunol.1502060
85. Wang J, Deobald K, Re F. Gasdermin D protects from melioidosis through pyroptosis and direct killing of bacteria. *J Immunol.* (2019) 202:3468–73. doi: 10.4049/jimmunol.1900045
86. Wang W, Shao Y, Li S, Xin N, Ma T, Zhao C, et al. Caspase-11 plays a protective role in pulmonary acinetobacter baumannii infection. *Infect Immun.* (2017) 85:e00350–17. doi: 10.1128/IAI.00350-17
87. Wang J, Shao Y, Wang W, Li S, Xin N, Xie F, et al. Caspase-11 deficiency impairs neutrophil recruitment and bacterial clearance in the early stage of pulmonary Klebsiella pneumoniae infection. *Int J Med Microbiol.* (2017) 307:490–6. doi: 10.1016/j.ijmm.2017.09.012
88. Cerqueira DM, Pereira MS, Silva AL, Cunha LD, Zamboni DS. Caspase-1 but not caspase-11 Is required for NLRC4-mediated pyroptosis and restriction of infection by flagellated legionella species in mouse macrophages and *in vivo*. *J Immunol.* (2015) 195:2303–11. doi: 10.4049/jimmunol.1501223
89. Simpson A, Martinez FD. The role of lipopolysaccharide in the development of atopy in humans. *Clin Exp Allergy.* (2010) 40:209–23. doi: 10.1111/j.1365-2222.2009.03391.x
90. Zasłona Z, Flis E, Wilk MM, Carroll RG, Palsson-McDermott EM, Hughes MM, et al. Caspase-11 promotes allergic airway inflammation. *Nat Commun.* (2020) 11:1055. doi: 10.1038/s41467-020-14945-2
91. Bonfield TL, Panuska JR, Konstan MW, Hilliard KA, Hilliard JB, Ghnaim H, et al. Inflammatory cytokines in cystic fibrosis lungs. *Am J Respir Crit Care Med.* (1995) 152(6 Pt 1):2111–8. doi: 10.1164/ajrccm.152.6.8520783
92. Rimessi A, Bezzerri V, Patergnani S, Marchi S, Cabrini G, Pinton P. Mitochondrial Ca2+-dependent NLRP3 activation exacerbates the Pseudomonas aeruginosa-driven inflammatory response in cystic fibrosis. *Nat Commun.* (2015) 6:6201. doi: 10.1038/ncomms7201
93. Mahenthiralingam E, Campbell ME, Speert D. Nonmotility P, and phagocytic resistance of Pseudomonas aeruginosa isolates from chronically colonized patients with cystic fibrosis. *Infect Immun.* (1994) 62:596–605. doi: 10.1128/IAI.62.2.596-605.1994
94. Jain M, Ramirez D, Seshadri R, Cullina JF, Powers CA, Schulert GS, et al. Type III secretion phenotypes of Pseudomonas aeruginosa strains change during infection of individuals with cystic fibrosis. *J Clin Microbiol.* (2004) 42:5229–37. doi: 10.1128/JCM.42.11.5229-5237.2004
95. Huus KE, Joseph J, Zhang L, Wong A, Aaron SD, Mah TF, et al. Clinical isolates of pseudomonas aeruginosa from chronically infected cystic fibrosis patients fail to activate the inflammasome during both stable infection and pulmonary exacerbation. *J Immunol.* (2016) 196:3097–108. doi: 10.4049/jimmunol.1501642
96. Beuzón CR, Méresse S, Unsworth KE, Ruíz-Albert J, Garvis S, Waterman SR, et al. Salmonella maintains the integrity of its intracellular vacuole through the action of SifA. *EMBO J.* (2000) 19:3235–49. doi: 10.1093/emboj/19.13.3235
97. Creasey EA, Isberg RR. The protein SdhA maintains the integrity of the Legionella-containing vacuole. *Proc Natl Acad Sci USA.* (2012) 109:3481–6. doi: 10.1073/pnas.1121286109
98. Ge J, Gong YN, Xu Y, Shao F. Preventing bacterial DNA release and absent in melanoma 2 inflammasome activation by a Legionella effector functioning in membrane trafficking. *Proc Natl Acad Sci USA.* (2012) 109:6193–8. doi: 10.1073/pnas.1117490109

99. Paciello I, Silipo A, Lembo-Fazio L, Curcurù L, Zumsteg A, Noël G, et al. Intracellular Shigella remodels its LPS to dampen the innate immune recognition and evade inflammasome activation. *Proc Natl Acad Sci USA.* (2013) 110:E4345–54. doi: 10.1073/pnas.1303641110
100. Wang X, Ribeiro AA, Guan Z, Abraham SN, Raetz CR. Attenuated virulence of a Francisella mutant lacking the lipid A 4'-phosphatase. *Proc Natl Acad Sci USA.* (2007) 104:4136–41. doi: 10.1073/pnas.0611606104
101. Kanistanon D, Powell DA, Hajjar AM, Pelletier MR, Cohen IE, Way SS, et al. Role of Francisella lipid A phosphate modification in virulence and long-term protective immune responses. *Infect Immun.* (2012) 80:943–51. doi: 10.1128/IAI.06109-11
102. Rebeil R, Ernst RK, Gowen BB, Miller SI, Hinnebusch BJ. Variation in lipid A structure in the pathogenic yersiniae. *Mol Microbiol.* (2004) 52:1363–73. doi: 10.1111/j.1365-2958.2004.04059.x
103. Lagrange B, Benaoudia S, Wallet P, Magnotti F, Provost A, Michal F, et al. Human caspase-4 detects tetra-acylated LPS and cytosolic Francisella and functions differently from murine caspase-11. *Nat Commun.* (2018) 9:242. doi: 10.1038/s41467-017-02682-y
104. Kobayashi T, Ogawa M, Sanada T, Mimuro H, Kim M, Ashida H, et al. The Shigella OspC3 effector inhibits caspase-4, antagonizes inflammatory cell death, and promotes epithelial infection. *Cell Host Microbe.* (2013) 13:570–83. doi: 10.1016/j.chom.2013.04.012
105. Chen R, Zeng L, Zhu S, Liu J, Zeh HJ, Kroemer G, et al. cAMP metabolism controls caspase-11 inflammasome activation and pyroptosis in sepsis. *Sci Adv.* (2019) 5:eaav5562. doi: 10.1126/sciadv.aav5562

10

High Nuclease Activity of Long Persisting *Staphylococcus aureus* Isolates within the Airways of Cystic Fibrosis Patients Protects Against NET-Mediated Killing

*Susann Herzog[1,2], Felix Dach[1,2], Nicole de Buhr[3], Silke Niemann[1], Jannik Schlagowski[1], Diego Chaves-Moreno[4], Claudia Neumann[1], Jonas Goretzko[5], Vera Schwierzeck[6], Alexander Mellmann[6], Angelika Dübbers[7], Peter Küster[8], Holger Schültingkemper[8], Ursula Rescher[5], Dietmar H. Pieper[4], Maren von Köckritz-Blickwede[3] and Barbara C. Kahl[1,2]**

[1] *Institute of Medical Microbiology, University Hospital Münster, Münster, Germany,* [2] *Interdisciplinary Center for Clinical Research, Münster, Germany,* [3] *Institute of Physiological Chemistry, University of Veterinary Medicine Hannover, Hanover, Germany,* [4] *Helmholtz Center for Infection Research, Helmholtz Association of German Research Centers (HZ), Brunswick, Germany,* [5] *Center for Molecular Biology of Inflammation (ZMBE), Institute of Medical Biochemistry, University of Münster, Münster, Germany,* [6] *Institute of Hygiene, University Hospital Münster, Münster, Germany,* [7] *Department of Pediatrics, University Hospital Münster, Münster, Germany,* [8] *Department of Pediatrics, Clemenshospital, Münster, Germany*

***Correspondence:**
Barbara C. Kahl
kahl@uni-muenster.de

Staphylococcus aureus is one of the first and most prevalent pathogens cultured from the airways of cystic fibrosis (CF) patients, which can persist there for extended periods. Airway infections in CF patients are characterized by a strong inflammatory response of highly recruited neutrophils. One killing mechanism of neutrophils is the formation of neutrophil extracellular traps (NETs), which capture and eradicate bacteria by extracellular fibers of neutrophil chromatin decorated with antimicrobial granule proteins. *S. aureus* secretes nuclease, which can degrade NETs. We hypothesized, that *S. aureus* adapts to the airways of CF patients during persistent infection by escaping from NET-mediated killing via an increase of nuclease activity. Sputum samples of CF patients with chronic *S. aureus* infection were visualized by confocal microscopy after immuno-fluorescence staining for NET-specific markers, *S. aureus* bacteria and overall DNA structures. Nuclease activity was analyzed in sequential isogenic long persisting *S. aureus* isolates, as confirmed by whole genome sequencing, from an individual CF patient using a FRET-based nuclease activity assay. Additionally, some of these isolates were selected and analyzed by qRT-PCR to determine the expression of *nuc1* and regulators of interest. NET-killing assays were performed with clinical *S. aureus* isolates to evaluate killing and bacterial survival depending on nuclease activity. To confirm the role of nuclease during NET-mediated killing, a clinical isolate with low nuclease activity was transformed with a nuclease expression vector (pCM28*nuc*). Furthermore, two sputa from an individual CF patient were subjected to RNA-sequence analysis to evaluate the activity of nuclease *in vivo*. In sputa, *S. aureus* was associated to extracellular DNA structures. Nuclease activity in clinical *S. aureus* isolates increased in a time-and phenotype-dependent manner. In the clinical isolates, the expression of *nuc*1 was inversely correlated to the activity of *agr* and was independent of *saeS*. NET-mediated killing was significantly higher in *S. aureus* isolates with low compared to isolates with high nuclease activity. Importantly, transformation of the clinical isolate with low nuclease activity with pCM28*nuc* conferred protection against NET-mediated killing confirming the beneficial role of nuclease for protection against NETs. Also, nuclease expression in *in vivo* sputa was high, which underlines the important role of nuclease within the highly inflamed CF airways. In conclusion, our data show that *S. aureus* adapts to the neutrophil-rich environment of CF airways with increasing nuclease expression most likely to avoid NET-killing during long-term persistence.

Keywords: Cystic fibrosis, *Staphylococcus aureus*, neutrophil extracellular traps, nuclease, adaptation, NET-mediated killing

INTRODUCTION

Cystic fibrosis (CF) is an autosomal recessive disease with mutations in the CF transmembrane conductance regulator (CFTR) gene causing a life-limiting multisystemic disease (1). Due to CFTR mutations, a dehydrated thickened airway surface fluid impairs mucociliary clearance and leads to chronic recurrent bacterial airway infections, which result in the decline of lung function and a reduced life expectancy (1, 2). *Staphylococcus aureus* is one of the most common bacterial pathogens in young CF patients that can persist for several years thereby causing high inflammatory responses in CF patient airways (3–5).

One of the hallmarks of CF lung disease is an exaggerated airway inflammation caused by excessive recruitment of dysfunctional neutrophils and accumulation of pro-inflammatory agents, which in turn fail to eradicate bacteria (6). Within the airways, neutrophils try to kill pathogens by different killing mechanisms such as phagocytosis with the release of oxidants and degrading enzymes during degranulation, and the formation of neutrophil extracellular traps (NETs) (7), which were previously described to be abnormal in CF (8, 9). In detail, bacterial digestion in the neutrophilic phagolysosome in CF is reduced by the lack of membranous chloride transport due to CFTR mutations causing defective intraphagolysosomal HOCL production and reduced chlorination of bacterial proteins (9). Moreover, cytosolic pH acidifies and leads to a massive release of antimicrobial enzymes from granules such as myeloperoxidase and neutrophil elastase and lactoferrin (10). The high concentration of neutrophilic defense peptides contributes additionally to the destruction of airway and lung tissue in CF (11, 12). It has been shown, that in the context of CF lung disease, NET formation by neutrophils is enhanced (13). Besides antimicrobial components of the neutrophil granules, NETs consist of extracellular DNA fibers released by chromatin decondensation and subsequent rupture of the nuclear membrane to capture and kill various pathogens (7, 11). Recently, the presence of NETs within CF airways has been shown and has been associated with poor pulmonary function assumingly driven by NET-mediated inflammation and increased amounts of thickened mucus (14, 15). *S. aureus* is not only a potent inducer of NETs (7, 16), but has also the potential to degrade NETs by the secretion of nuclease (17). We hypothesized, that in the airways of CF patients *S. aureus* will adapt to NET-mediated killing by increasing nuclease activity in long-persisting isolates. First, we used fresh sputa from patients with chronic *S. aureus* airway infection to visualize NETs by immuno-fluorescence and confocal microscopy. Next, we determined nuclease activity of sequential and isogenic clinical *S. aureus* CF isolates by DNase agar plates and a FRET-based assay to evaluate nuclease activity. Since the expression of nuclease confers escape from NET-mediated killing to *S. aureus*, NET-killing assays of isolates with different nuclease activity were performed. To confirm the specific effect of nuclease regarding NET-mediated killing, a clinical *S. aureus* isolate with low nuclease activity was transformed with a plasmid that expresses wild-type nuclease, and tested in the NET-killing assay. To verify the role of nuclease *in vivo*, two independent sputa of an individual CF patient were used for RNA sequence analysis.

Our data revealed, that (i) NET-structures were visible in CF sputa and that *S. aureus* was in close proximity to NETs, (ii) nuclease activity of isogenic sequential isolates of one individual patient increased significantly during persistence, (iii) isolates with high nuclease activity were protected against NET-mediated killing, (iv) protection against NET-mediated killing was caused by higher nuclease activity, and that (v) nuclease was highly expressed in sputa of an individual CF patient.

RESULTS

Extracellular DNA Entraps *S. aureus* Bacteria in CF Sputum Samples

To examine, if NET- formation occurs in the airways of CF patients with chronic *S. aureus* infection, confocal microscopy of stained sputum was performed and confirmed the presence of high amounts of NETs (**Figures 1A,B,E,F**). Furthermore, fluorescence microscopy revealed *S. aureus* being mostly entangled in extracellular DNA structures (**Figures 1C,D,G,H**), while there were also bacteria visible in an environment without NETs.

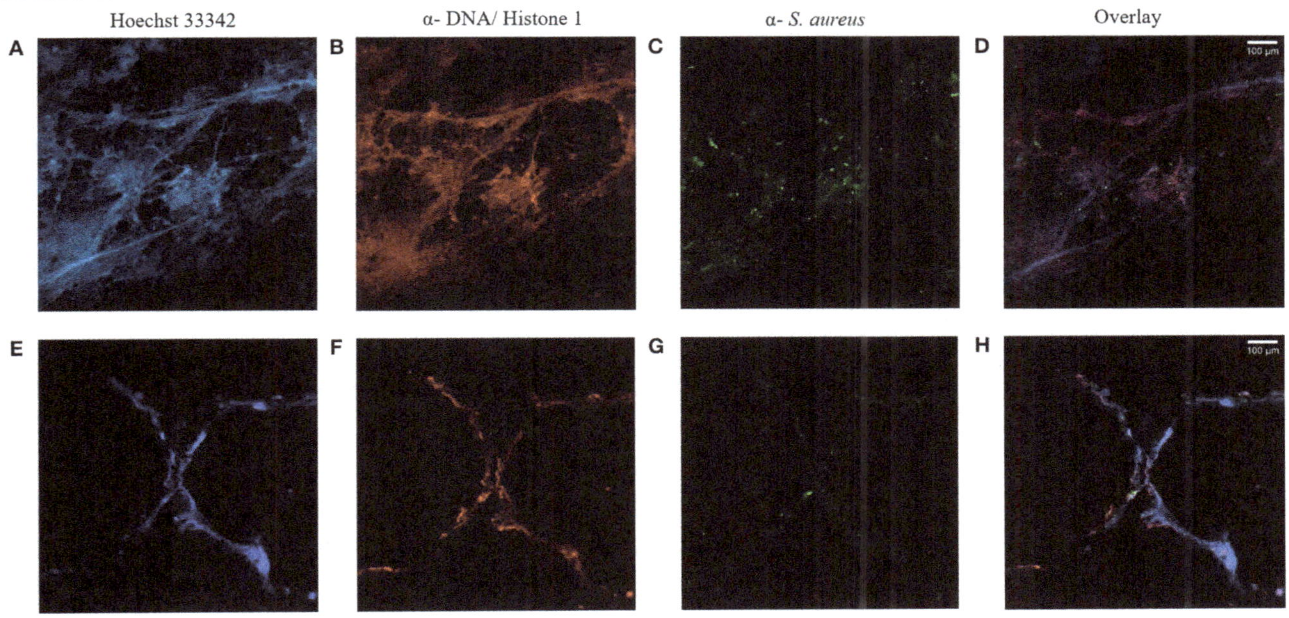

FIGURE 1 | CF sputum samples visualized by immunofluorescence staining and confocal microscopy. Staining of two sputa (**A–D** and **E–H**) of two different CF patients with chronic *S. aureus* infection. Nuclei and DNA structures (blue, **A,E**) and DNA-histone-1-complexes (red, **B,F**) are visible, whereas antibody-mediated staining specifically identifies *S. aureus* (green, **C,G**). Microscopy reveals NET-structures with *S. aureus* attached to it, but also with *S. aureus* without NET-binding **(D,H)**. Subsequent changes of color balance for color intensification were performed with ImageJ.

Nuclease Activity of *S. aureus* Correlates With Long-Term Persistence

To assess adaptation of *S. aureus* during long-term persistence regarding nuclease activity, 111 *S. aureus* isolates, which were recovered during 14 years of persistence from the airways of an individual CF patient (CF patient 1, **Table 1**), were further investigated. These isolates belonged predominantly to *spa*-type t617, showing that this patient was infected with one dominant *S. aureus* clone throughout persistence. Clonality of isolates was also confirmed by whole genome sequencing of 7 selected isolates (**Figure 2**). An initial approach for the categorization of nuclease activity of these *S. aureus* isolates was conducted on DNase agar plates (**Figures 3A–E**) (18) revealing an increase of nuclease activity in late compared to early *S. aureus* isolates (**Figures 3C,D**, **Figure Supplementary 1**). Moreover, the capability to degrade DNA was also seen to be phenotype-related in *S. aureus*. Strains with a normal phenotype showed larger clearing zones around colonies compared to small colony variants (SCVs), where no DNA degradation was detected around single colonies (**Figure 3D**). To quantify nuclease activity, all 111 *S. aureus* isolates were subjected to the nuclease FRET assay (19) showing a significant increase of nuclease activity in late isolates after 11 years of persistence (**Figure 4**). These results were confirmed by qRT-PCR analysis, which demonstrated a significant increase of *nuc*1 expression after 11 years of *S. aureus* persistence (**Figure 5**). Also, *nuc*2 expression revealed a significant increase after 7 years of persistence (**Figure Supplementary 2**). However, *nuc*2 expression (**Figure Supplementary 2**) was much lower than *nuc*1 expression (**Figure 5**).

Inverse Expression Pattern of Nuclease and *agr*

Seven clinical *S. aureus* strains (**Figure 4**: 17, 47, 80, 81, 86, 87, and 110) from one individual CF patient were subjected to qRT-PCR to analyze expression of *nuc*1 in relation to potential regulators of *S. aureus* nuclease (**Figure 6**). The results of *nuc*1 expression were in accordance to the results of nuclease activity by the nuclease FRET assay. Since *S. aureus* nuclease was shown to be SaeRS-regulated (20), transcription of *saeS* was determined for clinical isolates with low and high nuclease activity. Surprisingly, no alterations in *saeS* expression were observed for *S. aureus* isolates dependent of either low or high nuclease expression (**Figure 6**). Also, *eap*, a protein, which has been shown to be under the control of *saeRS* (21), was only very low expressed without any association to nuclease expression in all 7 clinical isolates. Interestingly, RNAIII, the effector molecule of the major virulence regulator *agr* (22), was higher expressed in *S. aureus* isolates with low *nuc*1 expression, whereas decreased RNAIII expression was observed in isolates with high nuclease expression (**Figure 6**) indicating an inhibiting role of *agr* in nuclease expression in the clinical isolates. Interestingly, whole genome sequencing revealed two subsequent non-synonymous SNPs in *agrA* of those *S. aureus* isolates with decreased RNAIII transcription and increased nuclease activity (**Table 2**).

Nuclease Activity Differs in CF Patients

To assess, if an increase in nuclease activity is a common adaptation pattern in other CF patients with long-term *S. aureus* persistence, 29 *S. aureus* strain pairs (early and late isolate) of

TABLE 1 | Clinical *S. aureus* isolates of CF patients used in this study.

Patient	Year of recovery	Sample site			*spa*-type
		Nose	Throat	Sputum	
1	2001	1,3	2,4,5,17		t617
1	2002		6		t499
1	2002	7	8,9,16		t617
1	2003		11		t499
1	2003	10,12,15	13,14		t617
1	2004	19,20,22,25	18,21,23,24		t617
1	2005	28–31,33	26,27,32		t617
1	2005		34		t930
1	2006	35, 37, 38, 41, 42, 44, 45	36,39,40,43,46	47	t617
1	2007			49	t930
1	2007			48,50–52	t617
1	2008			53	t930
1	2008			54	t034
-	2009		55–61	62	t617
-	2010			63–66	t617
-	2011			67–70,72,74,75	t617
-	2011			71	t002
-	2011			73	t230
-	2012		79–81	76–78,82–92	t617
-	2013		101	93–95, 97,99,100	t617
1	2013		96		t930
1	2013			98	t121
1	2014			102	t1459
1	2014			103–108	t617
1	2015			109–111	t617
2	2016			881*,912*	t034

*Isolates are numbered in chronological order of recovery. The year of recovery is presented, as well as the sample site of which isolates were recovered from the patient and the identified spa-type. NET killing experiments were performed with isolates from two different CF patients. Isolate no. 17 and no. 81 with low and high nuclease activity were recovered from one individual CF patient (underlined). Isolate no. 881 and 912 (marked with *) with low and high nuclease activity were recovered from another CF patient, respectively (**Figure Supplementary 3**). Isolate no. 17 was further transformed with the pCM28nuc plasmid and underwent NET killing analysis, whereby no. 81 served as the comparison strain with high nuclease activity.*

different CF patients were analyzed by the nuclease FRET assay. Seven of these 29 late *S. aureus* isolates revealed a significant increase of nuclease activity (**Figure 7**), whereas in 10 late isolates a significant decrease of nuclease activity and in 11 late strains, no change in nuclease activity was observed (**Figure 7**).

Higher Nuclease Activity Facilitates Increased Survival of *S. aureus* Interacting With NETs

Since secretion of nuclease facilitates evasion from NETs (17), we assessed survival of *S. aureus* isolates with high and low nuclease activity in interaction with NETs. After 90 min, the

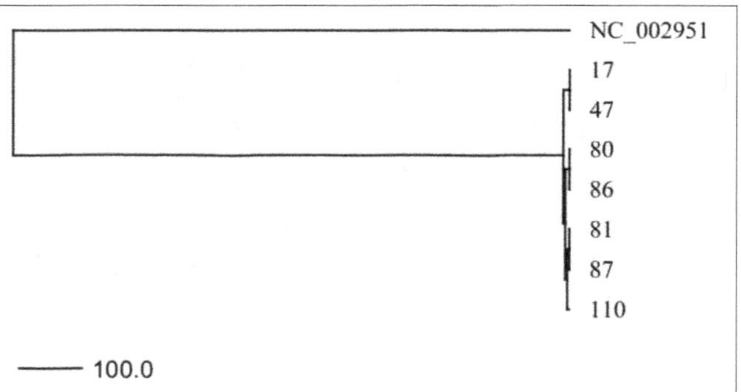

FIGURE 2 | UPGMA-tree based on the cgMLST allelic profiles of 7 clinical *S. aureus* isolates. The phylogenetic tree demonstrates the relationship of 7 *S. aureus* isolates, which were collected over 14 years. The tree was drawn to scale with branches given in absolute alleles distances.

S. aureus isolate with low nuclease activity (**Table 1**, no. 17 and 881) was significantly more affected by NET-mediated killing than the isolate with high nuclease activity (**Table 1**, no. 81 and 912; **Figure 8**, **Figure Supplementary 3**). In detail, the survival of the isolate with low nuclease activity was 54.7% in comparison to 74.9% of survival of the isolate with high nuclease activity (**Figure 8**). To confirm the role of nuclease in the context of NET-mediated killing on bacterial survival, the *S. aureus* isolate with low nuclease activity (**Table 1**, no. 17) was transformed with the nuclease expressing plasmid pCM28*nuc* (**Table 3**), which resulted in increased nuclease activity for the transformed strain (**Figure 9**). Similar to our previous results (**Figure 8**, **Figure Supplementary 3**), the CF isolate with low nuclease activity was killed to a significant higher extent than the corresponding late isolate with high nuclease activity after 90 min of NET interaction (**Figure 10**). In line with these results, the NET-killing capacity of the transformed strain was comparable to the late isolate with high nuclease activity (**Figure 10**). Interestingly, after 90 min of co-incubation with NETs, the bacterial survival of the transformed isolate with former low nuclease activity was higher than after 30 min of co- incubation, indicating that the high activity of nuclease conferred protection against NET-mediated killing and even allowed replication of bacteria as also observed for the late isolate in **Figure 10**.

Nuclease Expression *in vivo* in Sputa

To determine the role of nuclease expression *in vivo*, we collected two different sputa from one individual CF patient, who was persistently infected by *S. aureus*, and subjected this sputum to RNA-Seq analysis (**Figure 11**). The comparison of normalized transcription of *nuc* and other important virulence regulators and virulence factors against housekeeping (hk) genes revealed a high relative expression of *nuc* in both sputa, which was only surpassed by the expression of protein A (*spa*). The third highest transcript levels were obtained for *saeS*, which has been shown to be a regulator of *nuc* (20), while levels of adhesins (*fnbA*, *fnB*, *clfA*, and partially *clfB*) were low in both analyzed sputa (**Figure 11**). The obtained results of *in vivo* RNA-Seq analysis indicate the importance of nuclease during *in vivo S. aureus* airway infection.

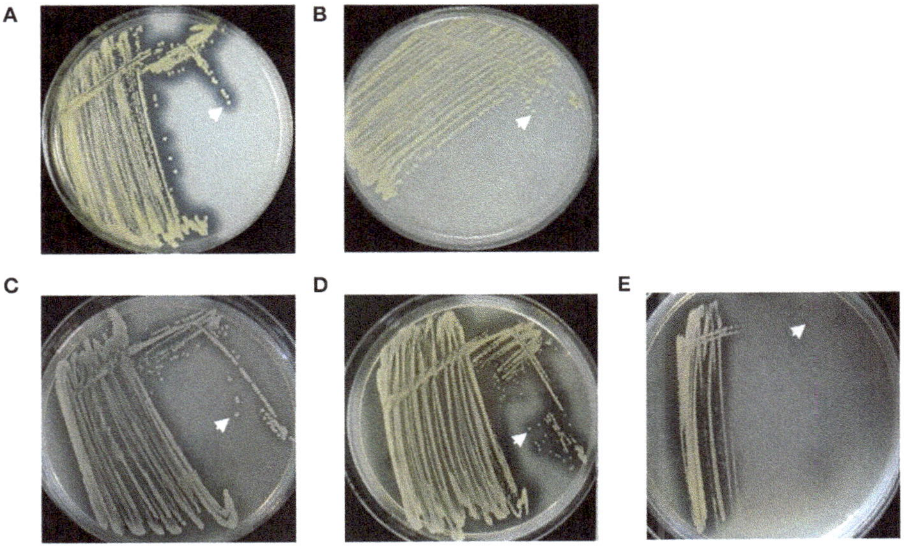

FIGURE 3 | Nuclease activity in different *S. aureus* strains analyzed by DNase agar plates. **(A)** *S. aureus* strain AH1263, positive control, showed large clearing zones (white arrow) around colonies. **(B)** *S. aureus* strain AH1680 (Δ*nuc*), negative control, presented without clearing zones (white arrow). **(C)** The early CF *S. aureus* isolate showed small clearing zones around colonies (white arrow), whereas **(D)** the late isolate revealed large clearing zones around colonies (white arrow). **(E)** *S. aureus* small colony variants (SCVs) did not reveal clearing zones around single colonies (white arrow).

DISCUSSION

Airway infections in CF lung disease are associated with strong inflammatory responses characterized by a domination of neutrophils (6), which can use different strategies to combat invading pathogens. Recently, NET-formation, also known as NETosis, within the airways of CF patients gained interest and it has been shown that abundant NETosis and NET- related markers in CF airway fluids occur (14, 26, 27). Most of these studies evaluated NET-formation in regard to *P. aeruginosa* airway infection in CF patients (15, 27–29). To our knowledge, there are no data about NET-formation and *S. aureus* in the context of CF. Therefore, we assessed, if sputum of patients with chronic *S. aureus* airway infections contain NETs. Several sputa of CF patients were stained for extracellular DNA structures characteristic for NETs and for *S. aureus*. As shown in two sputum samples exemplarily (**Figure 1**), *S. aureus* bacteria were visible in close proximity to NET- structures, but also without relation to NETs indicating that not all *S. aureus* bacteria are entangled and killed by NETs in CF sputa and that some isolates may have escaped NET-mediated killing. Since secreted *S. aureus* nuclease facilitates escape from NETs (17), we hypothesized that nuclease activity in long-persisting isolates would differ in comparison to early isolates. Therefore, we tested nuclease activity of more than 100 sequential *S. aureus* isolates, which were collected during persistence in the airways of one individual CF patients during a 14-year period. Our results showed, that isolates with increased nuclease activity occurred not earlier than after 11 years of persistence and were selected during the later years of persistence (**Figure 4**). These results were confirmed by qRT-PCR of selected strains with differential nuclease activity (**Figure 5**). Isolates with increased nuclease activity were mostly isolated from sputa, while isolates with low nuclease activity were more likely isolated from nasal and throat swabs (**Figure 4**). The fact, that isolates with high nuclease activity were more likely isolated from sputa indicates that there is a greater chance of selection of isolates with high nuclease activity at a site where more neutrophils are present, which most likely perform NETs. However, after 11 years most *S. aureus* isolates displayed higher nuclease activity indicating a survival advantage and pathoadaptation of these isolates to the NET-rich airways in CF as it has been suggested also by Rahman and Gadjeva (30).

In addition, isolates with SCV phenotype revealed less nuclease activity compared to normal growing isolates. Such data are in line with our earlier results showing that SCVs are characterized by a down- regulated metabolism, which facilitate long-term persistence (31, 32). Therefore, increased nuclease activity does not seem to be of importance for long-term survival for SCVs. Moreover, since SCVs mostly occur in mixed cultures with normal *S. aureus*, the secreted nuclease of the normal *S. aureus* might protect also SCVs from NET-mediated killing. Such assumption should be assessed in further NET-killing experiments with mixed cultures of normal and *S. aureus* SCVs.

As we investigated early/late *S. aureus* isolates from 29 different CF patients, only in the late isolates of 7 CF patients nuclease activity was significantly increased. However, considering the fact that nuclease increase in the sequential isolates of the described patient occurred only after 11 years of persistence, many of the studied late isolates might not have persisted long enough in the airways in order to adapt to NET-formation. Moreover, an increase in nuclease activity

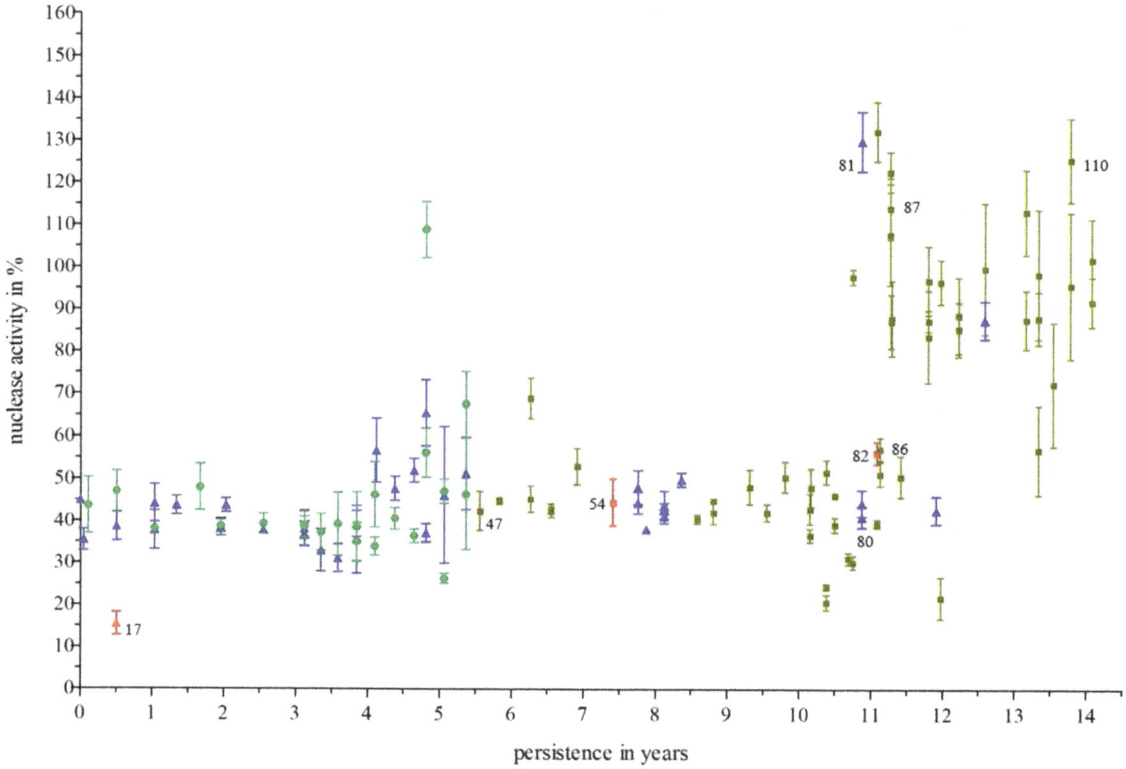

FIGURE 4 | Nuclease activity of *S. aureus* isolates during persistence. Nuclease activity was measured by the nuclease FRET assay (19). *S. aureus* isolates ($n = 111$) were recovered from the nose (green circles), throat (blue rectangles) and sputum (ochre squares) from one individual CF patient during long-term persistence of 14 years. There was a significant increase of nuclease activity after 11 years. Three clinical *S. aureus* isolates (17, 54, and 82; marked red) were selected for *nuc* expression analysis via qRT-PCR. Two isolates were further analyzed in NET-killing assays and used for transformation experiments representing a strain pair with low nuclease activity (no. 17) and high nuclease activity (no. 81), respectively. Technical replicates in the FRET assay: $n = 3$, biological replicates $n = 3$. For the calculation of significance, (i) isolates were grouped into nose, throat, and sputum samples and compared by the one- way analysis of variance (ANOVA) and Bonferroni's Post-Test, resulting in: nose vs. sputum $^{**}p \leq 0.01$; nose vs. throat had no significance, throat vs. sputum $^{***}p \leq 0.001$; (ii) regardless of sample site, isolates were grouped into early (0–7.039 years of persistence) and late (7.039–14.0.78 years of persistence). Both groups were compared using a two-tailed, unpaired student's *t*-test (result: $^{***}p \leq 0.001$).

especially occurred in *S. aureus* isolates recovered from sputa. Since not all late isolates of the tested 29 strains pairs were collected from sputa (**Table Supplementary 1**), this also might have influenced the results regarding the neutrophil domination in deeper CF airways, that is accompanied by a massive release of inflammatory agents (6, 33–35). Based on our findings, the observed enhancement of nuclease might be a result of a higher selective pressure for *S. aureus* present in lower airways compared to those that are present in nose or throat. Recently, Berends et al. showed resistance of *S. aureus* against NET-mediated entrapment and killing by the secretion of *S. aureus* nuclease (17). Therefore, we tested survival of NET-mediated killing of *S. aureus* isolates with high in comparison to low nuclease activity showing that *S. aureus* isolates with high nuclease activity were less killed by NETs compared to isolates with low nuclease activity. Such results indicate that *S. aureus* isolates with high nuclease activity were most likely selected in the airways of CF patients with high abundance of NET formation, which facilitate survival of *S. aureus* in this hostile environment. The beneficial role of high nuclease expression was confirmed by transformation of a clinical CF isolate with low nuclease with the nuclease expressing vector pCM28*nuc*. Survival of the transformed *S. aureus* strain during NET-killing was significantly increased compared to the corresponding isolate with low nuclease activity.

The fact that nuclease expression was also high in two *in vivo* sputum samples from one individual CF patient with persistent *S. aureus* airway infection as assessed by RNA-Seq analysis underscores the role of nuclease for the *in vivo* situation. Elucidating the transcriptome of *S. aureus* in the nasal niche by RNA-Seq analysis (36), the comparison of transcript levels of *S. aureus* recovered from CF sputum demonstrated higher expression of nuclease and the nuclease-regulating *saeS* component (20) compared to the nasal *S. aureus* isolate. The increase of *saeS* and *nuc* in CF compared to nasal isolates (36) underscores our hypothesis of *S. aureus* combating neutrophil-mediated eradication by the up-regulation of nuclease during adaptation to the highly inflammatory CF airways.

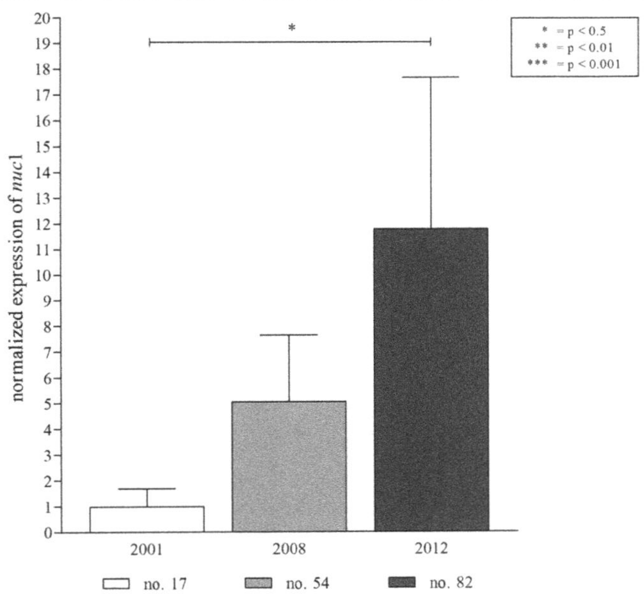

FIGURE 5 | Expression of *S. aureus nuc*1 in an early, intermediate and late *S. aureus* isolate from patient 1. For the assessment of *nuc* expression, isolates (**Figure 4**, in red) were grown in BHI medium until mid-logarithmic growth phase before RNA extraction. Expression of *nuc*1 increased significantly over time of *S. aureus* persistence. The obtained results are in line with the nuclease FRET assay detecting low nuclease activity for isolate no. 17 (2001, 15.9%), an intermediate activity for no. 54 (2008, 45.5%), and a high nuclease activity for the late isolate no. 82 (2012, 56.84%). Statistical analysis: two-tailed, unpaired student's *t*-test, error bars represent SD. Technical replicates $n = 2$, biological replicates $n = 3$.

If this high nuclease activity has an impact on macrophage viability during NET formation, especially regarding the concerted action of nuclease and adenosine synthase A as shown recently by Thammavonsga et al. (37), is an interesting aspect, which should be investigated in future experiments.

A first insight about the molecular mechanism of the increase in nuclease activity in the clinical isolates is given by the detected SNPs within *agrA*, which most likely caused down-regulation of RNAIII expression in late clinical isolates. *AgrA*-specific mutations have been previously shown by others (38, 39) to be responsible for a change in *agr* activity. Surprisingly, *saeRS*, which has been shown by others to positively regulate *nuc* (20, 21, 40) had no apparent impact on nuclease activity in these clinical isolates.

In conclusion, our data underline the importance of *S. aureus* nuclease activity during long-term airway infection of CF patients. In sputa of patients with chronic *S. aureus* infection, NET formation with entrapped *S. aureus* was apparent. In many CF patients, pathoadaptation of long-term persisting *S. aureus* isolates to the airways, where abundant NET formation is observed, was accomplished via increased nuclease activity. High nuclease activity conferred a survival advantage to *S. aureus* during NET-killing and high nuclease expression was determined in *in vivo* sputa from a CF patient chronically infected by *S. aureus*.

MATERIALS AND METHODS

Patients' and Volunteers' Specimens

The usage of sputum of CF patients and blood samples was approved by the Ethical Committee of the University Hospital Münster (no. 2018-466-f-S). Informed consent was given for blood samples by healthy volunteers and for sputa by CF patients.

Bacterial Strains and Growth Conditions

Clinical *S. aureus* isolates with the same or closely related *spa*-types ($n = 111$) from one individual CF patient, cultured from throat, nose, or sputum samples collected during a period of 14 years were used (**Table 1**). To assess adaptation regarding nuclease activity during persistence in more CF patients, *S. aureus* strain pairs of CF patients consisting of early and late isolates with at least 5 years of *S. aureus* persistence with identical or closely related *spa*-types were analyzed (**Table Supplementary 1**). These strain pairs were previously characterized in terms of virulence factor adaptation (23). All CF isolates and reference strains (**Table 3**) were cultivated on Columbia 5% blood agar plates (BD). Overnight cultures were grown in Brain Heart Infusion medium (BHI, Difco) at 37°C and 160 rpm. B2 medium was used for *S. aureus* plasmid transformation [modified after (41)]. To assess nuclease activity in qRT-PCR and NET-killing experiments, overnight cultures of *S. aureus* isolates in BHI were cultivated in fresh BHI medium for 4 h until mid-logarithmic growth phase starting from an OD_{578nm} of 0.1. For the nuclease FRET assay, *S. aureus* was cultured in 96-well-plates under the same conditions. The pCM28*nuc* plasmid was maintained in *S. aureus* AH1773 on tryptic soy agar (TSA, Difco) supplemented with 10 μg/ml chloramphenicol (CN).

spa-Typing of Clinical CF *S. aureus* Isolates

Molecular typing of sequential *S. aureus* isolates (**Table 1**) recovered from airway specimens (nose, throat, sputum) of an individual CF patient were performed by *spa*-typing (32, 42).

Whole Genome Sequencing of Clinical CF *S. aureus* Isolates

The clonal relationship of 7 *S. aureus* strains recovered from one individual CF patient (**Table 1**) was determined by whole genome sequencing (WGS) and subsequent core genome multilocus sequence typing (cgMLST). Genomic DNA of *S. aureus* isolates was purified using the MagAttract HMW DNA kit (Qiagen) following the manufacturer's instructions with the addition of 120 U Lysostaphin (Sigma-Aldrich). Clinical isolates were sequenced using Illumina technology and Nextera XT version 2 chemistry, with a 250-bp paired-end protocol on a MiSeq sequencer (Illumina). Quality trimming of fastq files (average base quality of 30, aiming for 100-fold coverage) and *de novo* assembly using SKESA (PMID: 30286803) were performed with SeqSphere$^+$ (version 6; Ridom GmbH, Münster, Germany) as described recently (43). Only genomes harboring ≥95% cgMLST targets of the *S. aureus* cgMLST scheme (44) passed quality control; otherwise, sequencing was repeated. For tree building using the unweighted pair group (UPGMA) method, the allelic

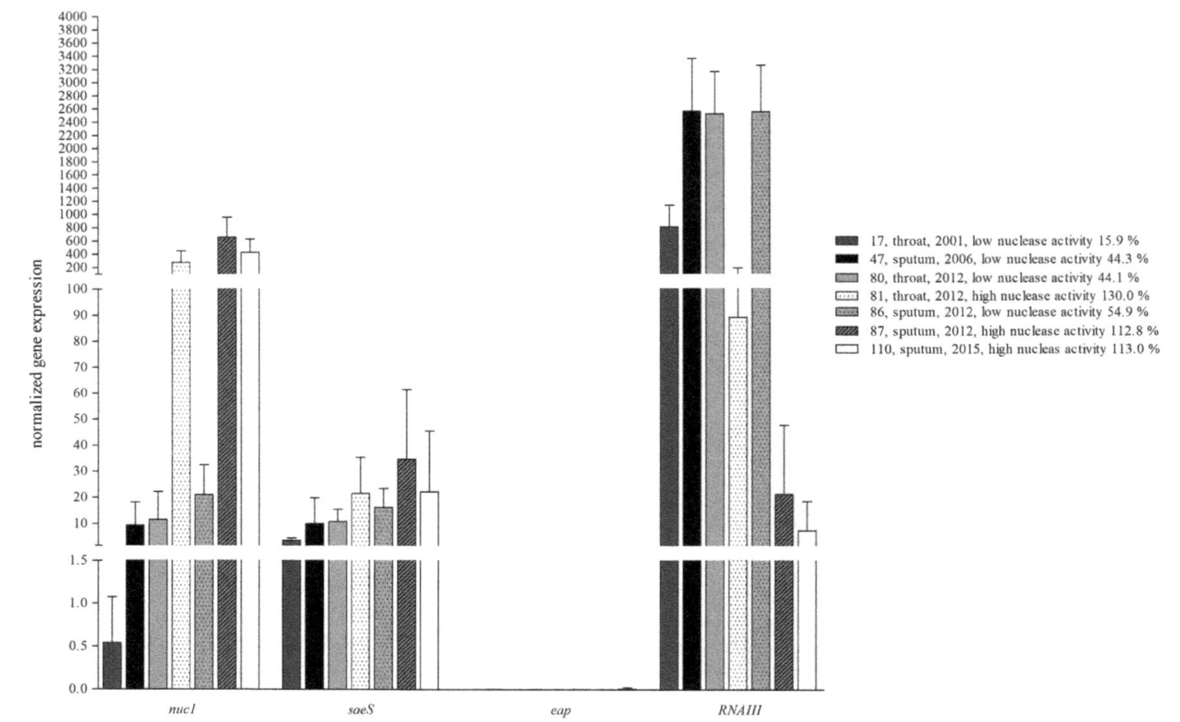

FIGURE 6 | Inverse expression pattern of nuclease and *agr*. Sequential clinical *S. aureus* isolates from one individual CF patient were grown in BHI until mid-logarithmic growth phase to determine *nuc1*, the potential *nuc* regulator *saeRS* (represented by *saeS*), *eap* as another *saeRS* regulated virulence factor and *RNAIII* as the effector gene of the *agr* regulon. *Nuc* expression was independent of *saeS*, but was inversely correlated with *agr*, while *eap* was only very low expressed. Isolates with low nuclease activity (17, 47, and 86) revealed high *RNAIII* expression, whereas isolates with high nuclease activity (81, 87, and 110) low *RNAIII* expression, respectively. Technical replicates $n = 3$, biological replicates $n = 4$.

TABLE 2 | Non-synonymous SNPs in agrA.

Gene	Target	Rel. position	NC_002951	Variant AA	17, 47	Isolates with variants	
						80, 86	81, 87, 110
agrA	SACOL2026	409	G	D→ Y	G	**T**	**T**
agrA	SACOL2026	520	C	H→ Y	C	C	**T**

Two subsequent non-synonymous SNPs were discovered in agrA of the clinical S. aureus isolates. Nuclease and RNAIII activity inversely correlated with the presence of both mutations.

profiles of up to 1, 861 core genome multilocus sequence typing (cgMLST) targets were used as described previously (45). To investigate molecular mechanisms associated with nuclease activity, the SeqSphere$^+$ software was used for SNP calling within the *agrA* gene.

Nuclease Test on DNase Agar

CF isolates and laboratory strains were streaked on DNase agar plates (Oxoid) and incubated for 17 h at 37°C. DNase agar plates were flooded with 1 N hydrochloric acid solution and evaluated qualitatively by the size of clearing zones around bacterial colonies as a result of DNA degradation by *S. aureus* nuclease. *S. aureus* strains AH1263 (wild-type) and AH1680 (Δ*nuc*-mutant) were used as negative and positive control, respectively (**Table 3**).

Nuclease FRET Assay

For the preparation of overnight cultures, single colonies of CF isolates and laboratory strains were inoculated in BHI medium in a 96-well-flat-bottomed microtiter plate with lid. AH1263 and AH1680 (**Table 3**) were used as negative and positive controls. The plate was incubated overnight for 16–18 h at 37°C using the TECAN Multireader. Overnight cultures were diluted to an OD_{578nm} of 0.1 in fresh BHI medium in a new 96-well-plate and incubated for another 4 h at 37°C in the TECAN Multireader. Analysis of nuclease activity in *S. aureus* strains was accomplished by the use of a molecular beacon as described recently (19). In brief, for analysis of nuclease activity, bacterial supernatants were collected and applied in 1:200 dilutions together with the molecular beacon (final concentration: 0.1 μM) into a black 96-well-plate. Nuclease

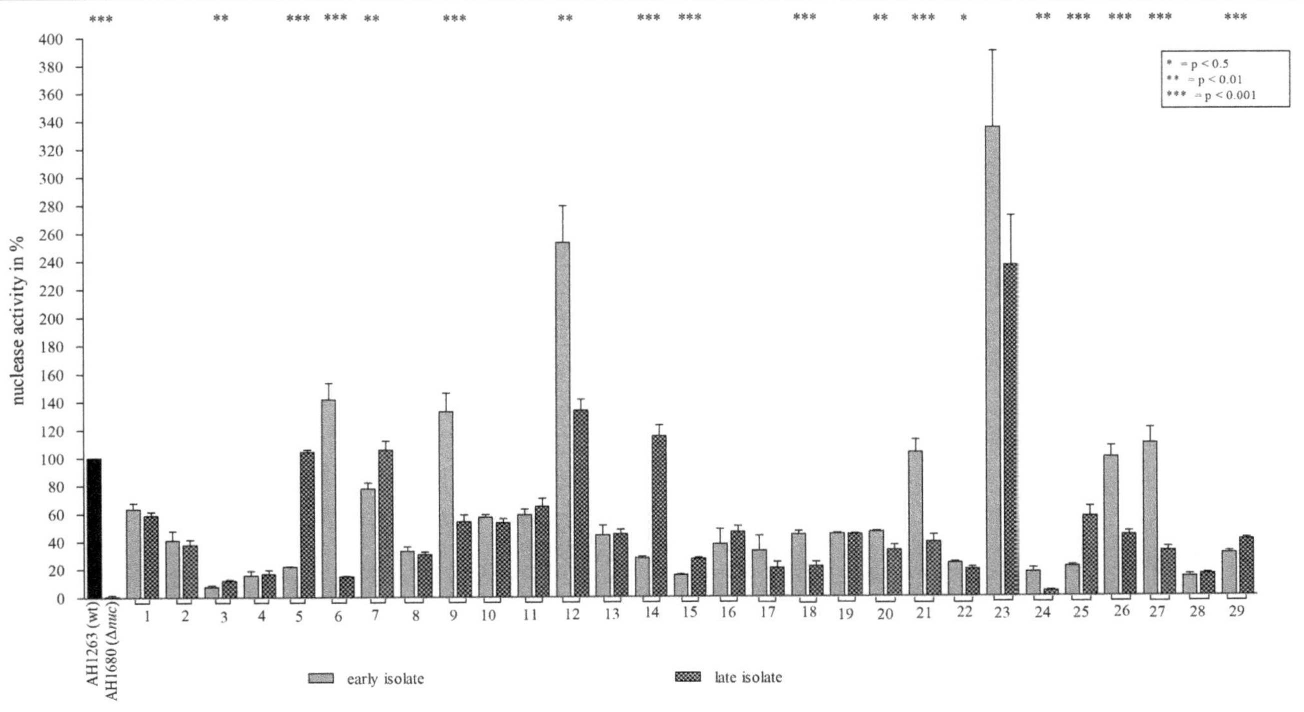

FIGURE 7 | Nuclease activity of different early/late *S. aureus* strain pairs. Nuclease activity of 29 *S. aureus* strain pairs (early, late) from different CF patients (23) were analyzed by the nuclease FRET assay. Regarding nuclease activity in late isolates, an increase was observed in 7 late strains (strain pairs 3, 5, 7, 14, 15, 25, and 29), a decrease in 10 (strain pairs 6, 9, 12, 18, 20, 21, 22, 24, 26, and 27) and an unchanged activity in 12 late strains. *S. aureus* strains AH1263 and AH1680 (Δ*nuc*) served as positive and negative control, respectively. Statistical comparisons: two-tailed, unpaired student's *t*-test, error bars represent SD. Technical replicates $n = 3$, biological replicates $n = 3$.

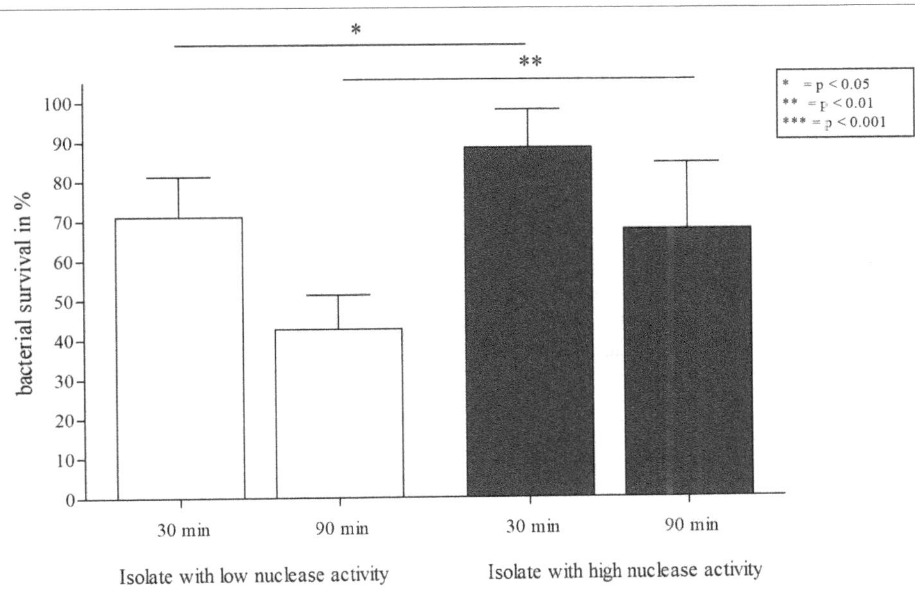

FIGURE 8 | NET-killing assay with *S. aureus* isolates from patient 1 with low/high nuclease activities. Survival rates (in %) after 30 and 90 min of incubation with NETs are depicted. A significant decrease of bacterial survival was observed for the (early) isolate with low nuclease activity (**Figure 4**, isolate 17) after 30 and 90 min of incubation with NETs in comparison to the corresponding (late) isolate with high nuclease activity (**Figure 4**, isolate 81). Statistical comparison of both *S. aureus* strains depending on incubation time: two-tailed, unpaired student's *t*-test, error bars represent SD. Statistical comparison of single *S. aureus* strains: two-tailed, paired student's *t*-test. Technical replicates $n = 2$, biological replicates $n = 6$.

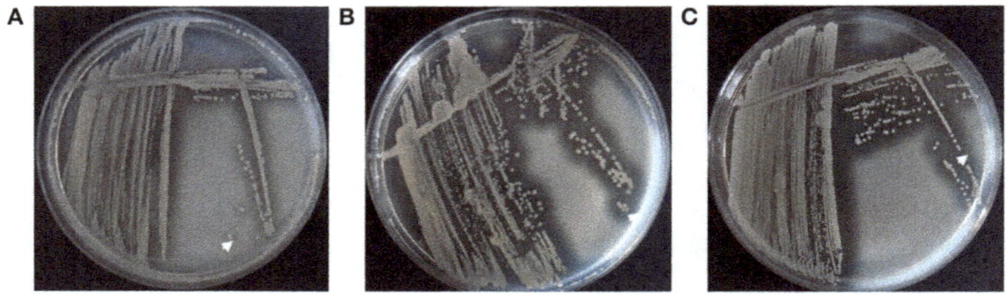

FIGURE 9 | Analysis of nuclease activity on DNase agar plates after the transformation of the early *S. aureus* isolate with low nuclease activity of patient 1 with the plasmid pCM28*nuc*. **(A)** The early *S. aureus* isolate with low nuclease activity (**Figure 4**, isolate17) shows minimal clearance zones (white arrow) around colonies. **(B)** The pCM28*nuc*-transformed early *S. aureus* isolate exhibits large clearance zones, **(C)** similar to the corresponding late *S. aureus* isolate with high nuclease activity (**Figure 4**, isolate 81).

TABLE 3 | *S. aureus* reference strains, plasmid and plasmid transformed strain used in this study.

Strain or plasmid	Description	References
AH1263	USA300 CA-MRSA ErmS (LAC), wild type strain	(24)
AH1680	AH1263 *nuc*:LtrB, Δ*nuc* mutant of wild type AH1263	(25)
pCM28*nuc*	*nuc*-complementing vector with chloramphenicol resistance	(25)
17 [pCM28*nuc*]	*S. aureus* strain with low nuclease activity transformed with pCM28*nuc*	This work

activity was determined as a kinetic measurement in 30 min intervals with excitation at 485/20 nm, emission at 528/20 nm under fast orbital shaking. Results were evaluated with the Gen5 best fit method. Nuclease activity was calculated in a growth-dependent manner to exclude impacts on actual nuclease activity by differing growth capacities of *S. aureus* CF strains in BHI medium. Growth- fitted nuclease activity was achieved by relative nuclease activity multiplied against a factor resulting from OD_{578nm} values of the analyzed CF strain, obtained after 4 h of incubation in fresh BHI, against the OD_{578nm} value of AH1263 (100% control).

qRT-PCR

Expression of both nucleases (*nuc*1, *nuc*2), *saeS, eap,* and *RNAIII* was assessed in the mid-logarithmic growth phase in BHI. RNA isolation, cDNA synthesis, and qRT-PCR were conducted as described (46). RNA samples were evaluated for successful DNA elimination by PCR using *S. aureus gmk* (guanylate monophosphate kinase) primers. The house-keeping genes *aroE* (Shikimate dehydrogenase NADP/H) and *gyrB* (DNA gyrase subunit B) served for normalization of nuclease gene expression. All primers used are described in **Table 4**.

Transformation of a CF *S. aureus* Isolate With Low Nuclease Activity

One selected *S. aureus* strain (no. 17, year 2001, throat, **Table 1**) with low nuclease activity was transformed with the pCM28*nuc* plasmid, containing the major *S. aureus* nuclease (*nuc*1) sequence. For the preparation of electro-competent cells, the CF isolate was cultivated in B2 medium (41) overnight. The culture was then diluted to OD_{578nm} of 0.5 in fresh B2 medium and incubated at 37°C, 160 rpm to OD_{578nm} of 0.6. Bacterial growth was stopped on ice and a pellet was harvested by centrifugation (3,000 × g for 10 min at RT). The pellet was consecutively washed in decreasing volumes of 4°C cold water before 4°C cold 10% glycerol was applied. For transformation, electro-competent cells of the CF isolate were mixed with 5 µl of the purified pCM28*nuc* plasmid (NEB Monarch Plasmid Miniprep Kit). Electroporation was executed by the Ec2 program of the BIORad MicroPulser Electroporator (Pulse 2.5 kV, number of impulse 1) in a 0.2 cm electroporation cuvette. After incubation in B2 medium for 2 h at 37°C and 350 rpm, screening for plasmid-positive colonies was performed by plating the mixture on TSA agar with 10 µg/ml chloramphenicol. The TSA plates were incubated at 37°C for 42 h. Colonies were verified for the acquisition of the pCM28*nuc* plasmid by PCR with nuclease specific primer (**Table 4**) after plasmid purification (NEB Monarch Plasmid 344 Miniprep Kit). Nuclease activities of the original and transformed CF isolate were compared by DNase agar plates as well as by the nuclease FRET assay (data not included).

NET-Killing Assay

Isogenic *S. aureus* isolates with low and high nuclease activity were analyzed using the NET-killing assay (17). Human neutrophils from healthy individuals were isolated from heparin-anticoagulated blood by gradient separation using PolymorphPrep (Abbott Diagnostics Technologies AS). Remaining erythrocytes were lysed with sterile water after the neutrophil pellet was purified with magnesium- and calcium-free 1 x Dulbecco's Phosphate Buffered Saline (DPBS). Isolated neutrophils were suspended in RPMI medium (Sigma-Aldrich)

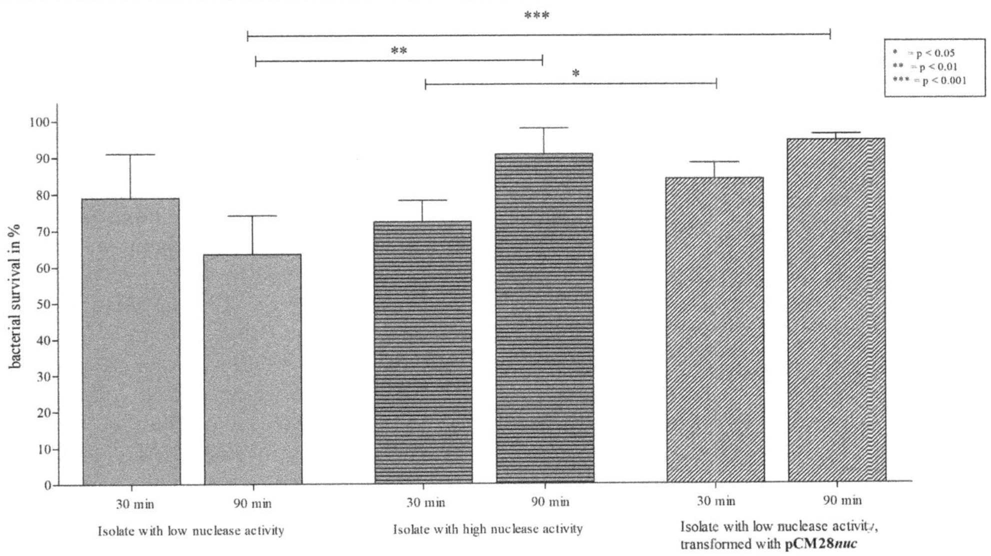

FIGURE 10 | NET-killing assay with an early *S. aureus* isolate with low nuclease activity of after transformation with pCM28*nuc*. Survival rates (in %) after 30 and 90 min of incubation with NETs are shown. A significant decrease of bacterial survival after 90 min is apparent for the isolate with low nuclease activity (**Figure 4**, isolate 17), compared to both isolates with enhanced nuclease activity. After 30 min, the survival rate for the isolate with high nuclease activity (**Figure 4**, isolate 81) is significantly lower than for the transformed strain. After 90 min, no difference in survival was observed for both *S. aureus* strains with high nuclease activity, but enhanced survival was shown for the two strains with high nuclease activity compared to the strain with low nuclease activity. Statistical comparison of *S. aureus* strains depending on incubation time: two-tailed, unpaired student's *t*-test, error bars represent SD. The comparison of single *S. aureus* strain pairs revealed no statistical differences (two-tailed, paired student's test). Technical replicates $n = 2$ and biological replicates $n = 7$ were performed.

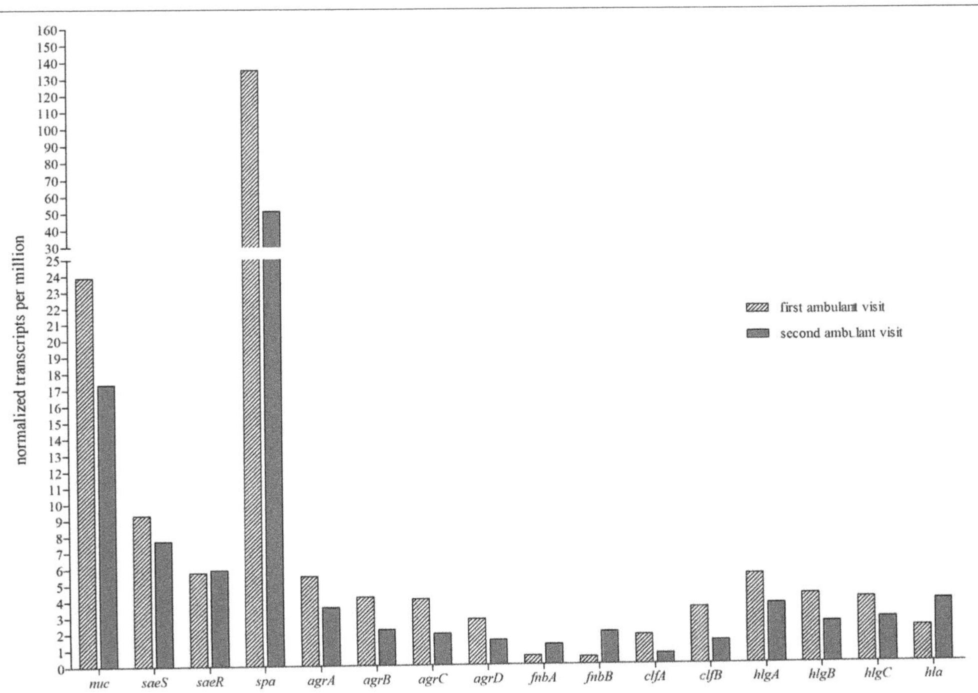

FIGURE 11 | RNA-Seq analysis of *in vivo* expression of nuclease and other important *S. aureus* virulence regulators and genes in sputa from one individual CF patient. Sputum samples were collected from a chronically infected CF patient at two visits and subjected to RNA-Seq analysis. Expression levels of nuclease (*nuc*), virulence regulators (*saeS, saeR, agrA, agrB, agrC,* and *agrD*), protein A (*spa*), fibronectin-binding proteins (*fnbA*, *fnbB*), clumping factor proteins (*clfA*, *clfB*), the subunits for γ-hemolysin (*hlgA*, *hlgB,* and *hlgC*) and α-hemolysin (*hla*) are shown as normalized transcripts per million (TPM). TPM levels of presented genes were normalized against TPM values 600 of the *S. aureus* housekeeping genes *aroE* and *gyrB*.

TABLE 4 | Primers used in qRT-PCR experiments.

Target	Sequence	References
aroE-fwd	5′-CTATCCACTTGCCATCTTTTAT-3′	(46)
aroE-rev	5′-ATGGCTTTAATATCACAATTCC-3′	
gmk-fwd	5′-AAGGTGCAAAGCAAGTTAGAA-3′	This work
gmk-rev	5′-CTTTACGCGCTTCGTTAATAC-3′	
gyrB-fwd	5′-AATTGAAGCAGGCTATGTGT-3′	(46)
gyrB-rev	5′-ATAGACCATTTTGGTGTTGG-3′	
nuc1-fwd	5′-AAGCTTTAGTTCGTCAAGGC-3′	This work
nuc1-rev	5′-TGAATCAGCGTTGTCTTCGC-3′	
nuc2-fwd	5′-TGGATGGTGATACATTTATTGC-3′	This work
nuc2-rev	5′-GTTTCACCGTTTCTGGCG-3′	
RNAIII-fwd	5′-ttcactgtgtcgataatcca-3′	(47)
RNAIII-rev	5′-tgatttcaatggcacaagat-3′	
eap-fwd	5′-AAGCGTCTGCCGCAGCTA-3′	(48)
eap-rev	5′-TGCATATGGAACATGGACTTTAGAA-3′	
saeS- fwd	5′-tcgaacgccacttgagc-3′	This work
saeS-rev	5′-ctatcgacattgctattagc-3′	

with 2% heat-inactivated fetal bovine serum (FBS, Fiebig). In 24-well-plates, 2 × 10^6 neutrophils/ml were incubated with 10 µg/ml cytochalasin D (Sigma-Aldrich) and 25 nM phorbol 12- myristate 13-acetate (PMA, Sigma-Aldrich) for 20 min at 37°C + 5% CO_2 prior infection. With a multiplicity of infection (MOI) of 2, *S. aureus* strains were applied as 4 × 106 bacteria/ml to RPMI medium (growth control) and activated neutrophils, respectively, and incubated at 37°C + 5% CO_2 for 30 min and 90 min. Bacterial strains were pre-cultured in BHI (overnight, for mid-logarithmic growth phase) as described above. The survival rates for each S. *aureus* strain were calculated in % by comparison of CFUs on blood agar plates of bacteria interacting with NET-forming neutrophils vs. bacteria in medium.

Sputum Staining

Visualization of DNA-related structures and *S. aureus* bacteria in sputa from different CF patients was realized with immuno-fluorescence staining (49, 50). After expectoration, fresh sputum was immediately streaked onto poly-D-lysine-coated slides and fixed in 4% methanol-free formaldehyde for 15 min. Fixed sputum was kept hydrated either in 50 ml reaction tubes with FBS or in a humidity chamber during the immuno-fluorescence staining process. After permeabilization with 0.5% Triton-X, the CF sputum was covered with blocking buffer (1% bovine serum albumin, 10% goat serum, 0.3 mol glycine, 0.1% Tween 20 in PBS) for 20 min to avoid non-specific binding of antibodies. Subsequently, the sputum was incubated with rabbit α-*S. aureus* (MyBioSource; 1:2,000 diluted) in blocking buffer for 45 min at room temperature (RT). After washing in fresh PBS, the corresponding secondary antibody α-rabbit Alexa Fluor 488 (Invitrogen, A11070; 1:500 diluted in blocking buffer) was added and incubated for 45 min at RT in the dark. The slide was washed and covered with blocking buffer for another 10 min. A second primary antibody, mouse α-DNA/Histone1 antibody (Merck; 1:1,100 diluted), was applied for 45 min at RT in the dark to visualize NET-specific DNA- structures. After washing in PBS, the secondary antibody α-mouse Alexa Fluor 568 (Invitrogen; 1:376,500 diluted) was added together with Hoechst 33342 (Invitrogen; 1:20,000 diluted) and incubated for 45 min at RT in the dark. Prolong Antifade Mountant (Invitrogen) was applied on the slide, covered by a 24 × 60 mm glass cover slip, and incubated overnight at RT. The slides were examined for NET-structures and *S. aureus* bacteria by fluorescence microscopy, using the ZEISS Observer Z1 microscope with a Plan-Neofluar 100x/1.3 Oil RMS objective and AxioVision Rel 4.8 software. For a more detailed acquisition of images, CF sputum was further analyzed by the Zeiss LSM800 microscope equipped with a Plan-Apochromat 63x/1.4 Oil DIC M27 objective and ZEN 2.3 software.

RNA Extraction and Sequencing Analysis of CF Sputa

Sputum of one CF patient, who is chronically colonized and infected by *S. aureus*, was collected at two different time points in 2016 and stored at −80°C until processing. Samples were gently mixed with an equivalent volume of Sputolysin (10%) and incubated during 30 min at 37°C on a ThermoMixer device. RNA extraction, library construction, sequencing analysis and data processing were conducted as described recently (36). Calculation of relative gene expression/normalization in transcripts per million (TPM) was based on the following formula:

$\frac{TPM\ gene\ of\ interest}{(TPMgyrB+TPM\ aroE)/2}$. The *S. aureus* genes *gyrB* and *aroE* served as housekeeping genes.

Statistical Analysis

Data were analyzed in GraphPad Prism 5. Nuclease activities of *S. aureus* isolates ($n = 111$) from one individual patient recovered from different sample sites were compared by (i) one-way analysis of variance (ANOVA) test, complemented by Bonferroni's Post-Test (ii) two-tailed, unpaired student's *t*-test. Nuclease activity and survival rates obtained by the NET-killing assays were compared by two-tailed, unpaired *t*-test. For the comparison of bacterial survival among *S. aureus* isolates, the two-tailed, paired *t*-test was used.

ETHICS STATEMENT

The studies involving human participants were reviewed and approved by Ethical Committee of the University Hospital Münster, Münster, Germany (2018-466-f-S). The patients/participants provided their written informed consent to participate in this study.

AUTHOR CONTRIBUTIONS

BK and SH designed the study. BK obtained the funding. SH performed and evaluated the majority of experiments and wrote the paper with the help of BK. FD established the FRET-based assay for the investigation of nuclease activity and analyzed *S. aureus* isolates from different CF patients. VS and AM performed whole genome sequencing and analyzed sequence data. DC-M and DP conducted and evaluated the RNA-Seq analysis of CF sputum. SN and CN gave theoretical and practical support with fluorescence microscopy and transformation with the pCM28nuc plasmid, respectively. NB and MK-B gave theoretical and practical support regarding the performance of NET killing assays and the immunofluorescence staining of CF sputa. JS performed *spa* typing of used *S. aureus* isolates. JG captured images of stained sputum samples using confocal microscopy under the scientific supervision of UR. AD, PK, and HS provided CF patient materials of which *S. aureus* isolates were recovered for this study, and sputum samples could be investigated on NETs. All authors read the paper.

ACKNOWLEDGMENTS

We thank Janina Treffon for the helpful communication and the providing of protocols regarding RNA isolation and qRT-analysis. Thanks to all CF patients and healthy individuals, who donated blood or sputum for research analysis.

REFERENCES

1. O'Sullivan BP, Freedman SD. Cystic fibrosis. *Lancet.* (2009) 373:1891–904. doi: 10.1016/S0140-6736(09)60327-5
2. Lipuma JJ. The changing microbial epidemiology in cystic fibrosis. *Clin Microbiol Rev.* (2010) 23:299–323. doi: 10.1128/CMR.00068-09
3. Cystic Fibrosis Foundation. *2017 Patient Registry: Annual Data Report.* Cystic Fibrosis Foundation Patient Registry (2017).
4. European Cystic Fibrosis Society Patient Registry (2018). *ECFSPR Annual Report 2016.* Available online at: www.ecfs.eu/ecfspr (accessed September 11, 2019).
5. Gangell C, Gard S, Douglas T, Park J, de Klerk N, Keil T, et al. Inflammatory responses to individual microorganisms in the lungs of children with cystic fibrosis. *Clin Infect Dis.* (2011) 53:425–32. doi: 10.1093/cid/cir399
6. Cohen TS, Prince A. Cystic fibrosis: a mucosal immunodeficiency syndrome. *Nat Med.* (2012) 18:509–19. doi: 10.1038/nm.2715
7. Brinkmann V, Reichard U, Goosmann C, Fauler B, Uhlemann Y, Weiss DS, et al. Neutrophil extracellular traps kill bacteria. *Science.* (2004) 303:1532–35. doi: 10.1126/science.1092385
8. Downey DG, Bell SC, Elborn JS. Neutrophils in cystic fibrosis. *Biol Chem.* (2007) 397:485–96. doi: 10.1515/hsz-2015-0271
9. Painter RG, Valentine VG, Lanson NA, Leidal K, Zhang Q, Lombard G, et al. CFTR expression in human neutrophils and the phagolysosomal chlorination defect in cystic fibrosis. *Biochemistry.* (2006) 45:10260–9. doi: 10.1021/bi060490t
10. Sagel SD, Sontag MK, Accurso FJ. Relationship between antimicrobial proteins and airway inflammation and infection in cystic fibrosis. *Pediatr Pulmonol.* (2009) 44:402–9. doi: 10.1002/ppul.21028
11. Law SM, Gray RD. Neutrophil extracellular traps and the dysfunctional innate immune response of cystic fibrosis lung disease: a review. *J Inflamm.* (2017) 14:29. doi: 10.1186/s12950-017-0176-1
12. Sly PD, Gangell CL, Chen L, Ware RS, Ranganathan S, Mott LS, et al. Risk factors for bronchiectasis in children with cystic fibrosis. *Survey Anesthesiol.* (2014) 58:82. doi: 10.1097/01.SA.0000443983.90197.36
13. Gray RD, Hardisty G, Regan KH, Smith M, Robb CT, Duffin R, et al. Delayed neutrophil apoptosis enhances NET formation in cystic fibrosis. *Thorax.* (2018) 73:134–44. doi: 10.1136/thoraxjnl-2017-210134
14. Manzenreiter R, Kienberger F, Marcos V, Schilcher K, Krautgartner WD, Obermayer A, et al. Ultrastructural characterization of cystic fibrosis sputum using atomic force and scanning electron microscopy. *J Cyst Fibros.* (2012) 11:84–92. doi: 10.1016/j.jcf.2011.09.008
15. Marcos V, Zhou-Suckow Z, Önder Yildirim A, Bohla A, Hector A, Vitkov L, et al. Free DNA in cystic fibrosis airway fluids correlates with airflow obstruction. *Mediat Inflamm.* (2015) 2015:408935. doi: 10.1155/2015/408935
16. Pilsczek FH, Salina D, Poon KKH, Fahey C, Yipp BG, Sibley CD, et al. A novel mechanism of rapid nuclear neutrophil extracellular trap formation in response to *Staphylococcus aureus. J Immunol.* (2010) 185:7413–25. doi: 10.4049/jimmunol.1000675
17. Berends ET, Horswill AR, Haste NM, Monestier M, Nizet V, von Köckritz-Blickwede M. Nuclease expression by *Staphylococcus aureus* facilitates escape from neutrophil extracellular traps. *J Innate Immun.* (2010) 2:576–86. doi: 10.1159/000319909
18. Disalvo JW. Desoxyrribonuclease and coagulase activity of micrococci. *Med Tech Bull.* (1958) 9:191–6.
19. Schilcher K, Andreoni F, Uchiyama S, Ogawa T, Schuepbach RA, Zinkernagel AS. Increased neutrophil extracellular trap-mediated *Staphylococcus aureus* clearance through inhibition of nuclease activity by clindamycin and immunoglobulin. *J Infect Dis.* (2014) 210:473–82. doi: 10.1093/infdis/jiu091
20. Olson ME, Nygaard TK, Ackermann L, Watkins RL, Zurek OW, Pallister KB, et al. *Staphylococcus aureus* nuclease is a *SaeRS*- dependent virulence factor. *Infect Immun.* (2013) 81:1316–24. doi: 10.1128/IAI.01242-12
21. Rogasch K, Rühmling V, Pané-Farré J, Höper D, Weinberg C, Fuchs S, et al. Influence of the two-component system SaeRS on global gene expression in two different *Staphylococcus aureus* strains. *J Bacteriol.* (2006) 188:7742–58. doi: 10.1128/JB.00555-06
22. Novick RP. Autoinduction and signal transduction in the regulation of *Staphylococcal* virulence. *Mol Microbiol.* (2003) 48:1429–49. doi: 10.1046/j.1365-2958.2003.03526.x
23. Hirschhausen N, Block D, Bianconi I, Bragonzi A, Birtel J, Lee JC, et al. Extended *Staphylococcus aureus* persistence in cystic fibrosis is associated with bacterial adaptation. *Int J Med Microbiol.* (2013) 303:685–92. doi: 10.1016/j.ijmm.2013.09.012
24. Boles BR, Thoendel M, Roth AJ, Horswill AR. Identification of genes involved in polysaccharide-independent *Staphylococcus aureus* biofilm formation. *PLoS ONE.* (2010) 5:e10146. doi: 10.1371/journal.pone.0010146
25. Kiedrowski MR, Kavanaugh JS, Malone CL, Mootz JM, Voyich JM, Smeltzer MS, et al. Nuclease modulates biofilm formation in community-associated methicillin-resistant *Staphylococcus aureus. PLoS ONE.* (2011) 6:e267. doi: 10.1371/journal.pone.0026714
26. Martínez-Alemán SR, Campos-García L, Palma-Nicolas JP, Hernández-Bello R, González GM, Sánchez-González A. Understanding the entanglement: Neutrophil Extracellular Traps (NETs) in cystic fibrosis. *Front Cell Infect Microbiol.* (2017) 7:104. doi: 10.3389/fcimb.2017.00104
27. Dwyer M, Shan Q, D'Ortona S, Maurer R, Mitchell R, Olesen H, et al. Cystic fibrosis sputum DNA has NETosis characteristics and neutrophil extracellular trap release is regulated by macrophage migration-inhibitory factor. *J Innate Immun.* (2014) 6:765–79. doi: 10.1159/000363242

28. Floyd M, Winn M, Cullen C, Sil P, Chassaing B, Yoo DG, et al. Swimming motility mediates the formation of neutrophil extracellular traps induced by flagellated *Pseudomonas aeruginosa*. *PLoS Pathog*. (2016) 12:e1005987. doi: 10.1371/journal.ppat.1005987
29. Young RL, Malcolm KC, Kret JE, Caceres SM, Poch KR, Nichols DP, et al. Neutrophil Extracellular Trap (NET)-mediated killing of *Pseudomonas aeruginosa:* evidence of acquired resistance within the CF airway, independent of CFTR. *PLoS ONE*. (2011) 6:e23637. doi: 10.1371/journal.pone.0023637
30. Rahman S, Gadjeva M. Does NETosis contribute to the bacterial pathoadaptation in cystic fibrosis? *Front Immunol.* (2014) 5:378. doi: 10.3389/fimmu.2014.00378
31. Kriegeskorte A, Block D, Drescher M, Windmüller N, Mellmann A, Baum C, et al. Inactivation of thyA in *Staphylococcus aureus* attenuates virulence and has a strong impact on metabolism and virulence gene expression. *Mbio*. (2014) 5:e01447-14. doi: 10.1128/mBio.01447-14
32. Kahl BC, Mellmann A, Deiwick S, Peters G, Harmsen D. Variation of the polymorphic region X of the protein A gene during persistent airway infection of cystic fibrosis patients reflects two independent mechanisms of genetic change in *Staphylococcus aureus*. *J Clin Microbiol*. (2005) 43:502–5. doi: 10.1128/JCM.43.1.502-505.2005
33. Birrer P, McElvaney NG, Rüdeberg A, Sommer CW, Liechti-Gallati S, Kraemer R, et al. Protease-antiprotease imbalance in the lungs of children with cystic fibrosis. *Am J Respir Crit Care Med*. (1994) 150:207–13. doi: 10.1164/ajrccm.150.1.7912987
34. Bonfield TL, Panuska JR, Konstan MW, Hilliard KA, Hilliard JB, Ghnaim H, et al. Inflammatory cytokines in cystic fibrosis lungs. *Am J Respir Crit Care Med*. (1995) 152(6 Pt 1):2111–8. doi: 10.1164/ajrccm.152.6.8520783
35. Cantin A. Cystic fibrosis lung inflammation: early, sustained, and severe. *Am J Respir Critic Care Med*. (1995) 151:939–41. doi: 10.1164/ajrccm/151.4.939
36. Chaves-Moreno D, Wos-Oxley ML, Jáuregui R, Medina E, Oxley AP, Pieper DH. Exploring the transcriptome of *Staphylococcus aureus* in its natural niche. *Sci Rep*. (2016) 6:33174. doi: 10.1038/srep33174
37. Thammavongsa V, Missiakas DM, Schneewind O. *Staphylococcus aureus* degrades neutrophil extracellular traps to promote immune cell death. *Science*. (2013) 342:863–6. doi: 10.1126/science.1242255
38. Traber K, Novick R. A slipped-mispairing mutation in AgrA of laboratory strains and clinical isolates results in delayed activation of Agr and failure to translate δ- and α-haemolysins. *Mol Microbiol*. (2006) 59:1519–30. doi: 10.1111/j.1365-2958.2006.04986.x
39. Shopsin B, Eaton C, Wasserman GA, Mathema B, Adhikari RP, Agolory S. Mutations in Agr do not persist in natural populations of methicillin-resistant *Staphylococcus aureus*. *J Infect Dis*. (2010) 202:1593–9. doi: 10.1086/656915
40. Giraudo AT, Calzolari A, Cataldi AA, Bogni C, Nagel R. The sae locus of *Staphylococcus aureus* encodes a two-component regulatory system. *FEMS Microbiol Lett*. (1999) 177:15–22. doi: 10.1016/S0378-1097(99)00282-7
41. Augustin J, Götz F. Transformation of *Staphylococcus epidermidis* and other *Staphylococcal* species with plasmid DNA by electroporation. *FEMS Microbiol Lett*. (1990) 54:203–7. doi: 10.1111/j.1574-6968.1990.tb03997.x
42. Harmsen D, Claus H, Witte W, Rothgänger J, Claus H, Turnwald D, et al. Typing of methicillin-resistant *Staphylococcus aureus* in a university hospital setting by using novel software for *spa* repeat determination and database management. *J Clin Microbiol*. (2003) 41:5442–8. doi: 10.1128/JCM.41.12.5442-5448.2003
43. Mellmann A, Bletz S, Böking T, Kipp F, Becker K, Schultes A, et al. Real-time genome sequencing of resistant bacteria provides precision infection control in an institutional setting. *J Clin Microbiol*. (2016) 54:2874–81. doi: 10.1128/JCM.00790-16
44. Leopold SR, Goering RV, Witten A, Harmsen D, Mellmann A. Bacterial whole-genome sequencing revisited: portable, scalable, and standardized analysis for typing and detection of virulence and antibiotic resistance genes. *J Clin Microbiol*. (2014) 52:2365–70. doi: 10.1128/JCM.00262-14
45. Schwartbeck B, Birtel J, Treffon J, Langhanki L, Mellmann A, Kale D, et al. Dynamic *in vivo* mutations within the Ica operon during persistence of *Staphylococcus aureus* in the airways of cystic fibrosis patients. *PLoS Pathog*. (2016) 12:e1006024. doi: 10.1371/journal.ppat.1006024
46. Treffon J, Block D, Moche M, Reiss S, Fuchs S, Engelmann S, et al. Adaptation of *Staphylococcus aureus* to the airways of cystic fibrosis patients by the up-regulation of superoxide dismutase M and iron-scavenging proteins. *J Infect Dis*. (2018) 217:1453–61. doi: 10.1093/infdis/jiy012
47. Vaudaux P, Francois P, Bisognano C, Kelley WL, Lew DP, Schrenzel J, et al. Increased expression of clumping factor and fibronectin-binding proteins by HemB mutants of *Staphylococcus aureus* expressing small colony variant phenotypes. *Infect Immun*. (2002) 70:5428–37. doi: 10.1128/IAI.70.10.5428-5437.2002
48. Harraghy N, Kormanec J, Wolz C, Homerova D, Goerke C, Ohlsen K, et al. Sae is essential for expression of the staphylococcal adhesins Eap and Emp. *Microbiology*. (2005) 151(Pt 6):1789–800. doi: 10.1099/mic.0.27902-0
49. de Buhr N, von Köckritz-Blickwede M. How neutrophil extracellular traps become visible. *J Immunol Res*. (2016) 2016:4604713. doi: 10.1155/2016/4604713
50. Köckritz-Blickwede M, Chow O, Ghochani M, Nizet V. Visualization and functional evaluation of phagocyte extracellular traps. *Methods Microbiol*. (2010) 37:139–60. doi: 10.1016/S0580-9517(10)37007-3

11

Pf Bacteriophage and their Impact on Pseudomonas Virulence, Mammalian Immunity and Chronic Infections

***Patrick R. Secor*[1,2,3*], *Elizabeth B. Burgener*[4,5], *M. Kinnersley*[1], *Laura K. Jennings*[1,2], *Valery Roman-Cruz*[1,2], *Medeea Popescu*[5], *Jonas D. Van Belleghem*[5], *Naomi Haddock*[5], *Conner Copeland*[6], *Lia A. Michaels*[1], *Christiaan R. de Vries*[5], *Qingquan Chen*[5], *Julie Pourtois*[5], *Travis J. Wheeler*[3,6], *Carlos E. Milla*[4] and *Paul L. Bollyky*[5*]**

[1] Division of Biological Sciences, University of Montana, Missoula, MT, United States, [2] Center for Translational Medicine, University of Montana, Missoula, MT, United States, [3] Center for Biomolecular Structure and Dynamics, University of Montana, Missoula, MT, United States, [4] Department of Pediatrics, Center for Excellence in Pulmonary Biology, Stanford University, Stanford, CA, United States, [5] Division of Infectious Diseases and Geographic Medicine, Department of Medicine, Stanford University, Stanford, CA, United States, [6] Department of Computer Science, University of Montana, Missoula, MT, United States

***Correspondence:**
Patrick R. Secor
patrick.secor@mso.umt.edu
Paul L. Bollyky
pbollyky@stanford.edu

Pf bacteriophage are temperate phages that infect the bacterium *Pseudomonas aeruginosa*, a major cause of chronic lung infections in cystic fibrosis (CF) and other settings. Pf and other temperate phages have evolved complex, mutualistic relationships with their bacterial hosts that impact both bacterial phenotypes and chronic infection. We and others have reported that Pf phages are a virulence factor that promote the pathogenesis of *P. aeruginosa* infections in animal models and are associated with worse skin and lung infections in humans. Here we review the biology of Pf phage and what is known about its contributions to pathogenesis and clinical disease. First, we review the structure, genetics, and epidemiology of Pf phage. Next, we address the diverse and surprising ways that Pf phages contribute to *P. aeruginosa* phenotypes including effects on biofilm formation, antibiotic resistance, and motility. Then, we cover data indicating that Pf phages suppress mammalian immunity at sites of bacterial infection. Finally, we discuss recent literature implicating Pf in chronic *P. aeruginosa* infections in CF and other settings. Together, these reports suggest that Pf bacteriophage have direct effects on *P. aeruginosa* infections and that temperate phages are an exciting frontier in microbiology, immunology, and human health.

Keywords: bacteriophage, cystic fibrosis, wound, *Pseudomonas aeruginosa*, immunology, infection, Pf phage, Inovirus

INTRODUCTION

Pseud omonas aeruginosa (*Pa*) is a major human pathogen associated with chronic infections in wounds, burns, and nosocomial settings (1–5). *Pa* is responsible for extensive mortality and billions of dollars in health care costs (6–8). In recognition of this, *Pa* was recently listed as a critical priority pathogen by the World health Organization (WHO) (9).

Pa infections are highly problematic in cystic fibrosis (CF), an inherited disease associated with defective ion transport and the accumulation of thick, tenacious airway secretions. Individuals with CF are prone to chronic pulmonary infections that over time lead to poor lung function and increased mortality (10, 11).

Pa is particularly pathogenic in CF because of its ability to form robust biofilms (12–18). These are slimy conglomerates of polymers and microbial communities that allow *Pa* to colonize airways and other surfaces (19). *Pa* biofilms are especially tenacious and, once established, very difficult to clear.

Many antibiotics have limited penetration through biofilms (20, 21). Hence, bacteria encased within biofilms are able to tolerate antibiotic concentrations hundreds or thousands of times higher than planktonic bacteria (12, 22–24). Over time, this favors the emergence of antibiotic resistant bacteria (19, 25) and the predominance of multi-drug resistant (MDR) strains (15, 20, 26, 27). Individuals with CF are often infected with *Pa* strains that are resistant to whole classes of anti-pseudomonal antibiotics (28–30), including all oral antibiotic options (15, 31). *Pa* biofilms are also often composed of a heterogeneous bacterial population that includes individuals that are less susceptible to antibiotics, such as metabolically dormant persister cells (32).

Pa biofilms also contribute to immune evasion by defying phagocytic engulfment (33–38). Robust biofilm formation by *Pa* contributes to physical impedance of phagocytosis (39, 40) and biofilm polymers also have properties that contribute to immune evasion, including antagonism of complement-mediated opsonization [(35, 37, 41)]. *Pa* also resists efficient bacterial clearance by neutrophil extracellular traps (NETs) (42–44). These are networks of DNA and other polymers released from lysed neutrophils that entrap and destroy bacteria (45, 46). The ability to resist NET-mediated killing (NETosis) is highly strain dependent (42, 43). In the CF airway, ongoing robust immune activation and impaired bacterial clearance perpetuate a vicious cycle of inflammation (47–52).

In light of these effects on antibiotic tolerance and immune evasion, there is great interest in identifying novel biomarkers, virulence factors, and therapeutic targets associated with *Pa* biofilm infections.

Pf bacteriophages, filamentous Inoviruses produced by *Pa* (53, 54), have emerged as a new front in the fight against *Pa* biofilm infections. Here, we review the diverse and surprising ways that Pf phages contribute to the pathogenesis of chronic *Pa* infections in CF and other settings. First, we review the structure, genetics, and epidemiology of Pf phage. Next, we address how Pf phages contribute to *Pa* phenotypes including effects on biofilm formation, antibiotic resistance, and motility. Then, we examine data indicating that Pf modulates mammalian immunity at sites of bacterial infection. Finally, we discuss recent literature implicating Pf in chronic *Pa* infections in CF and other settings. The goal of this work is to provide a comprehensive and integrated resource for those interested in Pf biology and in phage contributions to bacterial pathogenesis.

Pa AND Pf BACTERIOPHAGES

Pf phages are Inoviruses, a genus of temperate, non-enveloped filamentous viruses. Inoviruses are broadly distributed across all biomes and infect both Gram-positive and Gram-negative bacterial species, and even some Archaea (54). While all lytic phage obligately lyse their bacterial hosts during propagation and most other lysogenic phage typically lyse their bacterial host at some point during their lifecycle, Inoviruses are unique in their ability to establish chronic infection cycles where virions are continuously extruded from the bacterial cell envelope without lysis (55).

Inoviruses like Pf are among the better characterized bacteriophages due to their extensive use in research and industry. Inoviruses are amenable to genetic manipulation and some species, such as M13 (*Escherichia coli*) are widely used in biotechnological applications, such as phage display (56) and as drug carriers (57). Pf phages are also a model system for studying the molecular mechanisms of nucleoprotein assembly and membrane transport (58–68).

In this section, we discuss Pf phage structure, genetics, and lifecycle. We then address the prevalence and diversity of Pf phages amongst *Pa* clinical isolates.

Pf Virion Structure

Pf virions are ~6–7 nm in diameter and vary in length from ~0.8–2 μm, depending on the strain and genome size in question. Like all Inoviruses, Pf virions are composed of thousands of copies of a single major coat protein (p8, CoaB in Pf) with minor coat proteins at either end involved in phage assembly and host recognition (**Figure 1**) (70–72). Structurally, Inoviruses can be subdivided into two classes based on helical symmetry. Class I Inoviruses are highly symmetrical and include species, such as Fd and M13, which infect *Escherichia coli*. Class II Inoviruses have a twisted, helical symmetry and include Pf phages (73).

Pf phages package a single-stranded circular DNA genome. While most viruses package their genetic material into the smallest conformation possible, Inoviruses like Pf package their genome in the most extended conformation possible. The orientation of the packaged ssDNA Pf phage genome is also unusual; the genome is packaged in a *P* DNA confirmation where the DNA bases are inverted and pointing outwards with the C-terminus of CoaB capsid proteins reaching through the bases to stabilize the backbones of the anti-parallel DNA strands (**Figure 1**) (74).

Pf virions are relatively stiff filaments with a long persistence length and an overall negative charge density comparable to dsDNA (75). At sufficiently high concentrations, Pf phages, like other filamentous viruses, spontaneously align and assemble liquid crystalline structures (76). The uniform length, diameter, and charge density has made Pf and other Inoviruses a popular model system to study the soft matter physics of colloidal liquid crystals (77) and an effective tool to measure dipolar couplings in NMR structure determinations (78, 79). We discuss how the ability of Pf phages to assemble liquid crystalline structures in biofilms and airway secretions impacts *Pa* infection pathogenesis in a subsequent section below.

Pf Genome Structure

Pf phages have a conserved core genome structure encoding genes necessary for DNA replication, virion assembly, and

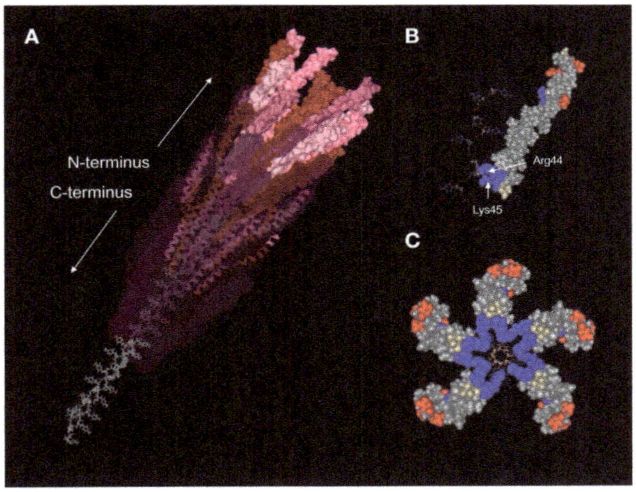

FIGURE 1 | Structure of the Pf1 virion. **(A)** Ribbon diagram with Van der Waals surface representation of a portion of the assembled Pf1 virion (PDBID: 1PFI) showing the helical arrangement of CoaB subunits around the P-form ssDNA viral genome. Subunit surface opacity is decreased along the length of the capsid to highlight the alpha-helical secondary structure of CoaB and the unique conformation of the DNA. Amino acids are colored according to charge, with positively-charged residues in blue, negatively-charged residues in red, and neutral residues in gray. **(B)** Space-filling model of a single CoaB subunit bound to a stretch of cytosines. Arg44 and Lys45 are situated on either side of the DNA backbone and act to stabilize it through electrostatic interactions. **(C)** Cross-sectional view of five CoaB subunits situated around the packaged viral genome. Amino acids are colored by charge as in **(B)**. Image adapted from reference (69).

morphogenesis. This is typically present in *Pa* as a prophage integrated into the bacterial chromosome (80). For this review, we refer to Pf gene names and numbers that correspond to the Pf4 prophage integrated into the chromosome of the reference strain *Pa* PAO1 (PA0715–PA0729) (**Figure 2**).

Characterized Pf genes in the core genome include *xisF4* (excisionase), c repressor gene (*pf4r*), *PA0720* (single-stranded DNA binding protein), *PA0723* (*coaB*, major coat protein), *PA0724* (*coaA*, minor coat protein), *PA0726* (morphogenesis protein), *PA0727* (replication initiation protein), and *PA0728* (*intF*, integrase). The functions of these genes are discussed in more detail below. The function of other genes in the Pf core genome remain to be characterized.

Accessory genes flank the core Pf genome (**Figure 2**) and are known as morons (they add more genes on) (81). While the functions of Pf phage morons are not well-characterized, other phage morons have been shown to reduce virulence factor production and inhibit *Pa* motility (82). Due to the presence of these accessory genes, the overall size of the Pf genome is variable amongst different Pf strains, ranging from ~7–12 kb.

The Pf Life Cycle

The events around initial infection of bacteria with Inoviruses has been reasonably well-characterized. Pf virions initiate infection by adsorbing to the tip of type IV pili, an extracellular appendage that mediates twitching motility in *Pa* (**Figure 3**) (83). Adsorption is mediated by the minor coat protein CoaA (PA0724), which is located on the end of the virion. The adsorbed virion is then drawn into the periplasm as the pili retracts where the phage coat protein CoaA contacts the secondary receptor TolA (72). TolA is part of the highly conserved Tol-Pal system that controls membrane integrity and invagination during cell division and is constitutively expressed and readily available for Pf phages to leverage to infect the host cell. CoaB capsid proteins are then drawn off the phage ssDNA genome and retained in the inner membrane while the ssDNA Pf genome is deposited into the cytoplasm. The ssDNA genome is then converted into a circular dsDNA replicative form (RF) by host enzymes and the RF serves as a template for transcription of phage genes.

At this point, the phage must decide whether it will initiate a chronic infection and produce progeny virions or initiate a lysogenic lifecycle and integrate into the bacterial chromosome as a prophage (80). If conditions favor Pf entering a lysogenic lifecycle after infecting a naïve bacterial host, the RF can be integrated into the bacterial chromosome as a prophage by the Pf-encoded site-specific tyrosine recombinase IntF (84).

Recent work has shed light on the molecular details for how Pf phages maintain lysogeny or initiate a chronic infection cycle. Like other phages, Pf phages respond to host stress. For example, Pf5 replication is strongly induced when the substrate binding protein DppA1 (involved in peptide utilization) is inactivated (85). Although the mechanism is not known, it is thought that Pf5 senses nutrient limitation of its host through DppA1 and in response, initiates the chronic infection cycle. Given the importance of Pf phages for Pa biofilm formation and pathogenesis discussed below, the further characterization of factors that drive production of Pf phages is likely to be an area of active research.

Pf phages, like several other phages, also respond to oxidative stress. When *Pa* is exposed to H_2O_2, cysteine residues in the OxyR transcriptional regulator are oxidized (86). Oxidized OxyR then binds to the Pf4 prophage between *PA0716* and *PA0719* (86). The binding of OxyR to this site likely suppresses the c repressor gene *pf4r*, which maintains lysogeny and confers immunity to superinfection by exogenous Pf virions. Pf4r promotes lysogeny and superinfection exclusion by repressing transcription of the Pf excisionase gene *xisF4* (84) (**Figure 2**).

When *pf4r* is suppressed, as it is by OxyR, or when sufficiently high titers of infecting Pf virions overwhelm Pf4r, as may happen during superinfection, XisF4 is free to promote the transcription of the operon encoding the replication initiator protein (PA0727) and IntF (84). The initiator protein binds to RF DNA at the origin of replication, recruits the host helicase UvrD and DNA polymerase III, and initiates rolling circle replication (87). Rolling circle replication not only produces new copies of the dsDNA RF, but also new ssDNA Pf genomes. The newly synthesized ssDNA genomes are quickly coated by numerous copies of the single stranded-binding protein PA0720, stabilizing and protecting the ssDNA species until it can be packaged into a new virion.

While the RF and ssDNA pools expand in the bacterial cytoplasm, structural Pf proteins, such as CoaB are produced. CoaB is translated with an N-terminal leader peptide that

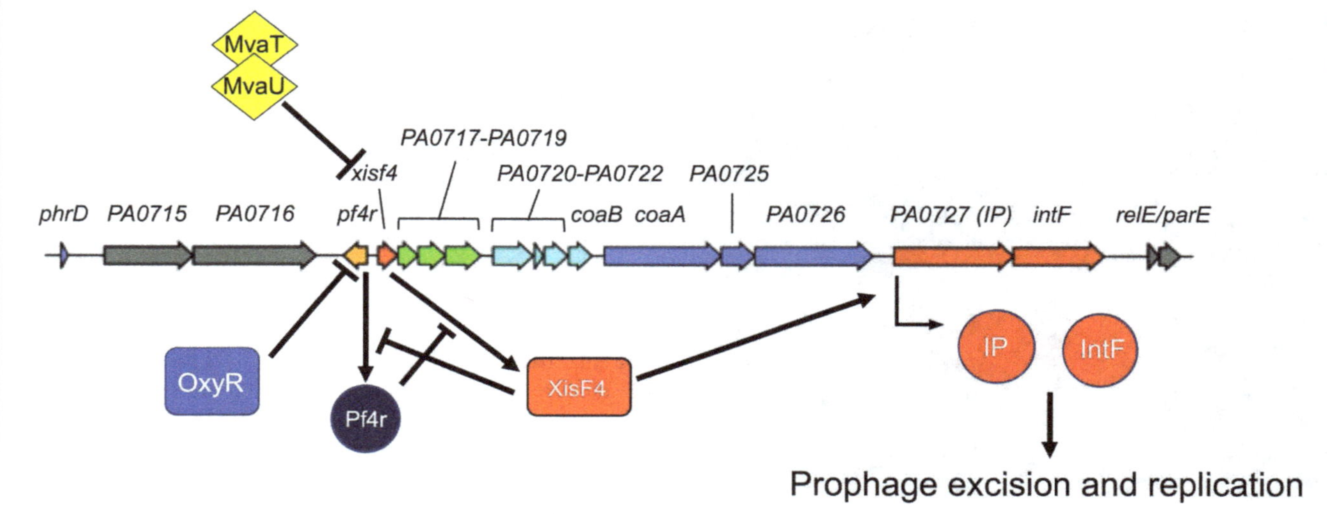

FIGURE 2 | Regulation of Pf replication decisions. The Pf4 prophage from *P. aeruginosa* strain PAO1 is shown. Colored genes correspond to the core Pf genome while gray genes are accessory genes that are variable from strain to strain (see **Figure 4** for more details). Pf4r (i.e., the c repressor) maintains lysogeny by repressing the excisionase *xisF4*. XisF4 promotes transcription of an operon encoding both the replication initiation protein PA0727 and integrase IntF. The transcriptional regulator OxyR suppresses *pf4r* while the global histone-nucleosome-like transcriptional regulators MvaT and MvaU suppress *xisF4*. **Figure 3** details events in the Pf lifecycle, such as genome replication and assembly of new virions.

targets the CoaB preprotein to the inner membrane. After CoaB is inserted in the inner membrane in the correct orientation, it is processed into its mature form by host Sec/YidC enzymes (88). CoaB monomers interact with membrane-associated morphogenesis machinery (which likely includes the morphogenesis protein PA0726) to package the ssDNA Pf genome. As CoaB is incorporated into the growing virion, PA0720 is displaced and the nascent phage particle is extruded through the cell envelope (**Figure 3**).

Superinfection of *Pa* by Pf Phages

Once extruded from the host cell, Pf virions likely encounter a host that is already lysogenized by a Pf prophage. This is especially true when bacterial densities are high, as they are in biofilms. Superinfection occurs when exogenous Pf virions successfully infect a bacterial cell already lysogenized by Pf. Even though Pf (and other Inoviruses) can replicate without lysing their bacterial host, Pf superinfection can result in bacterial lysis. At present it is unclear how Pf superinfection causes bacterial lysis. It is possible that during superinfection more Pf virions are produced than an individual host cell can handle. For example, CoaB monomers or other Pf proteins could accumulate in the inner membrane to sufficiently high levels such that the cytoplasmic membrane is destabilized.

Superinfection by Pf phages plays important roles in *Pa* biofilm development. Evaluation of the within-population genetic diversity of *Pa* PAO1 during biofilm formation revealed that the Pf4 population diversified at an evolutionary rate comparable to RNA viruses, far faster than the rest of the genome (89). In conjunction with the diversification of the Pf4 population, titers of superinfective Pf4 virions as high as 10^{11} plaque forming units per milliliter of biofilm effluent were observed. Interestingly, all mutations in Pf4 were within or upstream of the c repressor gene *pf4r,* suggesting that superinfective Pf phages lose the ability to self-regulate their replication. Lastly, the study by McElroy *et al.* also found that mutations in type IV pili genes also accumulated in *Pa* biofilm populations, most likely in response to selective pressures exerted by the expansion of the Pf phage population (89).

Pa can suppress Pf phage through the histone-like nucleoid-structuring (H-NS) proteins MvaT and MvaU (83). MvaT and MvaU are global regulators of gene expression and coordinately suppress AT-rich elements in the *Pa* genome (90). The *Pa* genome is G-C-rich (~66% GC content) and MvaT and MvaU offer a mechanism for *Pa* to incorporate xenogenic DNA (such as phages and other horizontally acquired genetic material with a relatively high AT-content) into its genome in a regulated way. Because MvaT and MvaU regulate the same target genes, *Pa* can tolerate the loss of either *mvaT* or *mvaU*; however, inactivation of both *mvaT* and *mvaU* is lethal to *Pa* (90). A transposon mutagenesis study discovered that the conditional depletion of MvaT in a Δ*mvaU* background induced Pf4 replication that resulted in the death of *Pa* (83). That study also demonstrated that Pf4 uses type IV pili as a cell surface receptor to initiate infection. Interestingly, when type IV pili were inactivated by deleting the *pilY* gene, depletion of MvaT in a Δ*mvaU* background was tolerated, even though the Pf4 prophage was induced and infectious Pf4 virions were produced (83). This observation indicates that superinfection was required to cause cell death.

These observations are consistent with a model where within *Pa* biofilms, populations of Pf phages with inactivated c repressor genes expand and Pf virions are produced in abundance. These virions could then superinfect *Pa* at a sufficiently high multiplicity of infection to overwhelm the superinfection

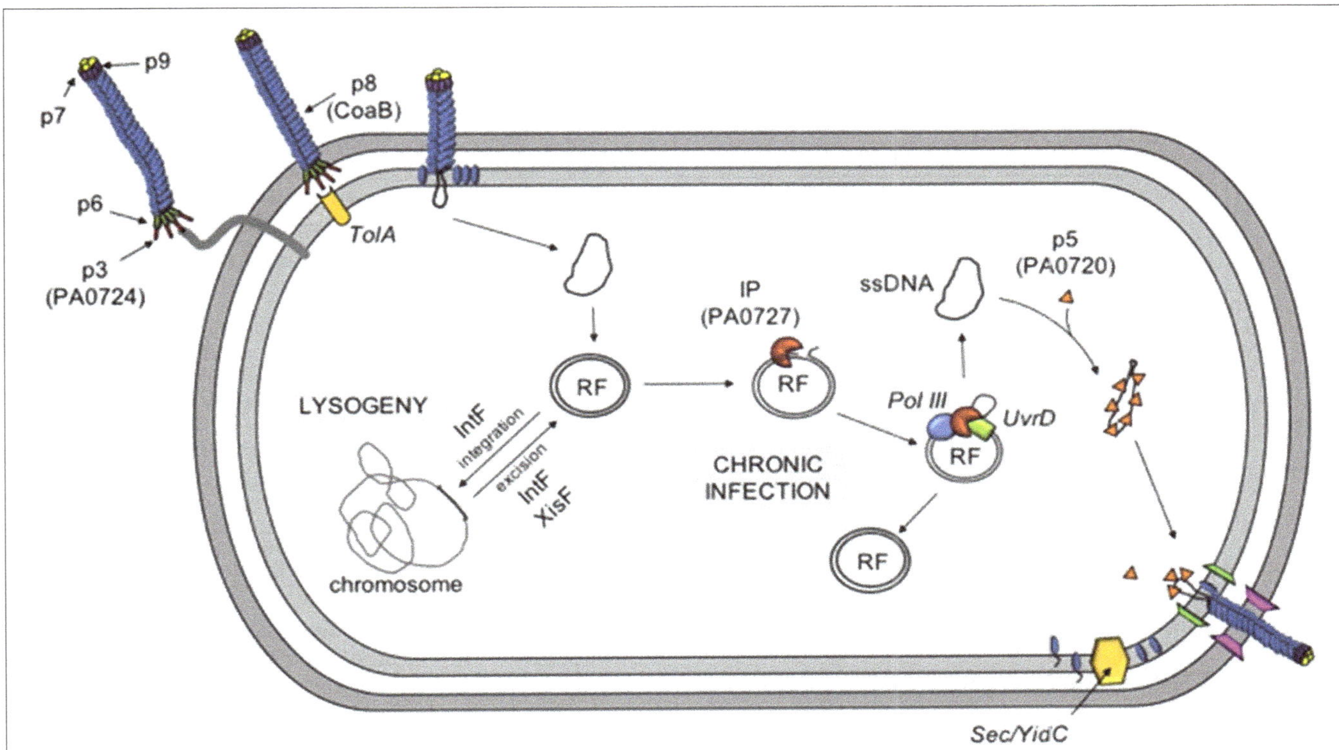

FIGURE 3 | The Pf life cycle. Pf infection is initiated when the minor coat protein p3 (PA0724) binds to type IV pili. Pilus retraction draws the phage into the periplasm where p3 binds the secondary receptor TolA. As the phage moves through the inner membrane, the major coat protein CoaB is removed and deposited in the inner membrane. The ssDNA genome is converted into a dsDNA replicative form (RF) and is either integrated into the host chromosome (lysogeny) or used to initiate a chronic infection. The phage initiator protein (IP, PA0727) and host enzymes (DNA polymerase III and UvrD) create additional copies of RF and the ssDNA infective form (IF) via rolling-circle replication. Newly-produced ssDNA molecules are then coated with protein p5 (PA0720) and targeted to the inner membrane where CoaB, which has been inserted into the inner membrane by the hist Sec/YidC machinery, replaces p5 as the virus is extruded through the cell envelope.

exclusion mechanism mediated by Pf4r proteins produced by the resident Pf prophage. Under these conditions, individuals with type IV pili mutations would be selected for as they would be resistant to Pf superinfection.

Pf Diversity and Prevalence Amongst *Pa* Isolates

Routine whole genome sequencing of *Pa* isolates has revealed that Pf prophages are prevalent amongst *Pa* isolates. In one study, out of 241 *Pa* strains, ~60% were lysogenized by Pf (80). Of 2,226 genomes available through the Pseudomonas Genome Database (91), 52% encoded a Pf prophage (92). A phylogenetic analysis of Pf prophage sequences revealed that most known Pf prophages encode their own integrase *intF* (**Figure 4**). However, Pf1, the first Pf strain isolated in 1966 (95), does not encode an intact integrase and replicates episomally (it cannot enter a lysogenic lifecycle). Strains of Pf that do not integrate into the bacterial chromosome would not be detected by whole genome sequencing. Therefore, the prevalence of Pf phages amongst *Pa* isolates is likely underestimated.

Many Pf prophages integrate into bacterial tRNA genes, as is true with other temperate phages (96). For example, the Pf4 prophage infecting *Pa* strain PAO1 integrates into the tRNA-Gly gene *PA0729.1*. It is worth noting that the subline strain MPAO1 harbors both Pf4 and a second similar Pf prophage designated Pf6 integrated into the tRNA-Met gene *PA4673.1* (97). Another example is Pf7, which is integrated into the tRNA-Met gene PSPA7_5361 in *Pa* strain PA7. Some Pf strains, however, integrate into other genomic locations. Strain Pf5, which infects *Pa* strain PA14, integrates between the C32 tRNA thiolase (*PA14_48870*) and *dnaJ* (*PA14_49040*). Other Pf prophages integrate into a homologous site in other strains of *Pa* including Pf-LES, which infects *Pa* epidemic strain LES58 (80) and an unclassified Pf strain infecting *Pa* strain 19660 (91).

We have observed that several strains of *Pa* are infected by multiple Pf prophages. This is in contrast to many species of phages (e.g., lambda) where, due to superinfection exclusion mechanisms, a preexisting phage prevents secondary infections by the same or closely related phage. As noted above, MPAO1 harbors both Pf4 and Pf6. Other strains, such as *Pa* B10W harbors three Pf prophages. Two of the three Pf prophages integrated into the B10W chromosome are genetically distinct from each other (**Figure 4**) indicating that the Pf prophages of BW10 were obtained from distinct infections by different strains of Pf phages along with potential duplications of the same Pf prophage. Given the roles Pf phages play in biofilm formation and infection

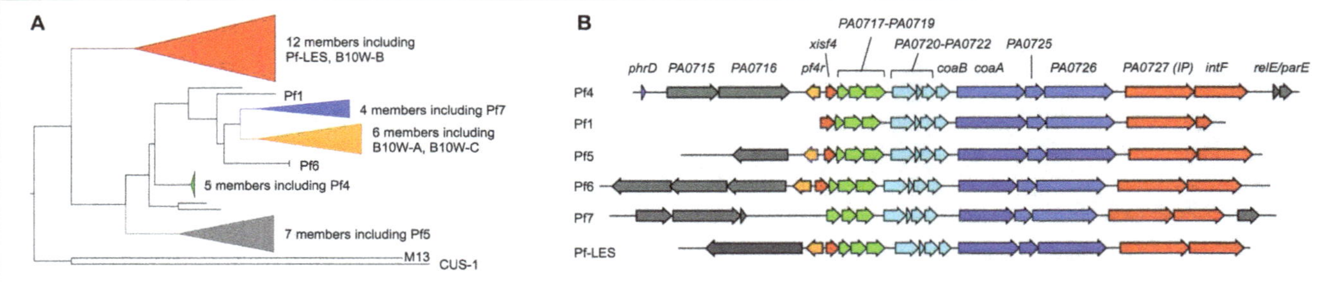

FIGURE 4 | Phylogenic analysis of Pf prophages. **(A)** Forty representative full-length Pf prophage instances were manually collected from the Pseudomonas Genome Database (91). Two DNA sequences encoding Protein III (PA0724) from Inovirus strains M13 and CUS-1 (*E. coli*) were added to serve as an outgroup for phylogenetic rooting. A multiple sequence alignment of these viral sequences was produced using MAFFT (93) (v7.215, default parameters), then manually trimmed to include only the well-aligned region containing Pf phage core proteins. A maximum-likelihood estimate of the strain phylogeny was produced with FastTree (94) (v2.1.3, default parameters), and visualized with FigTree (v1.4.4). **(B)** Representative full-length Pf prophage sequences were manually collected from the Pseudomonas Genome Database. Strain Pf4 was used as a reference; open reading frames identified in other Pf strains were color-coded based on genome location relative to Pf4. Gray genes indicate variable moron sequences (see text) outside of the core Pf genome.

pathogenesis (see below), it would be interesting to compare the fitness of *Pa* strains lysogenized by a single Pf prophage compared to strains lysogenized with several Pf phages.

Pf EFFECTS ON *Pa* PHENOTYPES AND FITNESS

Infection of the CF airway with *Pa* starts with planktonic (free living), variants often originating from the environment. Over time, as bacteria adapt to the CF airway, they environment, they form a biofilm (98). In this section we address the contribution of Pf phages to *Pa* biofilm formation and to other phenotypes involved in *Pa* pathogenicity.

Pf Phages and Small Colony Variant (SCV) Morphology

In *Pa* PAO1 biofilms, bacterial cells shed from the biofilm display a small colony variant (SCV) morphology after they are grown on solid agar (99–101). The production of SCVs is correlated with the emergence of superinfective Pf4 phage. SCVs revert back to a "fuzzy" wild-type colony morphology after subculture in Pf phage-free lysogeny broth (101), indicating that the SCV morphology is a phenotypic response to Pf superinfection and not due to heritable mutations. Because Pf superinfection both suppresses type IV pili-mediated twitching motility and induces a severe growth lag in *Pa*, it is possible that the SCV morphology associated with chronic Pf infection is a result of reduced growth coupled to inhibited twitching motility. The emergence of SCVs from *Pa* biofilms appears to be variable amongst *Pa* strains—*Pa* PA14 biofilms do not shed cells that form SCVs even though Pf5 virions were present at high densities in PA14 biofilms (102). The underlying mechanism for this discrepancy is unknown, but it may relate to the different integration sites of Pf4 and Pf5 and/or the different moron genes encoded by Pf4 and Pf5 (**Figure 4B**).

Pf Phages and *Pa* Biofilm Formation

Upregulation of Pf phage genes are a common feature of *Pa* biofilms, as found in a metanalysis of transcriptional data from *Pa* biofilms grown under various laboratory settings (103). In addition to gene expression data, *Pa* biofilms grown under different conditions (dripflow, chemostat, colony biofilms, etc.), are all associated with the production of abundant superinfective Pf phages at titers as high as 10^{11} PFU/ml (89, 99, 100, 104). Furthermore, semiviscous (105) and anaerobic conditions (106) that mimic environments in biofilms and in late-stage CF-airways were found to induce Pf phages, although the mechanisms behind these induction cues are unknown. Collectively, these observations indicate that Pf phages are consistently induced in *Pa* biofilms, raising the possibility that Pf phages play important roles in biofilm formation. Indeed, Pf phages contribute to *Pa* biofilms in diverse and surprising ways.

The formation of a biofilm is initiated by bacterial attachment to a surface followed by the formation of microcolonies (107). As microcolonies differentiate and grow, voids form in the middle of these microcolonies that are created by cell lysis (100). Cell lysis is accompanied by the release of DNA into the extracellular space (eDNA), which adds structural integrity to the biofilm (108). The presence of superinfective Pf phages in the biofilm effluent correlates with cell lysis and eDNA release prior to the dispersion phase of the biofilm lifecycle (109, 110) (**Figure 5**). To this point, when Pf4 prophage was deleted from the *Pa* PAO1 chromosome, bacterial lysis and eDNA release were not observed (99). Bacterial lysis and eDNA release caused by superinfective Pf phages appears to be a regulated process; the two-component regulator BfmR was reported to suppress Pf phage-mediated cell lysis through PhdA (PA0691), an antitoxin homolog in the Phd (prevent-host-death) family of proteins (111). Deleting *bfmR* caused the premature induction of superinfective Pf phages, increased bacterial lysis and eDNA release, phenotypes opposite to the ΔPf4 prophage mutant. It is possible that PhdA induces Pf replication by interacting with the ParE plasmid stabilization system encoded by Pf4 (**Figure 4B**) (110). However, experimental evidence for this interaction is lacking.

The presence of Pf phages is also associated with phenotypes linked to the pathogenicity of *Pa* biofilms (**Figure 5**). Expectorated sputum from CF patients infected by *Pa* contain

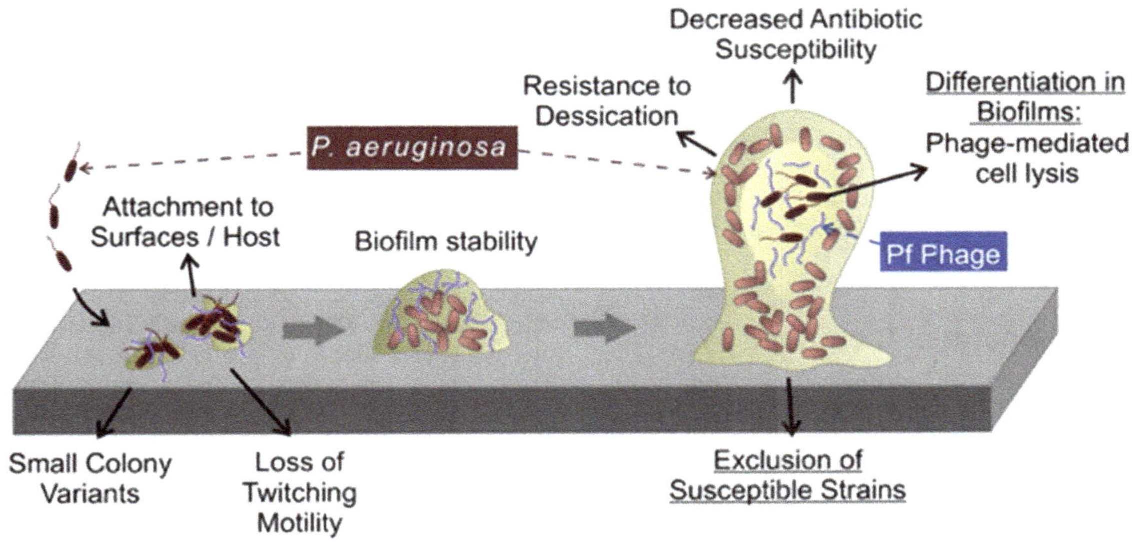

FIGURE 5 | Pf phages contribute to biofilm formation. During the early stages of biofilm formation, Pf phages promote bacterial adhesion to surfaces. During later stages, Pf phages serve as structural components in the biofilm matrix where they promote tolerance to desiccation and cationic antimicrobials. Superinfection by Pf phages (see text) promotes differentiation of the biofilm by inducing bacterial lysis in a subpopulation of cells deep within the biofi m.

$\sim 10^6$-10^9 Pf virions per ml (92, 101). Filamentous Pf phages can dramatically increase the viscosity of CF airway polymers, such as mucin and DNA (92, 101). Furthermore, Pf phage-producing biofilms are more adherent to surfaces compared to *Pa* not producing Pf virions (92, 99–101). Thus, Pf virions could benefit *Pa* infecting CF airways by reducing bacterial clearance from the lung. Consistent with this idea, *Pa* superinfected by Pf established a non-invasive infection phenotype in a mouse model of pneumonia and did not disseminate from the lung whereas *Pa* not producing Pf virions disseminated to distal tissues, suggesting that Pf phages contribute to the establishment of conditions that promote localized chronic infection (112). Other filamentous phages, such as MDAΦ that infects *Neisseria meningitidis* likewise promotes adhesion to epithelial cells promoting host colonization (113). Thus, filamentous phages may play key roles in host colonization and infection initiation in various bacterial infections.

Rice *et al.* demonstrated that biofilms formed by the Pf phage-deficient mutant ΔPf4 were more sensitive to disruption by the detergent SDS relative to the parental strain *Pa* PAO1 lysogenized by Pf4 (99), suggesting that filamentous Pf phages contribute to the structural integrity of biofilms. As discussed above, Pf phages are stiff, negatively charged filaments that spontaneously assemble liquid crystalline structures. Our previous work revealed that Pf virions accumulate in the biofilm matrix where they spontaneously align and give the biofilm matrix liquid crystalline properties (101, 114). Bacteria living in a liquid crystalline biofilm matrix were resistant to desiccation, possibly because the highly ordered liquid crystalline matrix was better able to retain water compared to non-crystalline matrices. Furthermore, the negative charge carried by Pf phages facilitates the binding and sequestration of cationic aminoglycoside antibiotics and cationic antimicrobial peptides (92, 101). This binding capacity was enhanced when Pf phages were in the liquid crystalline phase, allowing *Pa* to tolerate otherwise lethal doses of cationic antibiotics (101, 114). In clinical settings, tolerance to antimicrobials could promote the emergence of individuals with fixed antibiotic resistance, thus limiting treatment options and promoting chronic infection. Indeed, filamentous bacteriophages are associated with chronic *Pa* lung infections and antibiotic resistance in CF (92). Because all Inoviruses are composed of acidic coat proteins, filamentous bacteriophages may be an overlooked structural component of the biofilm matrix in other bacterial species.

Other ways that Pf phages could benefit *Pa* biofilms is by excluding susceptible strains (104). Consistent with this, recent work demonstrates that *Pa* isolates collected from older CF patients tend to be lysogenized by Pf compared to isolates collected earlier in disease (92). This observation raises the possibility that *Pa* strains not harboring Pf prophages may be replaced by strains lysogenized by Pf as the disease progresses to later stages. Future studies investigating the role of Pf phages in the establishment and maintenance of *Pa* lineages in chronic CF airway infections may provide insight into how *Pa* dominates CF airway infections.

Pf EFFECTS ON MAMMALIAN IMMUNITY

There is increasing interest in the impact of phages on human immunology. This trend parallels the resurgence of efforts to develop phage therapies to treat chronic/multidrug-resistant bacterial infections (115, 116) as well as the rapid expansion of research into endogenous phages residing on and within the human host (117–119). Much of this work has focused on CF and the viral pathogens of *Pa* (120, 121).

In this section, we discuss what is known about Pf and its impact on mammalian immunity. First, we discuss Pf and its impact on phagocytosis and bacterial clearance. Next, we address Pf effects on cytokine production and the inflammatory milieu. Finally, we discuss how Pf biology relates to what is known about mammalian immunity and other endogenous and exogenous phages and highlight the outstanding questions around these interactions.

Pf Effects on Bacterial Clearance by Phagocytes

The ability of *Pa* to establish residency and persist in the human lung is dependent upon the bacterium's efficacy at evading innate immune attacks, particularly neutrophil- and alveolar macrophage-mediated anti-bactericidal defenses (122–126). *Pa* must also contend with multiple pattern-recognition receptors (PRRs) including Toll-like receptors 4 (TLR4), 5 (TLR5), and 9 (TLR9) that recognize bacterial pathogen-associated molecular patterns (PAMP) molecules including lipopolysaccharide (LPS) (127, 128), flagellin (128, 129), and DNA containing CpG motifs (130), respectively. PAMP-mediated stimulation of phagocytosis is the primary host defense against *Pa* infection, as evidenced by the fact that both animal models and people with defects in phagocytic cell function are highly susceptible to *Pa* infection (125, 131, 132).

Pa possess a diverse set of virulence factors that impede phagocytosis by both neutrophils and macrophages (38, 133). Many of these factors impact the machinery of phagocytosis, including inflammatory cytokine production, cellular recruitment, and bacterial engulfment (38, 134, 135). These effects on phagocytic clearance contribute to *Pa* immune evasion and persistence within infected tissues (136).

We recently reported that Pf directly inhibits phagocytosis and bacterial clearance (137). Pf causes a significant decrease in the number of *Pa* phagocytosed by murine-derived dendritic cells (DC), macrophages, and human U937-derived and primary macrophages (137). Additionally, murine phagocytes exposed to Pf4 phagocytosed fewer dead *E. coli* particles compared to saline controls, indicating that the inhibitory effects of Pf on phagocytosis are not limited to engulfment of *Pa* (137).

Pf phage also influence bacterial phenotypes in ways that are likely to prevent efficient phagocytosis. As discussed above, some strains of Pf phage contribute to the emergence of SCV strains (99, 110) which are known to drive exopolysaccharide-dependent resistance to macrophage phagocytosis (138). Furthermore, Pf contributions to biofilm formation, adhesiveness, and increased polymer viscosity could be expected to interfere with phagocytosis given that biofilms formed by *Pa* and other organisms are known to prevent opsonization and engulfment of the bacteria within (38, 139–141). Finally, the same structural attributes that promote liquid crystal assembly by Pf phages also drives bacterial aggregation (142) and loss of motility (112), features associated with diminished phagocytosis (135). We discuss reduced phagocytic uptake of bacteria through the lens of CF in later sections.

Pf Effects on Cytokine Production and the Inflammatory Milieu

Inflammatory cytokines are critical to host immune clearance of *Pa*. It is well-established that TNF in particular plays a crucial role in stimulating phagocytosis (143, 144) and in polarizing macrophages toward an M1 phenotype associated with efficient bacterial clearance.

We recently reported that Pf phages are associated with decreased cellular production of TNF (137). These effects were associated with enhanced type 1 interferon levels. Consistent with a critical role for TNF in bacterial clearance, we observed that supplemental TNF could correct Pf effects on phagocytosis and bacterial clearance *in vivo* (137). Pf also suppressed the production of other cytokines and chemokines important for bacterial clearance, including CXCL1 and IL-17. Conversely, Pf increased production of IL-12 and type 1 interferon (112, 137). Fd phage, an *Inovirus* that infects *E. coli*, did not affect TNFa production or phagocytosis (137). The differences in the immunomodulatory properties of Pf and fd phages is unclear, but may relate to differences in coat protein/virion structure or amino acid composition.

Pf-dependent modulation of cytokine production by immune cells was associated with intracellular uptake of Pf phage. We reported that Pf is taken up by human and mouse macrophages, B cells, and dendritic cells within endosomal vesicles. These results are consistent with reports that other phages are internalized by mammalian cells, though those reports mostly implicated phagocytosis rather than endocytosis (145, 146). Further, there are indications that large numbers of phages are directionally transcytosed across epithelial layers into system circulation (147), raising the possibility that phages regularly modulate immune responses and impact human health and disease.

We observed that intracellular Pf phage reduce TNF production by triggering the viral pattern recognition receptor TLR3. In bone-marrow derived macrophages (BMDMs) from $TLR2^{-/-}$, $TLR9^{-/-}$, and $MyD88^{-/-}$ mice, Pf phage reduced TNF upon LPS stimulation, but in $TRIF^{-/-}$, $TLR3^{-/-}$, and $IFNAR^{-/-}$ BMDMs, Pf phage had no significant effect on TNF production (137).

Pf also impacts the polarization of macrophages in the inflammatory milieu. *Pa* PAO1 superinfected with Pf4 caused decreased expression of genes associated with pro-inflammatory M1 macrophage polarization, including Nos2, IL-12, and IFN-g; along with increased expression of cytokines associated with anti-inflammatory M2 macrophage polarization, including IL-10, Nos1, and Arg1 (112, 148). Together with the aforementioned effects on cytokine production, these data indicate that internalization of Pf phages triggers anti-viral pattern recognition receptors that antagonize antibacterial immunity (**Figure 6**).

The Emerging Picture of Phage/Immune Interactions

While our review here has focused on Pf phage, there is a growing body of literature on phage/immune interactions, primarily in the context of phage therapy. Much of that work is outside of the scope of this review and there are several recent, excellent summaries of that research (149–151). Nonetheless, it is worth

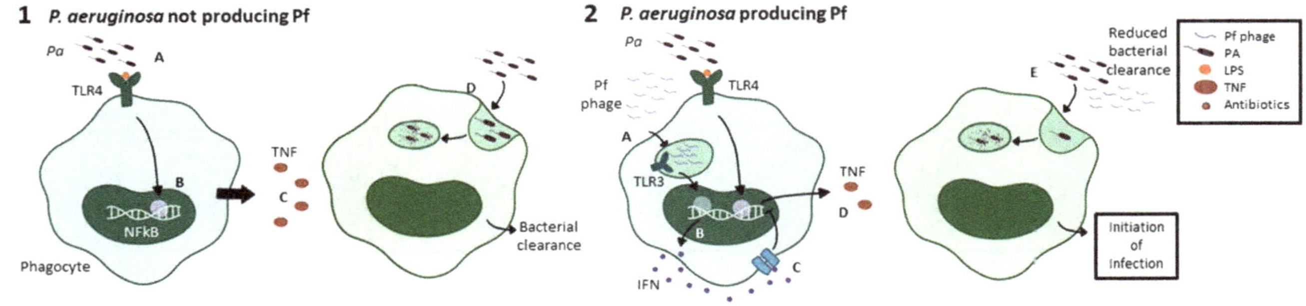

FIGURE 6 | Pf phages trigger viral pathogen recognition pathways leading to reduced phagocytosis. Phagocytosis is the major way that *Pa* infections are cleared by the immune system. In the absence of Pf phages, *Pa*-derived LPS is recognized by TLR4 on the surface of alveolar macrophages (**1**A), triggering NFkB activation and pro-inflammatory cytokine production (**1**B). TNF, a major pro-inflammatory effector, is secreted as a result (**1**C). This drives *Pa* phagocytosis by alveolar macrophages, leading to bacterial clearance (**1**D). In the presence of a *Pa* strain that produces Pf phages, phage particles are internalized in endosomes (**2**A), triggering TLR3 activation and production of interferons (**2**B). IFNα/β binds IFNAR on the cell surface (**2**C) and negatively regulates pro-inflammatory cytokine production, decreasing TNF secretion (**2**D). This results in decreased phagocytic engulfment of *Pa* (**2**E). Together, this supports a model where intracellular Pf phage triggers viral pattern recognition pathways that antagonize bacterial clearance.

addressing the commonalities and differences of this larger body of work in relation to Pf phages.

The finding that Pf suppresses phagocytosis contrasts with reports that lytic phages promote phagocytosis and interact synergistically with phagocytes (152–156). There are also suggestions that some species of phage may promote the opsonization of bacteria by adhering to the bacterial surface and acting as a target for antibody binding (157). In addition, there are reports that phages may be induced when their bacterial host is phagocytosed, lysing the bacteria and promoting clearance (149, 158). Together, these data suggest that lytic phages may promote opposite effects on bacterial clearance compared to Pf. The mechanistic basis for the differences and similarities seen between lytic and lysogenic phages is unclear, particularly since lytic phage are also internalized by eukaryotic cells (159). However, there are recent examples; enteric Caudovirales phages (tailed phages that package linear dsDNA) initially purified for therapeutic use were found to stimulate increased production of pro-inflammatory cytokines (119). In the context of inflammatory bowel diseases, these phages directly exacerbated disease. While further, direct comparisons are needed, these distinctions could be important for the future prospects of lytic phage therapy.

While the impact on bacterial clearance may differ, the impact of cytokine production and the inflammatory milieu appears to be more similar. Studies with lytic phage have generally reported similar, anti-inflammatory effects *in vitro* (160–162) as well as *in vivo* (163, 164). In particular, lytic phage may also dampen the inflammatory effects of LPS and other bacterial products (165, 166). This stands in contrast to some data implicating other, endogenous eukaryotic viruses in chronic inflammation (167) and, it has been theorized, in protection against pathogenic viral infections (168).

THE IMPACT OF Pf PHAGE ON *Pa* INFECTIONS IN CF AND OTHER SETTINGS

Recent reports have implicated Pf phage in clinical outcomes associated with *Pa* infections. Here, we discuss this literature and the potential role of Pf phage in CF lung infections. First, we discuss the links between Pf and clinical outcomes in CF. Next, we discuss the development of vaccines that target Pf to prevent infections with *Pa* and the implications of our work on lytic phage therapy. Finally, we address the relevance of our work on filamentous phage to studies on the lung microbiome.

Pf Phage in CF Airway Infections

CF is a genetic disease where the cystic fibrosis transmembrane conductance regulator (CFTR) gene is mutated. In healthy individuals, the CFTR protein is expressed highly on the apical surface of epithelial cells. In people with CF, CFTR is absent or dysfunctional leading to an imbalance of chloride secretion and sodium absorption which causes dehydration of the airway surface (169–171). Without well-hydrated airway surface liquid, impaired ciliary beating and mucous transport lead to mucus stasis and buildup of viscous mucous in the airways. This in turn sets off a vicious cycle of bacterial infection and neutrophil dominated inflammation, resulting in severe and progressive obstructive pulmonary disease with significant morbidity and mortality (172, 173).

Lung disease in CF begins early in life with recurrent and chronic bacterial infections (172, 174). As the disease progresses, the airways of most patients with CF become colonized by *Pa* (175). In its early stages, *Pa* is intermittently recovered in respiratory cultures, before progressing to a chronic state (176, 177). By adulthood, nearly 60% of CF patients have chronic *Pa* infections (178, 179). Over time, *Pa* becomes a driving force in clinical outcomes in CF lung infections. Chronic endobronchial infection with *Pa* is associated with poor lung function, increased frequency of symptomatic episodes of pulmonary exacerbation, and increased mortality (180–183). While *Pa* eradication antibiotic protocols are now standard of care, success is unfortunately variable and not sustained (184, 185).

We recently identified an association between chronic *Pa* infections in CF patients and Pf phage. In 474 samples collected from a cohort of 34 Danish CF patients infected with Pa,

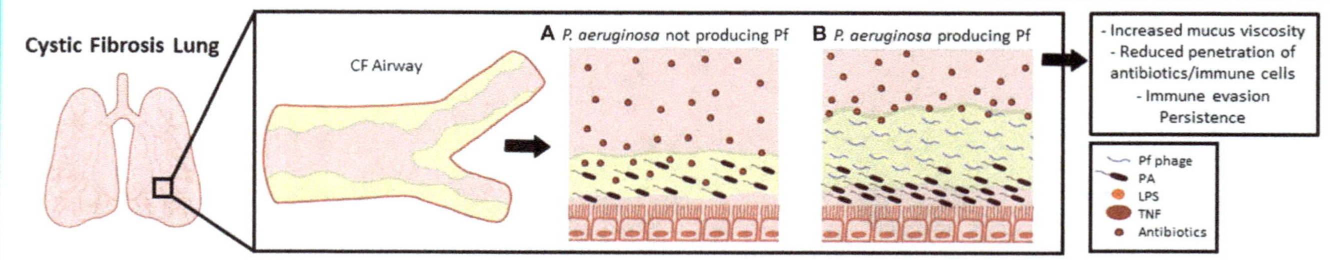

FIGURE 7 | Pf phages contribute to the pathogenesis of *Pa* airway infections in CF. The thick mucus coating the airways in a CF lung facilitates colonization with *Pa* and other bacterial pathogens. Even in the absence of Pf phages, *Pa* forms tenacious biofilms which protect bacterial cells from phagosomal clearance and resist penetration by antibiotics **(A)**. However, Pf phages when present organize the polymer-rich biofilm into crystalline, higher order structures **(B)**, This drives sputum viscosity, adhesiveness, and resistance to desiccation. It also enhances the antibiotic tolerance and immune evasion of bacterial colonies within biofilms, thereby contributing to increased bacterial burden. In this way Pf phages enhance the pathogenesis of *Pa* airway infections in CF.

we found that 44.5% were positive for Pf phage (92). In a cross-sectional study of 58 *Pa* positive CF patients followed at the Stanford CF Clinic, 36% were Pf phage positive. In this cohort, detection of Pf phage was associated with older age, advanced lung disease, worse disease exacerbations, and antibiotic resistance (92). As additional evidence for the damaging effects of these altered responses, we also observed a correlation between the presence of Pf in sputum and the activity of the neutrophil enzyme Elastase (186), a known marker of airway destruction and bronchiectasis in CF. Further, we found that immune dysfunction correlates of the presence of Pf with sputum cytokine profiling revealing higher levels of IL12p70 and lower levels of ENA78, RESISTIN and TRAIL (186). These changes suggest disrupted immune function in response to infection (187–192). Broadly speaking, these data are consistent with the enhanced virulence associated with Pf production in a mouse model of *Pa* lung infection and with reports by ourselves and others describing contributions of Pf to chronic infection phenotypes (99, 101, 110, 112).

The effects of Pf on clinical outcomes were also associated with an increased rate of genetically-encoded antibiotic resistance to several anti-pseudomonal antibiotics—particularly aztreonam, amikacin, and meropenem. These same antibiotics were also sequestered by Pf phage *in vitro* whereas ciprofloxacin was not (92) (**Figure 7**). This raises the intriguing possibility that over time, treatment with these antibiotics favors the acquisition of Pf(+) strains of *Pa*. Consistent with this, we observed that only 1 of 11 pediatric patients in our cohort was Pf(+), whereas 20 of 46 adult patients were (92). Further, 10 of 10 CF patients who underwent lung transplantation were Pf(+) (101). In light of these data, we have proposed that *Pa* strains that produce Pf phage may have a selective advantage and be disproportionately represented in the lungs of older patients with CF. These data also suggest that it may be possible to use the presence of Pf phage to inform antibiotic choices.

These findings in *Pa*-infected CF patients echo the results of our recent investigations into the role of Pf phages in *Pa* chronic wound infections. In a prospective cohort study of 113 patients with wound infections we found that *Pa* was detected in 37 patients and that 25 of these (68%) were positive for Pf phage. Pf(+) strains of *Pa* were more likely than Pf(−) strains to be present in chronic wounds (137).

Together, these data suggest that Pf phages may contribute to clinical outcomes in *Pa* infections in CF as well as in other clinical contexts.

The Development of Therapies That Target Pf Phages to Prevent *Pa* Infections

An effective vaccine against *Pa* would represent an important component in our armamentarium against this deadly bacterium. To date, there are no FDA approved vaccines for the prevention of *Pa* infections, though several are in various stages of development (193). Most of the vaccine candidates that have been evaluated have been against major components of *Pa* itself, including LPS, exopolysaccharides, extracellular and outer membrane proteins, flagella, or pili (193). Given the prevalence of Pf amongst *Pa* clinical isolates and its contribution to immune evasion and biofilm formation (92, 137), Pf represents an attractive and novel target for immunization against *Pa*.

The ability of antibodies to neutralize bacteriophages has been described and phage neutralizing antibodies have been detected in the sera of several species (151, 194, 195). Studies of sera from patients receiving phage therapy against *Staphylococcus aureus* showed the production of antibodies against the phages in question (196). In a different study, sera collected from healthy individuals contained neutralizing antibodies against naturally occurring bacteriophage (151, 197). On the other hand, other studies did not find evidence of phage targeted antibodies in phage therapy recipients (198). It may be that some phage are more antigenic than others in certain hosts, though the lack of standardized methodologies for these studies may also be a factor underlying these heterogenous results.

Our recent work demonstrated that immunization against Pf provided protection against *Pa* infections in mice. Immunization was performed using a peptide derived from the CoaB coat protein of Pf phage conjugated to the carrier protein keyhole limpet hemocyanin (KLH). Mice vaccinated with this novel formulation were able to clear *Pa* infection challenges more often than unvaccinated mice. Similar rates of clearance were obtained in the setting of passive immunization with monoclonal antibodies developed against the CoaB peptide. Further, anti-CoaB monoclonal antibodies (mAB) were effective in promoting opsonization of *Pa* (137). These data suggest that Pf phage is a potential candidate for a preventative vaccine against *Pa*.

Much work remains to be done before such vaccines could become a realistic possibility. In particular, the effectiveness of this strategy against clinical isolates, it's specificity for *Pa*, and a detailed mechanism of action in regards to how it promotes bacterial clearance will all be necessary. Nonetheless, the prospect of such a vaccine is enticing. It is tempting to consider that this could be administered to individuals diagnosed with CF before they develop chronic *Pa* infections. Similarly, individuals with diabetes could be immunized before they develop their first *Pa* wound infection.

The Relevance of Pf Studies for Lytic Phage Therapy

With the rising prevalence of antibiotic-resistant bacteria, novel approaches to deal with bacterial infections are an urgent need (199). Phage therapy is the application of bacteria-specific viruses to combat uncontrolled and undesired bacteria, such as those associated with infectious disease (200). Phage therapy for *Pa* infections has more than 50 years of history but there is a recent resurgence of interest in this approach (201–203). There are several potential advantages of phage therapy that make it an appealing alternative or adjunct to conventional antibiotics. These include the lytic activity of the phages, auto dosing, low inherent toxicity, minimal disruption of normal flora, narrower potential for inducing resistance, lack of cross-resistance with antibiotics, rapid discovery, formulation and application versatility, and effects on biofilm clearance (204). There nonetheless remain many potential issues that need to be addressed, including demonstrations of safety and efficacy in double-blinded, case controlled clinical trials.

One important potential consideration is the nature of the immunological response induced by phages. As briefly summarized above, there are some suggestions that phage-mediated effects on the inflammatory milieu are generally well-tolerated without major side effects [(119, 137, 151, 155, 161, 205)]. However, this remains to be examined in a rigorous and systematic manner, ideally in the context of parallel evaluations of safety and efficacy. A better understanding of the interactions of phage—host—human interactions will provide valuable insight into predicting the outcome of phage therapy (151).

Data on filamentous, lysogenic phage are of unclear relevance for phage therapy studies. As noted above, diverse phage seem to be have broadly non-inflammatory effects. However, to our knowledge lytic phage have not been reported to be directly immune suppressive in the way that Pf phages are reported to be. Indeed, there are reasons to think that the effects of lytic vs. temperate phage on local immunity may prove to be quite distinct. Not only are the viruses in question different genetically and phenotypically, but lytic phage are likely to be encountered in the context of bacterial detritus from lysed cells whereas Pf phage may not. It is also unclear to what extent different phage are taken up intracellularly or trigger viral PRRs. Clearly the comparative effects of different phage is an important question for future research. In the meantime, in the absence of evidence, we favor a cautious approach to extrapolating results from work on Pf phages to other phages.

Pf Phages in the Context of the Larger Lung Phageome

The virome is increasingly recognized as an integral part of the human microbiome, interacting with other members of the microbial community to shape host phenotypes (206). Bacteriophages make up a majority of this virome (207), but their impact on the larger microbial community within the lung and on lung health remain understudied. New sequencing methods have made metagenomics a more affordable and reliable approach to doing so (208) but substantial technical barriers remain (209, 210).

The lung phageome may be distinct in different disease states. One study suggested that in healthy individuals, the composition of the sputum phageome is highly heterogenous and may reflect organisms in inhaled air or oral flora. In contrast, the sputum phageome of in CF individuals was highly similar (211, 212). Given recent findings regarding microbial heterogeneity within different lung regions of CF patients (213), it may be important to revisit the question of the lung phageome with more in depth sampling regimens. Nonetheless, this common footprint is remarkable. It may be that selective bacterial growth conditions lead to common, relatively stable microbial community compositions over time (212, 214) with metabolic activities that reflect host characteristics (211, 214, 215). Supporting this idea, Willner et al. found that the viral community in the lungs of a CF patient's non-CF spouse shared taxonomy with the CF virome but had the metabolic profile of a non-CF virome (211).

The contributions of Pf phages to the overall lung microbiome are undefined but potentially substantial. The impact of Pf phages on biofilm formation, antibiotic sequestration, virulence factors, and modulation of immunity described above are likely to influence not only *Pa* phenotypes but also the overall ecology of the lung.

Pf phages can also affect the flow of resources within the biofilm. We reported that Pf phages impact the growth of fungal organisms, specifically Aspergillus and Candida. As noted above, Pf phages bind to free iron through charge-based interactions, much in the same way that they sequester antibiotics, and this deprives fungi of this critical resource (216, 217). We also reported that Pf phages change the material properties of biofilms, making them far more viscous (101). In addition to increasing the tenacity and thickness of CF sputum, this is also likely to impact the movement and distribution of microbes within the biofilm. It seems probable that we are only scratching the surface of the ways in which Pf phages may influence microbial ecology.

Future studies of the lung microbiome in Pf(+) and Pf(−) subjects are likely to be highly informative. The integrated, simultaneous study of both bacterial and phage communities, including prophages and their induction (218) will be important.

CONCLUDING REMARKS AND AREAS FOR FUTURE INVESTIGATION

Several themes emerge from this review. The relationship between Pf phages and *Pa* appears to be highly evolved and is clearly an important factor in *Pa* fitness. Despite the substantial energetic cost of producing so many phage particles, Pf phages are nonetheless common among *Pa* strains in multiple contexts, including in the CF lung.

Pf phage also contribute to *Pa* pathogenesis in multiple models, tissues, and human disease contexts. In the context of CF lung infections, Pf phages contribute to the impaired bacterial clearance and heightened inflammation that are characteristic of the disease. It seems likely that Pf contributions to antibiotic tolerance are a major driver in this setting. However, Pf effects on biofilm formation, antibiotic tolerance, microbial ecology, and immune modulation may be important as well.

It may be possible to exploit this biology for therapeutic gain. The anti-Pf vaccine discussed here is the clearest example of this. However, other applications are also possible. For example, the presence of Pf phages may also have potential to inform antibiotic treatment regimens. Manipulating the relationships between bacterial pathogens and their phages may also be an exciting therapeutic frontier.

Much about Pf phage biology remains unknown. While Pf phages are relatively well-characterized compared to most other phages, much remains unknown about their biology. In particular, the function of many Pf phage genes, the factors that govern Pf production, and the impact of Pf phages on *Pa* virulence factors are all promising areas of study that are likely to play important roles in *Pa* pathogenesis.

While the molecular details of the Pf lifecycle are reasonably well-defined, many questions remain regarding how the Pf lifecycle intersects with the functioning of their bacterial host. One obvious gap in our knowledge is the function of the uncharacterized genes in the core Pf genome. Another understudied aspect of Pf biology is their ability to bind not only cationic antimicrobials, but also multivalent cations like iron (75, 216, 217). Iron is a limiting nutrient at infection sites and the ability of Pf phages to bind and sequester this essential nutrient may have important implications in infection pathogenesis. Lastly, the ability of these filamentous phages to assemble liquid crystals in the extracellular environment likely has implications for the host-pathogen interactions.

The evolutionary origins of phage/mammalian host interactions are unclear. Recent work revealed that the (cGAS)-STING pathway, an innate antiviral defense mechanism in animals, has evolutionary roots with bacterial anti-phage defense mechanisms (219). Thus, phages may be triggering ancient highly conserved immune responses in animal cells. It seems unlikely that Pf phage evolved to manipulate mammalian immunity, given that mammals are not a natural host for *Pa*. Instead, it may be that these effects of Pf on animal immune systems enable *Pa* to likewise avoid predation by phagocytic predators, such as amoeba in the environment. Similar effects on amoeba predation have been hypothesized for other *Pa* factors that impact mammalian phagocytosis, including exotoxins, alginate secretion, and the regulation of motility (136).

The relationship between Pf and *Pa* may also be dynamic and in flux. Bacteria-phage relationships can evolve from parasitic interactions to mutualistic relationships over time with the most extreme examples giving rise to new bacterial functions. Examples include the type VI secretion system (220) and pyocins (221) of *Pa*. The Pf prophage may likewise eventually evolve from an independent virus into a bacterial operon encoding a filamentous structural element of the extracellular biofilm matrix that also has immunomodulatory properties.

Many outstanding questions remain to be addressed in regards to the impact of phage on mammalian immunity. Inoviruses like Pf are widespread amongst bacteria (54) and it is unclear whether the immune effects outlined here for Pf are present in association with other filamentous phage. There are some hints that this may be the case. M13 filamentous phages produced by *E. coli* can be internalized *in vivo* (222) and *in vitro* (223). As mentioned above, a filamentous phage (MDAφ) produced by *N. meningitidis* may likewise increase host-cell colonization, bacterial aggregation, and virulence (113). Given the extensive heterogeneity between and even within Inoviruses (54), it seems likely that here again further investigation will reveal substantial differences.

Relatively little is known about adaptive immune responses to Pf and other phages. Most studies suggest that humoral immunity (antibodies) against phage exists and is rapidly induced upon exposure to phage (194, 196, 197, 224, 225); the impact of these on phage therapy is an active area of investigation and may be particularly important for phage therapy (226).

In summary, Pf phages are an exciting frontier in microbiology, immunology, and human health. Further investigations are likely to yield additional insights into both *Pa* pathogenesis as well as novel therapeutic and prophylactic treatments.

AUTHOR CONTRIBUTIONS

PS, EB, MK, LJ, VR-C, MP, JV, NH, CC, LM, CV, QC, JP, TW, CM, and PB all contributed to the writing, graphics, and editing of this work.

FUNDING

PS was supported by NIH grants R01AI138981 and K22AI125282. PS and TW were supported by NIH grant P20GM103546. JV and CV were supported by grant T32 AI007502-22. PB was supported by grants R21AI133370, R21AI133240, R01AI12492093, grants from Stanford SPARK, the Falk Medical Research Trust, and the Cystic Fibrosis Foundation (CFF). MP was supported by a NSFGRF grant. EB was supported by grant T32 HL129970 and the Stanford Maternal Child Health Research Institute. CM was supported by grant R01 HL148184 and Ross Mosier CF Laboratories Research Fund.

REFERENCES

1. Casemore DP. Foodborne protozoal infection. *Lancet*. (1990) 336:1427–32. doi: 10.1016/0140-6736(90)93115-6
2. Lipsky BA, Berendt AR, Deery HG, Embil JM, Joseph WS, Karchmer AW, et al. Diagnosis and treatment of diabetic foot infections. *Clin Infect Dis*. (2004) 39:885–910. doi: 10.1086/424846
3. Tredget EE, Shankowsky HA, Rennie R, Burrell RE, Logsetty S. Pseudomonas infections in the thermally injured patient. *Burns*. (2004) 30:3–26. doi: 10.1016/j.burns.2003.08.007
4. Gardner SE, Frantz RA. Wound bioburden and infection-related complications in diabetic foot ulcers. *Biol Res Nurs*. (2008) 10:44–53. doi: 10.1177/1099800408319056
5. Jarbrink K, Ni G, Sonnergren H, Schmidtchen A, Pang C, Bajpai R, et al. Prevalence and incidence of chronic wounds and related complications: a protocol for a systematic review. *Syst Rev*. (2016) 5:152. doi: 10.1186/s13643-016-0329-y
6. Morales E, Cots F, Sala M, Comas M, Belvis F, Riu M, et al. Hospital costs of nosocomial multi-drug resistant *Pseudomonas aeruginosa* acquisition. *BMC Health Serv Res*. (2012) 12:122. doi: 10.1186/1472-6963-12-122
7. Sansgiry SS, Joish VN, Boklage S, Goyal RK, Chopra P, Sethi S. Economic burden of *Pseudomonas aeruginosa* infection in patients with cystic fibrosis. *J Med Econ*. (2012) 15:219–24. doi: 10.3111/13696998.2011.638954
8. Blanchette CM, Noone JM, Stone G, Zacherle E, Patel RP, Howden R, et al. Healthcare cost and utilization before and after diagnosis of *Pseudomonas aeruginosa* among patients with non-cystic fibrosis bronchiectasis in the U.S. *Med Sci*. (2017)5:20. doi: 10.3390/medsci50 40020
9. Tacconelli E, Carrara E, Savoldi A, Harbarth S, Mendelson M, Monnet DL, et al. Discovery, research, and development of new antibiotics: the WHO priority list of antibiotic-resistant bacteria and tuberculosis. *Lancet Infect Dis*. (2018) 18:318–27. doi: 10.1016/S1473-3099(17)30753-3
10. Folkesson A, Jelsbak L, Yang L, Johansen HK, Ciofu O, Hoiby N, et al. Adaptation of *Pseudomonas aeruginosa* to the cystic fibrosis airway: an evolutionary perspective. *Nat Rev Microbiol*. (2012) 10:841–51. doi: 10.1038/nrmicro2907
11. Malhotra S, Hayes D Jr, Wozniak DJ. Cystic Fibrosis and *Pseudomonas aeruginosa*: the Host-Microbe Interface. *Clin Microbiol Rev*. (2019) 32:e00138-18. doi: 10.1128/CMR.00138-18
12. Costerton JW, Stewart PS, Greenberg EP. Bacterial biofilms: a common cause of persistent infections. *Science*. (1999) 284:1318–22. doi: 10.1126/science.284.5418.1318
13. Jesaitis AJ, Franklin MJ, Berglund D, Sasaki M, Lord CI, Bleazard JB, et al. Compromised host defense on *Pseudomonas aeruginosa* biofilms: characterization of neutrophil and biofilm interactions. *J Immunol*. (2003) 171:4329–39. doi: 10.4049/jimmunol.171.8.4329
14. Moreau-Marquis S, Stanton BA, O'Toole GA. *Pseudomonas aeruginosa* biofilm formation in the cystic fibrosis airway. *Pulm Pharmacol Ther*. (2008) 21:595–9. doi: 10.1016/j.pupt.2007.12.001
15. Hirsch EB, Tam VH. Impact of multidrug-resistant *Pseudomonas aeruginosa* infection on patient outcomes. *Expert Rev Pharmacoecon Outcomes Res*. (2010) 10:441–51. doi: 10.1586/erp.10.49
16. Hoiby N, Ciofu O, Bjarnsholt T. *Pseudomonas aeruginosa* biofilms in cystic fibrosis. *Future Microbiol*. (2010) 5:1663–74. doi: 10.2217/fmb.10.125
17. Zhao G, Hochwalt PC, Usui ML, Underwood RA, Singh PK, James GA, et al. Delayed wound healing in diabetic (db/db) mice with *Pseudomonas aeruginosa* biofilm challenge: a model for the study of chronic wounds. *Wound Repair Regen*. (2010) 18:467–77. doi: 10.1111/j.1524-475X.2010.00608.x
18. Percival SL, Suleman L, Vuotto C, and Donelli, G. Healthcare-associated infections, medical devices and biofilms: risk, tolerance and control. *J Med Microbiol*. (2015) 64(Pt 4):323–34. doi: 10.1099/jmm.0.000032
19. Ishida H, Ishida Y, Kurosaka Y, Otani T, Sato K, Kobayashi H. *In vitro* and *in vivo* activities of levofloxacin against biofilm-producing *Pseudomonas aeruginosa*. *Antimicrob Agents Chemother*. (1998) 42:1641–5. doi: 10.1128/AAC.42.7.1641
20. Hoiby N, Bjarnsholt T, Givskov M, Molin S, Ciofu O. Antibiotic resistance of bacterial biofilms. *Int J Antimicrob Agents*. (2010) 35:322–32. doi: 10.1016/j.ijantimicag.2009.12.011
21. Bjarnsholt T. The role of bacterial biofilms in chronic infections. *APMIS Suppl*. (2013). (136):1–51. doi: 10.1111/apm.12099
22. Ciofu O, Bagge N, Hoiby N. Antibodies against beta-lactamase can improve ceftazidime treatment of lung infection with beta-lactam-resistant *Pseudomonas aeruginosa* in a rat model of chronic lung infection. *APMIS*. (2002) 110:881–91. doi: 10.1034/j.1600-0463.2002.1101207.x
23. Parsek MR, Singh PK. Bacterial biofilms: an emerging link to disease pathogenesis. *Annu Rev Microbiol*. (2003) 57:677–701. doi: 10.1146/annurev.micro.57.030502.090720
24. Chiang WC, Nilsson M, Jensen PO, Hoiby N, Nielsen TE, Givskov M, et al. Extracellular DNA shields against aminoglycosides in *Pseudomonas aeruginosa* biofilms. *Antimicrob Agents Chemother*. (2013) 57:2352–61. doi: 10.1128/AAC.00001-13
25. Meers P, Neville M, Malinin V, Scotto AW, Sardaryan G, Kurumunda R, et al. Biofilm penetration, triggered release and *in vivo* activity of inhaled liposomal amikacin in chronic *Pseudomonas aeruginosa* lung infections. *J Antimicrob Chemother*. (2008) 61:859–68. doi: 10.1093/jac/dkn059
26. Drenkard E, Ausubel FM. Pseudomonas biofilm formation and antibiotic resistance are linked to phenotypic variation. *Nature*. (2002) 416:740–3. doi: 10.1038/416740a
27. Levin-Reisman I, Ronin I, Gefen O, Braniss I, Shoresh N, Balaban NQ. Antibiotic tolerance facilitates the evolution of resistance. *Science*. (2017) 355:826–30. doi: 10.1126/science.aaj2191
28. Obritsch MD, Fish DN, MacLaren R, Jung R. Nosocomial infections due to multidrug-resistant *Pseudomonas aeruginosa*: epidemiology and treatment options. *Pharmacotherapy*. (2005) 25:1353–64. doi: 10.1592/phco.2005.25.10.1353
29. Lister PD, Wolter DJ, Hanson ND. Antibacterial-resistant *Pseudomonas aeruginosa*: clinical impact and complex regulation of chromosomally encoded resistance mechanisms. *Clin Microbiol Rev*. (2009) 22:582–610. doi: 10.1128/CMR.00040-09
30. Chmiel JF, Aksamit TR, Chotirmall SH, Dasenbrook EC, Elborn JS, LiPuma JJ, et al. Antibiotic management of lung infections in cystic fibrosis. I The microbiome, methicillin-resistant *Staphylococcus aureus*, gram-negative bacteria, and multiple infections. *Ann Am Thorac Soc*. (2014) 11:1120–9. doi: 10.1513/AnnalsATS.201402-050AS
31. Bassetti M, Vena A, Croxatto A, Righi E, Guery B. How to manage *Pseudomonas aeruginosa* infections. *Drugs Context*. (2018) 7:212527. doi: 10.7573/dic.212527
32. Grassi L, Di Luca M, Maisetta G, Rinaldi AC, Esin S, Trampuz A, et al. Generation of persister cells of *Pseudomonas aeruginosa* and *Staphylococcus aureus* by chemical treatment and evaluation of their susceptibility to membrane-targeting agents. *Front Microbiol*. (2017) 8:1917. doi: 10.3389/fmicb.2017.01917
33. Buret A, Cripps AW. The immunoevasive activities of *Pseudomonas aeruginosa*. Relevance for cystic fibrosis. *Am Rev Respir Dis*. (1993) 148:793–805. doi: 10.1164/ajrccm/148.3.793
34. Leid JG, Willson CJ, Shirtliff ME, Hassett DJ, Parsek MR, Jeffers AK. The exopolysaccharide alginate protects *Pseudomonas aeruginosa* biofilm bacteria from IFN-gamma-mediated macrophage killing. *J Immunol*. (2005) 175:7512–8. doi: 10.4049/jimmunol.175.11.7512
35. Morris MR, Doull IJ, Dewitt S, Hallett MB. Reduced iC3b-mediated phagocytotic capacity of pulmonary neutrophils in cystic fibrosis. *Clin Exp Immunol*. (2005) 142:68–75. doi: 10.1111/j.1365-2249.2005.02893.x
36. Anderson GG, O'Toole GA. Innate and induced resistance mechanisms of bacterial biofilms. *Curr Top Microbiol Immunol*. (2008) 322:85–105. doi: 10.1007/978-3-540-75418-3_5
37. Mishra M, Byrd MS, Sergeant S, Azad AK, Parsek MR, McPhail L, et al. *Pseudomonas aeruginosa* Psl polysaccharide reduces neutrophil phagocytosis and the oxidative response by limiting complement-mediated opsonization. *Cell Microbiol*. (2012) 14:95–106. doi 10.1111/j.1462-5822.2011.01704.x
38. Alhede M, Bjarnsholt T, Givskov M, Alhede M. *Pseudomonas aeruginosa* biofilms: mechanisms of immune evasion. *Adv Appl Microbiol*. (2014) 86:1–40. doi: 10.1016/B978-0-12-800262-9.00001-9

39. Vishwanath S, Ramphal R, Guay CM, DesJardins D, Pier GB. Respiratory-mucin inhibition of the opsonophagocytic killing of *Pseudomonas aeruginosa*. *Infect Immun.* (1988) 56:2218–22. doi: 10.1128/IAI.56.9.2218-2222.1988
40. Hansch GM, Brenner-Weiss G, Prior B, Wagner C, Obst U. The extracellular polymer substance of *Pseudomonas aeruginosa*: too slippery for neutrophils to migrate on? *Int J Artif Organs.* (2008) 31:796–803. doi: 10.1177/039139880803100907
41. Boucher JC, Yu H, Mudd MH, Deretic V. Mucoid *Pseudomonas aeruginosa* in cystic fibrosis: characterization of muc mutations in clinical isolates and analysis of clearance in a mouse model of respiratory infection. *Infect Immun.* (1997) 65:3838–46. doi: 10.1128/IAI.65.9.3838-3846.1997
42. Young RL, Malcolm KC, Kret JE, Caceres SM, Poch KR, Nichols DP, et al. Neutrophil extracellular trap (NET)-mediated killing of *Pseudomonas aeruginosa*: evidence of acquired resistance within the CF airway, independent of CFTR. *PLoS ONE.* (2011) 6:e23637. doi: 10.1371/journal.pone.0023637
43. Shan Q, Dwyer M, Rahman S, Gadjeva M. Distinct susceptibilities of corneal *Pseudomonas aeruginosa* clinical isolates to neutrophil extracellular trap-mediated immunity. *Infect Immun.* (2014) 82:4135–43. doi: 10.1128/IAI.02169-14
44. Yoo DG, Winn M, Pang L, Moskowitz SM, Malech HL, Leto TL, et al. Release of cystic fibrosis airway inflammatory markers from *Pseudomonas aeruginosa*-stimulated human neutrophils involves NADPH oxidase-dependent extracellular DNA trap formation. *J Immunol.* (2014) 192:4728–38. doi: 10.4049/jimmunol.1301589
45. Brinkmann V, Zychlinsky A. Neutrophil extracellular traps: is immunity the second function of chromatin? *J Cell Biol.* (2012) 198:773–83. doi: 10.1083/jcb.201203170
46. Baums CG, von Kockritz-Blickwede M. Novel role of DNA in neutrophil extracellular traps. *Trends Microbiol.* (2015) 23:330–1. doi: 10.1016/j.tim.2015.04.003
47. Bonfield TL, Panuska JR, Konstan MW, Hilliard KA, Hilliard JB, Ghnaim H, et al. Inflammatory cytokines in cystic fibrosis lungs. *Am J Respir Crit Care Med.* (1995) 152(6 Pt 1):2111–8. doi: 10.1164/ajrccm.152.6.85 20783
48. Hartl D, Latzin P, Hordijk P, Marcos V, Rudolph C, Woischnik M, et al. Cleavage of CXCR1 on neutrophils disables bacterial killing in cystic fibrosis lung disease. *Nat Med.* (2007) 13:1423–30. doi: 10.1038/nm1690
49. Mayer-Hamblett N, Aitken ML, Accurso FJ, Kronmal RA, Konstan MW, Burns JL, et al. Association between pulmonary function and sputum biomarkers in cystic fibrosis. *Am J Respir Crit Care Med.* (2007) 175:822–8. doi: 10.1164/rccm.200609-1354OC
50. Elizur A, Cannon CL, Ferkol TW. Airway inflammation in cystic fibrosis. *Chest.* (2008) 133:489–95. doi: 10.1378/chest.07-1631
51. Ulrich M, Worlitzsch D, Viglio S, Siegmann N, Iadarola P, Shute JK, et al. Alveolar inflammation in cystic fibrosis. *J Cyst Fibros.* (2010) 9:217–27. doi: 10.1016/j.jcf.2010.03.001
52. Sagel SD, Wagner BD, Anthony MM, Emmett P, Zemanick ET. Sputum biomarkers of inflammation and lung function decline in children with cystic fibrosis. *Am J Respir Crit Care Med.* (2012) 186:857–65. doi: 10.1164/rccm.201203-0507OC
53. Salmond GP, Fineran PC. A century of the phage: past, present and future. *Nat Rev Microbiol.* (2015) 13:777–86. doi: 10.1038/nrmicro3564
54. Roux S, Krupovic M, Daly RA, Borges AL, Nayfach S, Schulz F, et al. Cryptic inoviruses revealed as pervasive in bacteria and archaea across Earth's biomes. *Nat Microbiol.* (2019) 4:1895–906. doi: 10.1038/s41564-019-0510-x
55. Rakonjac J, Bennett NJ, Spagnuolo J, Gagic D, Russel M. Filamentous bacteriophage: biology, phage display and nanotechnology applications. *Curr Issues Mol Biol.* (2011) 13:51–76.
56. Mimmi S, Maisano D, Quinto I, Iaccino E. Phage display: an overview in context to drug discovery. *Trends Pharmacol Sci.* (2019) 40:87–91. doi: 10.1016/j.tips.2018.12.005
57. Ju Z, Sun W. Drug delivery vectors based on filamentous bacteriophages and phage-mimetic nanoparticles. *Drug Deliv.* (2017) 24:1898–908. doi: 10.1080/10717544.2017.1410259
58. Raoult D, Perrin G, Hechemy KE, Vestris G, San-Kale M. [Meningitis from Lyme disease, diagnosed in Marseilles]. *Presse Med.* (1985) 14:1615.
59. Colovic R, Jankovic R, Popovic M, Krivokapic Z. [Desmoid tumors]. *Srp Arh Celok Lek.* (1987) 115:605–8.
60. Rao S, Coleman PS. Control of DNA replication and cell growth by inhibiting the export of mitochondrially derived citrate. *Exp Cell Res.* (1989) 180:341–52. doi: 10.1016/0014-4827(89)90062-1
61. Nambudripad R, Stark W, Opella SJ, Makowski L. Membrane-mediated assembly of filamentous bacteriophage Pf1 coat protein. *Science.* (1991) 252:1305–8. doi: 10.1126/science.1925543
62. Welsh LC, Symmons MF, Marvin DA. The molecular structure and structural transition of the alpha-helical capsid in filamentous bacteriophage Pf1. *Acta Crystallogr D Biol Crystallogr.* (2000) 56(Pt 2):137–50. doi: 10.1107/S0907444999015334
63. Tsuboi M, Kubo Y, Ikeda T, Overman SA, Osman O, Thomas GJJr. Protein and DNA residue orientations in the filamentous virus Pf1 determined by polarized Raman and polarized FTIR spectroscopy. *Biochemistry.* (2003) 42:940–50. doi: 10.1021/bi020566v
64. Thiriot DS, Nevzorov AA, Zagyanskiy L, Wu CH, Opella SJ. Structure of the coat protein in Pf1 bacteriophage determined by solid-state NMR spectroscopy. *J Mol Biol.* (2004) 341:869–79. doi: 10.1016/j.jmb.2004.06.038
65. Goldbourt A, Gross BJ, Day LA, McDermott AE. Filamentous phage studied by magic-angle spinning NMR: resonance assignment and secondary structure of the coat protein in Pf1. *J Am Chem Soc.* (2007) 129:2338–44. doi: 10.1021/ja066928u
66. Park SH, Marassi FM, Black D, Opella SJ. Structure and dynamics of the membrane-bound form of Pf1 coat protein: implications of structural rearrangement for virus assembly. *Biophys J.* (2010) 99:1465–74. doi: 10.1016/j.bpj.2010.06.009
67. Straus SK, Scott WR, Schwieters CD, Marvin DA. Consensus structure of Pf1 filamentous bacteriophage from X-ray fibre diffraction and solid-state NMR. *Eur Biophys J.* (2011) 40:221–34. doi: 10.1007/s00249-010-0640-9
68. Clinical toxicology II. Clinical toxicology II. Strategies for clinical laboratory management: horizontal and vertical integration in hospital laboratories. *Clin Lab Med.* (1990) 10:441–641.
69. Lorieau JL, Day LA, McDermott AE. Conformational dynamics of an intact virus: order parameters for the coat protein of Pf1 bacteriophage. *Proc Natl Acad Sci USA.* (2008) 105:10366–71. doi: 10.1073/pnas.0800405105
70. Virus Taxonomy. Ninth report of the international committee on taxonomy of viruses. In: King AMQ, Adams MJ, Carstens EB, Lefkowitz EJ, editors. *Virus Taxonomy.* San Diego, CA: Elsevier (2012). p. 1281–325.
71. Marvin DA, Symmons MF, Straus SK. Structure and assembly of filamentous bacteriophages. *Prog Biophys Mol Biol.* (2014) 114:80–122. doi: 10.1016/j.pbiomolbio.2014.02.003
72. Hay ID, Lithgow T. Filamentous phages: masters of a microbial sharing economy. *EMBO Rep.* (2019) 20:1–24. doi: 10.15252/embr.201847427
73. Day LA, Marzec CJ, Reisberg SA, Casadevall A. DNA packing in filamentous bacteriophages. *Annu Rev Biophys Biophys Chem.* (1988) 17:509–39. doi: 10.1146/annurev.bb.17.060188.002453
74. Liu DJ, Day LA. Pf1 virus structure: helical coat protein and DNA with paraxial phosphates. *Science.* (1994) 265:671–4. doi: 10.1126/science.8036516
75. Janmey PA, Slochower DR, Wang YH, Wen Q, Cebers A. Polyelectrolyte properties of filamentous biopolymers and their consequences in biological fluids. *Soft Matter.* (2014) 10:1439–49. doi: 10.1039/c3sm50854d
76. Dogic Z, Fraden S. Ordered phases of filamentous viruses. *Curr Opin Colloid Interface Sci.* (2006) 11:47–55. doi: 10.1016/j.cocis.2005.10.004
77. Dogic Z. Filamentous phages as a model system in soft matter physics. *Front Microbiol.* (2016) 7:1013. doi: 10.3389/fmicb.2016.01013
78. Zweckstetter M, Bax A. Characterization of molecular alignment in aqueous suspensions of Pf1 bacteriophage. *J Biomol NMR.* (2001) 20:365–77. doi: 10.1023/A:1011263920003
79. Tomar S, Green MM, Day LA. DNA-protein interactions as the source of large-length-scale chirality evident in the liquid crystal behavior of filamentous bacteriophages. *J Am Chem Soc.* (2007) 129:3367–75. doi: 10.1021/ja068498d
80. Knezevic P, Voet M, Lavigne R. Prevalence of Pf1-like (pro)phage genetic elements among *Pseudomonas aeruginosa* isolates. *Virology.* (2015) 483:64–71. doi: 10.1016/j.virol.2015.04.008
81. Cumby N, Davidson AR, Maxwell KL. The moron comes of age. *Bacteriophage.* (2012) 2:225–8. doi: 10.4161/bact.23146

82. Tsao YF, Taylor VL, Kala S, Bondy-Denomy J, Khan AN, Bona D, et al. Phage morons play an important role in *Pseudomonas aeruginosa* phenotypes. *J Bacteriol.* (2018) 200:e00189-18. doi: 10.1128/JB.00189-18
83. Castang S, Dove SL. Basis for the essentiality of H-NS family members in *Pseudomonas aeruginosa. J Bacteriol.* (2012) 194:5101–9. doi: 10.1128/JB.00932-12
84. Li Y, Liu X, Tang K, Wang P, Zeng Z, Guo Y, et al. Excisionase in Pf filamentous prophage controls lysis-lysogeny decision-making in *Pseudomonas aeruginosa. Mol Microbiol.* (2019) 111:495–513. doi: 10.1111/mmi.14170
85. Lee Y, Song S, Sheng L, Zhu L, Kim JS, Wood TK. Substrate binding protein DppA1 of ABC transporter DppBCDF increases biofilm formation in *Pseudomonas aeruginosa* by inhibiting Pf5 prophage lysis. *Front Microbiol.* (2018) 9:30. doi: 10.3389/fmicb.2018.00030
86. Wei Q, Minh PN, Dotsch A, Hildebrand F, Panmanee W, Elfarash A, et al. Global regulation of gene expression by OxyR in an important human opportunistic pathogen. *Nucleic Acids Res.* (2012) 40:4320–33. doi: 10.1093/nar/gks017
87. Martinez E, Campos-Gomez J. Pf Filamentous phage requires UvrD for replication in *Pseudomonas aeruginosa. mSphere.* (2016) 1:e00104-15. doi: 10.1128/mSphere.00104-15
88. Chen M, Samuelson JC, Jiang F, Muller M, Kuhn A, Dalbey RE. Direct interaction of YidC with the Sec-independent Pf3 coat protein during its membrane protein insertion. *J Biol Chem.* (2002) 277:7670–5. doi: 10.1074/jbc.M110644200
89. McElroy KE, Hui JG, Woo JK, Luk AW, Webb JS, Kjelleberg S, et al. Strain-specific parallel evolution drives short-term diversification during *Pseudomonas aeruginosa* biofilm formation. *Proc Natl Acad Sci USA.* (2014) 111:E1419–27. doi: 10.1073/pnas.1314340111
90. Castang S, McManus HR, Turner KH, Dove SL. H-NS family members function coordinately in an opportunistic pathogen. *Proc Natl Acad Sci USA.* (2008) 105:18947–52. doi: 10.1073/pnas.0808215105
91. Winsor GL, Griffiths EJ, Lo R, Dhillon BK, Shay JA, Brinkman FS. Enhanced annotations and features for comparing thousands of Pseudomonas genomes in the Pseudomonas genome database. *Nucleic Acids Res.* (2016) 44:D646–53. doi: 10.1093/nar/gkv1227
92. Burgener EB, Sweere JM, Bach MS, Secor PR, Haddock N, Jennings LK, et al. Filamentous bacteriophages are associated with chronic Pseudomonas lung infections and antibiotic resistance in cystic fibrosis. *Sci Transl Med.* (2019) 11:eaau9748. doi: 10.1126/scitranslmed.aau9748
93. Katoh K, Kuma K, Miyata T, Toh H. Improvement in the accuracy of multiple sequence alignment program MAFFT. *Genome Inform.* (2005) 16:22–33. doi: 10.1093/nar/gki198
94. Price MN, Dehal PS, Arkin AP. FastTree 2–approximately maximum-likelihood trees for large alignments. *PLoS ONE.* (2010) 5:e9490. doi: 10.1371/journal.pone.0009490
95. Takeya K, Amako K. A rod-shaped Pseudomonas phage. *Virology.* (1966) 28:163–5. doi: 10.1016/0042-6822(66)90317-5
96. Canchaya C, Fournous G, Brussow H. The impact of prophages on bacterial chromosomes. *Mol Microbiol.* (2004) 53:9–18. doi: 10.1111/j.1365-2958.2004.04113.x
97. Klockgether J, Munder A, Neugebauer J, Davenport CF, Stanke F, Larbig KD, et al. Genome diversity of *Pseudomonas aeruginosa* PAO1 laboratory strains. *J Bacteriol.* (2010) 192:1113–21. doi: 10.1128/JB.01515-09
98. Mauch RM, Jensen PO, Moser C, Levy CE, Hoiby N. Mechanisms of humoral immune response against *Pseudomonas aeruginosa* biofilm infection in cystic fibrosis. *J Cyst Fibros.* (2018) 17:143–52. doi: 10.1016/j.jcf.2017.08.012
99. Rice SA, Tan CH, Mikkelsen PJ, Kung V, Woo J, Tay M, et al. The biofilm life cycle and virulence of *Pseudomonas aeruginosa* are dependent on a filamentous prophage. *ISME J.* (2009) 3:271–82. doi: 10.1038/ismej.2008.109
100. Webb JS, Thompson LS, James S, Charlton T, Tolker-Nielsen T, Koch B, et al. Cell death in *Pseudomonas aeruginosa* biofilm development. *J Bacteriol.* (2003) 185:4585–92. doi: 10.1128/JB.185.15.4585-4592.2003
101. Secor PR, Sweere JM, Michaels LA, Malkovskiy AV, Lazzareschi D, Katznelson E, et al. Filamentous bacteriophage promote biofilm assembly and function. *Cell Host Microbe.* (2015) 18:549–59. doi: 10.1016/j.chom.2015.10.013
102. Mooij MJ, Drenkard E, Llamas MA, Vandenbroucke-Grauls CM, Savelkoul PH, Ausubel FM, et al. Characterization of the integrated filamentous phage Pf5 and its involvement in small-colony formation. *Microbiology.* (2007) 153(Pt 6):1790–8. doi: 10.1099/mic.0.2006/003533-0
103. Folsom JP, Richards L, Pitts B, Roe F, Ehrlich GD, Parker A, et al. Physiology of *Pseudomonas aeruginosa* in biofilms as revealed by transcriptome analysis. *BMC Microbiol.* (2010) 10:294. doi: 10.1186/1471-2180-10-294
104. Whiteley M, Bangera MG, Bumgarner RE, Parsek MR, Teitzel GM, Lory S, et al. Gene expression in *Pseudomonas aeruginosa* biofilms. *Nature.* (2001) 413:860–4. doi: 10.1038/35101627
105. Yeung AT, Torfs EC, Jamshidi F, Bains M, Wiegand I, Hancock RE, et al. Swarming of *Pseudomonas aeruginosa* is controlled by a broad spectrum of transcriptional regulators, including MetR. *J Bacteriol.* (2009) 191:5592–602. doi: 10.1128/JB.00157-09
106. Platt MD, Schurr MJ, Sauer K, Vazquez G, Kukavica-Ibrulj I, Potvin E, et al. Proteomic, microarray, and signature-tagged mutagenesis analyses of anaerobic *Pseudomonas aeruginosa* at pH 6.5, likely representing chronic, late-stage cystic fibrosis airway conditions. *J Bacteriol.* (2008) 190:2739–58. doi: 10.1128/JB.01683-07
107. Stoodley P, Sauer K, Davies DG, Costerton JW. Biofilms as complex differentiated communities. *Annu Rev Microbiol.* (2002) 56:187–209. doi: 10.1146/annurev.micro.56.012302.160705
108. Whitchurch CB, Tolker-Nielsen T, Ragas PC, Mattick JS. Extracellular DNA required for bacterial biofilm formation. *Science.* (2002) 295:1487. doi: 10.1126/science.295.5559.1487
109. Rice AR, Hamilton MA, Camper AK. Movement, replication, and emigration rates of individual bacteria in a biofilm. *Microb Ecol.* (2003) 45:163–72. doi: 10.1007/s00248-002-1028-x
110. Webb JS, Lau M, Kjelleberg S. Bacteriophage and phenotypic variation in *Pseudomonas aeruginosa* biofilm development. *J Bacteriol.* (2004) 186:8066–73. doi: 10.1128/JB.186.23.8066-8073 2004
111. Petrova OE, Schurr JR, Schurr MJ, Sauer K. The novel *Pseudomonas aeruginosa* two-component regulator BfmR controls bacteriophage-mediated lysis and DNA release during biofilm development through PhdA. *Mol Microbiol.* (2011) 81:767–83. doi 10.1111/j.1365-2958.2011.07733.x
112. Secor PR, Michaels LA, Smigiel KS, Rohani MG, Jennings LK, Hisert KB, et al. Filamentous bacteriophage produced by *Pseudomonas aeruginosa* alters the inflammatory response and promotes noninvasive infection *in vivo*. *Infect Immun.* (2017) 85:IAI.00648-16. doi: 10.1128/IAI.00648-16
113. Bille E, Meyer J, Jamet A, Euphrasie D, Barnier JP, Brissac T, et al. A virulence-associated filamentous bacteriophage of Neisseria meningitidis increases host-cell colonisation. *PLoS Pathog.* (2017) 13:e1006495. doi: 10.1371/journal.ppat.1006495
114. Secor PR, Jennings LK, Michaels LA, Sweere JM, Singh PK, Parks WC, et al. Biofilm assembly becomes crystal clear - filamentous bacteriophage organize the *Pseudomonas aeruginosa* biofilm matrix into a liquid crystal. *Microb Cell.* (2015) 3:49–52. doi: 10.15698/mic2016.01.475
115. El Haddad L, Harb CP, Gebara MA, Stibich MA, Chemaly RF. A systematic and critical review of bacteriophage therapy against multidrug-resistant ESKAPE organisms in humans. *Clin Infect Dis.* (2019) 69:167–78. doi: 10.1093/cid/ciy947
116. Gordillo Altamirano FL, Barr JJ. Phage therapy in the postantibiotic era. *Clin Microbiol Rev.* (2019) 32:e00066-18. doi: 10.1128/CMR.00066-18
117. Manrique P, Bolduc B, Walk ST, van der Oost J, de Vos WM, Young MJ. Healthy human gut phageome. *Proc Natl Acad Sci USA.* (2016) 113:10400–5. doi: 10.1073/pnas.1601060113
118. Bollyky PL, Secor PR. The Innate Sense of Bacteriophages. *Cell Host Microbe.* (2019) 25:177–9. doi: 10.1016/j.chom.2019.01.020
119. Gogokhia L, Buhrke K, Bell R, Hoffman B, Brown DG, Hanke-Gogokhia C, et al. Expansion of bacteriophages is linked to aggravated intestinal inflammation and colitis. *Cell Host Microbe.* (2019) 25:285–99.e288. doi: 10.1016/j.chom.2019.01.008
120. Hraiech S, Bregeon F, Rolain JM. Bacteriophage-based therapy in cystic fibrosis-associated *Pseudomonas aeruginosa* infections: rationale and current status. *Drug Des Devel Ther.* (2015) 9:3653–63. doi: 10.2147/DDDT.S53123
121. Waters EM, Neill DR, Kaman B, Sahota JS, Clokie MRJ, Winstanley C, et al. Phage therapy is highly effective against chronic lung

infections with *Pseudomonas aeruginosa*. *Thorax*. (2017) 72:666–7. doi: 10.1136/thoraxjnl-2016-209265

122. Hashimoto S, Pittet JF, Hong K, Folkesson H, Bagby G, Kobzik L, et al. Depletion of alveolar macrophages decreases neutrophil chemotaxis to Pseudomonas airspace infections. *Am J Physiol*. (1996) 270(5 Pt 1):L819–28. doi: 10.1152/ajplung.1996.270.5.L819
123. Allen L, Dockrell DH, Pattery T, Lee DG, Cornelis P, Hellewell PG, et al. Pyocyanin production by *Pseudomonas aeruginosa* induces neutrophil apoptosis and impairs neutrophil-mediated host defenses *in vivo*. *J Immunol*. (2005) 174:3643–9. doi: 10.4049/jimmunol.174.6.3643
124. Alhede M, Bjarnsholt T, Jensen PO, Phipps RK, Moser C, Christophersen L, et al. *Pseudomonas aeruginosa* recognizes and responds aggressively to the presence of polymorphonuclear leukocytes. *Microbiology*. (2009) 155(Pt 11):3500–8. doi: 10.1099/mic.0.031443-0
125. Koh AY, Priebe GP, Ray C, Van Rooijen N, Pier GB. Inescapable need for neutrophils as mediators of cellular innate immunity to acute *Pseudomonas aeruginosa* pneumonia. *Infect Immun*. (2009) 77:5300–10. doi: 10.1128/IAI.00501-09
126. Raoust E, Balloy V, Garcia-Verdugo I, Touqui L, Ramphal R, Chignard M. *Pseudomonas aeruginosa* LPS or flagellin are sufficient to activate TLR-dependent signaling in murine alveolar macrophages and airway epithelial cells. *PLoS ONE*. (2009) 4:e7259. doi: 10.1371/journal.pone.0007259
127. Maldonado RF, Sa-Correia I, Valvano MA. Lipopolysaccharide modification in Gram-negative bacteria during chronic infection. *FEMS Microbiol Rev*. (2016) 40:480–93. doi: 10.1093/femsre/fuw007
128. Faure E, Kwong K, Nguyen D. *Pseudomonas aeruginosa* in chronic lung infections: how to adapt within the host? *Front Immunol*. (2018) 9:2416. doi: 10.3389/fimmu.2018.02416
129. Smith EE, Buckley DG, Wu Z, Saenphimmachak C, Hoffman LR, D'Argenio DA, et al. Genetic adaptation by *Pseudomonas aeruginosa* to the airways of cystic fibrosis patients. *Proc Natl Acad Sci USA*. (2006) 103:8487–92. doi: 10.1073/pnas.0602138103
130. Benmohamed F, Medina M, Wu YZ, Maschalidi S, Jouvion G, Guillemot L, et al. Toll-like receptor 9 deficiency protects mice against *Pseudomonas aeruginosa* lung infection. *PLoS ONE*. (2014) 9:e90466. doi: 10.1371/journal.pone.0090466
131. Andrews T, Sullivan KE. Infections in patients with inherited defects in phagocytic function. *Clin Microbiol Rev*. (2003) 16:597–621. doi: 10.1128/CMR.16.4.597-621.2003
132. Kurahashi K, Sawa T, Ota M, Kajikawa O, Hong K, Martin TR, et al. Depletion of phagocytes in the reticuloendothelial system causes increased inflammation and mortality in rabbits with *Pseudomonas aeruginosa* pneumonia. *Am J Physiol Lung Cell Mol Physiol*. (2009) 296:L198–209. doi: 10.1152/ajplung.90472.2008
133. Jensen PO, Givskov M, Bjarnsholt T, Moser C. The immune system vs. *Pseudomonas aeruginosa* biofilms. *FEMS Immunol Med Microbiol*. (2010) 59:292–305. doi: 10.1111/j.1574-695X.2010.00706.x
134. Kunert A, Losse J, Gruszin C, Huhn M, Kaendler K, Mikkat S, et al. Immune evasion of the human pathogen *Pseudomonas aeruginosa*: elongation factor Tuf is a factor H and plasminogen binding protein. *J Immunol*. (2007) 179:2979–88. doi: 10.4049/jimmunol.179.5.2979
135. Amiel E, Lovewell RR, O'Toole GA, Hogan DA, Berwin B. *Pseudomonas aeruginosa* evasion of phagocytosis is mediated by loss of swimming motility and is independent of flagellum expression. *Infect Immun*. (2010) 78:2937–45. doi: 10.1128/IAI.00144-10
136. Lovewell RR, Patankar YR, Berwin B. Mechanisms of phagocytosis and host clearance of *Pseudomonas aeruginosa*. *Am J Physiol Lung Cell Mol Physiol*. (2014) 306:L591–603. doi: 10.1152/ajplung.00335.2013
137. Sweere JM, Van Belleghem JD, Ishak H, Bach MS, Popescu M, Sunkari V, et al. Bacteriophage trigger antiviral immunity and prevent clearance of bacterial infection. *Science*. (2019) 363:eaat9691. doi: 10.1126/science.aat9691
138. Malone JG. Role of small colony variants in persistence of *Pseudomonas aeruginosa* infections in cystic fibrosis lungs. *Infect Drug Resist*. (2015) 8:237–47. doi: 10.2147/IDR.S68214
139. Kondo Y, Imai M. Effect of glutaraldehyde on renal tubular function. II Selective inhibition of Cl- transport in the hamster thin ascending limb of Henle's loop. *Pflugers Arch*. (1987) 408:484–90. doi: 10.1007/BF0058 5073
140. Pier GB, Coleman F, Grout M, Franklin M, Ohman DE. Role of alginate O acetylation in resistance of mucoid *Pseudomonas aeruginosa* to opsonic phagocytosis. *Infect Immun*. (2001) 69:1895–901. doi: 10.1128/IAI.69.3.1895-1901.2001
141. Mulcahy LR, Isabella VM, Lewis K. *Pseudomonas aeruginosa* biofilms in disease. *Microb Ecol*. (2014) 68:1–12. doi: 10.1007/s00248-013-0297-x
142. Secor PR, Michaels LA, Ratjen A, Jennings LK, Singh PK. Entropically driven aggregation of bacteria by host polymers promotes antibiotic tolerance in *Pseudomonas aeruginosa*. *Proc Natl Acad Sci USA*. (2018) 115:10780–5. doi: 10.1073/pnas.1806005115
143. Collins JM, Monty KJ. Cysteine biosynthesis in Salmonella typhimurium: the presence of ATP-sulfurylase and APS-kinase in various cysteine-requiring mutants. *Can J Biochem*. (1975) 53:1118–21. doi: 10.1139/o75-153
144. Lee JH, Del Sorbo L, Khine AA, de Azavedo J, Low DE, Bell D, et al. Modulation of bacterial growth by tumor necrosis factor-alpha *in vitro* and *in vivo*. *Am J Respir Crit Care Med*. (2003) 168:1462–70. doi: 10.1164/rccm.200302-303OC
145. Aronow R, Danon D, Shahar A, Aronson M. Electron microscopy of *in vitro* endocytosis of T2 phage by cells from rabbit peritoneal exudate. *J Exp Med*. (1964) 120:943–54. doi: 10.1084/jem.120.5.943
146. Wenger SL, Turner JH, Petricciani JC. The cytogenetic, proliferative and viability effects of four bacteriophages on human lymphocytes. *In Vitro*. (1978) 14:543–9. doi: 10.1007/BF02616097
147. Nguyen S, Baker K, Padman BS, Patwa R, Dunstan RA, Weston TA, et al. Bacteriophage Transcytosis Provides a Mechanism To Cross Epithelial Cell Layers. *MBio*. (2017) 8:e01874-17. doi: 10.1128/mBio.01874-17
148. Shapouri-Moghaddam A, Mohammadian S, Vazini H, Taghadosi M, Esmaeili SA, Mardani F, et al. Macrophage plasticity, polarization, and function in health and disease. *J Cell Physiol*. (2018) 233:6425–40. doi: 10.1002/jcp.26429
149. Gorski A, Miedzybrodzki R, Borysowski J, Dabrowska K, Wierzbicki P, Ohams M, et al. Phage as a modulator of immune responses: practical implications for phage therapy. *Adv Virus Res*. (2012) 83:41–71. doi: 10.1016/B978-0-12-394438-2.00002-5
150. Krut O, Bekeredjian-Ding I. Contribution of the Immune Response to Phage Therapy. *J Immunol*. (2018) 200:3037–44. doi: 10.4049/jimmunol.1701745
151. Van Belleghem JD, Dabrowska K, Vaneechoutte M, Barr JJ, and Bollyky PL. Interactions between Bacteriophage, Bacteria, and the Mammalian Immune System. *Viruses*. (2018) 11:10. doi: 10.3390/v11010010
152. Tiwari BR, Kim S, Rahman M, Kim J. Antibacterial efficacy of lytic Pseudomonas bacteriophage in normal and neutropenic mice models. *J Microbiol*. (2011) 49:994–9. doi: 10.1007/s12275-011-1512-4
153. Pincus NB, Reckhow JD, Saleem D, Jammeh ML, Datta SK, Myles IA. Strain specific phage Treatment for *Staphylococcus aureus* infection is influenced by host immunity and site of infection. *PLoS ONE*. (2015) 10:e0124280. doi: 10.1371/journal.pone.0124280
154. Leung CYJ, Weitz JS. Modeling the synergistic elimination of bacteria by phage and the innate immune system. *J Theor Biol*. (2017) 429:241–52. doi: 10.1016/j.jtbi.2017.06.037
155. Roach DR, Leung CY, Henry M, Morello E, Singh D, Di Santo JP, et al. Synergy between the host immune system and bacteriophage is essential for successful phage therapy against an acute respiratory pathogen. *Cell Host Microbe*. (2017) 22:38–47.e34. doi: 10.1016/j.chom.2017.06.018
156. Letrado P, Corsini B, Diez-Martinez R, Bustamante N, Yuste JE, Garcia P. Bactericidal synergism between antibiotics and phage endolysin Cpl-711 to kill multidrug-resistant pneumococcus. *Future Microbiol*. (2018) 13:1215–23. doi: 10.2217/fmb-2018-0077
157. Kaur S, Harjai K, Chhibber S. Bacteriophage-aided intracellular killing of engulfed methicillin-resistant *Staphylococcus aureus* (MRSA) by murine macrophages. *Appl Microbiol Biotechnol*. (2014) 98:4653–61. doi: 10.1007/s00253-014-5643-5
158. Jonczyk-Matysiak E, Lusiak-Szelachowska M, Klak M, Bubak B, Miedzybrodzki R, Weber-Dabrowska B, et al. The effect of bacteriophage preparations on intracellular killing of bacteria by phagocytes. *J Immunol Res*. (2015) 2015:482863. doi: 10.1155/2015/482863
159. Lehti TA, Pajunen MI, Skog MS, Finne J. Internalization of a polysialic acid-binding *Escherichia coli* bacteriophage into eukaryotic neuroblastoma cells. *Nat Commun*. (2017) 8:1915. doi: 10.1038/s41467-017-02057-3

160. Weber-Dabrowska B, Zimecki M, Mulczyk M. Effective phage therapy is associated with normalization of cytokine production by blood cell cultures. *Arch Immunol Ther Exp. (Warsz).* (2000) 48:31–7.
161. Van Belleghem JD, Clement F, Merabishvili M, Lavigne R, Vaneechoutte M. Pro- and anti-inflammatory responses of peripheral blood mononuclear cells induced by *Staphylococcus aureus* and *Pseudomonas aeruginosa* phages. *Sci Rep.* (2017) 7:8004. doi: 10.1038/s41598-017-08336-9
162. Zhang L, Hou X, Sun L, He T, Wei R, Pang M, et al. *Staphylococcus aureus* bacteriophage suppresses LPS-induced inflammation in MAC-T bovine mammary epithelial cells. *Front Microbiol.* (2018) 9:1614. doi: 10.3389/fmicb.2018.01614
163. Miernikiewicz P, Dabrowska K, Piotrowicz A, Owczarek B, Wojas-Turek J, Kicielinska J, et al. T4 phage and its head surface proteins do not stimulate inflammatory mediator production. *PLoS ONE.* (2013) 8:e71036. doi: 10.1371/journal.pone.0071036
164. Park K, Cha KE, Myung H. Observation of inflammatory responses in mice orally fed with bacteriophage T7. *J Appl Microbiol.* (2014) 117:627–33. doi: 10.1111/jam.12565
165. Miedzybrodzki R, Switala-Jelen K, Fortuna W, Weber-Dabrowska B, Przerwa A, Lusiak-Szelachowska M, et al. Bacteriophage preparation inhibition of reactive oxygen species generation by endotoxin-stimulated polymorphonuclear leukocytes. *Virus Res.* (2008) 131:233–42. doi: 10.1016/j.virusres.2007.09.013
166. Miernikiewicz P, Klopot A, Soluch R, Szkuta P, Keska W, Hodyra-Stefaniak K, et al. T4 phage tail adhesin Gp12 counteracts LPS-induced inflammation *in vivo*. *Front Microbiol.* (2016) 7:1112. doi: 10.3389/fmicb.2016.01112
167. Foxman EF, Iwasaki A. Genome-virome interactions: examining the role of common viral infections in complex disease. *Nat Rev Microbiol.* (2011) 9:254–64. doi: 10.1038/nrmicro2541
168. Duerkop BA, Hooper LV. Resident viruses and their interactions with the immune system. *Nat Immunol.* (2013) 14:654–9. doi: 10.1038/ni.2614
169. Matsui H, Randell SH, Peretti SW, Davis CW, Boucher RC. Coordinated clearance of periciliary liquid and mucus from airway surfaces. *J Clin Invest.* (1998) 102:1125–31. doi: 10.1172/JCI2687
170. Kreda SM, Mall M, Mengos A, Rochelle L, Yankaskas J, Riordan JR, et al. Characterization of wild-type and deltaF508 cystic fibrosis transmembrane regulator in human respiratory epithelia. *Mol Biol Cell.* (2005) 16:2154–67. doi: 10.1091/mbc.e04-11-1010
171. Tarran R, Button B, Boucher RC. Regulation of normal and cystic fibrosis airway surface liquid volume by phasic shear stress. *Ann Rev Physiol.* (2006) 68:543–61. doi: 10.1146/annurev.physiol.68.072304.112754
172. Stoltz DA, Meyerholz DK, Pezzulo AA, Ramachandran S, Rogan MP, Davis GJ, et al. Cystic fibrosis pigs develop lung disease and exhibit defective bacterial eradication at birth. *Sci Transl Med.* (2010) 2:29ra31. doi: 10.1126/scitranslmed.3000928
173. Hartl D, Gaggar A, Bruscia E, Hector A, Marcos V, Jung A, et al. Innate immunity in cystic fibrosis lung disease. *J Cyst Fibros.* (2012) 11:363–82. doi: 10.1016/j.jcf.2012.07.003
174. Hoegger MJ, Fischer AJ, McMenimen JD, Ostedgaard LS, Tucker AJ, Awadalla MA, et al. Impaired mucus detachment disrupts mucociliary transport in a piglet model of cystic fibrosis. *Science.* (2014) 345:818–22. doi: 10.1126/science.1255825
175. FitzSimmons SC. The changing epidemiology of cystic fibrosis. *J Pediatr.* (1993) 122:1–9. doi: 10.1016/S0022-3476(05)83478-X
176. Johansen HK, Høiby N. Seasonal onset of initial colonisation and chronic infection with *Pseudomonas aeruginosa* in patients with cystic fibrosis in Denmark. *Thorax.* (1992) 47:109–11. doi: 10.1136/thx.47.2.109
177. Burns JL, Gibson RL, McNamara S, Yim D, Emerson J, Rosenfeld M, et al. Longitudinal assessment of *Pseudomonas aeruginosa* in young children with cystic fibrosis. *J Infect Dis.* (2001) 183:444–52. doi: 10.1086/318075
178. Cystic Fibrosis Foundation (2016). *Cystic Fibrosis Foundation Patient Registry 2015 Annual Data Report.*
179. UK Cystic Fibrosis Registry (2017). *UK Cystic Fibrosis Registry Annual Data Report 2016.*
180. Nixon GM, Armstrong DS, Carzino R, Carlin JB, Olinsky A, Robertson CF, et al. Clinical outcome after early *Pseudomonas aeruginosa* infection in cystic fibrosis. *J Pediatr.* (2001) 138:699–704. doi: 10.1067/mpd.2001.112897
181. Rosenfeld M, Gibson RL, McNamara S, Emerson J, Burns JL, Castile R, et al. Early pulmonary infection, inflammation, and clinical outcomes in infants with cystic fibrosis. *Pediatr Pulmonol.* (2001) 32:356–66. doi: 10.1002/ppul.1144
182. Konstan MW, Morgan WJ, Butler SM, Pasta DJ, Craib ML, Silva SJ, et al. Risk factors for rate of decline in forced expiratory volume in one second in children and adolescents with cystic fibrosis. *J Pediatr.* (2007) 151:134–9, 139.e131. doi: 10.1016/j.jpeds.2007.03.006
183. Emerson J, McNamara S, Buccat AM, Worrell K, Burns JL. Changes in cystic fibrosis sputum microbiology in the United States between 1995 and 2008. *Pediatr Pulmonol.* (2010) 45:363–70. doi: 10.1002/ppul.21198
184. Doring G, Flume P, Heijerman H, Elborn JS, Consensus Study G. Treatment of lung infection in patients with cystic fibrosis: current and future strategies. *J Cyst Fibros.* (2012) 11:461–79. doi: 10.1016/j.jcf.2012.10.004
185. Mogayzel PJJr, Naureckas ET, Robinson KA, Brady C, Guill M, Lahiri T, et al. Cystic Fibrosis Foundation pulmonary guideline. pharmacologic approaches to prevention and eradication of initial Pseudomonas aeruginosa infection. *Ann Am Thorac Soc.* (2014) 11:1640–50. doi: 10.1513/AnnalsATS.201404-166CC
186. Burgener EB, Yacob AA, Bollyky P, Milla CE. 99 Pf bacteriophage (Pf) in *Pseudomonas aeruginosa* (Pa) biofilms is associated with increased elastase in the sputum of patients with cystic fibrosis (CF). *J Cystic Fibrosis.* (2017) 16:S90. doi: 10.1016/S1569-1993(17)30463-0
187. Chang MS, McNinch J, Basu R, Simonet S. Cloning and characterization of the human neutrophil-activating peptide (ENA-78) gene. *J Biol Chem.* (1994) 269:25277–82.
188. Koch AE, Kunkel SL, Harlow LA, Mazarakis DD, Haines GK, Burdick MD, et al. Epithelial neutrophil activating peptide-78: a novel chemotactic cytokine for neutrophils in arthritis. *J Clin Invest.* (1994) 94:1012–8. doi: 10.1172/JCI117414
189. Bokarewa M, Nagaev I, Dahlberg L, Smith U, Tarkowski A. Resistin, an adipokine with potent proinflammatory properties. *J Immunol.* (2005) 174:5789–95. doi: 10.4049/jimmunol.174.9.5789
190. Cooper AM, Khader SA. IL-12p40: an inherently agonistic cytokine. *Trends Immunol.* (2007) 28:33–8. doi: 10.1016/j.it.2006.11.002
191. Schaefer U, Voloshanenko O, Willen D, Walczak H. TRAIL: a multifunctional cytokine. *Front Biosci* (2007) 12:3813–24. doi: 10.2741/2354
192. Dandachi N, Kelly NJ, Wood JP, Burton CL, Radder JE, Leme AS, et al. Macrophage elastase induces TRAIL-mediated tumor cell death through its carboxy-terminal domain. *Am J Respir Crit Care Med.* (2017) 196:353–63. doi: 10.1164/rccm.201606-1150OC
193. Priebe GP, Goldberg JB. Vaccines for *Pseudomonas aeruginosa*: A long and winding road. *Expert Rev Vaccines.* (2014) 3:507–19. doi: 10.1586/14760584.2014.890053
194. Jerne NK. Bacteriophage inactivation by antiphage serum diluted in distilled water. *Nature.* (1952) 169:117–8. doi: 10.1038/169117b0
195. Jerne NK. The presence in normal serum of specific antibody against bacteriophage T4 and its increase during the earliest stages of immunization. *J Immunol.* (1956) 76:209–16.
196. Zaczek M, Lusiak-Szelachowska M, Jonczyk-Matysiak E, Weber-Dabrowska B, Miedzybrodzki R, Owczarek B, et al. Antibody production in response to staphylococcal MS-1 phage cocktail in patients undergoing phage therapy. *Front Microbiol.* (2016) 7:1681. doi: 10.3389/fmicb.2016.01681
197. Dabrowska K, Miernikiewicz P, Piotrowicz A, Hodyra K, Owczarek B, Lecion D, et al. Immunogenicity studies of proteins forming the T4 phage head surface. *J Virol.* (2014) 88:12551–7. doi: 10.1128/JVI.02043-14
198. Bruttin A, Brussow H. Human volunteers receiving *Escherichia coli* phage T4 orally: a safety test of phage therapy. *Antimicrob Agents Chemother.* (2005) 49:2874–8. doi: 10.1128/AAC.49.7.2874-2878.2005
199. Levy SB, Marshall B. Antibacterial resistance worldwide: causes, challenges and responses. *Nat Med.* (2004) 10:S122–9. doi: 10.1038/nm1145
200. Summers WC. Bacteriophage therapy. *Annu Rev Microbiol.* (2001) 55:437–51. doi: 10.1146/annurev.micro.55.1.437
201. Bertoye A, Gaillard L, Courtieu AL. [Adapted bacteriophages in the treatment of infections caused by antibiotic-resistant microorganisms]. *J Med Lyon.* (1959) 40:465–71.

202. Soothill J. Use of bacteriophages in the treatment of *Pseudomonas aeruginosa* infections. *Expert Rev Anti Infect Ther.* (2013) 11:909–15. doi: 10.1586/14787210.2013.826990
203. Chang RY, Wong J, Mathai A, Morales S, Kutter E, Britton W, et al. Production of highly stable spray dried phage formulations for treatment of *Pseudomonas aeruginosa* lung infection. *Eur J Pharm Biopharm.* (2017) 121:1–13. doi: 10.1016/j.ejpb.2017.09.002
204. Loc-Carrillo C, Abedon ST. Pros and cons of phage therapy. *Bacteriophage.* (2011) 1:111–4. doi: 10.4161/bact.1.2.14590
205. Shiley JR, Comfort KK, Robinson JB. Immunogenicity and antimicrobial effectiveness of *Pseudomonas aeruginosa* specific bacteriophage in a human lung *in vitro* model. *Appl Microbiol Biotechnol.* (2017) 101:7977–85. doi: 10.1007/s00253-017-8504-1
206. Cadwell K. The virome in host health and disease. *Immunity.* (2015) 42:805–13. doi: 10.1016/j.immuni.2015.05.003
207. Pride DT, Salzman J, Haynes M, Rohwer F, Davis-Long C, White RAIII, et al. Evidence of a robust resident bacteriophage population revealed through analysis of the human salivary virome. *ISME J.* (2012) 6:915–26. doi: 10.1038/ismej.2011.169
208. Yang J, Yang F, Ren L, Xiong Z, Wu Z, Dong J, et al. Unbiased parallel detection of viral pathogens in clinical samples by use of a metagenomic approach. *J Clin Microbiol.* (2011) 49:3463–9. doi: 10.1128/JCM.00273-11
209. Carding SR, Davis N, Hoyles L. Review article: the human intestinal virome in health and disease. *Aliment Pharmacol Ther.* (2017) 46:800–15. doi: 10.1111/apt.14280
210. Enault F, Briet A, Bouteille L, Roux S, Sullivan MB, Petit MA. Phages rarely encode antibiotic resistance genes: a cautionary tale for virome analyses. *ISME J.* (2017) 11:237–47. doi: 10.1038/ismej.2016.90
211. Willner D, Furlan M, Haynes M, Schmieder R, Angly FE, Silva J, et al. Metagenomic analysis of respiratory tract DNA viral communities in cystic fibrosis and non-cystic fibrosis individuals. *PLoS ONE.* (2009) 4:e7370. doi: 10.1371/journal.pone.0007370
212. Dickson RP, Huffnagle GB. The lung microbiome: new principles for respiratory bacteriology in health and disease. *PLoS Pathog.* (2015) 11:e1004923. doi: 10.1371/journal.ppat.1004923
213. Jorth P, Staudinger BJ, Wu X, Hisert KB, Hayden H, Garudathri J, et al. Regional isolation drives bacterial diversification within cystic fibrosis lungs. *Cell Host Microbe.* (2015) 18:307–19. doi: 10.1016/j.chom.2015.07.006
214. Fodor AA, Klem ER, Gilpin DF, Elborn JS, Boucher RC, Tunney MM, et al. The adult cystic fibrosis airway microbiota is stable over time and infection type, and highly resilient to antibiotic treatment of exacerbations. *PLoS ONE.* (2012) 7:e45001. doi: 10.1371/journal.pone.0045001
215. Huang YJ, LiPuma JJ. The microbiome in cystic fibrosis. *Clin Chest Med.* (2016) 37:59–67. doi: 10.1016/j.ccm.2015.10.003
216. Penner JC, Ferreira JAG, Secor PR, Sweere JM, Birukova MK, Joubert LM, et al. Pf4 bacteriophage produced by *Pseudomonas aeruginosa* inhibits *Aspergillus fumigatus* metabolism via iron sequestration. *Microbiology.* (2016) 162:1583–94. doi: 10.1099/mic.0.000344
217. Nazik H, Joubert LM, Secor PR, Sweere JM, Bollyky PL, Sass G, et al. Pseudomonas phage inhibition of *Candida albicans. Microbiology.* (2017) 163:1568–77. doi: 10.1099/mic.0.000539
218. James CE, Davies EV, Fothergill JL, Walshaw MJ, Beale CM, Brockhurst MA, et al. Lytic activity by temperate phages of *Pseudomonas aeruginosa* in long-term cystic fibrosis chronic lung infections. *ISME J.* (2015) 9:1391–8. doi: 10.1038/ismej.2014.223
219. Cohen D, Melamed S, Millman A, Shulman G, Oppenheimer-Shaanan Y, Kacen A, et al. Cyclic GMP-AMP signalling protects bacteria against viral infection. *Nature.* (2019) 574:691–5. doi: 10.1038/s41586-019-1605-5
220. Mougous JD, Cuff ME, Raunser S, Shen A, Zhou M, Gifford CA, et al. A virulence locus of *Pseudomonas aeruginosa* encodes a protein secretion apparatus. *Science.* (2006) 312:1526–30. doi: 10.1126/science.1128393
221. Hockett KL, Renner T, Baltrus DA. Independent co-option of a tailed bacteriophage into a killing complex in pseudomonas. *MBio.* (2015) 6:e00452. doi: 10.1128/mBio.00452-15
222. Costantini TW, Putnam JG, Sawada R, Baird A, Loomis WH, Eliceiri BP, et al. Targeting the gut barrier: identification of a homing peptide sequence for delivery into the injured intestinal epithelial cell. *Surgery.* (2009) 146:206–12. doi: 10.1016/j.surg.2009.05.007
223. Ivanenkov V, Felici F, Menon AG. Uptake and intracellular fate of phage display vectors in mammalian cells. *Biochim Biophys Acta.* (1999) 1448:450–62. doi: 10.1016/S0167-4889(98)00162-1
224. Ochs HD, Davis SD, Wedgwood RJ. Immunologic responses to bacteriophage phi-X 174 in immunodeficiency diseases. *J Clin Invest.* (1971) 50:2559–68. doi: 10.1172/JCI106756
225. Kamme C. Antibodies against staphylococcal bacteriophages in human sera. I Assay of antibodies in healthy individuals and in patients with staphylococcal infections. *Acta Pathol Microbiol Scand B Microbiol Immunol.* (1973) 81:741–8. doi: 10.1111/j.1699-0463.1973.tb02269.x
226. Hodyra-Stefaniak K, Miernikiewicz P, Drapala J, Drab M, Jonczyk-Matysiak E, Lecion D, et al. Mammalian host-versus-phage immune response determines phage fate *in vivo*. *Sci Rep.* (2015) 5:14802. doi: 10.1038/srep14802

12

Inactivation of FOXA2 by Respiratory Bacterial Pathogens and Dysregulation of Pulmonary Mucus Homeostasis

*Woosuk Choi, Shawn Choe and Gee W. Lau**

Department of Pathobiology, University of Illinois at Urbana-Champaign, Urbana, IL, United States

***Correspondence:**
Gee W. Lau
geelau@illinois.edu

Forkhead box (FOX) proteins are transcriptional factors that regulate various cellular processes. This minireview provides an overview of FOXA2 functions, with a special emphasis on the regulation airway mucus homeostasis in both healthy and diseased lungs. FOXA2 plays crucial roles during lung morphogenesis, surfactant protein production, goblet cell differentiation and mucin expression. In healthy airways, FOXA2 exerts a tight control over goblet cell development and mucin biosynthesis. However, in diseased airways, microbial infections and proinflammatory responses deplete FOXA2 expression, resulting in uncontrolled goblet cell hyperplasia and metaplasia, mucus hypersecretion, and impaired mucociliary clearance of pathogens. Furthermore, accumulated mucus clogs the airways and creates a niche environment for persistent microbial colonization and infection, leading to acute exacerbation and deterioration of pulmonary function in patients with chronic lung diseases. Various studies have shown that FOXA2 inhibition is mediated through induction of antagonistic EGFR and IL-13R-STAT6 signaling pathways as well as through posttranslational modifications induced by microbial infections. An improved understanding of how bacterial pathogens inactivate FOXA2 may pave the way for developing therapeutics that preserve the protein's function, which in turn, will improve the mucus status and mucociliary clearance of pathogens, reduce microbial-mediated acute exacerbation and restore lung function in patients with chronic lung diseases.

Keywords: chronic lung diseases, mucus homeostasis, mucociliary clearance, FOXA2, EGFR, STAT6, MUC5AC, MUC5B

INTRODUCTION

The *Forkhead* (*fox*) genes encode evolutionarily-conserved transcriptional regulators characterized by a winged-helix DNA-binding domain (DBD), called the forkhead box. Members of the FOX family have divergent roles, including embryonic development, cell survival, proliferation, differentiation, and energy homeostasis (1). Initially discovered in *Drosophila melanogaster,* a mutation in the *fox* gene generated a homeotic transformation of foregut into head that originates the nomenclature "forked head" (2). Over 100 FOX members have been identified, with 50 human *fox* genes cataloged into 19 subgroups from FOXA to FOXS (3). The FOXA subclass was the first discovered in mammals (4).

STRUCTURE AND FUNCTION OF FOXA2

FOXA1, FOXA2, and FOXA3 were originally identified in rat liver, the so-called hepatocyte nuclear factor 3 (HNF3)-α, -β, and -γ, respectively (4). The conserved domains of FOXA2 were originally analyzed (2), and the DBD was found to be the most evolutionarily conserved among the FOXA members, with an unique AKT/PKB phosphorylation site at the threonine (Thr)156 (5). The DBD of FOXA is structurally similar to H1/H5 linker histones capable of unwinding chromatin, which enables the recruitment of other transcriptional cofactors to the promoter (6, 7). The C-terminus of FOXA interacts with histones H3/H4 within nucleosome to support the opening of chromatin by the DBD (8). FOXA members regulate the expression of target genes by displacing histones from chromatin and serving as transcription factors at the enhancer region of the promotor (9, 10).

MODULATION OF FOXA2 ACTIVITY BY POST-TRANSLATIONAL MODIFICATIONS

FOXA transcription factors are abundantly expressed in liver and regulate metabolic homeostasis (4). During hypoglycemia, low plasma insulin activates FOXA2 to elevate the transcription of genes encoding metabolic enzymes involved in fatty acid oxidation and ketogenesis, supplying energy for gluconeogenesis and maintaining brain function, respectively. However, excess blood glucose elevates plasma insulin, which inactivates FOXA2 and decreases the expression of enzymes involved in gluconeogenesis (11, 12). This is supported by studies that show inactivation of hepatic FOXA2 in hyperinsulinemic *ob/ob* and *db/db* mice and in diet-induced obese mice (13). Insulin promotes nuclear export of FOXA2 through AKT-mediated phosphorylation at Thr156 (**Figures 1A,B**) (5). Cells expressing the phosphorylation-deficient FOXA2-T156A are unresponsive to insulin-induced AKT, resulting in constitutive nuclear localization. Interestingly, DNA-binding ability of FOXA2 is not altered by insulin and phosphorylation-deficiency, suggesting that phosphorylation at Thr156 does not regulate transcriptional activity. Further study indicates that in the presence of insulin, phosphorylation at Thr156 inactivates transcriptional function and induces nuclear exclusion of FOXA2. Nuclear export of FOXA2 is dependent upon nuclear export factor CRM1, which recognizes the leucin-rich NES consensus sequence $LX_{2,3}$(L/I/V/F/M)$X_{2,3}LX$(L/I) within amino acids 106-111 (LSPSLS) of FOXA2 (14). In contrast, others have reported that FOXA2 is constitutively localized to the nucleus, independent of the metabolic conditions (15, 16). The aforementioned discrepancies might be caused by distinct experimental conditions, including differences in transgenic obese mouse strains, feeding conditions, and immortalized hepatic cell lines. Subsequently, it was revealed that FOXA2 function could be modulated by IKKα-mediated phosphorylation on Ser107/111 (**Figure 1A**) (17). Both Thr156 and Ser107/111 residues are located within the nuclear localization signal domain and the nuclear export signal domain, respectively (**Figure 1A**), implying that phosphorylation of these residues dictates subcellular localization of FOXA2 (14).

Acetylation and deacetylation also compete to modulate the transcriptional activity of FOXA2. Insulin induces the SIRT1 deacetylase to deacetylate Lys259 on FOXA2 (**Figure 1A**), which attenuates target gene expression and increases export from the nuclei in hepatocytes. In contrast, glucagon induces FOXA2 acetylation through P300 acetyltransferase, which leads to nuclear accumulation and increased expression of target genes (12). The acetylation-deficient FOXA2-K259R has attenuated DNA binding ability, and is sequestered to the cytoplasm for degradation. As discussed above, FOXA2-T156A is sequestered in the nucleus; however, hepatic cells transfected with *FOXA2-T156A-K259R* exhibit similar phenotype to those transfected with *FOXA2-K259R*, suggesting that acetylation/deacetylation diminish phosphorylation event, and therefore, confer a dominant phenotype (12). Interestingly, it has been reported that during nutrient-deprivation, deacetylation by SIRT1 only attenuates FOXA2's transcriptional activity but not its nuclear export for degradation by the proteasome (11).

Sumoylation and ubiquitination also compete for maintenance and degradation of FOXA2 (18) Sumoylation of the Lys6 by PIAS stabilizes FOXA2's transcriptional activity. In contrast, polyubiquitination facilitates FOXA2 degradation by proteasome. Sumoylation-resistance FOXA2-K6R is more susceptible to ubiquitination and rapid degradation, suggesting that additional lysine residues might be ubiquitinated. Notably, although sumoylation increases both stability and transcriptional activity of FOXA2, nuclear localization is not affected.

ROLE OF FOXA2 IN LUNG DEVELOPMENT AND HOMEOSTASIS

FOXA2 is required for lung development. During mouse embryogenesis, FOXA2 is initially expressed in the primitive streak and in the node on embryonic day 6.5 (E6.5), inducing gastrulation. By E7.5, FOXA2 is highly expressed in both mesoderm and endoderm, and thereafter, persistently expressed throughout development and in adult endoderm-derived tissues, including the lung (19). After E10-E11, lung morphogenesis is facilitated by the spatiotemporal expression of FOXA2 restricted to respiratory epithelium. By E12.5, mouse embryo develops conducting airways and alveolar epithelial cells, and forms lung buds during late embryonic development (20). In contrast, *FOXA2* null mouse embryo shows lethality on E11-E12, with severe defects in all three germ layers before the initiation of lung morphogenesis (21). The conditional loss of FOXA2 on E12.5 disrupts branching formation and airway epithelial cell differentiation, resulting in the dilation of distal airways. In addition, postnatal (PN) lungs of *foxa1* null allele and lung epithelium-specific *foxa2* depleted mice ($foxa1^{-/-}/foxa2^{\Delta/\Delta}$) exhibit regressed formation of alveolar and peripheral lung saccules by PN day 3 (PN3), and extensive airspace enlargement with mucin glycoprotein overexpression by PN10–PN20 (20).

In postnatal lungs, FOXA2 is constitutively expressed in subsets of respiratory epithelial cells and transcriptional

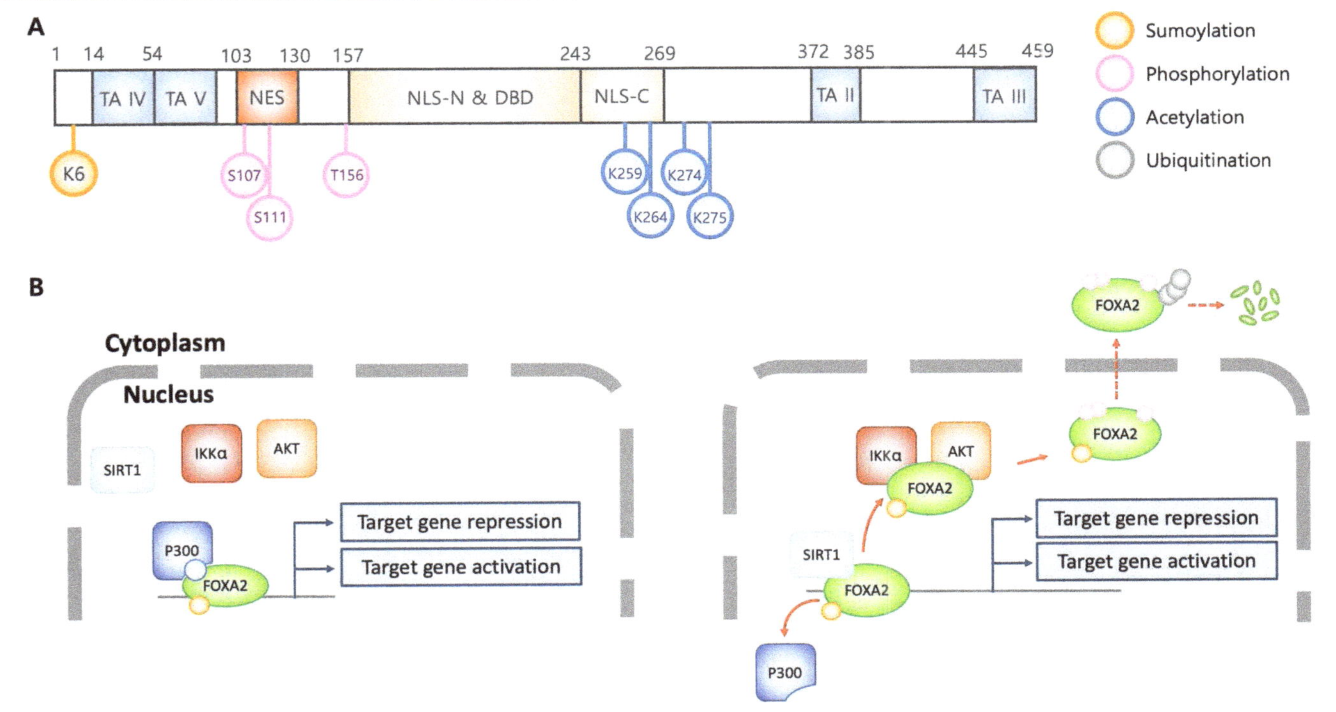

FIGURE 1 | Structural and functional characteristics of FOXA2 in association with posttranslational modification. **(A)** Schematic diagram of FOXA2 (adapted from J Biol Chem 2009, 284:24816-24; and Mol Cell Biol 1992, 12:3723-3732). Diagram shows functional domains of FOXA2. Colorized circles indicate post-translationally modified amino acid residues which alter FOXA2 functions. TA, transactivation domain; NES, nuclear export signal; NLS, Nuclear localization signal; DBD, DNA binding domain; K, lysine; S, serine; T, threonine. **(B)** Regulation of transcriptional activity and stability of FOXA2 by posttranslational modifications. Acetylation by P300 allows FOXA2 to be functionally active. In contrast, SIRT1 deacetylates FOXA2, leading to nuclear export via AKT and IKKα-mediated phosphorylation, and subsequently, ubiquitination and degradation. Sumoylation enhances the stability of nuclear FOXA2, which is diminished by ubiquitination, resulting in FOXA2 degradation.

controlled genes encoding club cell specific protein CC10 (22), surfactant proteins (SP) (23), thyroid transcription factor-1 (TTF-1) (24), and mucins MUC5AC and MUC5B (25, 26). Pulmonary surfactant is composed of 90% phospholipids and 10% proteins, including SP-A, SP-B, SP-C, and SP-D secreted by the type II alveolar cells and non-ciliated terminal bronchiolar Club cells. Together with phospholipids, SP-B and SP-C provide critical surface tension-lowering properties that reduce the work of breathing and maintain airspace patency. FOXA2$^{\Delta/\Delta}$ mice show significantly reduced SP-B expression with deteriorating respiratory distress syndrome (27). In contrast to upregulation of CC10, SFTPB, and TTF-1, FOXA2 represses the transcription of mucin genes. Conditional deletion of FOXA2 in the mouse respiratory epithelium causes airspace enlargement, goblet cell hyperplasia, increased mucin expression and neutrophil infiltration (25). Collectively, the aforementioned studies indicate crucial roles of FOXA2 in regulating embryonic lung development and postnatal lung homeostasis.

FOXA2 AND MUCUS HOMEOSTASIS

The apical surface of healthy airways is covered by the airway surface liquid (ASL) composed of mucin glycoproteins, antimicrobial peptides and proteins, innate immune cells, signaling molecules, and enzymes (28). ASL is bilayer, with the periciliary layer sandwiched between the top mucus gel layer and the bottom airway epithelium, forming the "gel-on-brush" structure (29) (**Figure 2A**). The periciliary layer is filled with hydrogel that provides space for ciliary beating and supports mucociliary clearance. Within the mobile mucus layer, MUC5AC and MUC5B are the predominant mucins that provide viscosity and gel-forming properties to mucus, trapping inhaled pathogens and irritants. Mucins also keep moisture in the airway epithelium (30), which help to maintain the periciliary layer and mucociliary clearance. MUC5AC is produced by the goblet cells while MUC5B is expressed in submucosal glands of trachea and bronchi, and in surface secretory cells throughout the airway down to the level of preterminal bronchioles (31, 32). MUC5AC-overexpressing mice are more resistant to PR8/H1N1 influenza virus (33). Similarly, MUC5B-deficient mice are more susceptible to lung infection with increased mortality caused by ensuing bacteremia (34).

FOXA2 deficiency causes pulmonary eosinophilia, recruitment of inflammatory immune cells and upregulation of IL-4, IL-13, IL-33, CCL-17, and CCL-20 that promote Th2 cell differentiation, goblet cell hyperplasia and metaplasia, and mucus hypersecretion (25, 35). These suggest that FOXA2 regulates airway mucus homeostasis by counteracting the effects of IL-4 and IL-13 (36, 37). Metaplastic effects of IL-4 and IL-13 are mediated through the STAT6 (35) and its downstream

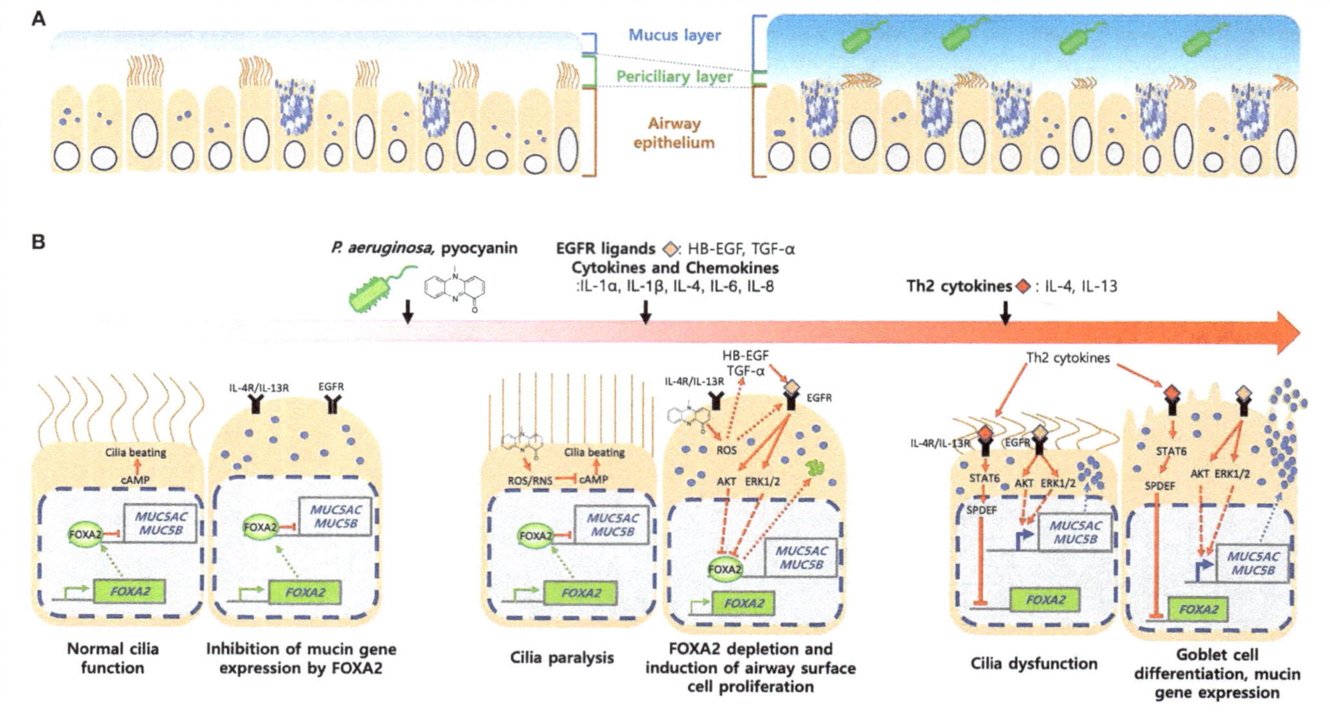

FIGURE 2 | Induction of mucus hypersecretion by *P. aeruginosa* pyocyanin. **(A)** Composition of mucus layers in heathy and diseased airways. **(B)** *P. aeruginosa* and its virulence factors, especially pyocyanin, stimulate excessive ROS, chemokines and cytokines and, ligands that activate IL-4R/IL-13R-STAT6-SPDEF, and EGFR-AKT/ERK1/2-mediated signaling pathways. Both kinase cascades converged to inhibit FOXA2, resulting in over proliferation and differentiation of airway epithelial (ciliated and club) cells to mucus-secreting goblet cells. Excessive mucus and failure in the clearance exacerbates airway obstruction and microbial colonization and infection.

effector SPDEF (25, 38, 39). MUC5Ac and MUC5B expression is dependent on SPDEF (38, 40). IL-13-stimulated airway epithelial cells show decreased *FOXA2* transcript, a process mediated by SPDEF (41). Conditional induction of SPDEF within transgenic mouse airways downregulates the *foxa2* gene, resulting in goblet cell hyperplasia (39). These findings indicate that FOXA2 and SPDEF compete to regulate the expression of MUC5AC and MUC5B.

Th2 cytokines also amplify the mucus-inducing EGFR signaling, which is highly activated in cystic fibrosis (CF), chronic obstructive pulmonary disease (COPD) and asthma (42, 43). In response to IL-4, IL-5, and IL-13, bronchial epithelial and immune cells produce ligands (EGF, TGF-α, amphiregulin) that induce EGFR in an autocrine manner (41, 44–46), which subsequently, activates the downstream cRAF-MEK-ERK and PI3K-AKT signaling cascades that inhibit FOXA2 and increase MUC5AC and MUC5B production (47). Interestingly, these pathways have distinct effects, with PI3K-AKT augments cell proliferation while cRAF-MEK-ERK directly enhances goblet cell metaplasia and mucin synthesis (48).

Notch signaling regulates cell-cell communication and differentiation of airway basal cells into secretory and ciliated cells (49). Both Notch1 and Notch2 are required for goblet cell development (50, 51). Interestingly, Notch ligands promotes goblet cell metaplasia independent of the IL-13R-STAT6 axis. It is unknown if Notch induction depletes FOXA2 expression during goblet cell development in diseased airways.

Interestingly, *MUC5B* gene transcription is differentially-regulated by FOXA2. Inhibition of FOXA2 by bacterial pathogens elevates MUC5B expression (26, 52–54). In contrast, FOXA2 positively regulates MUC5B expression in both idiopathic pulmonary fibrosis (55) and asthma (56), most likely caused by polymorphism in the *MUC5B* promoter (57). Additionally, inhibition of FOXA2 by IL-13 results in different inhibitory kinetics on *MUC5B* expression in the air-liquid interface (ALI) culture of airway cells vs. in mouse lungs (41), suggesting that additional mediators may modulate mucin production in an intact lung. Collectively, these findings suggest that regulatory activity of FOXA2 on *MUC5B* may vary, depending on disease context and additional interacting factors.

FOXA2 INACTIVATION BY RESPIRATORY BACTERIAL PATHOGENS

As previously discussed, excessive mucus causes airway obstruction, narrowing and airflow limitation in chronic lung diseases. Significantly, FOXA2 expression is depleted in airways of patients with bronchopulmonary dysplasia, bronchiectasis (25), and asthma (58). Cigarette smoking, the most important etiologic agent in COPD, directly suppress FOXA2 expression (59). Accumulated mucus allows microbes to thrive, resulting in persistent inflammation, acute exacerbation (60), and lung function impairment (61), with increased morbidity, and mortality (62). Among the bacterial pathogens, *Staphylococcus aureus* and *Pseudomonas aeruginosa (PA)* are the most important in young CF patients, but in adulthood, *PA* predominates (63). *Chlamydophila pneumoniae* and *Mycoplasma pneumoniae* are the most important in asthma induction and acute exacerbation (64). *Streptococcus pneumoniae*, *Haemophilus influenza*, and *Moraxella catarrhalis* are the most common in COPD. However, in advanced stages of COPD, *PA*, *M. pneumoniae*, *H. parainfluenzae*, and *Klebsiella pneumoniae* predominate. Acquisition of *PA* increases episodes of acute exacerbation, especially in COPD patients who received antibiotics and those who require mechanical ventilation. Significantly, a subset of these patients becomes chronically-infected with *PA* (65).

For the remainder of this review, we will focus on the FOXA2 inactivation by *PA* (**Figures 2A,B**). *PA* forms biofilms in the mucus-rich environments and becomes more resistant to antibiotics and phagocytic clearance. *PA* virulence factors, including pyocyanin (26, 52, 66, 67), LPS (68), flagellin (69, 70), alginate (71) and protease (72) induce mucus overproduction.

Among these aforementioned virulence factors, the tricyclic phenazine pyocyanin, is the most robust mucus inducer (73). Pyocyanin is zwittwerionic, which ionizes at physiological pH, penetrates cell membrane, and increases both intracellular reactive oxygen species (ROS) and nitrogen species (RNS) (74–76). Redox cycling of pyocyanin with intracellular electron donors and acceptors generates ROS/RNS (76, 77). Persistent oxidative stress causes dysfunction of ion pumps, antioxidant proteins and cellular reducing agents, resulting in cytotoxicity (78, 79).

Pyocyanin is important for lung infections (80) and recoverable at 0.1 mM concentrations from both COPD and CF sputa (81). Additionally, the levels of pyocyanin within sputa negatively-correlates with the function of CF lungs (82). Pyocyanin interferes with ciliary beating and mucus transport (81), induces bronchoconstriction (83), and decreases mucus velocity (84, 85). Mouse lungs chronically-exposed to pyocyanin develop goblet cell hyperplasia and metaplasia, peribronchial fibrosis, and alveolar airspace destruction, accompanied by polarization from initially a Th1 response toward a Th2 response dominated by IL-4 and IL-13 secreted by activated macrophages and $CD4^+$ T cells, with concomitant influx of neutrophils (52, 66). Many of these pathological features resemble the airways of FOXA2-deficient mice (25). Further studies in the both primary and immortalized human airway cells and in mice demonstrate that pyocyanin depletes FOXA2 expression by activating antagonistic EGFR-PI3K-AKT, EGFR-MEK-ERK and IL-13R-STAT6-SPDEF pathways, resulting in goblet cell hyperplasia and metaplasia and excessive mucins (52, 66). Additionally, pyocyanin activates EGFR directly through ROS or indirectly by inducing the release of proinflammatory cytokines and EGFR ligands from airway cells (86). ROS/RNS generated by pyocyanin post-translationally modify FOXA2 and reduce its binding affinity to the *MUC5B* promoter. Glutathione restores the expression of FOXA2, which inhibits the transcription of *MUC5AC* and *MUC5B* (26). Collectively, these results suggest that pyocyanin inactivates FOXA2 through EGFR-PI3K-AKT, EGFR-MEK-ERK, and IL-13R-STAT6-SPDEF signaling, and post-translational modification of FOXA2.

As for the remaining *PA* virulence factors, LPS activates the Src-dependent Ras-p38MAPK-pp90rsk pathway, leading to mucin overproduction (68). Flagellum binds asialoGM1 and induces a signaling cascade, leading to cleavage of PIP2 by PLC, formation of IP3, Ca^{2+} mobilization, phosphorylation of ERK1/2, and finally, transcription of the *MUC2* gene (70). Flagellum also activates mucin biosynthesis through the NF-κB induced by TLR5-IL-8 signaling (69). The mechanisms underlying mucin induction by exoproteases (72), alginate (71), and their association to FOXA2 inactivation remain uncharacterized.

FOXA2 appears to be an evolutionally-conserved target of inactivation. Besides *PA*, we have shown that *M. pneumoniae* inactivates FOXA2 by inducing both STAT3-STAT6 and EGFR signaling, resulting in overexpression of airway mucins (53). Additional evidences are found in canine species. Because of genetic predisposition and exposure to environmental pollutants and infectious agents, older dogs, especially of smaller breeds, develop lung diseases similar to those in humans. Our recent study in dogs with COPD and chronic bronchitis indicate that infection by *PA* and *Bordetella bronchiseptica*, and by viral-bacterial combination activate the antagonistic STAT6 and EGFR signaling to inhibit FOXA2, resulting in goblet cell hyperplasia and metaplasia and mucus hypersecretion (16).

SUMMARY

Although many aspects of mucus biology have been explored as therapeutic targets, few drugs are available because of inefficacy and adverse effects (87). Despite its importance, FOXA2 has not been targeted for the development of novel mucoregulators, perhaps due to the complexity in gene regulation, post-translational modifications, and toxicity associated with its regulation of multiple cellular processes. Recently, the peptide ADEL (Ala-Asp-Glu-Leu) was found to relieve bacterial-mediated inflammation and improve lung function while boosting FOXA2 expression (88). Additionally, GLP-1 analogs were shown to reduce mortality and improve lung function in mice with acute obstructive lung disease (89). Our latest results indicate that the GLP-1 analog Exenatide restores FOXA2-regulated airway mucus homeostasis through the GLP1R-PKA-PPARγ-phosphatase signaling, by dephosphorylating key kinases within both STAT6 and EGFR cascades (90). Some factors need to be considered before repurposing the GLP-1 analogs. Systemically-administered GLP-1 analogs could suppress appetite (91). Because patients with muco-obstructive diseases (e.g., CF, COPD) commonly experience inappetence, and in the case of CF patients, nutrient malabsorption (92, 93), GLP-1 analogs may adversely impact the health status of these patients. To minimize systemic toxicity, direct aerosolization should be considered. Also, co-prescribing steroids and appetite stimulants with GLP-1 analogs may boost positive outcome. Finally, detailed mechanistic characterization of how these drugs restore FOXA2 function may lead to new methods of controlling excessive mucus, lowering bacterial burden and improving the quality of life in patients with chronic lung diseases.

AUTHOR CONTRIBUTIONS

WC, SC, and GL co-wrote the manuscript.

REFERENCES

1. Carlsson P, Mahlapuu M. Forkhead transcription factors: key players in development and metabolism. *Dev Biol.* (2002) 250:1–23. doi: 10.1006/dbio.2002.0780
2. Costa R, Grayson D, Darnell J. Multiple hepatocyte-enriched nuclear factors function in the regulation of transthyretin and alpha 1-antitrypsin genes. *Mol Cell Biol.* (1989) 9:1415–25. doi: 10.1128/MCB.9.4.1415
3. Kaestner KH, Knöchel W, Martínez DE. Unified nomenclature for the winged helix/forkhead transcription factors. *Genes Dev.* (2000) 14:142–6. doi: 10.1101/gad.14.2.142
4. Lai E, Prezioso VR, Smith E, Litvin O, Costa RH, Darnell J. HNF-3A, a hepatocyte-enriched transcription factor of novel structure is regulated transcriptionally. *Genes Dev.* (1990) 4:1427–36. doi: 10.1101/gad.4.8.1427
5. Wolfrum C, Besser D, Luca E, Stoffel M. Insulin regulates the activity of forkhead transcription factor Hnf-3 /Foxa-2 by Akt-mediated phosphorylation and nuclear/cytosolic localization. *Proc Natl Acad Sci. USA.* (2003) 100:11624–9. doi: 10.1073/pnas.1931483100
6. Clark KL, Halay ED, Lai E, Burley SK. Co-crystal structure of the HNF-3/fork head DNA-recognition motif resembles histone H5. *Nature.* (1993) 364:412. doi: 10.1038/364412a0
7. Zaret K, Caravaca J, Tulin A, Sekiya T. Nuclear mobility and mitotic chromosome binding similarities between pioneer transcription factor FoxA and linker histone H1. *Cold Spring Harbor Symp Quant Biol.* (2010) 219–26. doi: 10.1101/sqb.2010.75.061
8. Cirillo LA, Lin FR, Cuesta I, Friedman D, Jarnik M, Zaret KS. Opening of compacted chromatin by early developmental transcription factors HNF3 (FoxA) and GATA-4. *Mol Cell.* (2002) 9:279–89. doi: 10.1016/S1097-2765(02)00459-8
9. Zaret KS, Carroll JS. Pioneer transcription factors: establishing competence for gene expression. *Genes Dev.* (2011) 25:2227–41. doi: 10.1101/gad.176826.111
10. Iwafuchi-Doi M, Zaret KS. Pioneer transcription factors in cell reprogramming. *Genes Dev.* (2014) 28:2679–92. doi: 10.1101/gad.253443.114
11. Westerheide SD, Van Gent R, Di Sanza C, Van Den Broek NJF, Fleskens V, Veenstra A, et al. SIRT1 mediates FOXA2 breakdown by deacetylation in a nutrient-dependent manner. *PLoS ONE.* (2014) 9:e98438. doi: 10.1371/journal.pone.0098438
12. Von meyenn F, Porstmann T, Gasser E, Selevsek N, Schmidt A, Aebersold R, et al. Glucagon-induced acetylation of Foxa2 regulates hepatic lipid metabolism. *Cell Metab.* (2013) 17:436–47. doi: 10.1016/j.cmet.2013.01.014
13. Wolfrum C, Shih DQ, Kuwajima S, Norris AW, Kahn CR, Stoffel M. Role of Foxa-2 in adipocyte metabolism and differentiation. *J Clin Invest.* (2003) 112:345–56. doi: 10.1172/JCI18698
14. Howell JJ, Stoffel M. Nuclear export-independent inhibition of Foxa2 by insulin. *J Biol Chem.* (2009) 284:24816–24. doi: 10.1074/jbc.M109.042135
15. Steneberg P, Rubins N, Bartoov-Shifman R, Walker MD, Edlund H. The FFA receptor GPR40 links hyperinsulinemia, hepatic steatosis, and impaired glucose homeostasis in mouse. *Cell Metab.* (2005) 1:245–58. doi: 10.1016/j.cmet.2005.03.007
16. Zhang L, Rubins NE, Ahima RS, Greenbaum LE, Kaestner KH. Foxa2 integrates the transcriptional response of the hepatocyte to fasting. *Cell Metab.* (2005) 2:141–8. doi: 10.1016/j.cmet.2005.07.002
17. Liu M, Lee D-F, Chen C-T, Yen C-J, Li L-Y, Lee H-J, et al. IKKα activation of NOTCH links tumorigenesis via FOXA2 suppression. *Mol Cell.* (2012) 45:171–84. doi: 10.1016/j.molcel.2011.11.018
18. Belaguli NS, Zhang M, Brunicardi FC, Berger DH. Forkhead box protein A2 (FOXA2) protein stability and activity are regulated by sumoylation. *PLoS ONE.* (2012) 7:e48019. doi: 10.1371/journal.pone.0048019
19. Burtscher I, Lickert H. Foxa2 regulates polarity and epithelialization in the endoderm germ layer of the mouse embryo. *Development.* (2009) 136:1029–38. doi: 10.1242/dev.028415
20. Wan H, Dingle S, Xu Y, Besnard V, Kaestner KH, Ang S-L, et al. Compensatory roles of Foxal and Foxa2 during lung morphogenesis. *J Biol Chem.* (2005) 280:13809–16. doi: 10.1074/jbc.M414122200
21. Weinstein DC, I Altaba AR, Chen WS, Hoodless P, Prezioso VR, Jessell TM, et al. The winged-helix transcription factor HNF-3β is required for notochord development in the mouse embryo. *Cell.* (1994) 78:575–88. doi: 10.1016/0092-8674(94)90523-1
22. Chang A, Ramsay P, Zhao B, Park M, Magdaleno S, Reardon MJ, et al. Physiological regulation of uteroglobin/CCSP expression. *Ann N Y Acad Sci.* (2000) 923:181–92. doi: 10.1111/j.1749-6632.2000.tb05529.x
23. Bohinski RJ, Di Lauro R, Whitsett JA. The lung-specific surfactant protein B gene promoter is a target for thyroid transcription factor 1 and hepatocyte nuclear factor 3, indicating common factors for organ-specific gene expression along the foregut axis. *Mol Cell Biol.* (1994) 14:5671–81. doi: 10.1128/MCB.14.9.5671
24. Ikeda K, Shaw-White JR, Wert SE, Whitsett JA. Hepatocyte nuclear factor 3 activates transcription of thyroid transcription factor 1 in respiratory epithelial cells. *Mol Cell Biol.* (1996) 16:3626–36. doi: 10.1128/MCB.16.7.3626
25. Wan H, Kaestner KH, Ang S-L, Ikegami M, Finkelman FD, Stahlman MT, et al. Foxa2 regulates alveolarization and goblet cell hyperplasia. *Development.* (2004) 131:953–64. doi: 10.1242/dev.00966
26. Hao Y, Kuang Z, Xu Y, Walling BE, Lau GW. Pyocyanin-induced mucin production is associated with redox modification of FOXA2. *Respirat Res.* (2013) 14:82. doi: 10.1186/1465-9921-14-82
27. Wan H, Xu Y, Ikegami M, Stahlman MT, Kaestner KH, Ang S-L, et al. Foxa2 is required for transition to air breathing at birth. *Proc Natl Acad Sci USA.* (2004) 101:14449–54. doi: 10.1073/pnas.0404424101
28. Kato A, Schleimer RP. Beyond inflammation: airway epithelial cells are at the interface of innate and adaptive immunity. *Curr Opin Immunol.* (2007) 19:711–20. doi: 10.1016/j.coi.2007.08.004
29. Button B, Cai L-H, Ehre C, Kesimer M, Hill DB, Sheehan JK, et al. A periciliary brush promotes the lung health by separating the mucus layer from airway epithelia. *Science.* (2012) 337:937–41. doi: 10.1126/science.1223012
30. Sheehan JK, Kesimer M, Pickles R. Innate immunity and mucus structure and function. *Novartis Foundation Symp.* (2006) 155:155–66. doi: 10.1002/9780470035399.ch13
31. Reid CJ, Gould S, Harris A. Developmental expression of mucin genes in the human respiratory tract. *Am J Respirat Cell Mol Biol.* (1997) 17:592–8. doi: 10.1165/ajrcmb.17.5.2798
32. Buisine M-P, Devisme L, Copin M-C, Durand-Réville M, Gosselin B, Aubert J-P, et al. Developmental mucin gene expression in the human respiratory tract. *Am J Respirat Cell Mol Biol.* (1999) 20:209–18. doi: 10.1165/ajrcmb.20.2.3259
33. Ehre C, Worthington EN, Liesman RM, Grubb BR, Barbier D, O'neal WK, et al. Overexpressing mouse model demonstrates the protective role of Muc5ac in the lungs. *Proc Natl Acad Sci USA.* (2012) 109:16528–33. doi: 10.1073/pnas.1206552109
34. Roy MG, Livraghi-Butrico A, Fletcher AA, Mcelwee MM, Evans SE, Boerner RM, et al. Muc5b is required for airway defence. *Nature.* (2014) 505:412–6. doi: 10.1038/nature12807
35. Chen G, Wan H, Luo F, Zhang L, Xu Y, Lewkowich I, et al. Foxa2 programs Th2 cell-mediated innate immunity in the developing lung. *J Immunol.* (2010) 184:6133–41. doi: 10.4049/jimmunol.1000223
36. Jain-Vora S, Wert SE, Temann U-A, Rankin JA, Whitsett JA. Interleukin-4 alters epithelial cell differentiation and surfactant homeostasis in the postnatal mouse lung. *Am J Respirat Cell Mol Biol.* (1997) 17:541–51. doi: 10.1165/ajrcmb.17.5.2883

37. Kuperman DA, Huang X, Koth LL, Chang GH, Dolganov GM, Zhu Z, et al. Direct effects of interleukin-13 on epithelial cells cause airway hyperreactivity and mucus overproduction in asthma. *Nat Med.* (2002) 8:885. doi: 10.1038/nm734
38. Park K-S, Korfhagen TR, Bruno MD, Kitzmiller JA, Wan H, Wert SE, et al. SPDEF regulates goblet cell hyperplasia in the airway epithelium. *J Clin Invest.* (2007) 117:978–88. doi: 10.1172/JCI29176
39. Chen G, Korfhagen TR, Xu Y, Kitzmiller J, Wert SE, Maeda Y, et al. SPDEF is required for mouse pulmonary goblet cell differentiation and regulates a network of genes associated with mucus production. *J Clin Invest.* (2009) 119:2914–24. doi: 10.1172/JCI39731
40. Chen G, Volmer AS, Wilkinson KJ, Deng Y, Jones LC, Yu D, et al. Role of Spdef in the regulation of Muc5b expression in the airways of naive and mucoobstructed mice. *Am J Respirat Cell Mol Biol.* (2018) 59:383–96. doi: 10.1165/rcmb.2017-0127OC
41. Zhen G, Park SW, Nguyenvu LT, Rodriguez MW, Barbeau R, Paquet AC, et al. IL-13 and epidermal growth factor receptor have critical but distinct roles in epithelial cell mucin production. *Am J Respirat Cell Mol Biol.* (2007) 36:244–53. doi: 10.1165/rcmb.2006-0180OC
42. Burgel P, Nadel J. Epidermal growth factor receptor-mediated innate immune responses and their roles in airway diseases. *Eur Respirat J.* (2008) 32:1068–81. doi: 10.1183/09031936.00172007
43. Lai HY, Rogers DF. Mucus hypersecretion in asthma: intracellular signalling pathways as targets for pharmacotherapy. *Curr Opin Allergy Clin Immunol.* (2010) 10:67–76. doi: 10.1097/ACI.0b013e328334643a
44. Booth BW, Adler KB, Bonner JC, Tournier F, Martin LD. Interleukin-13 induces proliferation of human airway epithelial cells *in vitro* via a mechanism mediated by transforming growth factor-α. *Am J Respirat Cell Mol Biol.* (2001) 25:739–43. doi: 10.1165/ajrcmb.25.6.4659
45. Burgel PR, Lazarus SC, Tam DCW, Ueki IF, Atabai K, Birch M, et al. Human eosinophils induce mucin production in airway epithelial cells via epidermal growth factor receptor activation. *J Immunol.* (2001) 167:5948–54. doi: 10.4049/jimmunol.167.10.5948
46. Okumura S, Sagara H, Fukuda T, Saito H, Okayama Y. FcεRI-mediated amphiregulin production by human mast cells increases mucin gene expression in epithelial cells. *J Allergy Clin Immunol.* (2005) 115:272–9. doi: 10.1016/j.jaci.2004.10.004
47. Jorissen RN, Walker F, Pouliot N, Garrett TP, Ward CW, Burgess AW. Epidermal growth factor receptor: mechanisms of activation and signalling. *EGF Receptor Family.* (2003) 284:33–55. doi: 10.1016/B978-012160281-9/50004-9
48. Tyner JW, Kim EY, Ide K, Pelletier MR, Roswit WT, Morton JD, et al. Blocking airway mucous cell metaplasia by inhibiting EGFR antiapoptosis and IL-13 transdifferentiation signals. *J Clin Invest.* (2006) 116:309–21. doi: 10.1172/JCI25167
49. Boucherat O, Morissette MC, Provencher S, Bonnet S, Maltais F. Bridging lung development with chronic obstructive pulmonary disease. Relevance of developmental pathways in chronic obstructive pulmonary disease pathogenesis. *Am J Respirat Crit Care Med.* (2016) 193:362–75. doi: 10.1164/rccm.201508-1518PP
50. Guseh JS, Bores SA, Stanger BZ, Zhou Q, Anderson WJ, Melton DA, et al. Notch signaling promotes airway mucous metaplasia and inhibits alveolar development. *Development.* (2009) 136:1751–9. doi: 10.1242/dev.029249
51. Danahay H, Pessotti AD, Coote J, Montgomery BE, Xia D, Wilson A, et al. Notch2 is required for inflammatory cytokine-driven goblet cell metaplasia in the lung. *Cell Reports.* (2015) 10:239–52. doi: 10.1016/j.celrep.2014.12.017
52. Hao Y, Kuang Z, Walling BE, Bhatia S, Sivaguru M, Chen Y, et al. *Pseudomonas aeruginosa* pyocyanin causes airway goblet cell hyperplasia and metaplasia and mucus hypersecretion by inactivating the transcriptional factor FoxA2. *Cell Microbiol.* (2012) 14:401–15. doi: 10.1111/j.1462-5822.2011.01727.x
53. Hao Y, Kuang Z, Jing J, Miao J, Mei LY, Lee RJ, et al. *Mycoplasma pneumoniae* modulates STAT3-STAT6/EGFR-FOXA2 signaling to induce overexpression of airway mucins. *Infect Immunity.* (2014) 82:5246–55. doi: 10.1128/IAI.01989-14
54. Choi W, Yang AX, Waltenburg MA, Choe S, Steiner M, Radwan A, et al. FOXA2 depletion leads to mucus hypersecretion in canine airways with respiratory diseases. *Cell Microbiol.* (2018) 21:e12957. doi: 10.1111/cmi.12957
55. Helling BA, Gerber AN, Kadiyala V, Sasse SK, Pedersen BS, Sparks L, et al. Regulation of MUC5B expression in idiopathic pulmonary fibrosis. *Am J Respirat Cell Mol Biol.* (2017) 57:91–9. doi: 10.1165/rcmb.2017-0046OC
56. Lachowicz-Scroggins ME, Finkbeiner WE, Gordon E, Yuan S, Zlock L, Bhakta NR, et al. Corticosteroid and long-acting ß-agonist therapy reduces epithelial goblet cell metaplasia. *Clin Exp Allergy.* (2017) 47:1534–45. doi: 10.1111/cea.13015
57. Seibold MA, Wise AL, Speer MC, Steele MP, Brown KK, Loyd JE, et al. A common MUC5B promoter polymorphism and pulmonary fibrosis. *N Engl J Med.* (2011) 364:1503–12. doi: 10.1056/NEJMoa1013660
58. Park SW, Verhaeghe C, Nguyenvu LT, Barbeau R, Eisley CJ, Nakagami Y, et al. Distinct roles of FOXA2 and FOXA3 in allergic airway disease and asthma. *Am J Respirat Crit Care Med.* (2009) 180:603–10. doi: 10.1164/rccm.200811-1768OC
59. Du C, Lu J, Zhou L, Wu B, Zhou F, Gu L, et al. MAPK/FoxA2-mediated cigarette smoke-induced squamous metaplasia of bronchial epithelial cells. *Int J Chronic Obstruct Pulmonary Dis.* (2017) 12:3341. doi: 10.2147/COPD.S143279
60. Tunney MM, Einarsson GG, Wei L, Drain M, Klem ER, Cardwell C, et al. Lung microbiota and bacterial abundance in patients with bronchiectasis when clinically stable and during exacerbation. *Am J Respirat Crit Care Med.* (2013) 187:1118–26. doi: 10.1164/rccm.201210-1937OC
61. Wilson C, Jones P, O'leary C, Hansell D, Cole P, Wilson R. Effect of sputum bacteriology on the quality of life of patients with bronchiectasis. *Eur Respirat J.* (1997) 10:1754–60. doi: 10.1183/09031936.97.10081754
62. Kreuter M, Cottin V. The threat in chronic lung diseases: acute exacerbations. *Eur Respiratory Soc.* (2017) 26:170075. doi: 10.1183/16000617.0075-2017
63. Riquelme SA, Ahn D, Prince A. *Pseudomonas aeruginosa* and *Klebsiella pneumoniae* adaptation to innate immune clearance mechanisms in the lung. *J Innate Immunity.* (2018) 10:442–54. doi: 10.1159/000487515
64. Resiliac J, Grayson MH. Epidemiology of infections and development of asthma. *Immunol Allergy Clin.* (2019) 39:297–307. doi: 10.1016/j.iac.2019.03.001
65. Döring G, Parameswaran IG, Murphy TF. Differential adaptation of microbial pathogens to airways of patients with cystic fibrosis and chronic obstructive pulmonary disease. *FEMS Microbiol Rev.* (2011) 35:124–46. doi: 10.1111/j.1574-6976.2010.00237.x
66. Caldwell CC, Chen Y, Goetzmann HS, Hao Y, Borchers MT, Hassett DJ, et al. *Pseudomonas aeruginosa* exotoxin pyocyanin causes cystic fibrosis airway pathogenesis. *Am J Pathol.* (2009) 175:2473–88. doi: 10.2353/ajpath.2009.090166
67. Xu Y, Duan C, Kuang Z, Hao Y, Jeffries JL, Lau GW. *Pseudomonas aeruginosa* pyocyanin activates NRF2-ARE-mediated transcriptional response via the ROS-EGFR-PI3K-AKT/MEK-ERK MAP kinase signaling in pulmonary epithelial cells. *PLoS ONE.* (2013) 8:e72528. doi: 10.1371/journal.pone.0072528
68. Li JD, Feng W, Gallup M, Kim JH, Gum J, Kim Y, et al. Activation of NF- B via a Src-dependent Ras-MAPK-pp90rsk pathway is required for Pseudomonas aeruginosa-induced mucin overproduction in epithelial cells. *Proc Natl Acad Sci USA.* (1998) 95:5718–23. doi: 10.1073/pnas.95.10.5718
69. Mohamed FB, Garcia-Verdugo I, Medina M, Balloy V, Chignard M, Ramphal R, et al. A crucial role of Flagellin in the induction of airway mucus production by *Pseudomonas aeruginosa*. *PLoS ONE.* (2012) 7:e39888. doi: 10.1371/journal.pone.0039888
70. Mcnamara N, Khong A, Mckemy D, Caterina M, Boyer J, Julius D, et al. ATP transduces signals from ASGM1, a glycolipid that functions as a bacterial receptor. *Proc Natl Acad Sci USA.* (2001) 98:9086–91. doi: 10.1073/pnas.161290898
71. Kishioka C, Okamoto K, Hassett DJ, De Mello D, Rubin BK. *Pseudomonas aeruginosa* alginate is a potent secretagogue in the isolated ferret trachea. *Pediatric Pulmonol.* (1999) 27:174–9. doi: 10.1002/(SICI)1099-0496(199903)27:3<174::AID-PPUL4>3.0.CO;2-A
72. Klinger JD, Tandler B, Liedtke C, Boat T. Proteinases of *Pseudomonas aeruginosa* evoke mucin release by tracheal epithelium. *J Clin Invest.* (1984) 74:1669–78. doi: 10.1172/JCI111583

73. Jeffries JL, Jia J, Choi W, Choe S, Miao J, Xu Y, et al. *Pseudomonas aeruginosa* pyocyanin modulates mucin glycosylation with sialyl-Lewisx to increase binding to airway epithelial cells. *Mucosal Immunol.* (2015) 9:1039–50. doi: 10.1038/mi.2015.119
74. Ran H, Hassett DJ, Lau GW. Human targets of Pseudomonas aeruginosa pyocyanin. *Proc Natl Acad Sci USA.* (2003) 100:14315–20. doi: 10.1073/pnas.2332354100
75. Gardner PR. Superoxide production by the mycobacterial and pseudomonad quinoid pigments phthiocol and pyocyanine in human lung cells. *Arch Biochem Biophy.* (1996) 333:267–74. doi: 10.1006/abbi.1996.0390
76. O'malley YQ, Reszka KJ, Spitz DR, Denning GM, Britigan BE. Pseudomonas aeruginosa pyocyanin directly oxidizes glutathione and decreases its levels in airway epithelial cells. *Am J Physiol.* (2004) 287:L94–103. doi: 10.1152/ajplung.00025.2004
77. Lau GW, Hassett DJ, Ran H, Kong F. The role of pyocyanin in *Pseudomonas aeruginosa* infection. *Trends Mol Med.* (2004) 10:599–606. doi: 10.1016/j.molmed.2004.10.002
78. O'malley YQ, Reszka KJ, Rasmussen GT, Abdalla MY, Denning GM, Britigan BE. The Pseudomonas secretory product pyocyanin inhibits catalase activity in human lung epithelial cells. *Am J Physiol.* (2003) 285:L1077–86. doi: 10.1152/ajplung.00198.2003
79. Schwarzer C, Fischer H, Kim E-J, Barber KJ, Mills AD, Kurth MJ, et al. Oxidative stress caused by pyocyanin impairs CFTR Cl- transport in human bronchial epithelial cells. *Free Rad Biol Med.* (2008) 45:1653–62. doi: 10.1016/j.freeradbiomed.2008.09.011
80. Lau GW, Ran H, Kong F, Hassett DJ, Mavrodi D. *Pseudomonas aeruginosa* pyocyanin is critical for lung infection in mice. *Infect Immunity.* (2004) 72:4275–8. doi: 10.1128/IAI.72.7.4275-4278.2004
81. Wilson R, Sykes D, Watson D, Rutman A, Taylor G, Cole P. Measurement of *Pseudomonas aeruginosa* phenazine pigments in sputum and assessment of their contribution to sputum sol toxicity for respiratory epithelium. *Infect Immunity.* (1988) 56:2515–7. doi: 10.1128/IAI.56.9.2515-2517.1988
82. Hunter RC, Klepac-Ceraj V, Lorenzi MM, Grotzinger H, Martin TR, Newman DK. Phenazine content in the cystic fibrosis respiratory tract negatively correlates with lung function and microbial complexity. *Am J Respirat Cell Mol Biol.* (2012) 47:738–45. doi: 10.1165/rcmb.2012-0088OC
83. Forteza R, Lauredo IT, Burch R, Abraham WM. Extracellular metabolites of *Pseudomonas aeruginosa* produce bronchoconstriction by different mechanisms. *Am J Respirat Crit Care Med.* (1994) 149:687–93. doi: 10.1164/ajrccm.149.3.8118638
84. Munro N, Barker A, Rutman A, Taylor G, Watson D, Mcdonald-Gibson W, et al. Effect of pyocyanin and 1-hydroxyphenazine on *in vivo* tracheal mucus velocity. *J Appl Physiol.* (1989) 67:316–23. doi: 10.1152/jappl.1989.67.1.316
85. Dormehl I, Ras G, Taylor G, Hugo N. Effect of *Pseudomonas aeruginosa*-derived pyocyanin and 1-hydroxyphenazine on pulmonary mucociliary clearance monitored scintigraphically in the baboon model. *Int J Rad Appl Instrument B Nucl Med Biol.* (1991) 18:455–9. doi: 10.1016/0883-2897(91)90105-T
86. Rada B, Gardina P, Myers TG, Leto TL. Reactive oxygen species mediate inflammatory cytokine release and EGFR-dependent mucin secretion in airway epithelial cells exposed to Pseudomonas pyocyanin. *Mucos Immunol.* (2011) 4:158–71. doi: 10.1038/mi.2010.62
87. Vallath S, Hynds RE, Succony L, Janes SM, Giangreco A. Targeting EGFR signalling in chronic lung disease: therapeutic challenges and opportunities. *Eur Respiratory Soc.* (2014) 44:513–22. doi: 10.1183/09031936.00146413
88. Khavinson VK, Tendler S, Vanyushin B, Kasyanenko N, Kvetnoy I, Linkova N, et al. Peptide regulation of gene expression and protein synthesis in bronchial epithelium. *Lung.* (2014) 192:781–91. doi: 10.1007/s00408-014-9620-7
89. Viby NE, Isidor MS, Buggeskov KB, Poulsen SS, Hansen JB, Kissow H. Glucagon-like peptide-1 (GLP-1) reduces mortality and improves lung function in a model of experimental obstructive lung disease in female mice. *Endocrinology.* (2013) 154:4503–11. doi: 10.1210/en.2013-1666
90. Choi W, Choe S, Lin J, Borchers MT, Kosmider B, Vassallo R, et al. Exendin-4 restores airway mucus homeostasis through the GLP1R-PKA-PPARγ-FOXA2-phosphatase signaling. *Mucosal Immunol.* (in press). doi: 10.1038/s41385-020-0262-1
91. Dailey MJ, Moran TH. Glucagon-like peptide 1 and appetite. *Trends Endocrinol Metab.* (2013) 24:85–91. doi: 10.1016/j.tem.2012.11.008
92. Nasr SZ, Drury D. Appetite stimulants use in cystic fibrosis. *Pediatric Pulmonol.* (2008) 43:209–19. doi: 10.1002/ppul.20766
93. Rawal G, Yadav S. Nutrition in chronic obstructive pulmonary disease: a review. *J Transl Intern Med.* (2015) 3:151–4. doi: 10.1515/jtim-2015-0021

13

Evidence for the Effect of Vaccination on Host-Pathogen Interactions in a Murine Model of Pulmonary Tuberculosis by *Mycobacterium tuberculosis*

Zyanya Lucia Zatarain-Barrón [1], Octavio Ramos-Espinosa [1], Brenda Marquina-Castillo [1], Jorge Barrios-Payán [1], Fernanda Cornejo-Granados [2], Otoniel Maya-Lucas [3], Gamaliel López-Leal [2], Camilo Molina-Romero [1], Richard M. Anthony [4], Adrián Ochoa-Leyva [2], Inti Alberto De La Rosa-Velázquez [5], Rosa Gloria Rebollar-Vega [5], Robin M. Warren [6], Dulce Adriana Mata-Espinosa [1], Rogelio Hernández-Pando [1*] and Dick van Soolingen [4]*

[1] Experimental Pathology Laboratory, Department of Pathology, Instituto Nacional de Ciencias Médicas y Nutrición "Salvador Zubirán", Mexico City, Mexico, [2] Departamento de Microbiología Molecular, Instituto de Biotecnología, Universidad Nacional Autónoma de México, Cuernavaca, Mexico, [3] Department of Genetics and Molecular Biology, Centro de Investigaciones y de Estudios Avanzados (CINVESTAV), Mexico City, Mexico, [4] Tuberculosis Reference Laboratory, National Institute for Public Health and the Environment (RIVM), Bilthoven, Netherlands, [5] Genomics Laboratory, Red de Apoyo a la Investigación (RAI), Universidad Nacional Autónoma de México – Instituto Nacional de Ciencias Médicas y Nutrición "Salvador Zubirán", Mexico City, Mexico, [6] Division of Molecular Biology and Human Genetics, Department of Biomedical Sciences DST/NRF Centre of Excellence for Biomedical Tuberculosis Research, MRC Centre for Molecular and Cellular Biology, Faculty of Health Sciences, Stellenbosch University, Tygerberg, South Africa

***Correspondence:**
Dulce Adriana Mata-Espinosa
dulmat@yahoo.com.mx
Rogelio Hernández-Pando
rhdezpando@hotmail.com

The global control of Tuberculosis remains elusive, anc Bacillus Calmette-Guérin (BCG) -the most widely used vaccine in history—has proven insufficient for reversing this epidemic. Several authors have suggested that the mass presence of vaccinated hosts might have affected the *Mycobacterium tuberculosis* (MTB) population structure, and this could in turn be reflected in a prevalence of strains with higher ability to circumvent BCG-induced immunity, such as the recent Beijing genotype. The effect of vaccination on vaccine-escape variants has been well-documented in several bacterial pathogens; however the effect of the interaction between MTB strains and vaccinated hosts has never been previously described. In this study we show for the first time the interaction between MTB Beijing-genotype strains and BCG-vaccinated hosts. Using a well-controlled murine model of progressive pulmonary tuberculosis, we vaccinated BALB/c mice with two different sub-strains of BCG (BCG-Phipps and BCG-Vietnam). Following vaccination, the mice were infected with either one of three selected MTB strains. Strains were selected based on lineage, and included two Beijing-family clinical isolates (strains 46 and 48) and a well-characterized laboratory strain (H37Rv). Two months after infection, mice were euthanized and the bacteria extracted from their lungs. We characterized the genomic composite of the bacteria before and after exposure to vaccinated hosts, and also characterized the local response to the bacteria by sequencing the lung transcriptome in animals during the infection. Results from this study show that the interaction within the lungs of the vaccinated hosts results in the selection of higher-virulence bacteria, specifically for the Beijing genotype strains 46 and 48. After exposure to the BCG-induced immune response, strains 46 and 48 acquire genomic mutations associated with several virulence factors. As a result, the bacteria collected from these vaccinated hosts have an increased ability for immune evasion, as shown in both the host transcriptome and the histopathology studies, and replicates far more efficiently compared to bacteria collected from unvaccinated hosts or to the original-stock strain. Further research is warranted to ascertain the pathways associated with the genomic alterations. However, our results highlight novel host-pathogen interactions induced by exposure of MTB to BCG vaccinated hosts.

Keywords: tuberculosis, BCG vaccination, Beijing genotype, virulence, lung transcriptome

INTRODUCTION

In 1921 the Bacillus Calmette-Guérin (BCG) vaccine, constituting of viable but attenuated *Mycobacterium bovis* bacteria, was introduced as the first and so far only tuberculosis (TB) preventive vaccine approved by the World Health Organization (WHO) (1). However, despite billions of individuals having been vaccinated in the past century, TB continues to pose a serious threat to global health. Recently, the WHO reported that TB accounts for ~10 million incident cases, 44% of which are concentrated in the South-East Asian region (2). Furthermore, TB is presently the most deadly infectious disease due to a single pathogen.

The BCG vaccine has been outstandingly successful in preventing severe forms of tuberculosis (meningeal and miliary). Nonetheless, the vaccine presents considerable shortcomings in terms of preventing pulmonary tuberculosis, with a considerable variability in efficacy, ranging from 0 to 75% in different regions of the world (3, 4). Hypotheses to explain this remarkable heterogeneity in efficacy include flaws in the design of long-term studies, genomic differences between the BCG daughter strains, and that BCG protection may differ by *Mycobacterium tuberculosis* (MTB) genotype (5–7). Indeed, the distribution of MTB genotypes differs significantly by geographic area (8), if BCG vaccination protects against some, but not all genotypes to the same extent (9) this may contribute to the success of specific genotypes. If so, there would be an ongoing selection of MTB genotypes with an increased ability to circumvent BCG-induced immunity, particularly in high prevalence countries with high vaccination coverage (5).

The most studied in this respect is the Beijing genotype (recently re-named Lineage 2), highly prevalent in South East Asia, the former Soviet Union, and South Africa (10, 11). The Beijing genotype is part of the modern MTB lineage, and is represented by often genetically highly conserved, widespread strains (12, 13). Moreover, Beijing strains have been significantly associated with the spread of multidrug resistant (MDR)-TB, although recent reports from patients in the Beijing area have challenged previous studies (14–16). Several studies have indicated Beijing strains may have selective advantages over other genotypes; they are more prevalent in young patients, and show high clonality, suggesting ongoing transmission, and are associated with rapid disease progression and unfavorable treatment outcomes (17–19). Moreover, studies in mice have shown that BCG vaccination protects less efficiently against infection by Beijing strains compared with other genotypes, and this impediment to the efficacy of BCG has been linked to a decrease in effector immunity in subjects infected by Beijing-genotype strains (20, 21).

Other factors may also come into play when dissecting the reasons behind the fact that vaccination alone as a prophylactic strategy has not been enough to reverse the TB epidemic. One such factor is the effect of vaccinated hosts on a microorganism's population structure. This effect has been described previously, particularly for "imperfect vaccines," which act by reducing the growth rate of a microorganism within a host, rather than preventing the infection process and spread to new humans (22). In such cases, higher vaccine coverage would consequentially more efficiently eliminate less virulent forms, driving the selection of microorganisms with a higher degree of virulence. These vaccine-adapted bacteria would possess competitive advantages compared with wild-type bacteria, potentially in both vaccine-naïve and vaccinated individuals (22).

In this study, we hypothesize that exposure to BCG-induced immunity may select vaccine-escape microorganism variants with a higher capacity for disease breakdown. If so, MTB bacilli would increase their virulence, as a function of changes in their genetic makeup, after exposure to BCG-induced immunity in vaccinated hosts. We tested this hypothesis in a syngeneic BALB/c mouse model of progressive pulmonary tuberculosis, by comparing the virulence of two Beijing genotype strains (and control strain H37Rv) before and after passage through BCG-vaccinated and non-vaccinated mice. The course of the disease in terms of pulmonary bacillary loads determined by colony forming units [CFUs]/mL, histopathology assessment of lung tissue and survival curves were used as parameters.

METHODS

MTB Strain Selection and Culture Conditions

An overview of the experimental design is portrayed in **Figure 1**. Strains were selected from a collection of clinical isolates from different regions of the world, considering diverse factors for strain selection including genotype and having been previously characterized using a murine model (23) (**Table 1**).

Stock bacteria from the selected strains (namely strains 1 [laboratory strain H37Rv; Euro-American lineage], 46 and 48 [Beijing lineage]) were grown in Middlebrook 7H9 broth (Difco Laboratories, Detroit, MI, USA) supplemented with glycerol, Tween-80, and OADC enrichment (containing oleic acid, albumin, dextrose, and catalase) at 35°C, 75 RPM. All cultures were monitored for optic density and obtained at mid log-phase. Bacterial viability was assessed using the LIVE/DEAD BacLight Bacterial Viability Kit (Invitrogen, Eugene, OR) for flow cytometry, following manufacturer's instructions. Briefly, liquid cultures were centrifuged at 10,000 × g for 15 min. The supernatant was removed and the pellet was re-suspended in 2 mL of 0.85% NaCl. One mL of this suspension was added to a new 50 mL tube containing 20 mL of 0.85% NaCl, and incubated at room temperature for 1 h. The sample was centrifuged at 10,000 × g for 15 min and re-suspended in 20 mL of 0.85% NaCl and centrifuged at 10,000 × g in order to remove any traces of growth medium. The pellet was re-suspended in a separate tube with 10 mL of 0.85% NaCl and 1 mL of this suspension was used for assessment of optic density using a spectrophotometer at 600 nm (OD600). The suspension was diluted 1:100 in filtered, sterile water and from this stock solution different dilutions were prepared in cytometer-compatible tubes in a total volume of 2 mL. Using a microfuge tube, a mixture was prepared with 35 μL

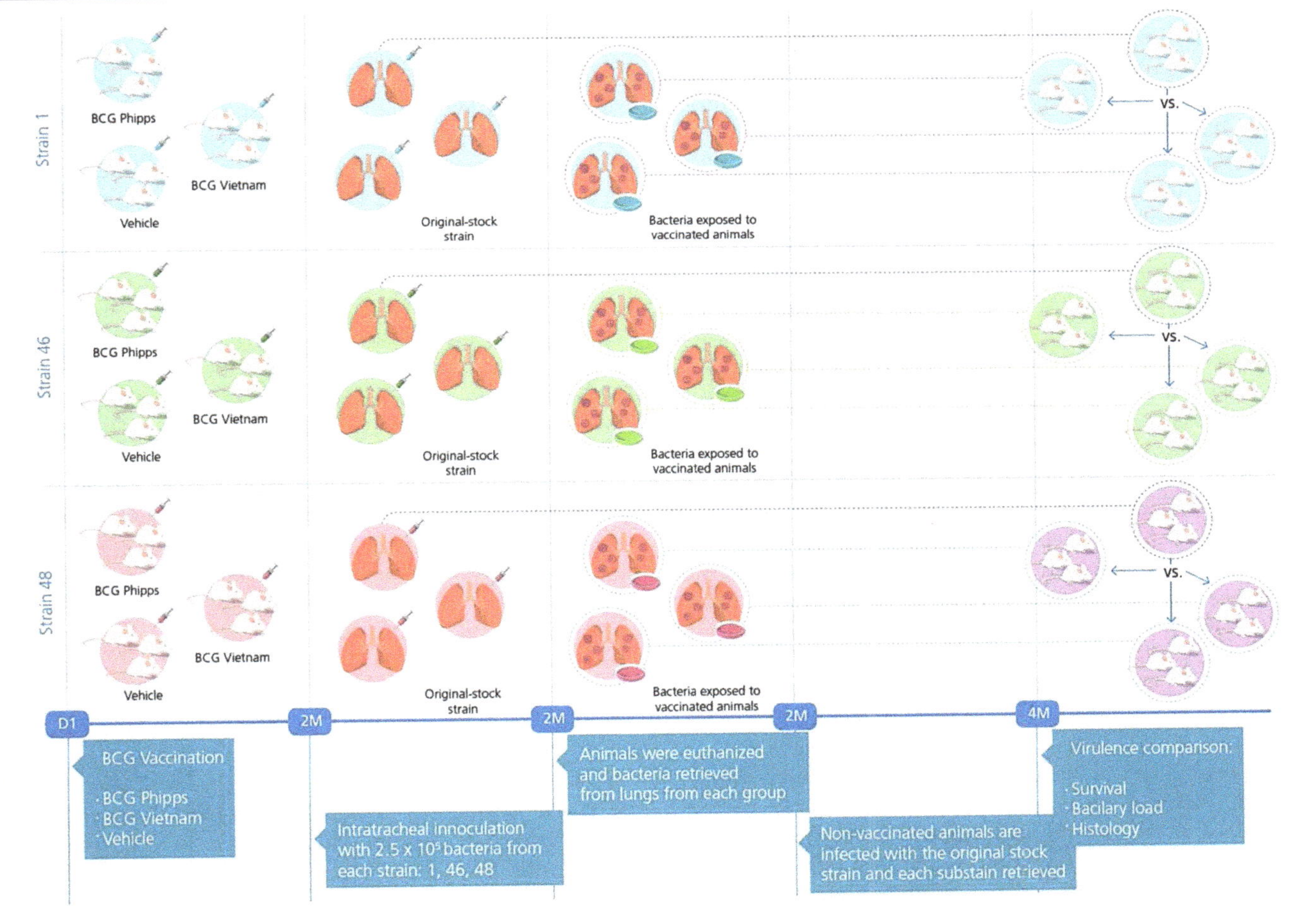

FIGURE 1 | Experimental strategy.

TABLE 1 | Bacterial strains selected for experimentation.

Code	Species	Genotype/code	Lineage	Country of origin	Cluster size
1	*M. tuberculosis*	Euro American	4	United States	n/a (reference strain H37Rv)
46	*M. tuberculosis*	Beijing Typical (2002-1612)	2	Vietnam	4
48	*M. tuberculosis*	Beijing Atypical Sublineage-1 (2697)	2	South Africa	1

of component A and 35 μL of component B. We added 6 μl of this mixture to each sample and mixed by pipetting. The mixture was incubated in the dark for 15 min at room temperature. Data were acquired using a cytometer using standard procedures. The kit contains both SYTO9 stain and propidium iodide, therefore bacteria are labeled red when dead and green when alive. All MTB strains were required to have >90% live cells in order to be stored and used for animal experimentation. Each strain was plated in serial dilutions in Middlebrook 7H10 agar in order to count the Colony Forming Units (CFUs) per mL and then stored at −80°C in individual aliquots.

Exposure of Original-Stock Bacteria to the Immune System of BCG-Vaccinated Mice

Groups of five male BALB/c mice 6–8 weeks old were immunized subcutaneously with either one of two different sub strains of BCG (BCG Phipps or BCG Vietnam, 8,000 live bacilli suspended in 50 μl PBS), for a control group, a third group of five mice received a subcutaneous injection of the vehicle solution, Phosphate-Buffered Saline (PBS). Two months post-immunization the mice in each group were challenged with the selected strains (1, 46, and 48) through the intratracheal route. Briefly, each mouse was anesthetized with sevofluorane in a gas chamber, immobilized and inoculated intratracheally using a stainless steel cannula with 0.1 mL of PBS containing 2.5 × 10^5 live bacteria. Mice were kept in vertical position until they fully recovered. Infected mice were kept in cages fitted with micro-isolators in groups of ≤ six animals per cage. All animal procedures were performed according to the national regulations on animal care and experimentation (NOM 062-ZOO-1999) after approval by the Animal Experimentation Committee at the National Institute of Medical Sciences and Nutrition México (PAT-1860-16/18-1).

Two months after challenge with bacterial strains, mice were euthanized by exsanguination while under anesthesia; lungs were extracted and immediately snap-frozen in liquid nitrogen. Each lung was homogenized in PBS-Tween-80 0.05% and serial dilutions were cultured in Middlebrook 7H10 agar medium at 37°C with 5% CO_2. Plates were reviewed every week to check for bacilli colony growth. Following 2–3 weeks (2 weeks for H37Rv, 3 weeks for both Beijing strains) after plating, three colonies were placed in 7H9 medium for colony growth and in blood-agar plates in order to ascertain MTB purity. Purity was also assessed at all time points further whenever the bacterial stocks were manipulated by plating a sample in blood-agar, and performing a Ziehl-Neelsen stain and gram stain in order to identify only ziehl-neelsen positive bacteria in all the samples. Any samples in which other microorganisms grew within the blood-agar or were identified using gram staining were disposed of accordingly. A total of three sub strains from each original strain were obtained from vaccinated and control animals: the first one was obtained from mice immunized with BCG Phipps, the second one from mice immunized with BCG Vietnam, and the third one from non-vaccinated, control mice. Growth curves were constructed with each of these sub strains (each assigned a suffix letter P, V, or S in order to reflect whether they had passed through mice vaccinated with BCG-Phipps [P], BCG-Vietnam [V], or Saline-control [S]) and bacilli were collected at the log-phase. All collected bacilli were assessed for viability as previously described. Following, they were seeded in Middlebrook 7H10 agar in serial dilutions in order to count the number of CFUs per mL and stored at −80°C.

Virulence Assessment

Tubes containing bacteria collected from all experimental groups (P, V, S) as well as the original-stock strain were thawed at 37°C and prepared in order to infect groups of 50 naïve, non-vaccinated, BALB/c mice following the same procedure previously described. Once infected, mice were monitored and then euthanized following the model of progressive pulmonary TB, which has been extensively described elsewhere (24). Briefly, five mice per group were euthanized by exsanguination after total anesthesia at days 1, 3, 7, 14, 21, 28, 60, and 120 following infection. Lungs from euthanized animals were extracted and stored according to their future use: 4 lungs were snap-frozen in liquid nitrogen for future CFU-assessment; 3 lungs were snap-frozen in liquid nitrogen for future RNA extraction; 3 lungs were instilled by the trachea with ethyl alcohol and stored in ethyl alcohol-filled tubes for histopathology evaluation. Methods for these assessments have been extensively reviewed elsewhere (25). Two independent experiments were performed with each set of strains.

Evaluation of Lung Bacillary Load Through CFU

The right lung from four of the euthanized animals in each time point was quickly removed after exsanguination and snap-frozen in liquid nitrogen. Lungs were progressively unfrozen and homogenized with a polytron (Kinematica, Lucerne, Switzerland) in tubes containing 1 ml PBS, Tween-80 0.05%. Dilutions of each homogenate were seeded in plates containing 7H10 medium. The plates were placed in incubators at 37°C with 5% CO_2 for 3 weeks. The number of colonies was counted and extrapolated to show data as number of CFU per mL of lung tissue.

Preparation of Lung Tissue for Histopathology Studies

The left lung from three of the euthanized animals in each time point was perfused through the trachea with ethyl alcohol (J:T Baker, Mexico City, México). Lungs were then dehydrated and embedded in paraffin, 4 μm sections were obtained and stained with haematoxylin and eosin in order to evaluate lung pathology. Histopathological parameters evaluated in this study included pneumonia (expressed as percentage of lung area affected); necrosis (expressed as percentage of lung area affected); average number of granulomas per lung ($n = 3$) and average size of granulomas (in μm^2). Definitions for each parameter have been previously established in this murine model, briefly pneumonia is defined as areas with inflammatory infiltrate that occupied alveolar lumens and alveolar-capillary interstitium. For the quantification of the area of granulomas, all the granulomas [defined as well-delimited nodular aggregates of lymphocytes and macrophages that can include dendritic cells and fibroblasts formed in response to persistent TB infection (24, 26)] were blind measured by a well-trained pathologist in the whole slide at 400X magnification. Necrosis was defined as Areas with total tissue architecture destruction with abundant cellular eosinophilic cytoplasmic debris, along with fragmented or karyorrhectic nuclei. Data is reported as the mean values ± SD from three different subjects at each time-point. All parameters were assessed using an automated image analyzer (QWin Leica, Milton Keynes, Cambridge, UK).

Statistical Analysis for Virulence Parameters

In order to determine statistical significance in the bacillary load and the histopathology studies we compared groups using a 2-way ANOVA followed by a Bonferroni posttest in order to determine significant differences among the groups ($p < 0.05$ was considered significant). The survival curves were evaluated using a Log-Rank test in order to find differences between the curves along the duration of the study. Each survival analysis was performed with 50 subjects per group, a total of 200 subjects per experimental set of strains (subjects were censured from the survival analysis at the time of euthanasia). All the statistical analysis was performed using GraphPad Prism Software (version 6.0, La Jolla, USA).

NGS-Sequencing and Bioinformatics

Bacterial gDNA was extracted from liquid cultures and libraries were constructed using the Illumina TruSeq DNA PCR-Free library prep kit (Illumina, San Diego USA, Cat. No. 20015962). Libraries were constructed starting with 2 µg of gDNA and sequenced in paired-end version (2 × 150 bases) using an Illlumina NextSeq500 equipment at the Biotechnology Institute (IBT, Cuernavaca, Mexico). A Beijing-genotype genome NITR203 (RefSeq: NC_021054.1) recently curated by the NCBI was used as a reference strain. Raw sequences were filtered and low quality reads were deleted using Trimmomatic (v 0.33) (27). As previously reported for Beijing-genomes, CLC Genomics Workbench version 10 was used in order to assemble the 4 sequenced strains. Details regarding genome assembly can be found in **Supplementary Table 1**.

In order to call variants, the Snippy V4.3.6 program was used, with the default setting. Following, the genome was annotated using Prokka (default settings) v1.13 (28). Variants were initially identified between each of the sequenced strains and the reference Beijing genome NITR203. All the variants which were shared between the original-stock strain and the vaccine-exposed strains when comparing with the reference strain were filtered out, and only those variants which were unique to the original-stock strain or to the vaccine-exposed strain were considered biologically relevant for comparison purposes. Unique variants were compared between the original strains and the vaccine-exposed strains which presented a virulence increase (46 vs. 46P, 48 vs. 48V). Further, variants were compared between the two vaccine-exposed strains (46P vs. 48V).

For RNAseq, RNA was extracted from lungs of infected mice at day 21 post-infection and quantified using Qubit; quality was assessed using a Bioanalyzer. Only samples with an RNA integrity number (RIN) >8.0 were used. Libraries were constructed using 1 µg of each RNA sample, using the TruSeq stranded mRNA kit (Illumina, San Diego, USA, 20020594). Libraries were sequenced in single end version (125 bases) in an Illumina HiSeq2500 equipment at the RAI (RAI, Mexico City, Mexico). Raw sequences were trimmed using Trimmomatic (v 0.33) (27). Following, reads were mapped using BWA_MEM (29), against the *Mus musculus* reference genome (GCA_000001635.8 GRCm38.p6). The read count was performed using htseq (30). The differential gene expression (DGE) was assessed using the bioconductor package DESeq2 (version 3.7) (31). The GO (Gene Ontology (GO) enrichment analysis for differentially regulated genes, which considers the functional hierarchy of the differentially expressed genes) and KEGG enrichment were evaluated using WebGestalt (32).

RESULTS

Virulence Assessment

Survival Rate

In order to test whether immunization exerted a change in the virulence in MTB bacilli exposed to vaccinated mice, groups of 50 naïve BALB/c mice were intratracheally infected with each of the following bacteria: original stock strain ($n = 50$), "P" strain ($n = 50$) isolated from the lungs of BCG Phipps vaccinated mice, "V" strain ($n = 50$) isolated from the lungs of BCG Vietnam vaccinated mice and control "S" strain ($n = 50$) isolated from the lungs of sham-vaccinated, control mice. Survival rates for animals infected with strain 1 (reference strain H37Rv) and vaccine-exposed variants (1P, 1V, and 1S) showed no significant differences (**Supplementary Figure 1A**). In contrast, animals infected by vaccine immunity-exposed Beijing genotype strain 46P had a significantly decreased survival compared with the original-stock strain 46 ($p < 0.0001$) (**Figure 2A**). Similarly, in the case of Beijing genotype strains 48, 48P, 48V, and 48S, animals infected with vaccine-exposed strain 48V had a significantly decreased survival when compared with the original-stock strain 48 ($p < 0.0001$) (**Figure 2B**).

Pulmonary Bacillary Load

To further assess the virulence level of the original-stock strains in comparison with the vaccine-exposed strains, the presence of colony forming units (CFU) were compared in lungs from animals infected by original-stock bacilli and vaccine-exposed bacilli. Lungs from animals infected with Euro-American genotype laboratory strain 1 (H37Rv) and vaccine-exposed strains 1P, 1V, and 1S showed no significant difference in terms of bacillary load on days 1, 3, 7, 21, 28, 60, and 120 post-infection (**Supplementary Figure 1B**), although we observed a four times lower bacillary load in lungs collected from animals infected by strain 1 (4.5×10^6 CFU/mL lung homogenate) compared with those infected by strain 1V (17.4×10^6 CFU/mL homogenate) on day 14 post-infection ($p < 0.01$). This difference did not correlate with survival or histological damage (**Supplementary Figure 1C**). However, in the case of Beijing strains 46, 46P, 46V, and 46S, we observed a significant difference in bacillary load at day 21 post infection when comparing lungs

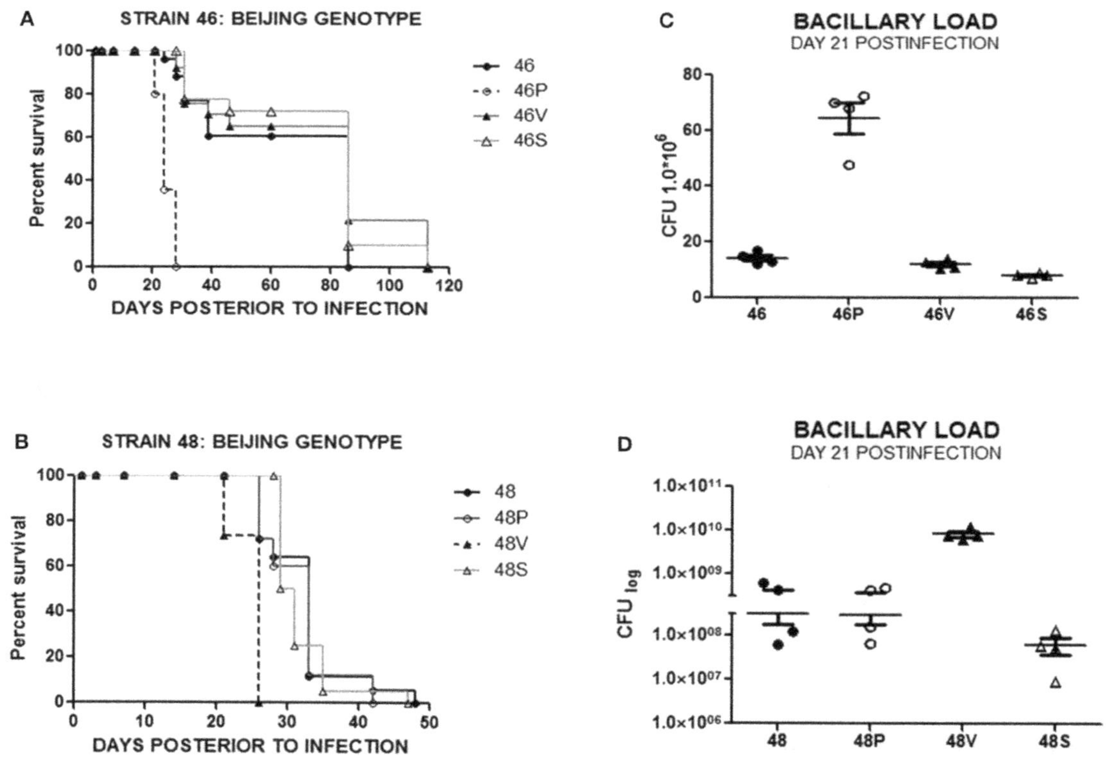

FIGURE 2 | (A) Survival rate for animals infected with strains 46, 46P, 46V, and 46 S ($n = 50$ subjects/strain). **(B)** Survival rate for animals infected with strains 48, 48P, 48V, and 48S ($n = 50$ subjects/strain). **(C)** Bacillary load in lungs from animals infected with strains 46, 46P, 46V, and 46S at day 21 postinfection. **(D)** Bacillary load in lungs from animals infected with strains 48, 48P, 48V, and 48S at day 21 postinfection.

obtained from animals infected by the original strain 46 (1.4×10^7 CFU/mL lung homogenate) and those infected with strain 46P (6.5×10^7 CFU/mL lung homogenate) at day 21 post-infection ($p < 0.001$) (**Figure 2C**). Similarly, Beijing-genotype strain 48 had a significantly lower bacillary load (3.1×10^8 CFU/mL lung homogenate) compared with vaccine-exposed strain 48V (8.3×10^9 CFU/mL lung homogenate) at day 21 post-infection ($p < 0.01$) (**Figure 2D**).

Histopathological Damage

The third virulence parameter evaluated was histopathological damage. Animals infected by strain H37Rv (Euro-American lineage) strain 1 and vaccine-exposed 1P, 1V, and 1S had pneumonia-type damage, which appeared at day 21 post-infection and increased throughout days 28, 60, and 120 post-infection. A significant difference in lung area affected by pneumonia was observed on day 120 between the original-stock strain 1 (52.6%) and the vaccine-exposed strain 1P (78.6%) ($p < 0.05$); nonetheless, this difference did not correlate with other parameters for evaluating virulence (**Supplementary Figure 1C**).

In correlation with the previously described parameters, animals infected by Beijing-genotype strains generally developed more pulmonary necrosis. Moreover, animals infected by strain 46 and vaccine-exposed strain 46P had a significantly different lung damage pattern (**Figure 3**). First, animals infected by vaccine-exposed strain 46P developed pneumonia earlier throughout the course of the disease, with initial small pneumonic areas appearing as early as day 14 postinfection compared with strain 46 (9.8 vs. 0%; $p < 0.001$), and gradually increasing throughout day 21 (20.9 vs. 13.2%; $p < 0.01$) and 28 (65.5 vs. 60.5%; $p > 0.05$) postinfection (**Figure 3A**). Although by day 28 the area affected by pneumonia was similar between animals infected by both strains, in the case of animals infected by strain 46P, these pneumonic areas were mostly occupied by areas of pulmonary necrosis, with large areas occupied by cellular debris and fragmented cells, along with an intensely acidophilic material in the extracellular space. When this parameter was measured, animals infected by strain 46P had a significantly larger lung percentage affected by necrosis at day 21 (11.6 vs. 2.5%; $p < 0.05$) and 28 (46.6 vs. 4.9%; $p < 0.001$) post-infection (**Figure 3B**). We also quantified the number and size of granulomas in animals infected by strains 46 and 46P (the strains which had showed significant differences in other virulence parameters) and identified that animals infected by vaccine-exposed strain 46P developed granulomas later compared with those infected with original strain 46 (average number of granulomas at days 7 [2 vs. 0; $p < 0.05$]; 14 [18.3 vs. 4.3; $p < 0.001$]; 21 [6.3 vs. 6.3; $p > 0.05$]; and 28 [3.0 vs. 1.3; $p > 0.05$]) (**Figure 3C**). Additionally, the size of the granulomas

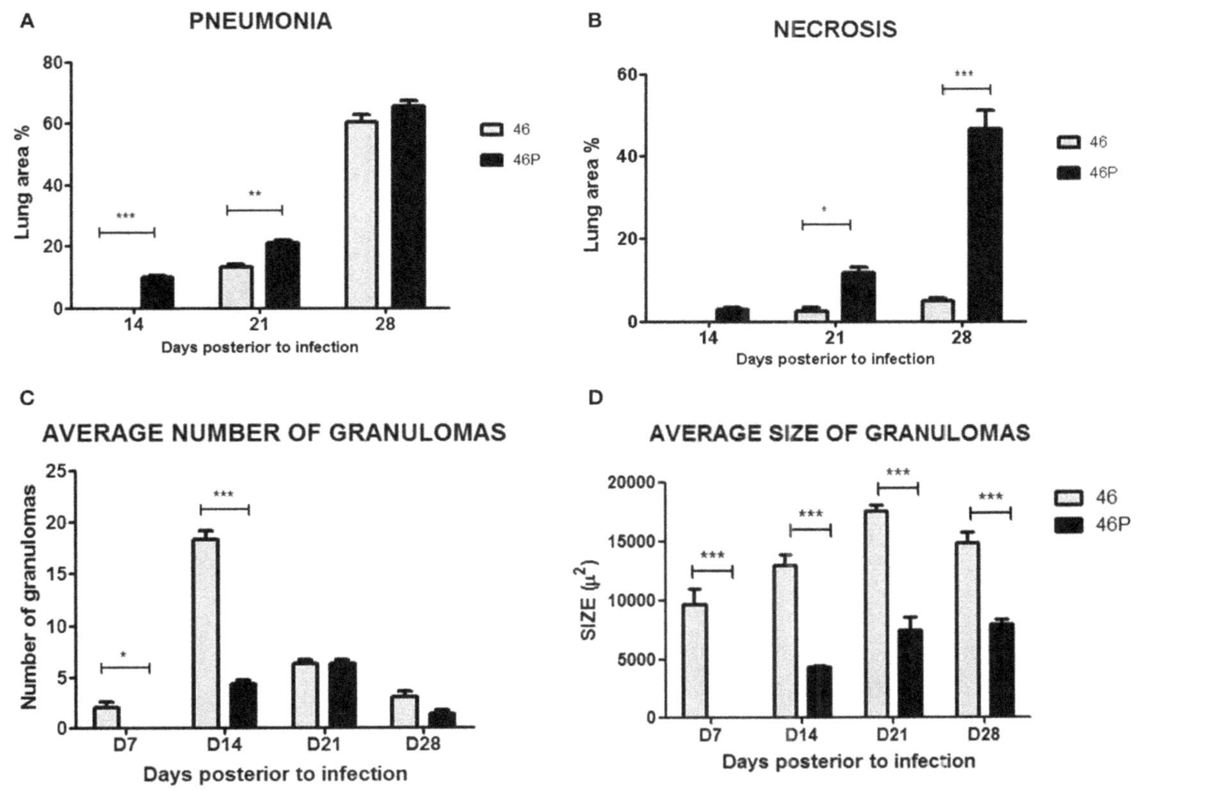

FIGURE 3 | (A) Lung area affected by pneumonia in animals infected by strain 46 and 46P. **(B)** Lung area affected by necrosis in animals infected by strain 46 and 46P. **(C)** Average number of granulomas in animals infected by strain 46 and 46P. **(D)** Average size of granulomas in animals infected by strains 46 and 46P. *$p<0.05$, **$p < 0.01$, ***$p < 0.001$.

was significantly smaller in animals infected by strain 46P compared with those infected with strain 46 (average size of granulomas at days 7 [9655.6 vs. 0%; $p < 0.001$]; 14 [12977.6 vs. 4324.0%; $p < 0.001$]; 21 [17522.4 vs. 7423.4%; $p < 0.001$]; and 28 [14915.4 vs. 7970.0%; $p < 0.001$]) (**Figure 3D**). Representative images of the areas of necrosis, pneumonia and of granulomas in animals infected by strains 46 and 46P can be found in **Figures 4, 5**.

The histological parameters in animals infected by Beijing-genotype strain 48 and vaccine-exposed strains 48P, 48V, and 48S were similar to those identified in the experiments with strain 46. Animals infected by vaccine-exposed strain 48V developed pneumonia earlier and with more extensive lung area compromised compared with animals infected by strain 48 [days 14 [2.2 vs. 0%]; 21 [44.9 vs. 27.8%; $p < 0.05$]; 28 [animals infected by strain 48V all suffered spontaneous death by this day vs. 43.2%] postinfection, respectively] (**Figure 6A**). In terms of necrosis, animals infected by strain 48V developed small areas of necrosis by day 14 postinfection (0.5 vs. 0%; $p > 0.05$), which were significantly greater by day 21 postinfection compared with those found in animals infected by strain 48 (42.9 vs. 8.4%; $p < 0.001$) (**Figure 6B**). This comparison cannot be made for day 28 postinfection since all animals infected by strain 48V had been deceased by this day. Similar to strain 46P, animals infected by vaccine-exposed strain 48V had a statistically significantly smaller number and average size of granulomas throughout the course of the infection (**Figures 6C,D**). Representative images of the areas of necrosis, pneumonia and of granulomas in animals infected by strains 48 and 48V can be found in **Figure 7** (animals infected with strain 48V all suffered spontaneous death before day 28 postinfection, therefore no images are available for the animals at this time point during the kinetics of the experiment).

Transcriptomic Profile

Among those bacteria which showed a significantly different disease phenotype from the virulence experiments (46 vs. 46P; 48 vs. 48V) we isolated RNA from the lungs of animals at day 21 postinfection (this day in both cases showed the highest difference in terms of survival, lung bacillary load and histological damage between the aforementioned strains). We identified a total of 41 up-regulated genes in the mice infected by strain 46 compared with those infected by strain 46P at day 21 post-infection (**Supplementary Table 2**). Furthermore, a total of 45 up-regulated genes were identified in mice infected by strain 48 compared with those infected by strain 48V at day 21 post-infection (**Supplementary Table 3**). A total of 8 genes were down-regulated in animals infected by strain 46 compared with those infected by strain 46P (**Supplementary Table 4**) and 69 genes were downregulated in animals infected by strain 48 compared with those infected by

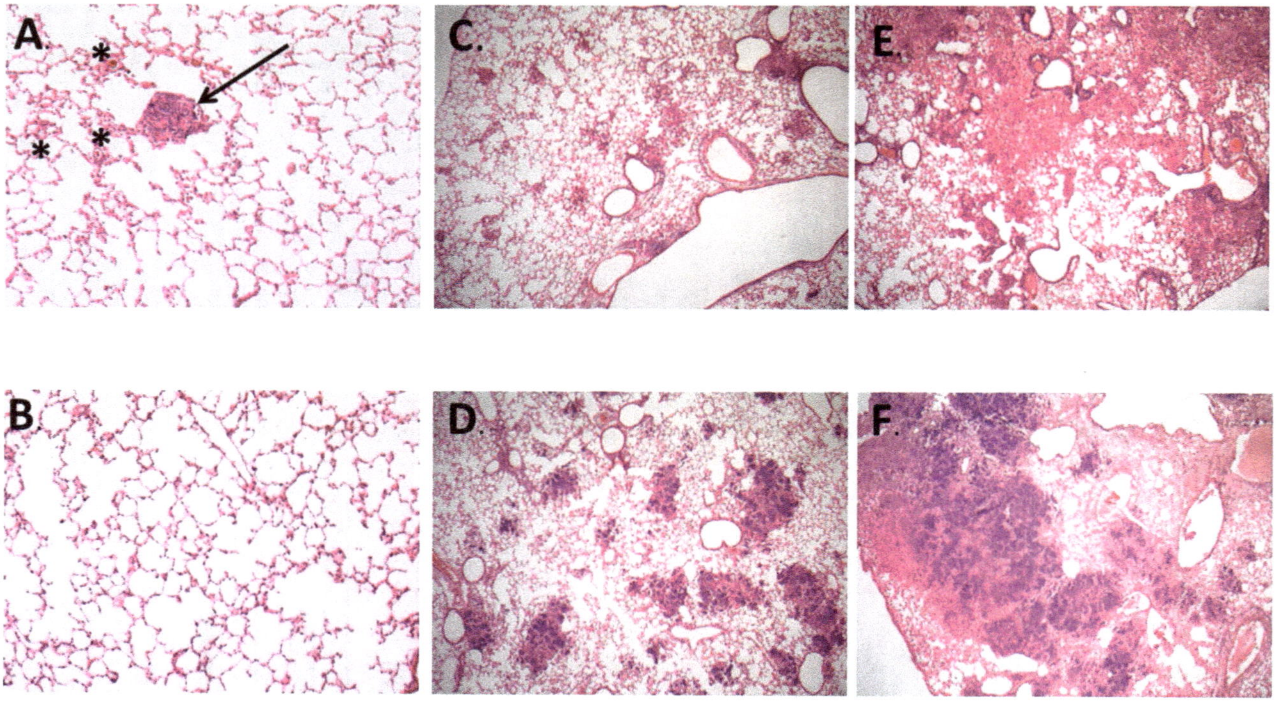

FIGURE 4 | Representative images of histopathological findings in animals infected by strain 46 and strain 46P. **(A)** Animals infected by strain 46 had early formation of granulomas (arrow) and interstitial inflammation, since day 7 post-infection (100X magnification). **(B)** Representative image of animals infected by strain 46P at day 7 postinfection, without formation of granulomas and very scarce if any interstitial inflammation (100X magnification). **(C)** On day 21 postinfection, animals infected by strain 46 had small pneumonic areas throughout the lung tissue (25X magnification). **(D)** Animals infected by strain 46P, instead, had larger pneumonic and necrotic areas by day 21 postinfection (25X magnification). **(E)** By day 28 postinfection, animals infected by strain 46 had larger, confluent pneumonic areas, with scarce areas with necrosis (25X magnification). **(F)** Contrary, animals infected by strain 46P had large areas of massive pulmonary necrosis which occupied most of the lung tissue (25X magnification). Stained with hematoxylin and eosin. * areas of interstitial inflammation.

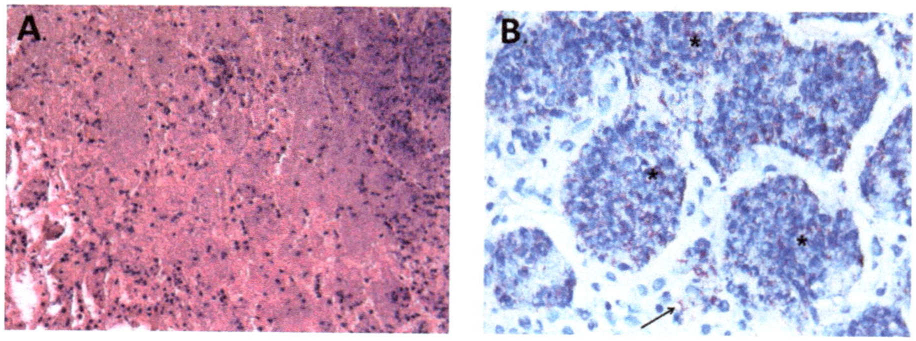

FIGURE 5 | (A) Representative image of pulmonary necrosis in animals infected by strain 46P on day 28 postinfection. The image shows the complete loss of pulmonary tissue architecture over large areas, with cellular debris, picnotic and fragmented nuclei and acidophilic material occupying the extracellular space (200X magnification). **(B)** Ziehl-Neelsen stain showing specific necrotic areas with the presence of large ammounts of acid-fast bacteria within the necrotic tissue (*) but also free in the interstitial space (arrow) (1000X magnification; stained with Ziehl-Neelsen).

strain 48V (**Supplementary Table 5**). Several biological processes were impacted with the up-regulation of genes relative to strains. For animals infected by strains 46 vs. 46P, up-regulated genes were significantly grouped in terms of immune-related processes, including genes related to immune response, leucocyte migration, leucocyte chemotaxis, response to stress, inflammatory response, acute inflammatory response, C-X-X chemokine binding, and interleukin-8 binding, among others (**Figure 8**). In the case of animals infected by strains 48 vs. 48V, up-regulated genes included those associated with immune processes, including immune system process, and immune response, leucocyte migration, positive regulation of leucocyte

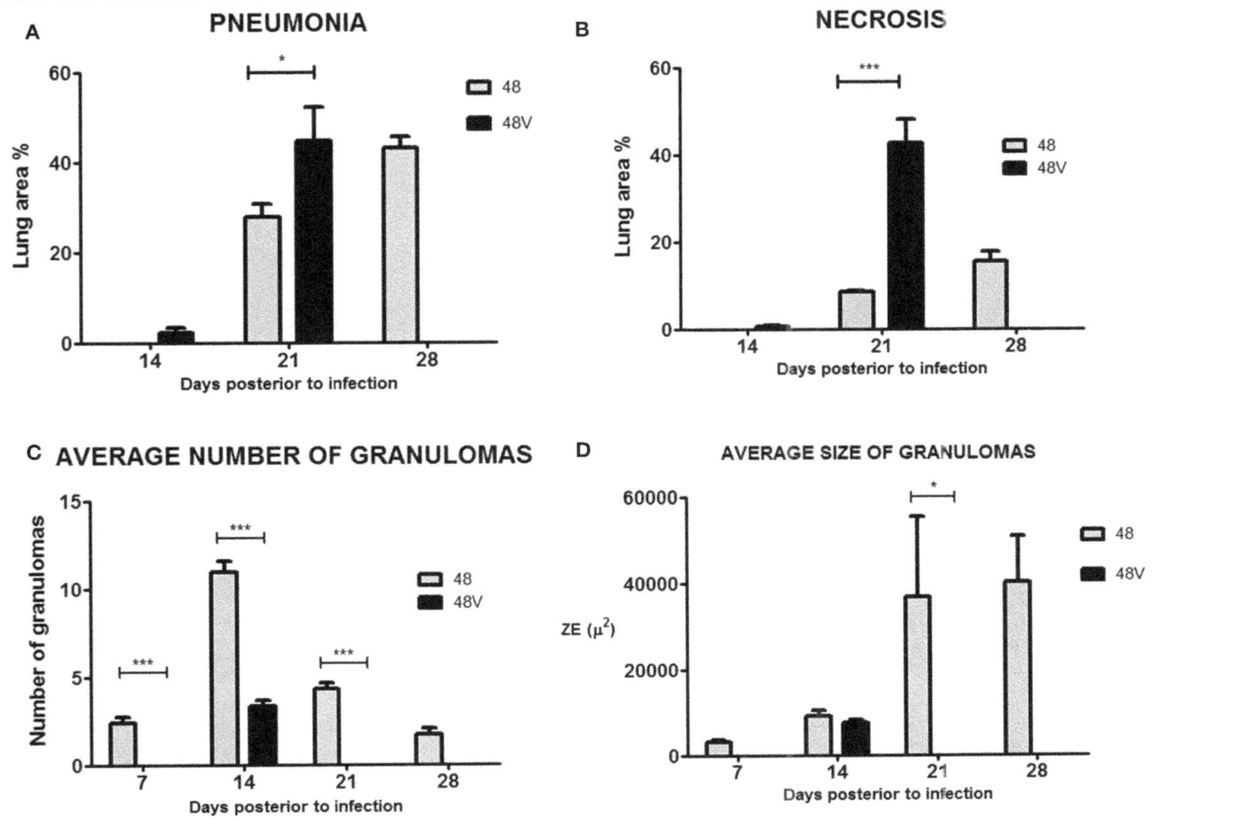

FIGURE 6 | (A) Lung area affected by pneumonia in animals infected by strain 48 and 48V. **(B)** Lung area affected by necrosis in animals infected by strain 48 and 48V. **(C)** Average number of granulomas in animals infected by strain 48 and 48V. **(D)** Average size of granulomas in animals infected by strains 48 and 48V. $^{*}p < 0.05$, $^{***}p < 0.001$.

activation, inflammatory response, and acute inflammatory response. Additionally other pathways were also enriched in the animals infected by these strains, including the up-regulation of collagen catabolic processes and lymph node development (**Figure 9**).

We identified several influenced pathways with differential gene expression in mice infected by the different Beijing-genotype bacilli. For animals infected with strain 46 vs. 46P, four pathways were enriched in terms of up-regulated genes (complement and coagulation cascades [$n = 4$]; cytokine-cytokine receptor interaction [$n = 5$]; hematopoietic cell lineage [$n = 3$]; and toll-like receptor signaling pathway [$n = 3$]). For animals infected by strains 48 vs. 48V, three pathways were enriched in terms of up-regulated genes (amoebiasis [$n = 3$]; cytokine-cytokine receptor interaction [$n = 4$]; and osteoclast differentiation [$n = 3$]). Interestingly, when comparing the animals infected by both bacterial sets (46 vs. 46P, 48 vs. 48V) we identified two up-regulated genes which were present in both cases. These included Glycoprotein-2 and Vanin-1.

Genomic Profile

When comparing the genome sequence from bacilli before and after passage through vaccinated mice, several mutations and other type of variants were observed. Variants were compared between the original strains and the vaccine-exposed strains (46 vs. 46P, 48 vs. 48V). Strain 46 had two unique mutations compared to strain 46P, while strain 46P had three mutations compared to strain 46. Strain 48 had five mutations compared to strain 48V, while strain 48V presented nine mutations compared to strain 48 (**Table 2**). Interestingly, when comparing the mutations present in both vaccine-exposed strains (46P vs. 48V) we identified one variant which was shared by both genomes. This variant was an inframe insertion present in a PE-family protein. The datasets for the sequenced genomes and lung transcriptomes in this project have been deposited as a Bioproject at NCBI and can be accessed through the project number PRJNA628024.

DISCUSSION

The WHO estimates that in the last two decades 43 million lives have been saved by improved TB control. Despite the encouraging data, we are still far from reaching the ambitious goals of the END-TB strategy, which include reducing global mortality attributable to TB by 95% in the year 2030. The current global trend shows only a 2% reduction in the number of TB deaths per year; however, a 17% yearly reduction would be required to achieve the WHO target. As such, it is strikingly clear

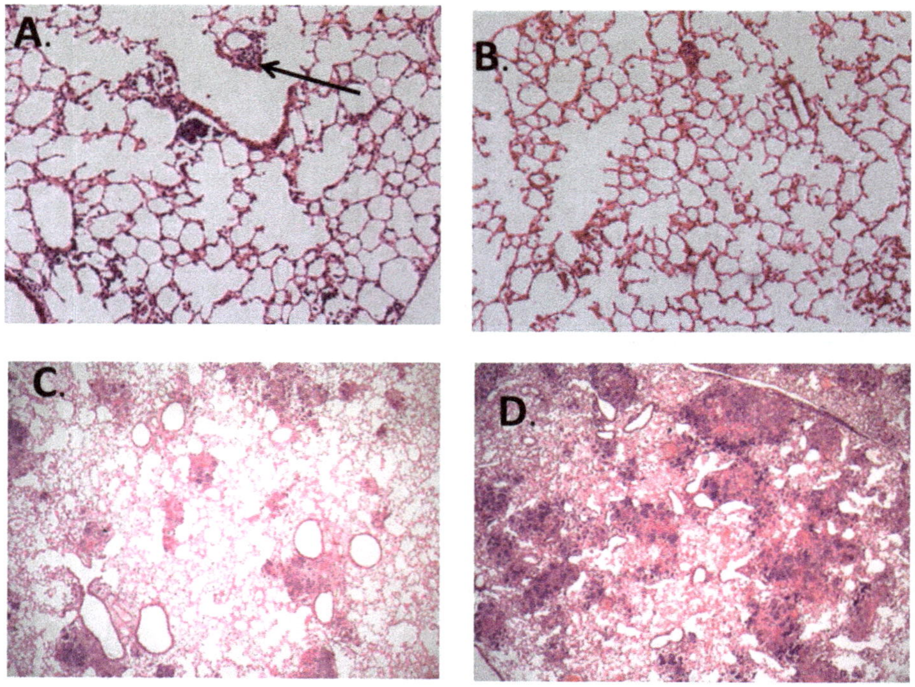

FIGURE 7 | Representative images of histopathological findings in animals infected by strain 48 and strain 48V. **(A)** Lung tissue from animal infected by strain 48 at day 14 postinfection, with formation of small granulomas and perivascular inflammation (arrow) (100X magnification). **(B)** Lung tissue from animal infected by strain 48V at day 14 postinfection shows scarce interstitial inflammation without granuloma formation (100X magnification). **(C)** Animals infected by strain 48 had small pneumonic and necrotic areas throughout the lung tissue by day 21 postinfection (25X magnification). **(D)** Animals infected by strain 48V developed large confluent areas of pulmonary necrosis by day 21 postinfection (25X magnification). Stained with hematoxylin and eosin.

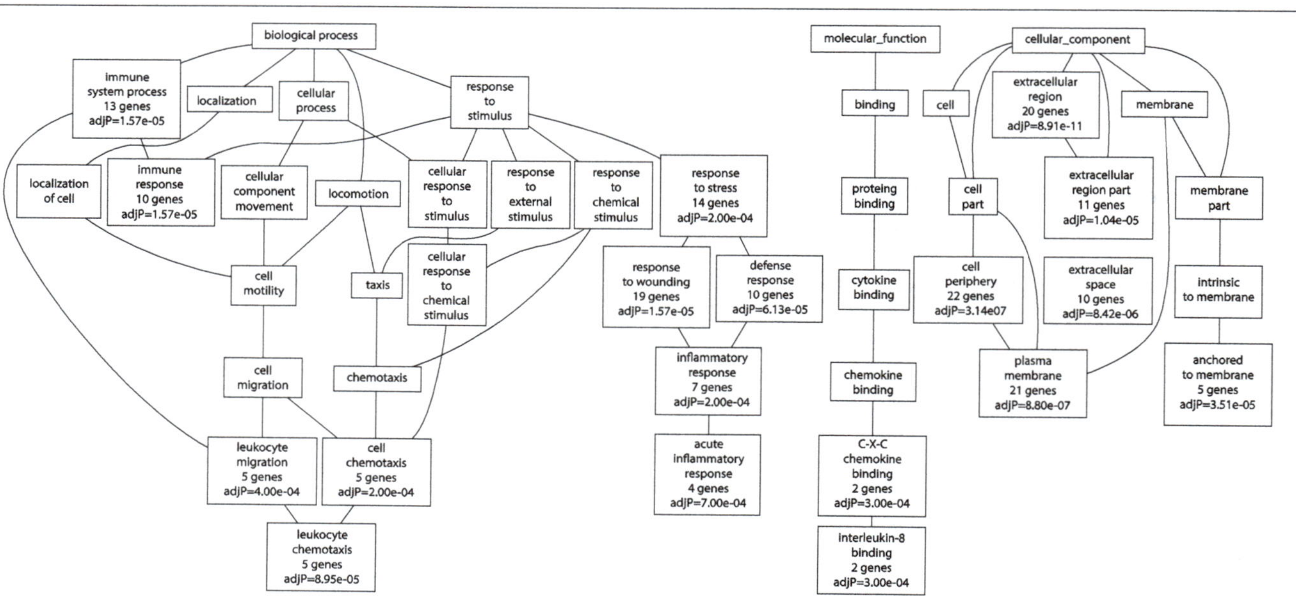

FIGURE 8 | Biological processes impacted by up-regulated genes in animals infected with strain 46 compared with animals infected with strain 46P at day 21 postinfection.

that ending TB will require "a surge in our efforts" (33). It has been almost a century since the BCG was introduced as, so far, the only vaccine to control TB (6), and although this was successful in several geographic regions, its limitations in terms of efficacy against pulmonary TB have become clear in the past decades. BCG vaccination has been shown to be highly cost-effective, and

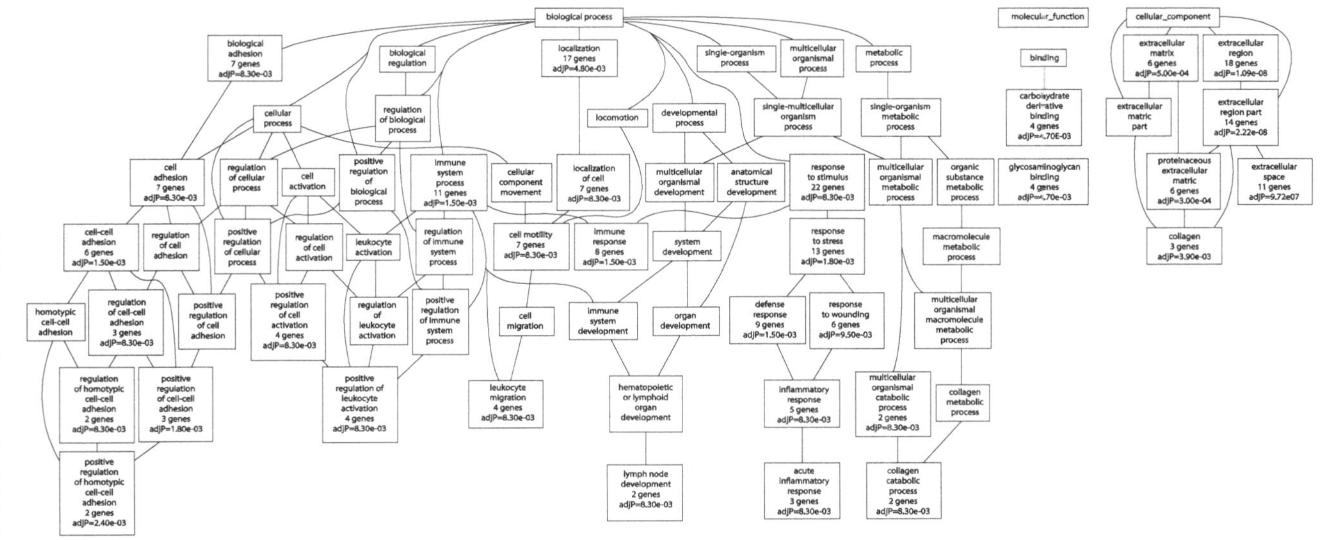

FIGURE 9 | Biological processes impacted by up-regulated genes in animals infected with strain 48 compared with animals infected with strain 48V at day 21 postinfection.

it has been consistently shown to prevent meningeal and miliary TB (34). Nonetheless, its ability to prevent pulmonary TB is much less well-established, particularly in the case of the Beijing genotype. It has been previously suggested that BCG could act as a selective pressure, favoring genetic and phenotypic changes which would in turn contribute to the dissemination of these conserved strains, however, experimental data to support this hypothesis had never before been presented (5).

In this study we present evidence stemming from a murine TB model, in which we directly evaluated the effect of BCG vaccination on the virulence of two Beijing genotype strains and a well-characterized MTB control strain, H37Rv. Interestingly, only Beijing-genotype strains (46 and 48) showed a significant increase in virulence after exposure to BCG-induced immunity. The presented data supports previous observations, in which Beijing-genotype strains have been identified as having adaptive advantages compared with other genotypes, including increased expression of α-crystallin and the *dosR* regulon gene, and induction of a deteriorated immune response in infected hosts (12, 35). Altogether, these characteristics lead to an increased virulence, evasion of host immune response and an increased capacity for latency and transmission (12).

As a consequence of vaccination, the immune system is primed to generate a significant arrangement of cells, cytokines and humoral factors to create a hostile environment against microorganisms. In the case of MTB, this pathogen can readily adapt to hostile environments including nutrient deficiency, high media acidity and even hypoxia (36). Despite the environment induced by BCG vaccination the infection, or even the disease, often cannot be prevented (22). During this process, the fittest bacteria may undergo adaptive evolution (37). Accordingly, mass vaccination may shift the previously existing balance between wild-type and vaccine-resistant strains to the latter (38). This is mainly the case when the level of induced immunity is inferior in terms of cross-reactivity compared with naturally-acquired immunity and the pathogen strain variability is high (38), such as with MTB (**Supplementary Figure 2**). Such shifts in bacterial populations, in order to "outsmart" their host have been previously studied (39). In a study performed in Dutch patients, researchers observed important polymorphisms in virulence factors of *Bordetella pertussis* after the introduction of whole-cell vaccination. Moreover, these polymorphisms allowed the bacteria to cause disease in hosts who had been previously vaccinated, since the polymorphisms conferred these vaccine-adapted strains with different virulence factors compared with those which were present in the strains used to prepare the vaccine (39). Interestingly, the authors in this study observed a statistically-significant inverse relation between the percentage of specific subtypes of the virulence factor P.69 present in the strains isolated from individuals, and their degree of vaccine-induced immunity. This finding highlights the fact that the shift in bacterial population from those which carry the identical virulence factor as in the vaccine strain (i.e., P.69A) to strains with non-vaccine-type P.69, has been very likely driven by vaccination. Thus, as previously discussed by van Loo Inge "like the use of antibiotics, vaccination can impose a strong selective force on populations of microorganisms, nevertheless long term, population-based, studies addressing the effect of vaccination are limited" (40). Among some of the earlier evidence, studies have reported that following the introduction of H. influenza vaccination, a small increase in incidence of invasive disease was observed (41). The population structure of the measles virus has likely also been affected by vaccination, and evidence shows that genes from pre-vaccination isolates have important variants which result in antigenic differences with pre-vaccination isolates as well as

TABLE 2 | Genome variants present in Beijing genotype bacilli before and after passage through BCG-vaccinated mice.

Strain	Number of variants	Type of variant	Sequence change	Product
46	2	Frameshift variant	c.545dupG p.Val183fs	Glycerol kinase
		Synonymous variant	c.169C>T p.Leu57Leu	ESAT-6-like protein EsxI
46P	3	Disruptive inframe insertion	c.3913_3914insGCACCGGCG p.Gly1304_Val1305insGlyThrGly	PE family protein
		Frameshift variant	c.1305_1306dupCC p.Gln436fs	PPE family protein PPE13
		Missense variant	c.812T>C p.Val271Ala	PE family protein
48	5	Conservative inframe insertion	c.2109_2110insGACGGTGGGGCC GGCGGCAACGGCGCC p.Ala703_Asn704insAspGlyGlyAlaG lyGlyAsnGlyAla	PE family protein
		Missense variant	c.3263G>T p.Gly1088Val	DNA-directed RNA polymerase subunit beta'
		Synonymous variant	c.1407_1410delTGGAinsCGGT p.471	PE family protein
		Synonymous variant	c.195C>T p.Ser65Ser	DUF222 domain-containing protein
		Synonymous variant	c.687T>C p.Gly229Gly	PE family protein
48V	9	Conservative inframe insertion	c.58_66dupTTGGCACTG p.Leu22_Ile23insLeuAlaLeu	LppP/LprE family lipoprotein
		Disruptive inframe deletion	c.483_500delCAACGGCGG CGCCGGCGG p.Asn162_Gly167del	hypothetical protein
		Disruptive inframe insertion	c.3913_3914insGCACCGGCG p.Gly1304_Val1305insGlyThrGly	PE family protein
		Frameshift variant and missense variant	c.4774_4777delAAGGinsGAGGT p.Lys1592fs	PE-PGRS family protein
		Missense variant	c.1416_1426delTGTGAGTAGTTinsCA TCAACAGTA p.ValSerSerSer473IleAsnSerThr	Hypothetical protein
		Missense variant	c.3259_3263delCGGGGinsTGGGT p.ArgGly1087TrpVal	DNA-directed RNA polymerase subunit beta'
		Synonymous variant	c.1407T>C p.Gly469Gly	PE family protein
		Synonymous variant	c.1713T>C p.Gly571Gly	PE family protein
		Synonymous variant	c.1809A>T p.Ala603Ala	Hypothetical protein

with vaccine-strain virus (42, 43). Recently, several mumps outbreaks have been identified in locations with high vaccine coverage (>95%), and results from molecular epidemiology studies suggest a higher prevalence of specific genotype viruses which have a substantial capacity to spread among vaccinated hosts. An epidemic wave reported in 2015 in Catalonia, for example, has been related to antigenic differences between the circulating and vaccine strains (termed immune escape) in addition to a waning immunity (44). Overall, results from different studies in a varied number of microorganisms suggest that circulating genotypes might be affected over time, and this in turn might advocate for a continuous evaluation of vaccine strain efficacy while considering the current molecular epidemiology scene.

Among the MTB genotype families the Beijing genotype is recognized for being particularly capable to evade the immune response (20). Some of these strains have managed, as reflected by multiple determinants, to cause serious illness in naïve as well as vaccinated individuals, creating a new risk in regions where TB had long ceased to be a serious public health threat (45). In this regard, one of the most interesting findings in our study is the fact that two MTB strains of the Beijing genotype showed a significant increase in virulence when exposed to vaccinated mice. This was not the case for the Euro-American genotype strain, highlighting the different response to vaccination amongst the different MTB lineages. Arguably, H37Rv is a lab adapted strain which might be unable to readily adapt under these circumstances. However, it is important to highlight that when both strains, 46 and 48, were exposed to sham-vaccinated mice, neither one of the sub strains (46S and 48S) had a hyper-virulent phenotype compared to the original-stock strain. This would suggest that the change in virulence is due to the vaccinated host, rather than other factors. Interestingly, the Beijing-genotype strains did not have the same response in terms of which BCG-substrain exposure produced differences in disease phenotype. In the case of strain 46, exposure to BCG-Phipps produced the higher-virulence strain: 46P; meanwhile in the case of strain 48, exposure to BCG-Vietnam produced the higher-virulence strain: 48V. Both BCG substrains were selected for this experiment because of previous characterization in which using laboratory strain H37Rv and other genotype strains, BCG-Phipps showed a higher degree of protective efficacy compared with BCG-Vietnam (46). Nonetheless, when these vaccinated animals were infected with strains 46 and 48, histopathological damage was different according to the infective strain and the BCG substrain used for immunization (**Supplementary Figure 3**). Interestingly, strain 46 was collected from the region of Vietnam, and therefore it is likely that this strain had historically been adapted to BCG-Vietnam vaccinated hosts, unlike strain 48, which was isolated from South Africa. The images would suggest that protection by BCG-Phipps is better in the case of strain 48, therefore likely leaving a higher number of escape variants in animals infected with BCG Vietnam, nonetheless this is a hypothesis and further studies are in course in order to characterize the factors underlying this observation. In such case, it is interesting to point out that, as previous studies have ascertained, BCG protection varies greatly according to vaccine substrain and also according to the particular infective strain, even among same-genotype isolates (46).

It is important to note that the initial experiments which evaluated virulence suggested a common mechanism by which the Beijing-genotype bacteria increased their virulence, as both strains 46P and 48V showed a similar virulence phenotype: both vaccine exposed strains showed similar survival rates, with 100% mortality 4 weeks post-infection; both vaccine-exposed strains produced extensive pulmonary necrosis instead of (or in addition to) the more common histopathological finding in this animal model (pneumonia), and both strains produced very little, if any, tissue damage and inflammation (perivascular and interstitial inflammation) and formation of granulomas during days 1-14 post-infection, as if going unrecognized by the host immune response (Additional images for histology patterns can be found in **Supplementary Figures 4, 5**). Nonetheless, the transcriptome pattern in lungs of animals infected by the Beijing-genotype strains differed considerably at day 21 post-infection. Animals infected by strains 46 and 46P differentially expressed several genes with known immune functions; for example the CD-14 antigen, a known co-receptor that binds microbial molecules in monocytes and macrophages. Previous studies using CD14 knockout mice infected with MTB have shown that these animals have a reduced inflammatory response, which protects them from lethality through the late course of infection (47). In the case of animals infected by strains 48 and 48V, differentially expressed genes included cytokine-like 1, a known chemotactic factor for monocytes and macrophages. This cytokine is similar to CCL2, which is known to increase macrophage and T cell accumulation in the lung, as well as mediate their organization during MTB infection (48), a finding which would suggest an explanation to the difference in early-phase inflammation in the lungs of these animals. Other differentially expressed genes in the lungs of animals infected by strains 46 and 46P included IL-33 as well as Interleukin 1 receptor (type 1). In the specific case of MTB, IL-33 has been shown to have protective effects in infected animals, as well as a therapeutic effect when given systemically post-infection (49). Interestingly, two genes were up-regulated in both Beijing-genotype infected animals, glycoprotein 2, which plays an important role in the innate immune response, and vanin 1, which in mice regulates the migration of T-cell progenitors to the thymus. Although the role of these factors during MTB infection remains unexplored, it is interesting to note that Vanin-1 has been previously studied in models with other microorganisms. In a previous study, vanin-1 was shown to control granuloma formation and macrophage polarization during *Coxiella burnetii* infection (50). In this study, the authors conclude that vanin-1 is a key component in shaping the nature and intensity of the immune response against infection, this derived from the fact that vanin-1 has a role in macrophage polarization toward an M2 phenotype, leading to a defective granuloma formation and reduced microbicidal response. Although this role in MTB infected mice has not been specifically studied, our results show that animals infected by these strains have a differential expression of Vanin-1 (both in the case of vaccine-exposed strains 46P and 48V), and this correlates with a decreased ability by the animals infected with these strains to form granulomas during the early phase of the disease (day 14) compared with animals infected by the original stock-strains (**Supplementary Figure 6**), and which limits granuloma size during the later stage (days 21–28). These results warrant future investigation into the role of Vanin-1 during MTB infection, and its potential therapeutic effect as an immune-modulator. It is important to highlight that the fold-change in these differentially-expressed genes ranged to 1.44 in the upper limit. Nonetheless, such changes in previous studies have been reported to provide clinically meaningful information (51), and therefore the biological significance of such changes cannot at this point be conclusively ascertained.

Lastly, with DNA sequencing we found virulence associated genetic mutations in vaccine-exposed strains compared with the original-stock strains. At this point, this data seems to support the hypothesis that these mutations are the result of selective pressure by the host's immune system, however, it is important to note that they might also be caused by random mechanisms, so further exploration should be considered before drawing conclusions. Although we found one shared mutation (Disruptive inframe insertion c.3913_3914insGCACCGGCG p.Gly1304_Val1305insGlyThrGly) between both hyper-virulent vaccine-exposed strains, it is at this point difficult to evaluate the potential biological effect of this in-frame insertion. Furthermore, this variant was observed in a sequence which encodes a PE-protein. PE along with PPE proteins make up to 10% of the coding regions in MBT genomes, and as can be seen in **Table 2**, several mutations identified fall in these coding regions. These proteins share a proline-glutamic acid (PE) or proline-proline-glutamic acid (PPE) motif, and although their specific function remains unknown, several authors suggest that they provide antigenic variation to the bacteria. The sequences are of a highly polymorphic nature, and therefore the biological relevance of the mutation present in both these strains should be further explored.

Overall, the experiments presented in this study present experimental evidence as to the role of vaccinated hosts in shaping the host-pathogen interactions. From our results, it could be suggested that hosts interact differently with pathogens with different degrees of virulence, despite their having a very similar genomic make-up. Pathogens on the other hand, are constantly adapting to a changing environment, and can alter how they are recognized by the host's immune system in order to survive in a vaccinated population. Nonetheless, we urge a cautious interpretation of these results, and call attention to the fact that this data stems from a murine TB model, and should therefore not be extrapolated to human populations at this stage. Nonetheless, this information could be considered in the urgent need to produce a higher-efficacy vaccine against TB. As in the case of *Bordetella pertussis*, it could be possible that we can counter the spread of these vaccine-adapted strains by introducing a different prophylactic strategy to which they have not yet developed adaptive mechanisms (39, 52, 53). The study presented here has several strengths, including the use of syngeneic mice in order to reduce inter-host variance, and the use of methodology to avoid artifacts during the genome comparison process, including the use of PCR-free methods to build the DNA-libraries for sequencing, as well as a depth of sequencing ranging from 475 to 715 in each of the sequenced strains. Nonetheless, it is important to highlight that the results should be interpreted in light of the limitations of the study, including a design which did not consider the sequencing of strains which did not portray a virulence change in the initial stage of the study (i.e., strains 45V, 48P, 46S, and 48S), and the fact that in this particular study only two MTB Beijing genomes were tested. Currently, further studies are underway which seek to evaluate this effect on the wide MTB genomic landscape, which should give more information and add valuable information. Last, it is important to once again highlight that the results from this murine model should provide information, but we do not encourage extrapolation of these results to the clinical setting. Rather, we are currently working to ascertain the effects of BCG vaccination on bacteria recovered from vaccinated and non-vaccinated individuals from a single transmission chain. Further information is needed using other experimental models in order to draw more robust conclusions.

As a closing remark, we emphatically stress that vaccination is currently the most cost-effective health intervention, and saves an estimated three million lives per year. However, BCG vaccination as the only prophylactic strategy approved by the WHO falls short of the current epidemiological needs, and therefore considerable efforts, both financial and intellectual, should be put forward in order to seek a more effective strategy, meanwhile optimal use of BCG as recommended by the WHO remains adamantly needed in light of the current world trends regarding tuberculosis incidence and mortality.

ETHICS STATEMENT

The animal study was reviewed and approved by Animal Experimentation Committee at the National Institute of Medical Sciences and Nutrition México (PAT-1860-16/18-1).

AUTHOR'S NOTE

Partial results from this study were presented at the Keystone Symposia held in Santa Fe, New Mexico, January 22–January 27, 2015. Abstract number: 3079.

AUTHOR CONTRIBUTIONS

ZZ-B performed the in vivo experiments, including mice euthanasia, CFU determination, lung tissue preparation and assessment of lung pathology. Additionally, she performed the molecular biology experiments (including RNA-seq and DNA-seq), and participated in the data analysis and interpretation, as well as manuscript writing and revision. OR-E performed molecular biology experiments and lung tissue preparation and assessment of lung pathology. DM-E planned, coordinated the study, prepared the bacterial strains and vaccines, determined lung bacillary load and analyzed and interpreted the data. BM-C aided in the performance of the molecular biology experiments. JB-P infected the mice and kept survival records. OM-L performed the bioinformatics analysis for the genomic data. FC-G and AO-L performed the genomic experiments and contributed with the data analysis. CM-R performed in vivo experiments including mice euthanasia and CFU determination. ID and RR-V performed the RNA and DNA libraries and the NGS. GL-L analyzed the RNA-Seq data and performed the GO and KEGG-pathways enrichments. RW donated the MTB bacilli for the experiments, and critically reviewed the manuscript. RH-P, RA, and DS planned and coordinated the study, interpreted the data, and critically reviewed the manuscript. All authors reviewed the manuscript prior to submission and approved the final version.

ACKNOWLEDGMENTS

ZZ-B gratefully acknowledges the scholarship from CONACYT to pursue her graduate studies. She would also like to express her deep gratitude to the graduate program in Biochemical Sciences at the National Autonomous University in Mexico (UNAM), for their continued support in this endeavour.

SUPPLEMENTARY MATERIAL

Supplementary Figure 1 | (A) Survival rate of animals infected with the original stock strain 1 (H37Rv) and vaccine-exposed strains 1P, 1V, and 1S. **(B)** Lung bacillary load in animals infected with the original stock strain 1 and vaccine exposed strains 1P, 1V, and 1S. **(C)** Percentage of lung area affected by pneumonia in animals infected with the original stock strain 1 and vaccine-exposed strains 1P, 1V, and 1S. $^{*}p < 0.05$, $^{**}p < 0.01$.

Supplementary Figure 2 | Emergence of vaccine-adapted microorganisms.

Supplementary Figure 3 | (A) BCG Phipps vaccinated animals infected by strain 46 presented by 2 months post-infection moderate areas of pulmonary pneumonia **(B)** BCG Vietnam vaccinated animals infected by strain 46 presented by 2 months post-infection moderate areas of pulmonary pneumonic areas. **(C)** BCG Phipps vaccinated animals infected by strain 48 had small pneumonic areas by 2 months postinfection, suggesting a good level of protection by this BCG substrain compared with **(D)** BCG Vietnam vaccinated animals infected with strain 48 show large areas of pneumonia by 2 months postinfection, highlighting a lower level of protection against this Beijing-genotype strain (48). Stained with haematoxylin and eosin, images taken at 25X.

Supplementary Figure 4 | Representative histological images from lungs of animals infected with strains 46, 46P, 46V, and 46S and euthanized on days 14, 21, and 28 post-infection. Animals infected by strain 46P show large areas of necrosis (*) compared with animals infected with the original-stock strain 46, or animals infected with strains 46V and 46S, which develop lung damage in the form of pneumonia (arrows). Stained with haematoxylin and eosin (Black bar in the first image corresponds to 500 μm).

Supplementary Figure 5 | Representative histological images from lungs of animals infected with strains 48, 48P, 48V, and 48S and euthanized on days 14, 21, and 28 post-infection. Lungs from animals infected with the original-stock strain 48 show interstitial, peribronchial, and perivascular inflammation (*) by day 14 post-infection. Contrary, lungs from animals infected by strain 48V show very scarce if any inflammatory infiltrate on day 14 post-infection. Lungs from animals which were infected by strain 48V and euthanized on day 21 post-infection show pneumonic and necrotic areas (arrows), in comparison with those infected by strain 48 on this same time-point, which show mostly pneumonia (dotted arrow), with very scarce or null necrosis. Stained with hematoxylin and eosin (black bar in the first image corresponds to 500 μm).

Supplementary Figure 6 | Representative granuloma from a subject infected by original stock strain 46, and sacrificed at day 7 postinfection. Stained with hematoxylin and eosin, 100X magnification.

Supplementary Table 1 | Genome assembly data.

Supplementary Table 2 | Up-regulated genes in the mice infected by strain 46 compared to those infected by strain 46P.

Supplementary Table 3 | Up-regulated genes in the mice infected by strain 48 compared to those infected by strain 48V.

Supplementary Table 4 | Down-regulated genes in the mice infected by strain 46 compared to those infected by strain 46P.

Supplementary Table 5 | Down-regulated genes in the mice infected by strain 48 compared to those infected by strain 48V.

REFERENCES

1. Wilson ME. Applying experiences from trials of bacille Calmette-Guerin vaccine. *Clin Infect Dis.* (2000) 30:S262–5. doi: 10.1086/313886
2. World Health Organization. *Global Tuberculosis Report.* Geneva: World Health Organization (2018).
3. Druszczynska M, Kowalewicz-Kulbat M, Fol M, Wlodarczyk M, Rudnicka W. Latent *M. tuberculosis* infection–pathogenesis, diagnosis, treatment and prevention strategies. *Pol J Microbiol.* (2012) 61:3–10. doi: 10.33073/pjm-2012-001
4. Luca S, Mihaescu T. History of BCG vaccine. *Maedica.* (2013) 8:53–8.
5. Abebe F, Bjune G. The emergence of Beijing family genotypes of *Mycobacterium tuberculosis* and low-level protection by bacille Calmette-Guerin (BCG) vaccines: is there a link? *Clin Exp Immunol.* (2006) 145:389–97. doi: 10.1111/j.1365-2249.2006.03162.x
6. Liu J, Tran V, Leung AS, Alexander DC, Zhu B. BCG vaccines: their mechanisms of attenuation and impact on safety and protective efficacy. *Hum Vaccin.* (2009) 5:70–8. doi: 10.4161/hv.5.2.7210
7. Poyntz HC, Stylianou E, Griffiths KL, Marsay L, Checkley AM, Mcshane H. Non-tuberculous mycobacteria have diverse effects on BCG efficacy against *Mycobacterium tuberculosis. Tuberculosis.* (2014) 94:226–37. doi: 10.1016/j.tube.2013.12.006
8. Gagneux S, Deriemer K, Van T, Kato-Maeda M, De Jong BC, Narayanan S, et al. Variable host-pathogen compatibility in *Mycobacterium tuberculosis. Proc Natl Acad Sci USA.* (2006) 103:2869–73. doi: 10.1073/pnas.0511240103
9. Borgdorff MW, Van Soolingen D. The re-emergence of tuberculosis: what have we learnt from molecular epidemiology? *Clin Microbiol Infect.* (2013) 19:889–901. doi: 10.1111/1469-0691.12253
10. Kremer K, Van-Der-Werf MJ, Au BK, Anh DD, Kam KM, Van-Doorn HR, et al. Vaccine-induced immunity circumvented by typical *Mycobacterium tuberculosis* Beijing strains. *Emerg Infect Dis.* (2009) 15:335–9. doi: 10.3201/eid1502.080795
11. Merker M, Blin C, Mona S, Duforet-Frebourg N, Lecher S, Willery E, et al. Evolutionary history and global spread of the *Mycobacterium tuberculosis* Beijing lineage. *Nat Genet.* (2015) 47:242–9. doi: 10.1038/ng.3195
12. Parwati I, Van Crevel R, Van Soolingen D. Possible underlying mechanisms for successful emergence of the *Mycobacterium tuberculosis* Beijing genotype strains. *Lancet Infect Dis.* (2010) 10:103–11. doi: 10.1016/S1473-3099(09)70330-5
13. Hanekom M, Gey Van Pittius NC, Mcevoy C, Victor TC, Van Helden PD, Warren RM. *Mycobacterium tuberculosis* Beijing genotype: a template for success. *Tuberculosis.* (2011) 91:510–23. doi: 10.1016/j.tube.2011.07.005
14. He GX, Wang HY, Borgdorff MW, Van Soolingen D, Van Der Werf MJ, Liu ZM, et al. Multidrug-resistant tuberculosis, People's Republic of China, 2007-2009. *Emerg Infect Dis.* (2011) 17:1831–8. doi: 10.3201/eid1710.110546
15. Liu Y, Jiang X, Li W, Zhang X, Wang W, Li C. The study on the association between Beijing genotype family and drug susceptibility phenotypes of *Mycobacterium tuberculosis* in Beijing. *Sci Rep.* (2017) 7:15076. doi: 10.1038/s41598-017-14119-z
16. Zhao LL, Li MC, Liu HC, Xiao TY, Li GL, Zhao XQ, et al. Beijing genotype of *Mycobacterium tuberculosis* is less associated with drug resistance in south China. *Int J Antimicrob Agents.* (2019) 54:766–70. doi: 10.1016/j.ijantimicag.2019.08.005
17. Glynn JR, Whiteley J, Bifani PJ, Kremer K, Van Soolingen D. Worldwide occurrence of Beijing/W strains of *Mycobacterium tuberculosis*: a systematic review. *Emerg Infect Dis.* (2002) 8:843–9. doi: 10.3201/eid0805.020002
18. Pang Y, Song Y, Xia H, Zhou Y, Zhao B, Zhao Y. Risk factors and clinical phenotypes of Beijing genotype strains in tuberculosis patients in China. *BMC Infect Dis.* (2012) 12:354. doi: 10.1186/1471-2334-12-354
19. Liu Q, Wang D, Martinez L, Lu P, Zhu L, Lu W, et al. *Mycobacterium tuberculosis* Beijing genotype strains and unfavourable treatment outcomes: a systematic review and meta-analysis. *Clin Microbiol Infect.* (2019) 26:180–8. doi: 10.1016/j.cmi.2019.07.016
20. Lopez B, Aguilar D, Orozco H, Burger M, Espitia C, Ritacco V, et al. A marked difference in pathogenesis and immune response induced by different *Mycobacterium tuberculosis* genotypes. *Clin Exp Immunol.* (2003) 133:30–7. doi: 10.1046/j.1365-2249.2003.02171.x
21. Ordway DJ, Shang S, Henao-Tamayo M, Obregon-Henao A, Nold L, Caraway M, et al. *Mycobacterium bovis* BCG-mediated protection against W-Beijing strains of *Mycobacterium tuberculosis* is diminished concomitant with the emergence of regulatory T cells. *Clin Vaccine Immunol.* (2011) 18:1527–35. doi: 10.1128/CVI.05127-11
22. Gandon S, Mackinnon M, Nee S, Read A. Imperfect vaccination: some epidemiological and evolutionary consequences. *Proc Biol Sci.* (2003) 270:1129–36. doi: 10.1098/rspb.2003.2370
23. Cornejo-Granados F, Zatarain-Barrón ZL, Cantu-Robles VA, Mendoza-Vargas A, Molina-Romero C, Sánchez F, et al. Secretome prediction of two *M. tuberculosis* clinical isolates reveals their high antigenic density and potential drug targets. *Front Microbiol* (2017) 8:128. doi: 10.3389/fmicb.2017.00128
24. Hernandez-Pando R, Orozcoe H, Sampieri A, Pavon L, Velasquillo C, Larriva-Sahd J, et al. Correlation between the kinetics of Th1, Th2 cells and pathology in a murine model of experimental pulmonary tuberculosis. *Immunology.* (1996) 89:26–33.

25. Marquina-Castillo B, Garcia-Garcia L, Ponce-De-Leon A, Jimenez-Corona ME, Bobadilla-Del Valle M, Cano-Arellano B, et al. Virulence, immunopathology and transmissibility of selected strains of *Mycobacterium tuberculosis* in a murine model. *Immunology.* (2009) 128:123–33. doi: 10.1111/j.1365-2567.2008.03004.x
26. Ramakrishnan L. Revisiting the role of the granuloma in tuberculosis. *Nat Rev Immunol.* (2012) 12:352–66. doi: 10.1038/nri3211
27. Bolger AM, Lohse M, Usadel B. Trimmomatic: a flexible trimmer for Illumina sequence data. *Bioinformatics.* (2014) 30:2114–20. doi: 10.1093/bioinformatics/btu170
28. Seemann T. Prokka: rapid prokaryotic genome annotation. *Bioinformatics.* (2014) 30:2068–9. doi: 10.1093/bioinformatics/btu153
29. Li H, Durbin R. Fast and accurate short read alignment with Burrows-Wheeler transform. *Bioinformatics.* (2009) 25:1754–60. doi: 10.1093/bioinformatics/btp324
30. Anders S, Pyl PT, Huber W. HTSeq–a Python framework to work with high-throughput sequencing data. *Bioinformatics.* (2015) 31:166–9. doi: 10.1093/bioinformatics/btu638
31. Love MI, Huber W, Anders S. Moderated estimation of fold change and dispersion for RNA-seq data with DESeq2. *Genome Biol.* (2014) 15:550. doi: 10.1186/s13059-014-0550-8
32. Wang J, Vasaikar S, Shi Z, Greer M, Zhang B. WebGestalt 2017: a more comprehensive, powerful, flexible and interactive gene set enrichment analysis toolkit. *Nucleic Acids Res.* (2017) 45:W130–7. doi: 10.1093/nar/gkx356
33. World Health Organization. *Bending the Curve - Ending TB: Annual Report 2017.* New Delhi: World Health Organization (2017).
34. Bloom BR, Atun R, Cohen T, Dye C, Fraser H, Gomez GB, et al. Tuberculosis. In: Rd, Holmes KK, Bertozzi S, Bloom BR, Jha P, editors. *Major Infectious Diseases.* Washington, DC: The International Bank for Reconstruction and Development/The World Bank (2017). p. 233–313.
35. Van Laarhoven A, Mandemakers JJ, Kleinnijenhuis J, Enaimi M, Lachmandas E, Joosten LA, et al. Low induction of proinflammatory cytokines parallels evolutionary success of modern strains within the *Mycobacterium tuberculosis* Beijing genotype. *Infect Immun.* (2013) 81:3750–6. doi: 10.1128/IAI.00282-13
36. Stokes RW, Waddell SJ. Adjusting to a new home: *Mycobacterium tuberculosis* gene expression in response to an intracellular lifestyle. *Future Microbiol.* (2009) 4:1317–35. doi: 10.2217/fmb.09.94
37. Engering A, Hogerwerf L, Slingenbergh J. Pathogen-host-environment interplay and disease emergence. *Emerg Microbes Infect.* (2013) 2:e5. doi: 10.1038/emi.2013.5
38. Mclean AR. Vaccines and their impact on the control of disease. *Br Med Bull.* (1998) 54:545–56. doi: 10.1093/oxfordjournals.bmb.a011709
39. Mooi FR, Van Oirschot H, Heuvelman K, Van Der Heide HG, Gaastra W, Willems RJ. Polymorphism in the *Bordetella pertussis* virulence factors P.69/pertactin and pertussis toxin in The Netherlands: temporal trends and evidence for vaccine-driven evolution. *Infect Immun.* (1998) 66:670–5. doi: 10.1128/IAI.66.2.670-675.1998
40. van Loo Inge HM. *Vaccine-Driven Evolution of Bordetella pertussis: Changes in Population Structure and Strain Fitness.* (2002). Available online at: https://dspace.library.uu.nl/bitstream/handle/1874/450/full.pdf?sequence=1
41. Urwin G, Krohn JA, Deaver-Robinson K, Wenger JD, Farley MM. Invasive disease due to *Haemophilus influenzae* serotype F: clinical and epidemiologic characteristics in the *H. influenzae* serotype b vaccine era. The *Haemophilus influenzae* Study Group. *Clin Infect Dis.* (1996) 22:1069–76. doi: 10.1093/clinids/22.6.1069
42. Rota PA, Bloom AE, Vanchiere JA, Bellini WJ. Evolution of the nucleoprotein and matrix genes of wild-type strains of measles virus isolated from recent epidemics. *Virology.* (1994) 198:724–30. doi: 10.1006/viro.1994.1086
43. Tamin A, Rota PA, Wang ZD, Heath JL, Anderson LJ, Bellini WJ. Antigenic analysis of current wild type and vaccine strains of measles virus. *J Infect Dis.* (1994) 170:795–801. doi: 10.1093/infdis/170.4.795
44. Barrabeig I, Antón A, Torner N, Pumarola T, Costa J, Domínguez À, et al. Mumps: MMR vaccination and genetic diversity of mumps virus, 2007-2011 in Catalonia, Spain. *BMC Infect Dis.* (2019) 19:954. doi: 10.1186/s12879-019-4496-z
45. Agerton TB, Valway SE, Blinkhorn RJ, Shilkret KL, Reves R, Schluter WW, et al. Spread of strain W, a highly drug-resistant strain of *Mycobacterium tuberculosis,* across the United States. *Clin Infect Dis.* (1999) 29:85–92; discussion: 93–5. doi: 10.1086/520187
46. Castillo-Rodal AI, Castanon-Arreola M, Hernandez-Pando R, Calva JJ, Sada-Diaz E, Lopez-Vidal Y. *Mycobacterium bovis* BCG substrains confer different levels of protection against *Mycobacterium tuberculosis* infection in a BALB/c model of progressive pulmonary tuberculosis. *Infect Immun.* (2006) 74:1718–24. doi: 10.1128/IAI.74.3.1718-1724.2006
47. Wieland CW, Van Der Windt GJ, Wiersinga WJ, Florquin S, Van Der Poll T. CD14 contributes to pulmonary inflammation and mortality during murine tuberculosis. *Immunology.* (2008) 125:272–9. doi: 10.1111/j.1365-2567.2008.02840.x
48. Domingo-Gonzalez R, Prince O, Cooper A, Khader SA. Cytokines and chemokines in *Mycobacterium tuberculosis* infection. *Microbiol Spectr.* (2016) 4:1–58. doi: 10.1128/microbiolspec.TBTB2-0018-2016
49. Pineros AR, Campos LW, Fonseca DM, Bertolini TB, Gembre AF, Prado RQ, et al. M2 macrophages or IL-33 treatment attenuate ongoing *Mycobacterium tuberculosis* infection. *Sci Rep.* (2017) 7:41240. doi: 10.1038/srep41240
50. Meghari S, Berruyer C, Lepidi H, Galland F, Naquet P, Mege JL. Vanin-1 controls granuloma formation and macrophage polarization in *Coxiella burnetii* infection. *Eur J Immunol.* (2007) 37:24–32. doi: 10.1002/eji.200636054
51. Wang S, He L, Wu J, Zhou Z, Gao Y, Chen J, et al. Transcriptional profiling of human peripheral blood mononuclear cells identifies diagnostic biomarkers that distinguish active and latent tuberculosis. *Front Immunol.* (2019) 18:10:2948. doi: 10.3389/fimmu.2019.02948
52. Dorji D, Mooi F, Yantorno O, Deora R, Graham RM, Mukkur TK. *Bordetella pertussis* virulence factors in the continuing evolution of whooping cough vaccines for improved performance. *Med Microbiol Immunol.* (2018) 207:3–26. doi: 10.1007/s00430-017-0524-z
53. Hovingh ES, Mariman R, Solans L, Hijdra D, Hamstra HJ, Jongerius I, et al. *Bordetella pertussis* pertactin knock-out strains reveal immunomodulatory properties of this virulence factor. *Emerg Microbes Infect.* (2018) 7:39. doi: 10.1038/s41426-018-0039-8

14

Production of Neutrophil Extracellular Traps Contributes to the Pathogenesis of *Francisella* tularemia

Sivasami Pulavendran[1†], Maram Prasanthi[1], Akhilesh Ramachandran[1], Rezabek Grant[1], Timothy A. Snider[1], Vincent T. K. Chow[2], Jerry R. Malayer[1] and Narasaraju Teluguakula[1†]*

[1] College of Veterinary Medicine, Oklahoma State University, Stillwater, Oklahoma, OK, United States, [2] Department of Microbiology and Immunology, School of Medicine, National University of Singapore, National University Health System, Singapore, Singapore

***Correspondence:**
Narasaraju Teluguakula
narasa@okstate.edu

[†] These authors have contributed equally to this work and share first authorship

Francisella tularensis(*Ft*) is a highly virulent, intracellular Gram-negative bacterial pathogen. Acute *Ft* infection by aerosol route causes pneumonic tularemia, characterized by nodular hemorrhagic lesions, neutrophil-predominant influx, necrotic debris, fibrin deposition, and severe alveolitis. *Ft* suppresses activity of neutrophils by impairing their respiratory burst and phagocytic activity. However, the fate of the massive numbers of neutrophils recruited to the infection site is unclear. Here, we show that *Ft* infection resulted in prominent induction of neutrophil extracellular traps (NETs) within damaged lungs of mice infected with the live attenuated vaccine strain of *Ft*(*Ft*-LVS), as well as in the lungs of domestic cats and rabbits naturally infected with *Ft*. Further, *Ft*-LVS infection increased lung myeloperoxidase (MPO) activity, which mediates histone protein degradation during NETosis and anchors chromatin scaffolds in NETs. In addition, *Ft* infection also induced expression of peptidylarginine deiminase 4, an enzyme that causes citrullination of histones during formation of NETs. The released NETs were found largely attached to the alveolar epithelium, and disrupted the thin alveolar epithelial barrier. Furthermore, *Ft* infection induced a concentration-dependent release of NETs from neutrophils *in vitro*. Pharmacological blocking of MPO reduced *Ft*-induced NETs release, whereas addition of H_2O_2 (a substrate of MPO) significantly augmented NETs release, thus indicating a critical role of MPO in *Ft*-induced NETs. Although immunofluorescence and electron microscopy revealed that NETs could efficiently trap *Ft* bacteria, NETs failed to exert bactericidal effects. Taken together, these findings suggest that NETs exacerbate tissue damage in pulmonary *Ft* infection, and that targeting NETosis may offer novel therapeutic interventions in alleviating *Ft*-induced tissue damage.

Keywords: *Francisella*, neutrophil extracellular traps, myeloperoxidase, NEtosis, alveolar injury

INTRODUCTION

Francisella tularensis(Ft) is a zoonotic, intracellular bacterial pathogen, known to cause the disease tularemia that affects major organs including lungs, liver, and spleen (1–3). *Ft* can transmit by direct skin contact or through mucosal, respiratory or gastrointestinal tract routes. The aerosol route of *Ft* infection causes pneumonic tularemia, a severe form of the disease with high fatality rates (4–6). Several studies support that aggravated immune response with massive neutrophils influx contribute to host tissue destruction and pathophysiology in *Ft* infection (7–9). Together with necrotic debris and bacteria, excessive neutrophils recruitment clogs the bronchioles and alveolar airspaces, results in granuloma formation (7, 10–12). It has been reported that induction of matrix metalloproteinase 9 (MMP 9) aggravates neutrophil influx and mortality in *Ft* infection and that mice lacking MMP 9 gene (MMP 9 $^{-/-}$) exhibit diminished neutrophils recruitment and improved survival in both vaccine strain of *Ft* (*Ft*-LVS) and also highly virulent Type A strain (SchuS4) infections (13). Although these findings implicate massive neutrophil influx in the pathogenesis of *Ft* infection, the fate of these neutrophils at the infection site is unknown. Further, mechanisms of how these infiltrated neutrophils contribute to *Ft* pathophysiology remain largely unexplored.

Both neutrophils and macrophages are targets for *Ft* infection (14, 15). Several studies have demonstrated that *Ft* parasitizes inside the neutrophils and disrupts their antimicrobial defense by suppressing neutrophil respiratory burst (15, 16). One proposed mechanism is that *Ft* inhibits assembly of NADPH oxidase enzyme complex, which is required for reactive oxygen species (ROS) generation, and by inhibiting neutrophil respiratory burst, it escapes from phagosomal lysis (17). Neutrophils are terminally differentiated and short-lived cells which undergo constitutive apoptosis. *Ft* infection has been shown to prolong their lifespan by inhibiting apoptotic signaling mechanism (18). Previous *in vitro* studies on *Ft*-neutrophil interactions have implicated in implicated impaired neutrophil function *in vitro*, but the activation status of the pulmonary sequestered neutrophils is unclear. Emerging evidence supports a potential role of excessive neutrophil influx, their activation and NETosis in the pathophysiology of various bacterial and viral diseases (19–23). NETs were initially discovered for their role in bacterial killing (24). However, we found that presence of excessive NETs in *Streptococcus pneumoniae (S. pneumoniae)* superinfection following influenza infection in mice does not reduce bacterial load, but augmented bacterial burden and aggravated pathology (19). During NETs formation, the released chromatin strands are decorated with toxic proteins such as histones, MPO and neutrophil elastase (NE), which contribute to host pathology (24). We have previously reported NETs embroiled with thin alveolar-capillary surfaces of the lungs during severe influenza and *S. pneumoniae* superinfection following influenza which mediate cytotoxic effects in alveolar epithelial and endothelial cells (19, 25). Further, our recent studies have identified extracellular histones as major mediators in NETs-induced tissue damage and organ failure (23).

Although massive neutrophil influx is implicated in *Ft* pathophysiology, there are hitherto no *in vivo* reports on NETs induction or their role in tissue damage during *Ft* infection. In the present study, we characterized the induction of NETs in *Ft*-LVS infected mice. Further, accumulation of NETs was also evaluated in clinically diagnosed *Ft*-positive domestic cats and rabbits. Our findings revealed induction of extensive NETs during *Ft* infection. We also found induction of NETosis, when mouse neutrophils were infected with *Ft*-LVS *in vitro*. The NETs induction was found to be dependent on MPO activity. Although *Ft* was found trapped in NETs during infection, NETs failed to show bactericidal effects against *Francisella*. These studies indicate that NETs release contributes to the lung pathology in *Ft* infection.

MATERIALS AND METHODS

Bacteria, Animals, and Ethics Approval

Live attenuated vaccine strain of *Francisella tularensis* LVS (*Ft*-LVS); and *Ft*-LVS-GFP (GFP labeled) American Type Culture Collection (ATCC, VA) were provided by Dr. Jerry Malayer. The bacteria were cultured on chocolate agar plates at 37°C in a 5% CO_2incubator. For bacterial counts, a serial 10-fold dilutions were made from a single colony in phosphate buffered saline (PBS) and colony forming units (CFU) were determined. For preparation of formalin-killed bacteria, the bacteria were incubated with 4% neutral buffered formalin for 1 h at 37°C and washed with PBS to remove formalin. BALB/c mice (6–8 weeks old) were used in this study. The animals were housed in microisolator cages in a BSL-2 animal facility. All animal experiments were approved by the Institutional Animal Care and Use Committee (IACUC) of Oklahoma State University (protocol number VM-17-36) and were performed in strict accordance with their recommendations.

Ft-Infected Clinical Samples

Severely ill domestic rabbits (n = 4) and cats (n = 3) were brought to the Oklahoma State University veterinary clinic with symptoms of high fever, diarrhea, nasal blood discharge, lethargy and respiratory complications. Animals were euthanized and performed necropsy analysis at Oklahoma Animal Disease and Diagnostic Laboratory (OADDL). Routine RT-PCR analysis on liver and spleen specimens identified *Francisella* positive infection. For histopathologic and NETs immunostaining analysis, lungs and liver tissues were fixed in neutral buffered formalin and embedded in paraffin. Uninfected rabbit lungs and liver samples (n = 3) were used as controls in this study.

Mice Infections

For all infections, animals were anesthetized with a mixture of ketamine (7.5 mg/kg) and xylazine (0.1 mg/kg) by intraperitoneal injection. The mice were then intranasally challenged with a lethal dose of about 1000 CFU of *Ft*-LVS in 50 µl diluted in sterile phosphate-buffered saline (PBS). Mock-inoculated control mice received equal volumes of PBS. The actual dose of the bacteria was confirmed by plating onto chocolate-agar and CFU were determined after 72 h. $N = 5$–7 mice were used in each group. Animals were monitored for clinical signs of weight loss, lethargy, and respiratory distress.

Histopathology Analysis

Following infection, mice were euthanized at 5 dpi, as infected animals exhibited severe clinical signs of illness with lethargy and respiratory distress. Lungs and other organs including liver, spleen, and heart were fixed in 4% formalin as described previously (23). Whole lungs from control and infected animals were fixed by the intratracheal instillation of 4% neutral-buffered formalin at 25-cm water gauge pressure and embedded in paraffin. In another set of experiments, lungs were lavaged with equal volumes of PBS as described earlier and bronchoalveolar lavage fluids were used to determine NETs release (25). A Semi-quantitative histology scores based on the lesions in the lungs, including tissue necrosis, lymphoid necrosis, Pyknotic debris, inflammation (neutrophil/macrophage/lymphocytes), alveolar damage, interstitial pneumonia, bronchopneumonia, nodular and hemorrhagic lesions, and accumulations of necrotic debris were analyzed by board certified pathologists in a blinded manner (23). For liver, scoring was based on tissue necrosis, lymphoid necrosis, Pyknotic debris, discrete/non-discrete granuloma formation and composition of degenerative, and non-degenerative neutrophil infiltrations. Histology scores were given as 0,No lesions; 1, Mild lesions; 2, Moderate lesions; and 3, Marked lesions. Similarly, pathologic analysis of lungs and liver sections from domestic *Ft*-positive cats, rabbits and uninfected rabbits were analyzed and scored in a blinded manner.

Bacterial Burden

A portion of the lung was homogenized in sterile PBS using mortar-pestle. The homogenate was centrifuged at $100 \times g$ for 10 min. A Serial 10-fold dilutions of the supernatants were prepared in sterile PBS. A 10-μl aliquots of serially diluted supernatants were plated onto chocolate-agar and quantification of the colonies was performed after 72 h incubation at 37°C as described above. The results were expressed as $\log_{10}$ CFU/milligram protein.

Immunohistochemistry Analysis

Mock or *Ft*-infected mouse lungs and liver samples were cut into 4-μm thick section and immunohistochemistry performed to detect NET release using antibodies against citH3 and MPO as described previously (26). Briefly, lung and liver sections were deparaffinized in xylene, permeabilized with 0.5% Triton X-100, and blocked with 3% fetal bovine serum. The sections were then incubated at 4°C overnight with 1:400 dilutions of primary antibodies, i.e., mouse anti–citH3 (Abcam, MA) or anti-MPO (Abcam, MA). After washing thrice with PBS, the slides were incubated with 1:500 dilutions of secondary antibodies conjugated to Alexa Fluor 488 or Alexa Fluor 546 (Molecular Probes, Eugene, OR, United States) at room temperature for 1 h. The slides were washed thrice with PBS, mounted in medium containing DAPI (Vector Laboratories, Burlingame, CA, United States) and examined using an Olympus fluorescence microscope. Similarly, *Ft*-positive domestic cats and rabbits and control rabbits were evaluated for induction of NETs formation in their lung and liver sections by immunostaining using anti-citH3 (Abcam, MA) and monoclonal anti-MPO antibodies (Abcam, MA).

For visualizing alveolar damage during *Ft* infection, mock, and *Ft*-infected mouse lung tissue sections were stained with primary antibodies against alveolar type I epithelial membrane marker (T1α, 1: 500, DSHB, University of Iowa, IA) and citH3 (1:400, Abcam, MA) and incubated overnight at 4°C. Lung sections were then labeled with secondary Alexa Fluor antibodies as described above.

Western Blot Analysis in the Cell-Free BAL Fluids

For collection of BAL, both mock infected and *Ft*-LVS infected mouse lungs were lavaged with equal volumes of phosphate buffered saline. The recovery of lavage fluids was more than 90% in all samples. All the western blots were carried out by loading equal volumes of BAL from control and infected animals. The samples were further centrifuged at 4000 rpm for 15 min to obtain cell-free BAL. For western blot analysis, equal volumes of BAL samples from control, infected and treatment groups were loaded, as described in our previous publications (26). The BAL fluids were analyzed for extracellular histones (H2A or H2B, 1:1000, Abcam, MA) and modified histones (citH3, 1:1000, Abcam, MA) by western blot as described previously (26). Lung injury was assessed by T1-α (1:1000, DSHB, University of Iowa). The release of peptidylarginine deiminase 4 (PAD4, 1:200, Santa Cruz, CA, United States) in the BAL was an indication of active NETosis during *Ft* infection. Densitometry on western blots carried out using Image J software (National Institutes of Health).

Measurement MPO Activity

MPO activity in the lung homogenates from mock infected, and *Ft* infected mice was performed as described previously (17). The MPO activity was determined using the formula: units/mg protein = $\Delta OD/\text{minute} \times 45.1$, expressed as U/mg protein lung (27). One unit of the enzyme is defined as the amount that consumes 1 μmol of H_2O_2 per minute.

Ft-Neutrophil Interaction Induces NETs *in vitro*

Mouse blood was collected in sodium citrate. Neutrophils were isolated as by MACS neutrophil isolation kit (Miltenyi Biotec Inc, CA) using Ly6G antibodies through a positive selection as described previously (25). The neutrophils purity was > 90%, determined by modified Giemsa staining. For *Ft*-neutrophil interaction, neutrophils were seeded at the density of 1×10^5 cells onto poly-D-lysine coated 12 mm size coverslips, placed in 24 well culture plates. For determining NETs induction during *Ft*-neutrophil interaction, *Ft*-LVS was added to the neutrophils at MOI of 10:1, 20:1, 30:1, 50:1, and 100:1 diluted in DMEM medium (Gibco, Invitrogen, CA) containing 1% mouse serum, for 4 h at 37°C in a 5% CO_2incubator. Neutrophils cultured without bacteria were used as control. To determine f viable *Ft* was required for NETs induction, neutrophils were incubated with formalin-killed *Ft*-LVS for 4 h. The NETs released were visualized using DAPI (nuclear dye) under fluorescence microscope at 400× magnification. Released NETs were also validated using NETs marker, lactoferrin (1:400, Sigma, MO) and immunocytochemistry was performed (26). We evaluated at least 5 fields on each slide to quantify the total positive cells showing NETs.

Scanning Electron Microscopy

Mouse neutrophils, isolated as described above, were cultured on to 12-mm coverslips, infected with *Ft*-LVS (1:20), and incubated for 4 h. Cells were fixed in 2.5% glutaraldehyde for 2 h and washed in 0.2 M Cacodylate buffer three times and stored at 4°C overnight. Samples were then post-fixed for 1 h in aqueous 1% osmium tetroxide, and washed three times in Cacodylate buffer. Cells were dehydrated through a graded ethanol series (50, 60, 70, 90, and 95%) and washed three times with absolute ethanol. Finally the samples were chemically dehydrated using hexamethyldisilazane, and air-dried. Dried cells were mounted onto aluminum stubs, grounded with silver paint, and then sputter coated with 3.5 nm gold. Samples were viewed in a FEI Quanta 600 FEG scanning electron microscope. For positive release of NETs, we stimulated neutrophils with Phorbol 12-myristate 13-acetate (PMA, 20 nM).

Effect of MPO Inhibitor or NADPH Oxidase Inhibitor or Hydrogen Peroxide (H_2O_2) on Ft-Induced NETs

Ft infection has been shown to inhibit ROS generation by inhibiting NADPH oxidase activity within 60 min (15). We previously demonstrated that NETs generation is induced by redox enzymes such as MPO and superoxide dismutase (SOD) (19). To determine the role of MPO in *Ft*-infected neutrophils (1:20 MOI) were incubated with or without a MPO inhibitor 4-aminobenzoic acid hydrazide (4-ABAH, 100 μM) or H_2O_2, a MPO substrate (180 μM). NETs release was observed after 4 h. *Ft*-mediated NADPH oxidase inhibition was reported until 60 min after infection (15). Since NETs were observed after 4 h and to test whether *Ft*-induced NETs release is independent of NADPH oxidase activity, *Ft*-infected neutrophils were incubated in the presence of Diphenyleneiodonium (DPI, 10 μM) to completely block NADPH oxidase activity and the release of NETs evaluated after 4 h. PMA at 20 nM concentration was used as a positive control for NETs induction. These experiments were repeated three times. A total of 5 fields were counted for NETs positive staining and expressed as the percentage of total NETs-positive cells in different conditions.

Microbicidal Activity of NETs

To determine if NETs have bactericidal activity against *Francisella*, mouse neutrophils were isolated as described above. Neutrophils were seeded onto poly-D-lysine coated coverslips as described above and incubated with *Francisella* at 20:1 ratio dilution. After infection, cultures were lysed with freeze/thaw cycles and 0.1% Triton-X 100 in PBS for 3 min. Neutrophil lysates were serially diluted in PBS and plated onto chocolate agar plates for bacterial counts. For control, *Francisella* seeded without neutrophils was used. Surviving colonies were counted after 72 h. Further, to examine if NETs induced during infection trap the *Ft* bacteria, neutrophils were infected with *Ft*-LVS-GFP. At 3 h post infection, cells were stained with DAPI. Bright field and green and blue fluorescence images were captured at 1000× using Olympus fluorescence microscope.

Impact of Antibiotic Ciprofloxacin Treatment on NETosis *in vitro*

To assess impact of antibiotic treatment on NETosis, mouse neutrophils were infected with *Ft*-LVS (1:20 MOI) and incubated with ciprofloxacin (10and 20 μg/ml) prepared in sterile PBS. After 4 h, cells were stained with nuclear dye, DAPI and determined NETs release was determined as described above. To assess if ciprofloxacin has direct impact on NETosis, neutrophils were pre-incubated with 20 μg/ml ciprofloxacin for 20 min, followed by stimulation with PMA (20 nM). NETs release was evaluated after 4 h.

Effect of Treatment Ciprofloxacin Treatment on Ft-LVS Infection in Mice

To further assess impact of ciprofloxacin on NETosis during Ft infection in mice, BALB/c mice were infected with 1000 CFU of *Ft*-LVS. Ciprofloxacin (30 mg/kg) was administered orally starting at 48 h post infection, twice daily and given for 3 days. Animals were sacrificed at 5 days post infection. Lungs were lavaged with equal volumes of PBS and NETosis was analyzed by evaluating BAL for released H2A, citH3 and PAD4 levels by western blot analysis as described above.

Statistical Analyses

All the data were expressed as the means ± SE. Statistical analyses were performed using Student's *t*-test or analysis of variance (ANOVA) using Excel or GraphPad Prism 7 software. A value of $p < 0.05$ was considered statistically significant.

RESULTS

Ft Infection in Mice Induces Widespread NETosis and Accumulation of Extracellular Histones

BALB/C mice were infected intranasally with 10^3 CFU of *Ft*-LVS or PBS (for mock infection) and euthanized at 5 dpi. Histopathology and release of NETs were evaluated by H&E staining, immunohistochemistry and western blot analysis. Mock-infected mouse lungs and liver did not show any pathologic lesions (**Figures 1A,C**). *Ft*-infected mouse lungs displayed widespread nodular hemorrhagic lesions with massive degenerative and non-degenerative neutrophilic influx, necrotic debris and fibrin deposition (**Figure 1B**). The liver tissue from *Ft*-infected mice displayed mild hepatic necrosis with degenerative neutrophil infiltrations (**Figure 1D**). A semi-quantitative lung pathology scoring revealed significant pathology in *Ft* infected

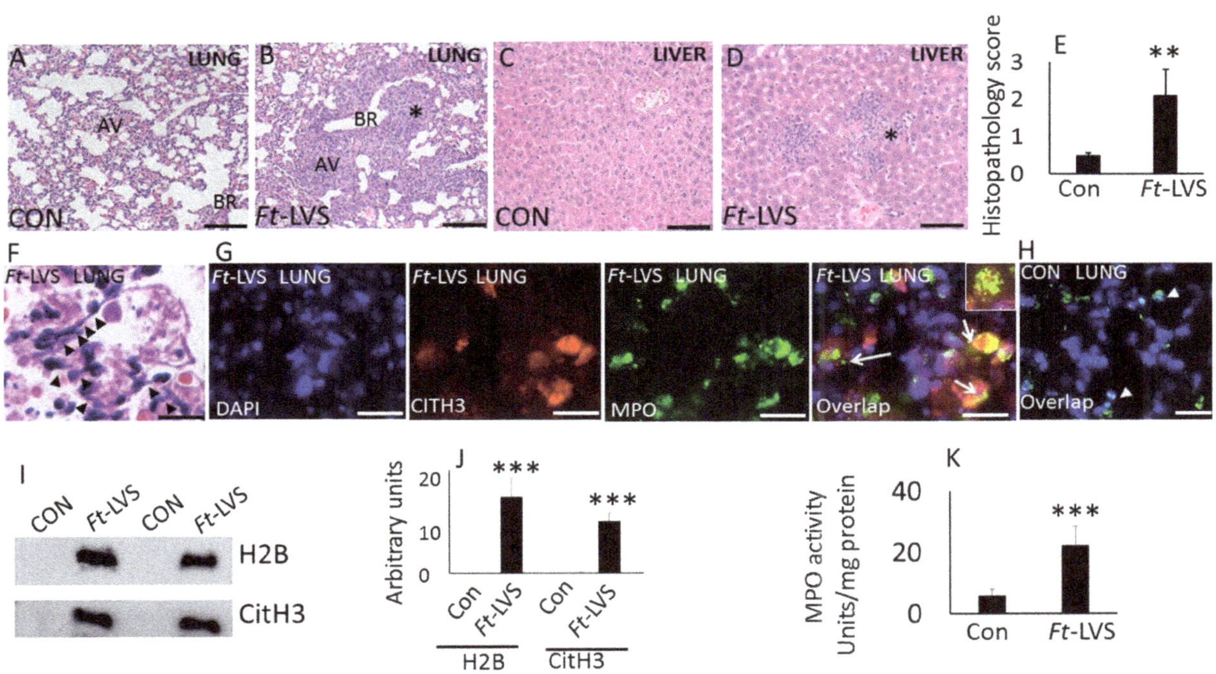

FIGURE 1 | *In vivo* evidence for NETs formation during Ft infection in mice. Paraffin-embedded lung tissues from mice challenged with lethal *Ft*-LVS were stained with hematoxylin-eosin or by immunofluorescence at 5 days post infection. **(A,B)** Mock-infected and *Ft*-LVS infected mouse lungs. *Ft-LVS* infected lungs displayed nodular hemorrhagic lesions with severe alveolar destruction and dense neutrophil influx (asterisk). **(C,D)** Histopathology of mock and *Ft*-LVS infected mouse liver. Liver displays hepatic necrosis with degenerative neutrophil infiltrations (asterisk) AV- alveoli; BR-bronchioles. **(E)** Semi-quantitative scoring of lung histopathology from control and *Ft*-LVS infected mice. **(F)** Extensive induction of NETs was detected in the alveoli (black arrow heads), within severely affected areas of infected lungs. **(G,H)** Immunostaining for NETs identified by co-localization of DNA (blue) with citrullinated H3 (citH3, red) and neutrophil granule marker MPO (green). Insert shows co-localization of citH3 with MPO, indicative of NETs release by lung neutrophils. **(I)** Detection of released NETs and extracellular histones in the BAL fluids by Western blot analysis. All the western blots were carried out by loading equal volumes of BAL from control and infected animals. **(J)** Densitometry analyses of histones H2B, and citH3. Control (Con) or *Ft*-LVS infected mice. **(K)** MPO activity in lung homogenates from control and infected mice. White arrows indicate NETs formation. Results are expressed as means ± SE. $N = 5$ in each group. Student's *t*-test was performed for comparing CitH3, H2B, and MPO densitometry values between control and *Ft*-LVS infected mice and *p* value of <0.05 was considered as significant. Scale bars: 40 μm **(A)**; 20 μm **(C–D)**. ** depicts $P < 0.01$, *** depicts $P < 0.001$ vs. control.

mice (**Figure 1E**). Intriguingly, prominent NETs release appeared individually or bundled within the areas of tissue damage, predominantly within nodular regions that were filled with neutrophils (**Figure 1F**). Owing to the processing and thin sectioning of fixed tissue, the release of NETs frequently appeared as elongated extensions with cellular origin or condensed small chromatin extensions from the neutrophils on H&E staining (**Figure 1F**). To validate the released NETs, we performed immunostaining that revealed the presence of citH3 and MPO co-localizing or appearing in the same cell depending on the status of the cells undergoing NETosis. The released NETs prominently appear within the affected regions of the lungs (**Figure 1G**). Prominent NETs release was observed in necrotic regions with discrete neutrophilic inflammations in the liver (**Supplementary Figure S1**). Mock-infected lungs did not show any staining for presence of citH3 or MPO (**Figure 1H**). To further validate the release of NETs in *Ft* infection, we performed western blot analysis of the BAL fluids collected from mock and *Ft* infected mice. Accumulation of histones (H2B) and modified histones (citH3, indicative of NETs release) was measured by western blot analysis (**Figure 1I**). Lungs were lavaged with equal volumes of PBS and the BAL densitometry analysis has shown significant accumulation of both extracellular histones and NETs in *Ft* infected lungs (**Figure 1J**). *Ft* infection of neutrophils has been shown to impair neutrophil activity and respiratory burst *in vitro* (15). To assess whether *Ft* infected lungs also exhibit impaired neutrophil activity *in vivo*, we measured lung MPO activities in mock and *Ft* infected mice. Interestingly, we found a fivefold increase in lung MPO activity (units per mg protein) in the lung homogenates of *Ft* infected mice (**Figure 1K**), thus indicating massive neutrophil influx.

The Released NETs Entangle With Alveolar Epithelium That Displays Membrane Disruption and Alveolar Damage

We have demonstrated earlier that the close attachment of NETs contribute significant cytopathic effect on alveolar epithelium and endothelium in influenza and *Streptococcus pneumoniae* superinfection following influenza challenge in mice (19). *Ft* bacteria interact with both type I and type II cells and induces

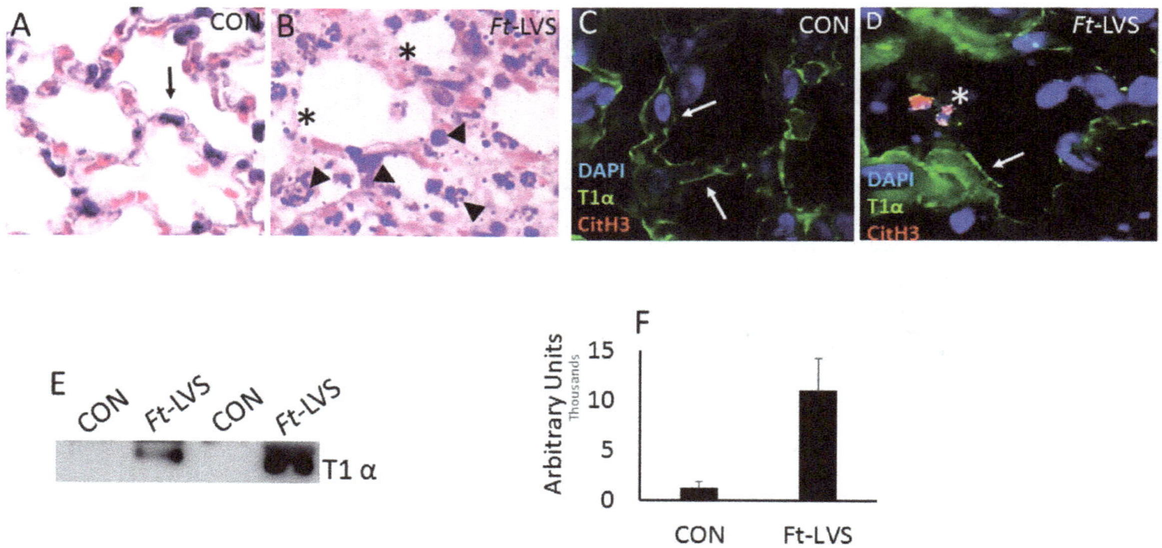

FIGURE 2 | *In vivo* accumulation of NETs within the damaged lungs and evidence for alveolar epithelial injury. **(A)** Mock-infected mice displayed normal alveolar structures (black arrow). **(B)** *Ft*-LVS infected mouse lungs on H&E staining showed released NETs (arrow head) attached onto the alveolus that shows disrupted epithelium (asterisk). **(C)** Mock-infected lungs show typical continuous staining for T1α on type I alveolar epithelium (white arrow). **(D)** *Ft*-LVS infected mouse lungs displayed disrupted alveolar epithelium (asterisk) upon close interaction with NETs (citH3 positive staining, red). Other areas of alveoli show normal epithelium shown as continuous staining for T1α (white arrow). DNA (blue) with citH3 (red), and T1α (green). White arrows indicate T1α staining and asterisks indicate damaged alveolar epithelial lining. **(E)** Western blot analysis for the release of T1α by analysis in BAL fluids. All the western blots were carried out by loading equal volumes of BAL from control and infected animals. **(F)** Densitometry analysis for T1α indicates significant alveolar epithelial injury in *Ft* infection. Results are expressed as means ± SE. Student's *t*-test was performed for comparing T1α densitometry values between control and *Ft*-LVS infected mice. $N = 5$ mice per group. Scale bars: 20 μm. ** depicts $P < 0.01$ vs. control.

cytotoxicity in type II cells, but not type I cells (28). To assess whether NETs interact with alveolar epithelium and trigger alveolitis, we evaluated less damaged areas showing normal alveolar architecture by histopathology and immunostaining analysis. As shown in **Figure 2A**, mock-infected mouse lungs displayed normal alveoli (black arrow) and immunostaining with Type I alveolar epithelial membrane marker, T1α that appears as continuous staining (**Figure 2C**, white arrow) on the membrane, as 95% of alveoli are covered with alveolar type I epithelium. Upon *Ft* infection, the released NETs show widespread attachment to the alveolar epithelium (**Figure 2B**, arrow head), which exhibited disrupted alveoli (**Figures 2B,D** asterisk). The areas that are adjacent to nodular regions appear normal with intact epithelial membrane staining (arrow). To further validate alveolar epithelial damage, we evaluated western blot and immunostaining for T1 α (a membrane protein of alveolar type I cell), which was significantly increased in infected mice (**Figures 2E,F**). These results indicate that the released NETs could contribute to collateral alveolar injury, which may exacerbate pathophysiology in *Ft* infection.

Ft Infected Domestic Cats and Rabbits Exhibit Severe Lung Pathology Associated With Extensive NETs Release

Severely ill domestic rabbits and cats with symptoms of high fever, lethargy, respiratory complications, diarrhea, and nasal blood discharge were brought to the Oklahoma State University veterinary clinic. Animals were euthanized, subjected to necropsy analysis, and *Ft* infection was confirmed by real-time PCR analysis of liver and spleen samples. We have included uninfected rabbit lung and live samples as controls. No pathologic lesions were observed in the lungs and liver samples collected from uninfected rabbits (**Figures 3A,C**). Histopathologic analysis of rabbit lungs revealed typical nodular and hemorrhagic lesions in *Ft*-positive rabbits (**Figure 3B**, asterisk). Necrotic foci were composed of degenerated neutrophils accompanied by cellular debris, abundant fibrin. In liver, hepatic architecture was multifocally effaced by discrete foci of coagulative necrosis of the liver (**Figure 3D**, asterisk). The necrotic foci consisted of dead, numerous non-degenerate and degenerate neutrophils, eosinophilic hepatocytes, and histiocytes (Kupffer cells). Three uninfected rabbits were included as controls in this study. Pathologic lesions in *Ft*-positive cats were similar to rabbits with widespread typical nodular and hemorrhagic lesions in the lungs; which often display discrete foci of necrosis and neutrophilic infiltrates (**Figure 3E**). The liver tissue was effaced by discrete foci of coagulative necrosis. The necrotic foci were comprised of dead, eosinophilic hepatocytes, numerous non-degenerate and degenerate neutrophils, and sparse hemorrhage and some fibrin strands (**Figure 3F**). Total histopathologic scores between control and *Ft*-positive rabbits are shown in **Figure 3G**. Intriguingly, prominent NETosis was observed in lung and liver tissue of both *Ft*-positive rabbits and cats. Histopathology analysis also showed

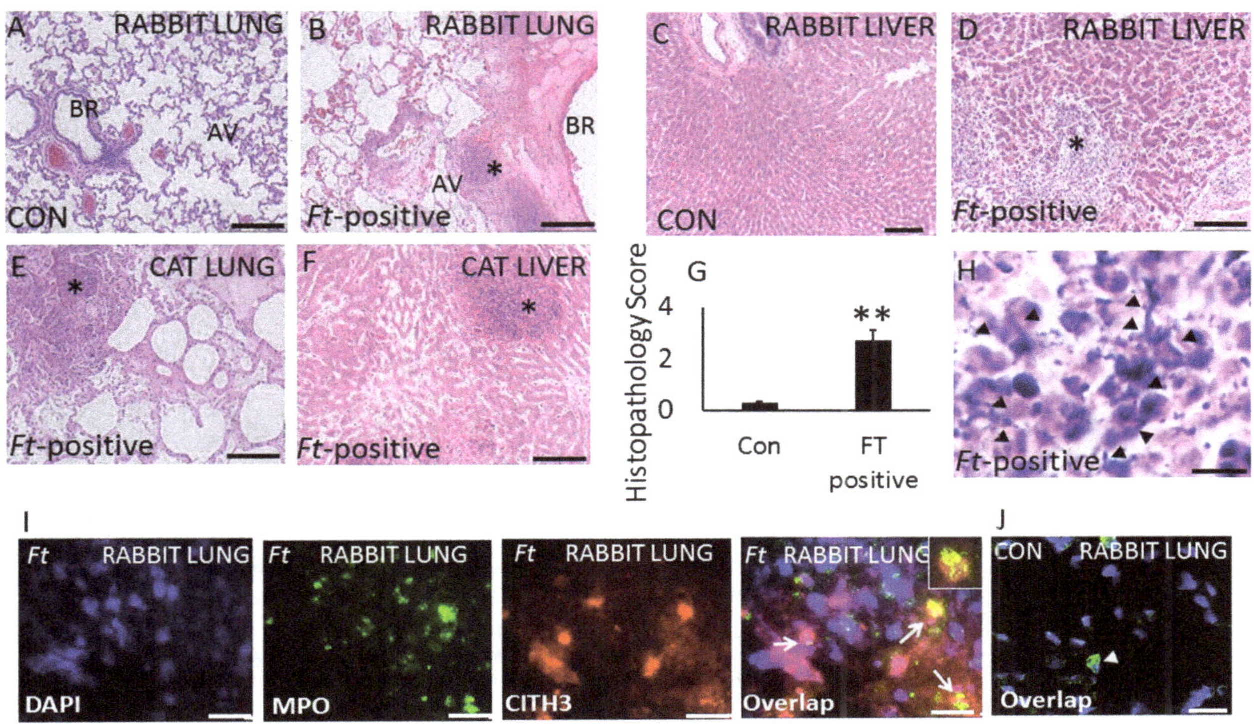

FIGURE 3 | Evidence for the induction of NETosis *in* Ft-positive rabbits and cats. **(A,B)**H&E images of lung, and liver samples from control rabbits. Severe alveolar damage and neutrophil influx (asterisk). **(C,D)** *Ft*-positive rabbits hepatic degeneration and dense neutrophil influx (asterisk) and **(E,F)** *Ft*-positive cats. Degeneration and dense neutrophil influx in the cat lung and liver (asterisk). **(G)** Semi-quantitative histopathology scores of control (Con) and *Ft*-positive rabbit lungs. **(H)** Extensive induction of NETs was detected within the alveoli (black arrow heads) within severely affected areas of the rabbit lungs. **(I,J)** Immunostaining for NETs formation in infected lungs. NETs were identified by co-localization of DNA (blue) with citH3 (red) and neutrophil granule marker MPO (green). Insert shows co-localization of citH3 with MPO indication of NETs release by lung neutrophils. $N = 4$ *Ft*-positive rabbits; 3 *Ft*-positive cats and 3 uninfected rabbits. Student's *t*-test was performed for comparing T1α densitometry values between control and *Ft*-LVS infected rabbits.Results are expressed as means ± SE. Scale bars: 20 μm. $^{**}P < 0.01$ vs. control.

NETs, which appeared as elongated extensions with cellular origin by H&E staining (**Figure 3H**). Immunostaining analysis for identification of NETs revealed prominent NETs in *Ft*-positive rabbit lungs, but not in uninfected rabbit lungs (**Figure 3I**). Prominent NETs appeared within the liver granulomas with discrete neutrophilic necrosis (**Supplementary Figure S2**) of *Ft*-positive rabbits. Control rabbit lungs did not show any staining for citH3 and MPO (**Figure 3J**).

Ft Induces NETs, Which Is Dependent on MOI of Infection *in vitro*

Mouse neutrophils were infected with different MOI (1:10, 1:20, 1:30, 1:50, and 1:100) of *Ft* for 4 h. The released NETs were identified by staining with DAPI (nuclear dye) to identify NETs. *Ft* infection induced NETs release by 4 h (**Figure 4A**) and NETs induction was enhanced with the increase in MOI of *Ft* infection (**Figure 4B**). However, at MOI of 1: 100 significant number of neutrophils exhibited disintegrated nuclei (**Figure 4A**, asterisk), but decrease in NETs release. The released NETs were confirmed by immunostaining analysis using a NETs marker, lactoferrin, which appeared as "beads on a string" staining on released NETs (**Figure 4C**). We have earlier found that released NETs trap bacteria in the extracellular environment (19, 29). To assess if NETs released during *Ft* infection interact with bacteria, we infected neutrophils with *Ft*-LVS-GFP, i.e. GFP-labeled bacteria. As shown in **Figures 5A–D**, the ingested bacteria were trapped in the NETs releasing from the neutrophils and bacteria were also present in the cytoplasm of the infected cell. These studies indicate that NETs occur during active ingestion of the bacteria. Although NETs appeared to trap the bacteria, we did not find bactericidal effects of NETs (**Figure 5E**). To further validate these results, we have performed scanning electron microscopy to identify *Ft-LVS* interaction with released NETs. We observed clusters or single bacterial cell attached to the NETs chromatin strands or trapped in NETs (**Figures 5F–I**). We have also included SEM of NETs released by neutrophils stimulated with Phorbol 12-myristate 13-acetate (PMA) (**Figure 5J**).

Active Bacterial Infection Required for NETs Formation

Earlier studies have shown that live bacterial infection is required for inhibition of phagocytic activity and formalin killed bacteria fails to prolong neutrophil life span or to delay apoptotic death in neutrophils. To assess whether live bacterial infection is essential for induction of NETosis, formalin killed *Ft*-LVS was

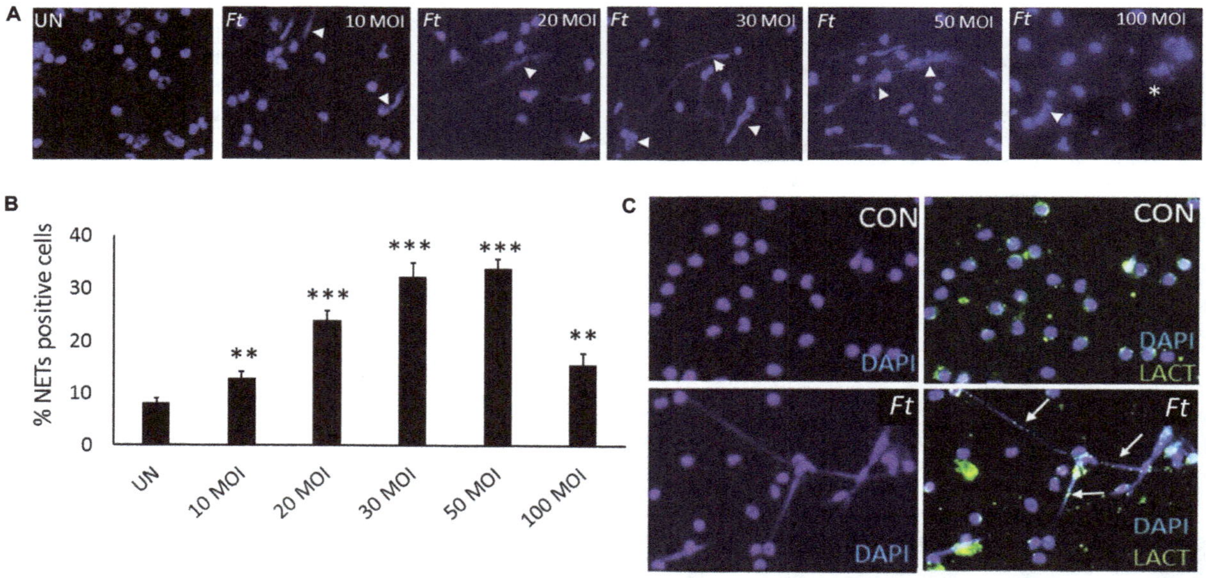

FIGURE 4 | Ft-infection induces NETosis *in vitro.* **(A)**Neutrophils were infected with different MOI of the *Ft*-LVS (1:10, 1:20, 1:30, 1:50, and 1:100) and NETs induction evaluated after 4 h by staining with DAPI, a nuclear dye (white arrow heads).**(B)** Significant induction of NETs release was observed upon *Ft*-LVS infection and NETs formation increased with the increase in MOI. **(C)** NETs release was validated using lactoferrin, which appeared as "green beads on strand" staining on chromatin fibers (white arrow). The values are average of three independent experiments. Results are expressed as means ± SE. Scale bars: 20 μm. One-way ANOVA with Tukey's multiple comparison was analyzed. ** depicts $P < 0.01$ and *** depicts $P < 0.001$vs. uninfected control.

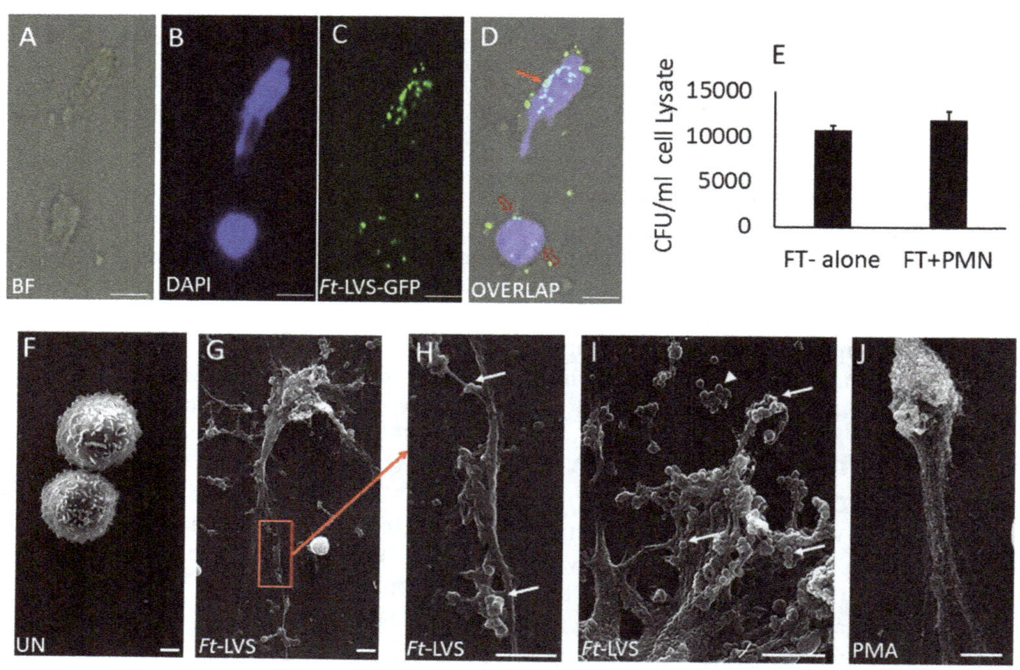

FIGURE 5 | NETs trap Ft-LVS bacteria, but fails to kill. To test whether NETs trap *Ft* bacteria, murine neutrophils were infected with green fluorescence protein (GFP) labelled *Ft* bacteria, *Ft*-LVS-GFP at MOI of 1:20. **(A–D)** Immunostaining analysis clearly demonstrates trapping of *Ft*-LVS-GFP bacteria in NETs. Red arrow shows *Ft* trapped in NETs. Red open arrow shows Ft in the cytoplasm. **(E)** However, no differences in CFU were found in the presence of NETs. **(F–I)** Scanning electron microscopy of NETs formed during Ft infection. **(J)** Positive control of NETs induction when neutrophils were stimulated with PMA. BF–bright field image. White arrow – bacteria attached to NETs. Arrow head – cluster of free bacteria not attached to NETs. The values are average of three independent experiments. Scale Bar for **A–D** = 20 μm; Scale Bar for **F–J** = 1 μm. Results are expressed as means ± SE.

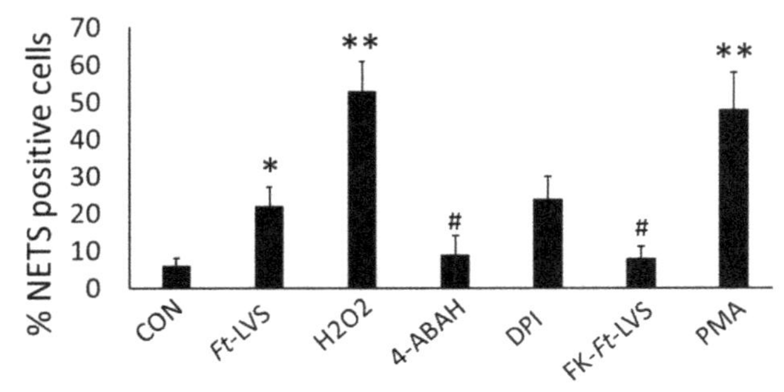

FIGURE 6 | Ft induced NETosis is dependent on MPO activity. Neutrophils were infected with *Ft*-LVS (1:20 MOI) and NETs induction evaluated by immunostaining for lactoferrin and counter stained with DAPI. *Ft*-induced NETosis require active bacterial infection. To test this, *Ft*-LVS was killed with formalin. Formalin killed (FK), FK-*Ft*-LVS fail to induce NETosis. Activation of MPO with its substrate, H_2O_2 significantly enhanced NETs release, while pharmacological blocking of MPO activity with 4-ABAH significantly inhibited *Ft*-LVS induced NETosis. Similarly, blocking NADPH oxidase with DPI did not show any difference compared to neutrophils infected with *Ft*-LVS alone infected neutrophils. PMA stimulation was used as positive control. One-way ANOVA with Tukey's multiple comparison was analyzed. $^{*}P < 0.05$ vs. control; $^{\#}P < 0.05$ and $^{**}P < 0.001$ vs.*Ft*-LVS.

incubated with neutrophils. The formalin-killed bacteria (FK-*Ft*-LVS) did not induce NETs, thus suggesting that NETosis is an active mechanism that requires bacterial phagocytosis by neutrophils. NETs induction by PMA showed significant induction of NETosis (**Figure 6**).

Ft-Induced NETs Is Dependent on MPO Activity

NADPH oxidase activity is required for generation of ROS during NETosis. Since *Ft* inhibits NADPH oxidase activity, we hypothesized a possibility for NADPH oxidase-independent NETs release during *Ft* infection. MPO and neutrophil elastase released from azurophilic granules anchor chromatin scaffolds in NETs, and mediate histone degradation during NETs formation (30, 31). Since we found significant induction of MPO activity in *Ft*-infected lungs, we asked whether MPO is critical in *Ft*-induced NETs formation. To test this, mouse neutrophils were infected with *Ft* in the presence or absence of pharmacological blocker of MPO (4-ABAH). Blocking with 4-ABAH significantly inhibited NETs release (**Figure 6**). To assess if induction of MPO activity potentiates NETosis, *Ft* infected neutrophils were incubated in the presence of a MPO substrate, H_2O_2. Interestingly, the addition of H_2O_2 significantly increased NETs release, thus indicating that activation of MPO potentiates NETs generation. To further assess NADPH oxidase independence in *Ft* induced NETs, neutrophils were incubated in the presence of NADPH oxidase inhibitor to completely abolish the NADPH oxidase activity. The addition of NADPH oxidase inhibitor also induces NETs release similar to *Ft*-alone group, suggesting that *Ft*-induced NETosis is NADPH oxidase independent. These findings indicate that MPO activity is critical in the release of NETs during *Ft* infection.

Effect of Antibiotic Ciprofloxacin on NETosis *in vivo* and *in vitro*

To assess impact of antibiotic treatment on NETosis, *Ft* infected neutrophils were incubated with different concentrations of ciprofloxacin. Significant decrease in NETs formation was observed compared to *Ft* infection (**Figure 7A**). To determine if ciprofloxacin has direct impact on NETosis, neutrophils were incubated with ciprofloxacin and stimulated with PMA. Ciprofloxacin incubation reduced PMA-induced NETs (**Figure 7B**). To further assess impact of ciprofloxacin on NETosis during *Ft* infection in mice, infected mice were treated with ciprofloxacin and analyzed for NETs release by western blot analysis. The antibiotic significantly abrogated NETs induction and release of extracellular histones, as evident by decreased H2A and citH3 levels (**Figures 7C–E**). Further ciprofloxacin treatment also reduced lung PAD4 levels (**Figures 7C,F**), thus indicating that antibiotic treatment significantly suppressed NETosis *in vivo*.

DISCUSSION

Our findings demonstrate that *Ft* infection triggers NETosis both *in vivo* and *in vitro*. The released NETs prominently appeared in the lungs and liver of *Ft*-LVS infected mice, and in clinically diagnosed *Ft*-positive domestic cats and rabbits. Although aggravated neutrophil influx has been associated with in host tissue injury in severe *Ft* infections, their role in *Ft* pathophysiology is not completely understood. Our findings reveal that neutrophils recruited at infection site exhibit high MPO activity and undergo NETopathic cell death during active *Ft* infection. The released chromatin strands released from NETs prominently appear within nodular hemorrhagic lesions, indicating a potential role of NETs in aggravating collateral tissue damage. We found that *Ft*-LVS infection in neutrophils induces NETs release *in vitro*. Further, *Ft*-LVS-induced NETs release required MPO activity and was independent of NADPH oxidase activity. Antibiotic treatment with ciprofloxacin significantly suppressed NETosis both *in vivo* and *in vitro*. These studies provide a novel basis for the role of NETs in *Ft* pathophysiology.

Previous studies have shown that *Ft* parasitizes inside the neutrophil and suppresses the neutrophil's antimicrobial defense by impairing respiratory burst, thus allowing the *Ft* to escape from phagosomal killing (15–18).*Ft*-mediated suppression of neutrophil respiratory burst occurs *via* disruption of NADPH oxidase enzyme complex that aids in bacterial survival in these immune cells (15, 32). Simultaneously, *Ft* also enhances neutrophil life-span by inhibiting their apoptotic signaling pathway *in vitro* (18, 33, 34). Although studies on *Ft*-neutrophil interactions implicate how *Ft* can suppresses host innate immune defense and neutrophil functionality *in vitro*, the fate of massive neutrophils that are recruited at the infection site remain poorly defined. Furthermore, activation status of these infiltrated neutrophils are so far unknown. Our studies have identified that lung-sequestered neutrophils are functionally active and generate NETs. We found strong immunostaining of NETs components (including citH3 and MPO) in the damaged lungs and liver of

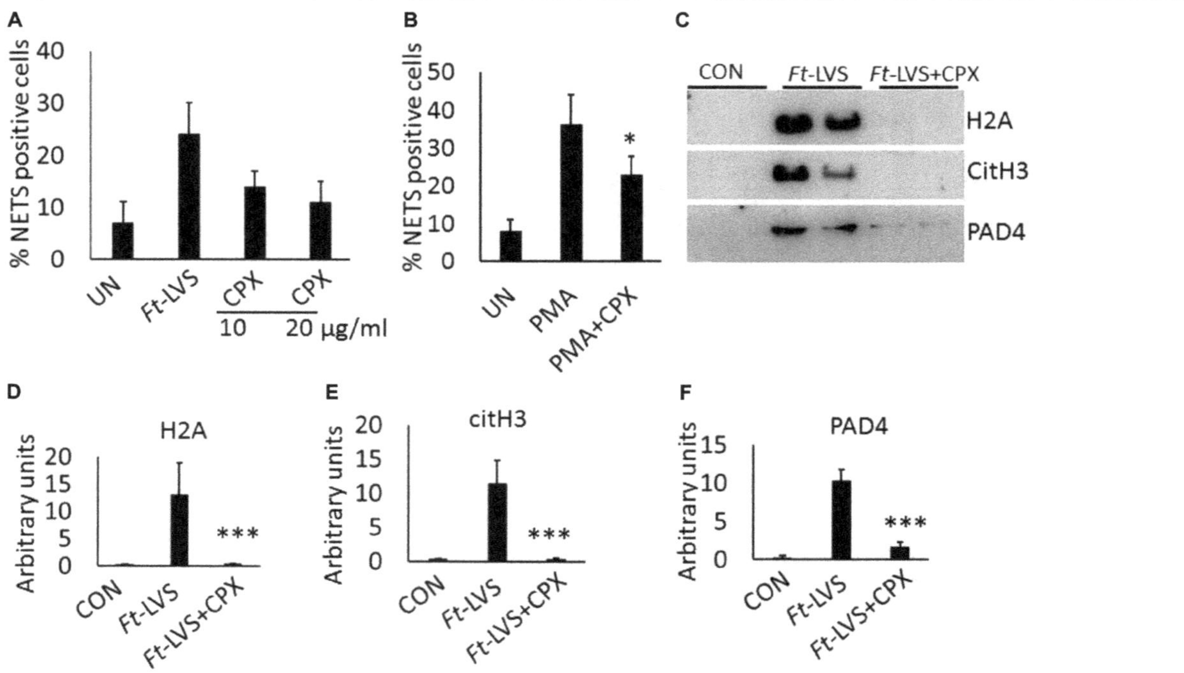

FIGURE 7 | Impact of ciprofloxacin on NETosis *in vitro* and *in vivo*. **(A)** Murine neutrophils were infected with *Ft*-LVS at 1:20 MOI in the presence of ciprofloxacin (10 and 20 µg/ml). The release of NETs was determined. **(B)** Effect of ciprofloxacin on PMA-induced NETosis. **(C)** Western blot analysis for the release of H2A, citH3, and PAD4 in BAL fluids of infected (10^3 CFU of *Ft*-LVS) and ciprofloxacin (30 mg/kg) treated BALB/c mice at 5 days post infection. All the western blots were carried out by loading equal volumes of BAL from control and infected animals. **(D–F)** Densitometry analysis of H2A, citH3 and PAD4 ($n = 4$). **(A,B)** The values are average of three independent experiments. Results are expressed as means ± SE. Student's *t*-test was performed for comparing T1α densitometry values between control and *Ft*-LVS infected mice and *p* value of <0.05 was considered as significant. *$P < 0.05$, vs.*Ft*-LVS or PMA, ***$P < 0.001$ vs.*Ft*-LVS.

mice infected with *Ft*-LVS as well as *Ft*-positive domestic rabbits and cats. It is also noted that only a subpopulation of neutrophils appeared to release NETs, since we also detected MPO positive neutrophils without citH3 staining with disintegrated nuclei that were possibly undergoing apoptosis or necrosis.

Neutrophil extracellular traps are formed as large extracellular web-like chromatin strands that were initially proposed as a defense mechanism against invading pathogens (24). However, excessive release of NETs aggravate tissue injury and death as reported in several clinical and disease conditions (20–22, 35, 36). Although aerosol route of *Ft* infection causes severe pneumonia tularemia pneumonia with high fatalities, the pathophysiology in this devastating respiratory disease is not yet completely understood (37). Careful examination of the *Ft*-infected mouse, domestic rabbit and cat lungs revealed that the NETs DNA fibers were frequently entangled to the alveolar epithelium, suggesting suggests that these structures may contribute to damage of thin alveolar-capillary barrier. There are several possibilities how these NETs could aggravate *Ft* pathophysiology. First, the close-proximity of the NETs fibers carrying toxic nuclear and granule proteins such as histones, MPO, MMPs, and neutrophil elastase could disrupt thin alveolar-capillary barrier, thereby enhancing the systemic spread of the bacteria (38). In support of this, we recently showed that extracellular histones induce cytotoxic response in alveolar epithelial cells *in vitro* and *in vivo*. Interestingly, despite presence of excessive NETs in dual-infected mice (*Streptococcus pneumoniae* superinfection, following influenza), aggravated alveolar disruption and augmented systemic spread of the bacteria were noted, thus suggesting that NETs-mediated injury could compromise alveolar function (19). Second, *Ft* infection of alveolar type II epithelial cells and alveolar macrophages triggers high induction of cytokines including IL-8, MCP-1, and IL-1β(28, 39). These chemoattractant cytokines potentially modulate inflammatory status in the lungs by attracting massive neutrophil influx and activation at the infection site. In addition, we report here that NETs released during *Ft* infection, entangle alveolar epithelial cells and disrupt thin alveolar epithelial bed. Indeed, the DNA fibers entangled with alveolar epithelium has been implicated in the pathophysiology of influenza, bacterial pneumonia and sepsis (19, 25, 40). These findings suggest that a cumulative effect of *Ft*-inflicted alveolar type II epithelial injury together with NETs-mediated alveolitis could contribute to widespread pathophysiology in severe *Ft* infections. Work is currently underway to further characterize mechanisms of *Ft*-induced NETs.

Next, to validate whether *Ft*-neutrophil interaction triggers NETosis, we infected neutrophils with different MOI of *Ft*-LVS. Our data has shown that *Ft* infection induces NETs release, which is dependent on MOI. The lack of NETs formation with formalin-killed *Ft* bacteria suggested that active bacterial infection is required for the formation of NETs. The mechanism of NETosis is a complex process and mediated by various factors. Previously, it has been shown that *Ft* infection disrupts assembly of gp91/p22*phox* or p47/p67*phox* domains in NADPH oxidase, and thereby impairs neutrophil respiratory burst and activity observed within 60 min after infection (15). Although activity of NADPH oxidase has been linked to NETs formation, it is not indispensible in forming the NETs as NADPH oxidase independent NETosis has been identified in *Staphylococcus aureus* infection (41). Moreover, NETs release was observed 4 h after *Ft* infection and NADPH oxidase activity during that time is unknown. To exclude the involvement of NADPH oxidase activity, *Ft*-infected neutrophils were inhibited by pharmacological drug against NADPH oxidase. Interestingly, blocking NADPH oxidase did not show any impact on NETs release indicating that *Ft* induced NETs release occurred independently of NADPH oxidase activity. Our studies have revealed that pharmacological blocking of MPO significantly reduced NETs generation, whereas induction of MPO activity by addition of H2O2 potentiated NETs release. Further studies are needed to determine whether *Ft* infection induces MPO expression or enhances its activity both *in vitro* and *in vivo*. Taken together these findings suggest that recruited neutrophils into the infection site potentially induce NETosis, which is dependent on MPO activity.

Antibiotic therapy is an effective treatment choice for *Ft* infections(42). The use of gentamycin and tetracyclins are effective *Ft*-treatments. However, some clinical reports have documented failures with relapse when these antibiotics were used (43, 44). On the other hand, gentamicin also inhibits neutrophil chemotaxis function (45). Although ciprofloxacin and doxycycline are recommended for milder forms of the disease, treatment with doxycycline is contraindicated in children under 8 years of age (46). These findings indicate that a better understanding of therapeutic effectiveness in antibiotic treatments and their association with host response is needed. The involvement of host-related pathogenesis in *Ft* infection is still not completely understood. Our studies indicate a possible mechanism how the excessive neutrophils could exacerbate pulmonary pathology in *Ft* infections. With our findings indicating extensive release of NETs and their pathogenic link in *Ft*-infection, we assessed the impact of antibiotic treatment on NETs. Interestingly, antibiotic treatment suppressed NETosis both *in vitro* and *in vivo* and we found direct inhibitory effect of ciprofloxacin in PMA-induced NETs release, suggesting a direct suppression of NETs formation by antibiotic treatment. This was further evident by decreased citH3 and PAD4 levels in infected lungs. One of the prominent characteristics of the NETs is to trap and kill the microbial pathogen in the extracellular environment. Interestingly, neutrophils infected with GFP-labeled *Ft* bacteria displayed a significant number of bacteria being trapped in the NETs chromatin fibers. However, no bactericidal effects were observed, thus suggesting that NETs induced during *Ft* infection can contribute to lung injury, but have limited bactericidal activity.

Taken together, these studies indicate that massive induction of NETs could significantly contribute to acute pulmonary damage in *Ft*-infection. Further, we found that massive neutrophils recruited at the infection site are functionally active and undergo NETosis. The released NETs attach and disrupt alveolar epithelial bed. We also found that *Ft*-infection induces NETs release *in vitro*. Furthermore, we document that NETs formation is an active process and is dependent on MPO activity. Hence, intervention strategies to inhibit NETosis or targeting MPO may have potential therapeutic impact to ameliorate the severe pulmonary pathology in severe *Ft* infections.

ETHICS STATEMENT

The animal study was reviewed and approved by the Institutional Animal Care and Use Committee (IACUC) of Oklahoma State University (protocol number VM-17-36).

AUTHOR CONTRIBUTIONS

SP, AR, JM, and NT contributed to conception and design of experiments. SP, MP, and NT acquired and analyzed the data. RG and TS contributed to histopathology analyses. NT, JM, and VC drafted and critically reviewed the manuscript.

SUPPLEMENTARY MATERIAL

FIGURE S1 | Immunostaining for NETs formation in infected mouse liver. NETs were identified by co-localization of DNA (blue) with citH3 (red) and neutrophil granule marker MPO (green).

FIGURE S2 | Immunostaining for NETs formation in infected rabbit liver. NETs were identified by co-localization of DNA (blue) with citH3 (red) and neutrophil granule marker MPO (green).

REFERENCES

1. Allen LA. Neutrophils: potential therapeutic targets in tularemia? *Front Cell Infect Microbiol.* (2013) 27:109. doi: 10.3389/fcimb.2013.00109
2. Sharma J, Mares CA, Li Q, Morris EG, Teale JM. Features of sepsis caused by pulmonary infection with *Francisella tularensis* Type A strain. *Microb Pathog.* (2011) 51:39–47. doi: 10.1016/j.micpath.2011.03.007
3. Pechous RD, McCarthy TR, Zahrt TC. Working toward the future: insights into *Francisella tularensis* pathogenesis and vaccine development. *Microbiol Mol Biol Rev.* (2009) 73:684–711. doi: 10.1128/MMBR.00028-09
4. Fritz DL, England MJ, Miller L, Waag DM. Mouse models of aerosol-acquired tularemia caused by *Francisella tularensis* types A and B. *Comp Med.* (2014) 64:341–50.
5. Sjostedt A. Tularemia: history, epidemiology, pathogen physiology, and clinical manifestations. *Ann N Y Acad Sci.* (2007) 1105:1–29. doi: 10.1196/annals.1409.009
6. World Health Organization. *Health Aspects of Chemical and Biological Weapons.* Geneva: World Health Organization (1970).
7. Mares CA, Ojeda SS, Morris EG, Li Q, Teale JM. Initial delay in the immune response to *Francisella tularensis* is followed by hypercytokinemia characteristic of severe sepsis and correlating with upregulation and release

of damage-associated molecular patterns. *Infect Immun.* (2008) 76:3001–10. doi: 10.1128/IAI.00215-08
8. Flick-Smith HC, Fox MA, Hamblin KA, Richards MI, Jenner DC, Laws TR, et al. Assessment of antimicrobial peptide LL-37 as a post-exposure therapy to protect against respiratory tularemia in mice. *Peptides.* (2013) 43:96–101. doi: 10.1016/j.peptides.2013.02.024
9. Chris AM, Ojeda SS, Morris EG, Li Q, Teale JM. Initial Delay in the immune response to *Francisella tularensis* is followed by hypercytokinemia characteristic of severe sepsis and correlating with upregulation and release of damage-associated molecular patterns. *Infect Immun.* (2008) 76:3001–10.
10. Evans ME, Gregory DW, Schaffner S, McGee ZA. Tularemia: a 30-year experience with 88 cases. *Medicine.* (1985) 64:251–69. doi: 10.1097/00005792-198507000-00006
11. Staples JE, Kubota KA, Chalcraft LG, Mead PS, Petersen JM. Epidemiologic and molecular analysis of human tularemia, United States, 1964-2004. *Emerg Infect Dis.* (2006) 12:1113–8. doi: 10.3201/eid1207.051504
12. Schricker RL, Eigelsbach HT, Mitten JQ, Hall WC. Pathogenesis of tularemia in monkeys aerogenically exposed to *Francisella tularensis* 425. *Infect Immun.* (1972) 5:734–44. doi: 10.1128/IAI.5.5.734-744.1972
13. Malik M, Bakshi CS, McCabe K, Catlett SV, Shah A, Singh R, et al. Matrix metalloproteinase 9 activity enhances host susceptibility to pulmonary infection with type A and B strains of *Francisella tularensis. J Immunol.* (2007) 178:1013–20. doi: 10.4049/jimmunol.178.2.1013
14. Anthony LD, Burke RD, Nano FE. Growth of *Francisella* spp. in rodent macrophages. *Infect Immun.* (1991) 59:3291–6. doi: 10.1128/IAI.59.9.3291-3296.1991
15. McCaffrey RL, Allen LA. *Francisella tularensis* LVS evades killing by human neutrophils via inhibition of the respiratory burst and phagosome escape. *J Leukoc Biol.* (2006) 80:1224–30. doi: 10.1189/jlb.0406287
16. Schwartz JT, Barker JH, Kaufman J, Fayram DC, McCracken JM, Allen L-AH. *Francisella tularensis* inhibits the intrinsic and extrinsic pathways to delay constitutive apoptosis and prolong human neutrophil lifespan. *J Immmunol.* (2012) 188:3351–63. doi: 10.4049/jimmunol.1102863
17. McCaffrey RL, Schwartz JT, Lindemann SR, Moreland JG, Buchan BW, Jones BD, et al. Multiple mechanisms of NADPH oxidase inhibition by type A and type B *Francisella tularensis. J Leukoc Biol.* (2010) 88:791–805. doi: 10.1189/jlb.1209811
18. Kinkead LC, Allen LA. Multifaceted effects of *Francisella tularensis* on human neutrophil function and lifespan. *Immunol Rev.* (2016) 273:266–81. doi: 10.1111/imr.12445
19. Anandi NM, Narasaraju T, Prashant R, Perumalsamy R, Tan KB, Wang S, et al. *In vivo* and *in vitro* studies on the roles of neutrophil extracellular traps during secondary pneumococcal pneumonia after primary pulmonary influenza infection. *Front Immunol.* (2013) 4:56. doi: 10.3389/fimmu.2013.00056
20. Tang BM, Shojaei M, Teoh S, Meyers A, Ho J, Ball TB, et al. Neutrophils-related host factors associated with severe disease and fatality in patients with influenza infection. *Nat Commun.* (2019) 10:3422. doi: 10.1038/s41467-019-11249-y
21. Ebrahimi F, Giaglis S, Hahn S, Blum CA, Baumgartner C, Kutz A, et al. Markers of neutrophil extracellular traps predict adverse outcome in community-acquired pneumonia: secondary analysis of a randomised controlled trial. *Eur Respir J.* (2018) 51:1701389. doi: 10.1183/13993003.01389-2017
22. Wartha F, Beiter K, Albiger B, Fernebro J, Zychlinsky A, Normark S, et al. Capsule and D-alanylated lipoteichoic acids protect Streptococcus pneumoniae against neutrophil extracellular traps. *Cell Microbiol.* (2007) 9:1162–71. doi: 10.1111/j.1462-5822.2006.00857.x
23. Ashar HK, Mueller NC, Rudd JM, Snider TA, Achanta M, Prasanthi M, et al. Role of extracellular histones in influenza virus pathogenesis. *Am J Pathol.* (2018) 188:135–48. doi: 10.1016/j.ajpath.2017.09.014
24. Brinkmann V, Reichard U, Goosmann C, Fauler B, Uhlemann Y, Weiss DS, et al. Neutrophil extracellular traps kill bacteria. *Science.* (2004) 303:1532–5. doi: 10.1126/science.1092385
25. Narasaraju T, Edwin Y, Perumal RS, Ng HH, Poh WP, Audrey-Ann L, et al. Excessive neutrophils and neutrophil extracellular traps contribute to acute lung injury of influenza pneumonitis. *Am J Pathol.* (2011) 179:199–210. doi: 10.1016/j.ajpath.2011.03.013
26. Pulavendran S, Rudd JM, Maram P, Thomas PG, Akhilesh R, Malayer JR, et al. Combination therapy targeting platelet activation and virus replication protects mice against lethal influenza pneumonia. *Am J Respir Cell Mol Biol.* (2019) 61:689–701. doi: 10.1165/rcmb.2018-0196OC
27. Narasaraju T, Ng HH, Phoon MC, Chow VTMCP-. 1 antibody treatment enhances damage and impedes repair of the alveolar epithelium in influenza pneumonitis. *Am J Respir Cell Mol Biol.* (2010) 42:732–43. doi: 10.1165/rcmb.2008-0423OC
28. Faron M, Fletcher JR, Rasmussen JA, Apicella MA, Jones BD. Interactions of *Francisella tularensis* with alveolar type II epithelial cells and the murine respiratory epithelium. *PLoS One.* (2015) 10:e0127458. doi: 10.1371/journal.pone.0127458
29. Anandi NM, Prashant R, Jiao H, Shi W, Kong BT, Liang Q, et al. Capsules of virulent pneumococcal serotypes enhance formation of neutrophil extracellular traps during in vivo pathogenesis of pneumonia. *Oncotarget.* (2016) 7:19327–40. doi: 10.18632/oncotarget.8451
30. Papayannopoulos V, Metzler KD, Hakkim A, Zychlinsky A. Neutrophil elastase and myeloperoxidase regulate the formation of neutrophil extracellular traps. *J Cell Biol.* (2010) 191:677–91. doi: 10.1083/jcb.201006052
31. Metzler Kathleen D, Goosmann C, Lubojemska A, Zychlinsky A, Papayannopoulos VA. Myeloperoxidase-containing complex regulates neutrophil elastase release and actin dynamics during NETosis. *Cell Rep.* (2014) 8:883–96. doi: 10.1016/j.celrep.2014.06.044
32. Kinkead LC, Whitmore LC, McCracken JM, Fletcher JR, Ketelsen BB, Kaufman JW, et al. Bacterial lipoproteins and other factors released by *Francisella tularensis* modulate human neutrophil lifespan: effects of a TLR1 SNP on apoptosis inhibition. *Cell Microbiol.* (2018) 20:e12795. doi: 10.1111/cmi.12795
33. Plzakova L, Kubelkova K, Krocova Z, Zarybnicka L, Sinkorova Z, Macela AB. cell subsets are activated and produce cytokines during early phases of *Francisella tularensis* LVS infection. *Microb Pathog.* (2014) 75:49–58. doi: 10.1016/j.micpath.2014.08.009
34. Celli J, Zahrt TC. Mechanisms of *Francisella tularensis* intracellular pathogenesis. *Cold Spring Harb Perspect Med.* (2013) 3:a010314. doi: 10.1101/cshperspect.a010314
35. Sivanandham R, Brocca-Cofano E, Krampe N, Falwell E, Venkatraman S, Ribeiro RM, et al. Neutrophil extracellular trap production contributes to pathogenesis in SIV-infected nonhuman primates. *J Clin Investigat.* (2018) 128:5178–83. doi: 10.1172/JCI99420
36. Wong SL, Demers M, Martinod K, Gallant M, Wang Y, Goldfine AB, et al. Diabetes primes neutrophils to undergo NETosis, which impairs wound healing. *Nat Med.* (2015) 21:815–9. doi: 10.1038/nm.3887
37. Twenhafel NA, Alves DA, Purcell BK. Pathology of inhalational *Francisella tularensis* spp. tularensis SCHU S4 infection in African green monkeys (Chlorocebus aethiops). *Vet Pathol.* (2009) 46:698–706. doi: 10.1354/vp.08-VP-0302-T-AM
38. Porto BN, Stein RT. Neutrophil extracellular traps in pulmonary diseases: too much of a good thing? *Front Immunol.* (2016) 7:311. doi: 10.3389/fimmu.2016.00311
39. Hall JD, Craven RR, Fuller JR, Pickles RJ, Kawula TH. *Francisella tularensis* replicates within alveolar type II epithelial cells in vitro and in vivo following inhalation. *Infect Immun.* (2007) 75:1034–9. doi: 10.1128/IAI.01254-06
40. Clark SR, Ma AC, Tavener SA, McDonald B, Goodarzi Z, Kelly MM, et al. Platelet TLR4 activates neutrophil extracellular traps to ensnare bacteria in septic blood. *Nat Med.* (2007) 13:463–9. doi: 10.1038/nm1565
41. Malachowa N, Kobayashi SD, Freedman B, Dorward DW, DeLeo FR. Staphylococcus aureus leukotoxin GH promotes formation of neutrophil extracellular traps. *J Immunol.* (2013) 191:6022–9. doi: 10.4049/jimmunol.1301821
42. Russell P, Eley SM, Fulop MJ, Bell DL, Titball RW. The efficacy of ciprofloxacin and doxycycline against experimental tularaemia. *J Antimicrob Chemother.* (1998) 41:461–5. doi: 10.1093/jac/41.4.461
43. Enderlin G, Morales L, Jacobs RF, Cross JT. Streptomycin and alternative agents for the treatment of tularemia: review of the literature. *Clin Infect Dis.* (1994) 19:42–7. doi: 10.1093/clinids/19.1.42

44. Lovell VM, Cho CT, Lindsey NJ, Nelson PL. *Francisella tularensis* meningitis: a rare clinical entity. *J Infect Dis.* (1986) 154:916–8. doi: 10.1093/infdis/154.5.916
45. Burgaleta C, Martínez-Beltrán J, Bouza E. Comparative effects of moxalactam and gentamicin on human polymorphonuclear leukocyte functions. *Antimicrob Agents Chemother.* (1982) 21:718–20. doi: 10.1128/AAC.21.5.718
46. Tarnvik A. *WHO Guidelines on Tularaemia.* (2007). Available online at: https://www.who.int/csr/resources/publications/WHO_CDS_EPR_2007_7.pdf?ua=1

15

Pulmonary Pathogens Adapt to Immune Signaling Metabolites in the Airway

*Sebastián A. Riquelme†, Tania Wong Fok Lung† and Alice Prince**

Department of Pediatrics, Columbia University Medical Center, New York, NY, United States

***Correspondence:**
Alice Prince
asp7@cumc.columbia.edu

†These authors have contributed equally to this work

A limited number of pulmonary pathogens are able to evade normal mucosal defenses to establish acute infection and then adapt to cause chronic pneumonias. Pathogens, such as *Pseudomonas aeruginosa* or *Staphylococcus aureus*, are typically associated with infection in patients with underlying pulmonary disease or damage, such as cystic fibrosis (CF) or chronic obstructive pulmonary disease (COPD). To establish infection, bacteria express a well-defined set of so-called virulence factors that facilitate colonization and activate an immune response, gene products that have been identified in murine models. Less well-understood are the adaptive changes that occur over time *in vivo*, enabling the organisms to evade innate and adaptive immune clearance mechanisms. These colonizers proliferate, generating a population sufficient to provide selection for mutants, such as small colony variants and mucoid variants, that are optimized for long term infection. Such host-adapted strains have evolved in response to selective pressure such as antibiotics and the recruitment of phagocytes at sites of infection and their release of signaling metabolites (e.g., succinate). These metabolites can potentially function as substrates for bacterial growth and but also generate oxidant stress. Whole genome sequencing and quantified expression of selected genes have helped to explain how *P. aeruginosa* and *S. aureus* adapt to the presence of these metabolites over the course of *in vivo* infection. The serial isolation of clonally related strains from patients with cystic fibrosis has provided the opportunity to identify bacterial metabolic pathways that are altered under this immune pressure, such as the anti-oxidant glyoxylate and pentose phosphate pathways, routes contributing to the generation of biofilms. These metabolic pathways and biofilm itself enable the organisms to dissipate oxidant stress, while providing protection from phagocytosis. Stimulation of host immune signaling metabolites by these pathogens drives bacterial adaptation and promotes their persistence in the airways. The inherent metabolic flexibility of *P. aeruginosa* and *S. aureus* is a major factor in their success as pulmonary pathogens.

Keywords: *Pseudomonas aeruginosa*, *Staphylococcus aereus*, succinate, fumarate, cystic fibrosis, COPD, immunometabolism, inflammation

INTRODUCTION

Pseudomonas aeruginosa and *Staphylococcus aureus* are major respiratory pathogens that activate airway inflammation to produce pneumonia. These pathogens express a number of specific virulence determinants that can directly damage host tissues. They also activate host inflammation that contributes to the damage via the release of proteases and ROS by recruited immune cells. Such opportunistic pathogens are common in the environment and when inadvertently inhaled are usually cleared by normal mucociliary function. An excessive inflammatory response and/or and especially virulent organisms result in the fulminant acute pneumonias with high mortality, as described for the toxin-producing methicillin-resistant *S. aureus* (MRSA) (1) and *P. aeruginosa* (2). More commonly, these pathogens adapt to the milieu within the airway and cause a more chronic infection. In individuals with genetic or acquired respiratory dysfunction, such as in cystic fibrosis (CF) and chronic obstructive pulmonary disease (COPD), these bacteria are able to colonize the respiratory tract, adapt to the milieu of the airway by altering their metabolic activity and through the selection of mutants that have enhanced fitness in the presence of inflammatory products and metabolites. Both *S. aureus* and *P. aeruginosa* undergo a gradual adaptation to the human airway, resulting in the production of biofilms that thwart opsonization by antibody or complement, inhibit phagocytosis, and create a barrier for antibiotic penetration. Although the mechanisms used by these pathogens to attach to the lung parenchyma and the genetics of their subsequent biofilm formation are well-known, exactly what triggers this adaptation remains less clear. In this review we discuss how *P. aeruginosa* and *S. aureus* have evolved mechanisms to adapt to the airway environment to cause acute and chronic lung infections.

ACQUISITION OF *P. AERUGINOSA* FROM THE ENVIRONMENT

P. aeruginosa are highly versatile opportunists with a large genome and tremendous metabolic flexibility (3). These organisms normally reside in an aquatic environment, in streams, soil, plants and readily contaminate hospital paraphernalia. *P. aeruginosa* enjoys genetic adaptability and readily acquires novel genes in response to selective pressure, such as those conferring antimicrobial resistance determinants as well as altering expression of its own gene products, such as its chromosomal β-lactamase *ampC*, as a response to antibiotics in the environment. This genetic flexibility has led to multi-drug resistance and designation by the CDC and WHO as an exceptionally important human pathogen (4). Within its large genome, *P. aeruginosa* retains numerous genes that are activated specifically in response to contact with eukaryotic hosts, and alter expression of numerous metabolic and secreted proteins. Some of these changes in gene expression are in direct response to host immune pressure, either to avoid phagocytic clearance or to exploit and respond to immune cell products.

The pathogenesis of airway infection by *P. aeruginosa* has been well-studied, driven in part by the unusual association of this specific pathogen with cystic fibrosis (5), infecting over 75% of CF patients and contributing substantially to their pulmonary disease (6). The longitudinal study of *P. aeruginosa* strains from CF patients over decades has provided a wealth of information detailing the geno-phenotypic adaptation of these organisms to the human lung and has been highly relevant to the pathogenesis of other airway opportunists. The organisms inadvertently inhaled from a contaminated environment express a number of gene products to initiate infection: flagella for bacterial motility, pili for attachment, siderophores to trap iron and micronutrients as well as proteases and toxins that generate substrates for bacterial growth (5). Each of these has associated immunogenicity and is recognized by a specific pattern recognition receptor that initiates host airway inflammation. Substantially different genes are activated later *in vivo* in response to the local milieu in the airway, particularly the presence of immunometabolites.

INNATE IMMUNE RESPONSES TO *P. AERUGINOSA*

LPS Induces the Release of Succinate, Activation of Inflammasomes, and IL-1β

LPS, lipopolysaccharide or endotoxin, is a major component of *P. aeruginosa* that activates immune signaling (7). Upon recognition of LPS by toll-like receptor 4 (TLR4), resident alveolar macrophages and neutrophils increase glycolysis, succinate oxidation and generation of reactive oxidative species (ROS) (8–10) (**Figure 1A**). When primed by LPS, mitochondria shunt succinate into the cytoplasm, which inhibits prolyl-hydroxylase activity (PHD) and enable the stabilization of HIF-1α (11) (**Figure 1A**). HIF-1α, in turn, induces expression of pro-IL-1β mRNA (8, 11). This transcript is translated into the inactive pro-IL-1β form, which by the action of caspases is cleaved. Mature IL-1β is then released into the extracellular milieu where it activates local and surveilling phagocytes that sense and increase their bactericidal activities.

These immune responses are generated by inflammasome activation. Inflammasomes are complexes of multiple proteins that function together to transduce the signals provided by K^+ fluxes, specific microbial gene products or DNA into the activation of pro-caspases (12). While the NLRC4 inflammasome recognizes *P. aeruginosa* type 3 secretion system (T3SS) toxins and flagellin monomers, NLRP3 senses cytoplasmic LPS (13–15). Through the activity of caspase-1, the substrate gasdermin D is cleaved and produces membrane pores resulting in a form of cell death termed pyroptosis and the leakage of intracellular contents, such as metabolites and cytokines such as IL-1β (16). The activation of local and recruited macrophages while important in initiating the clearance of *P. aeruginosa* also generates an environment with large amounts of the metabolic byproducts ROS and succinate.

Although the activation of the inflammasome and IL-1β release are major components of the host reaction to

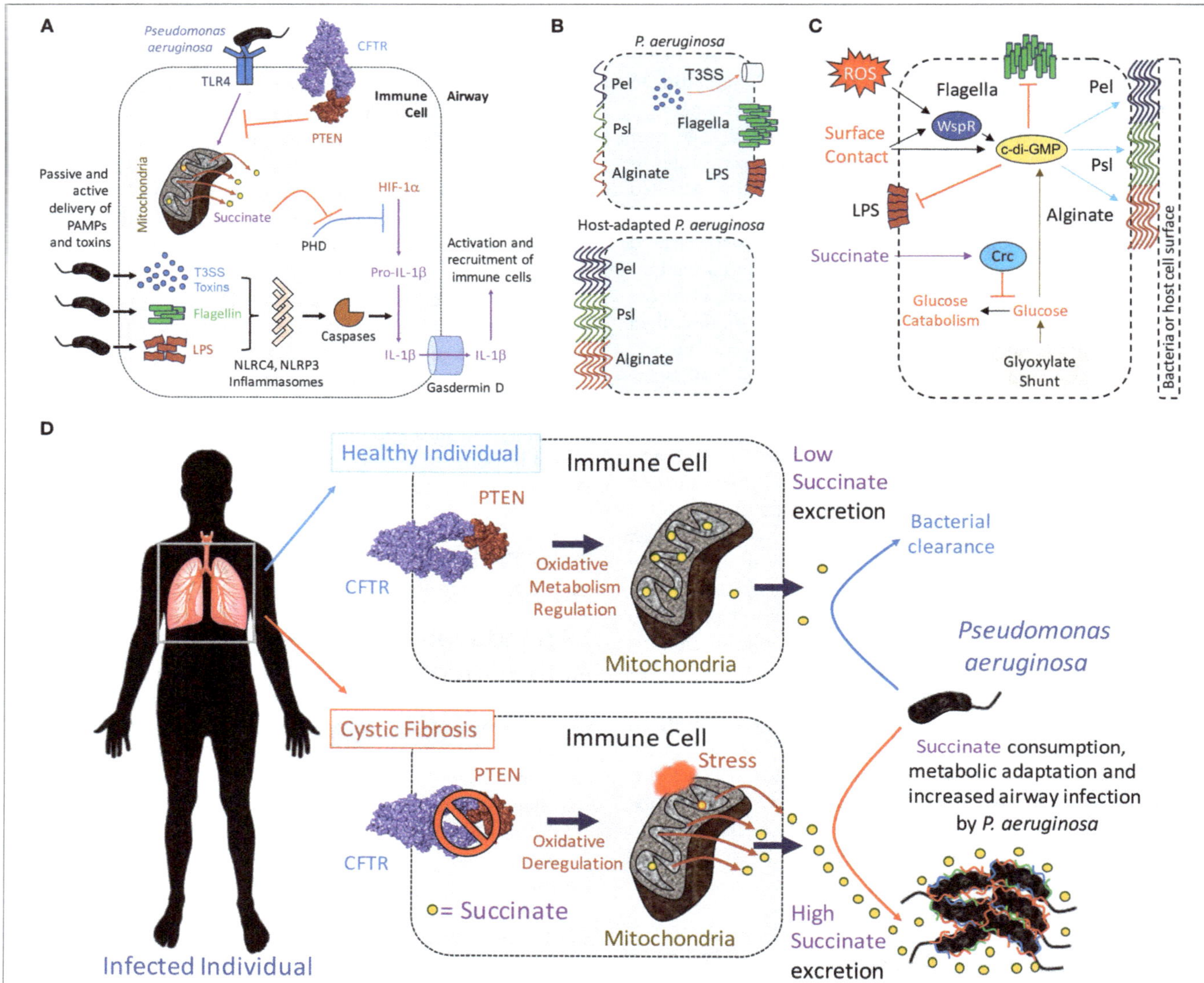

FIGURE 1 | The mitochondrial PTEN-succinate axis promotes *P. aeruginosa* airway infection. **(A)** Once interacting with surface TLR4 receptor, *P. aeruginosa* LPS triggers inflammation. Mitochondria become depolarized producing ROS and succinate (yellow circles). This is a tightly regulated process by the CFTR-PTEN complex, which signals through Akt and PI3Kγ/δ to suppress LPS-TLR4-driven inflammation. Succinate leaked into the cytoplasm inhibits PHD, which activates HIF-1α to induce production of pro-IL-1β. In parallel, *P. aeruginosa* release soluble LPS in the cytoplasm, flagellin or inject T3SS toxins. These activate different inflammasomes, priming caspases and cleavage of pro-IL-1β to produce IL-1β. Gasdermin D form pores in the cell membrane releasing mature IL-1β and causing cell death. Once extracellular, IL-1β induces recruitment of more immune cells to clear infection. **(B)** Laboratory and *P. aeruginosa* clinical strains derived from acutely infected patients (e.g., ICU) are more immunostimulatory than host-adapted isolates, such as in CF. **(C)** The immunosignaling metabolite succinate induces *crc*-dependent polysaccharide production by repressing glucose catabolism in *P. aeruginosa*. Extracellular ROS and surface contact also induce c-di-GMP generation, which promotes the synthesis of Pel, Psl and alginate and biofilm production. The pro-gluconeogenic glyoxylate shunt pathway contributes with extracellular polysaccharides production by shunting carbon atoms into glucose synthesis. **(D)** Insufficient CFTR-PTEN interaction induces excessive succinate release (yellow circles) by immune cells and *P. aeruginosa* airway adaptation. In healthy individuals (upper panel), the CFTR-PTEN complex regulates the oxidative state of mitochondria. In cystic fibrosis patients (lower panel), lack of membrane CFTR-PTEN induces mitochondrial deregulation, producing ROS and more succinate release. Cytoplasmic succinate is excreted into the extracellular milieu feeding *P. aeruginosa*. Succinate-stressed *P. aeruginosa* upregulate anti-oxidant genes, causing metabolic adaptation, extracellular polysaccharide synthesis (color lines) and biofilm production. Biofilm-producing *P. aeruginosa* attach to the airway parenchyma, which protects them from phagocytes, antibiotics and antibodies.

P. aeruginosa infection, the bacteria appear to thrive despite this response. Mice deficient for IL-1β receptor (IL-1R) or lacking the caspases that produce mature IL-1β exhibit decreased airway bacterial burden (17, 18). These findings suggest that these organisms have mechanisms to adapt to ROS and/or they can metabolize the succinate released from the macrophages, supporting ongoing proliferation despite host efforts of clearance through phagocytosis. Among a large number of carbon sources, succinate is a preferred substrate for *P. aeruginosa* metabolism (19–22).

Macrophage Release of Succinate Promotes Inflammation

Succinate in the airway promotes inflammation through several mechanisms. The release of succinate from LPS-activated macrophages not only contributes to HIF-1α and IL-1β production, it also generates ROS from its own oxidation by succinate dehydrogenase (SDH) (8). ROS can damage DNA in both the host and pathogen, increasing mutation rates and the selection of variants.

Mitochondrial and cytoplasmic succinate are released into the extracellular space by cell death or by active membrane transporters of the SCL13 family (23, 24). Once extracellular, succinate signals back through its SUNCR1 receptor (also known as GPR91), which boosts IL-1β production by activated phagocytes (25). How specifically the IL-1β-IL-1R signaling favors *P. aeruginosa* pulmonary infection is under active investigation. Substantial IL-1β release and induction of phagocyte pyroptosis may cause diminished bacterial engulfment and killing, facilitating extracellular bacterial proliferation. Constant IL-1β production in the site of infection is associated with more recruitment of pro-oxidant neutrophils, which can cause local tissue damage and cell dysfunction. IL-1β signaling, tissue fibrosis and activation of chronic mechanisms of cell repair (26, 27) are pathways associated with *P. aeruginosa* infection, as seen in CF and COPD. *In vitro* macrophages studies with the intracellular pathogen *Mycobacterium tuberculosis* have shown that IL-1β-IL-1R signaling restricts intracellular bacterial proliferation by inducing glycolysis (28). *P. aeruginosa* seems to evade this pathway, as it escapes from intracellular killing by inducing IL-1β-mediated autophagy (29), changes associated with reduced glycolysis (30). These studies suggest that pulmonary Gram-negative pathogens have evolved different intracellular survival mechanisms to exploit IL-1β signaling to cause disease. Thus, a major component of the innate immune response to *P. aeruginosa*, namely the release of succinate and IL-1β, may actually have beneficial consequences for these bacteria by forcing them to adapt and survive. Accumulating data suggest that host immunometabolites have a central role in the adaptation of virulent *P. aeruginosa* to enable chronic airway infection, as commonly seen in COPD and CF.

P. aeruginosa Type Three Toxins Target Host Defenses

In addition to LPS, there are many other *P. aeruginosa* gene products that activate innate immune signaling. The T3SS toxins are expressed by organisms initiating infection and have been specifically associated with fulminant pneumonia (2). The T3SS has been closely linked to the pathogenesis of acute pneumonia and the secreted virulence proteins termed effectors have multiple mechanisms that interrupt normal host metabolism, barrier and immune functions. Following pilin-mediated attachment, T3SS toxins such as exoenzyme S (ExoS) function to alter the polarization of the epithelial cell, subverting the actin cytoskeleton and perturbing epithelial tight junctions to enable bacterial invasion (31). ExoS, along with ExoT are synthetized as a bacterial response to exogenous oxidative stress and suppress neutrophil function by in turn inhibiting anti-bacterial ROS production. Both toxins affect Ras and PI3K, two key cell regulators involved in glycolysis and the generation of energy (32, 33) and cytoskeleton dynamics (34). ExoS ADP-ribosylates the signaling protein Ras, impairing its interaction with PI3K and the complex required to generate ROS by phagocytic NADPH-oxidase. ExoT also reduces PI3K function by ADP-ribosylation contributing to the deactivation of neutrophils. Thus, the activities of these toxins reflect a general theme that *P. aeruginosa* itself alters host metabolic activity which, in turn, enhances their ability to persist in the lung.

The T3SS toxins also inhibit epithelial repair, a process that diverts host metabolic functions. ExoT deregulates cell cytokinesis (35), a key process to repair damaged tissue that entails cytoskeleton remodeling and requires a substantial ATP expenditure derived from glycolysis (36). In addition to harboring an ADP-ribosyltransferase function in its C-terminus, ExoT is bifunctional and contains a GTPase-activating domain in its N-terminal portion. ExoT targets RhoA using its GTPase domain and syntaxin-2 using its ADP-ribosyltransferase domain in epithelial cells, cytoskeleton-coupled factors that direct early and late cytokinesis, respectively. Negative effects of ExoS and ExoT on pulmonary integrity not only affect epithelial cells, but also neutrophils, which undergo apoptosis following ExoT intoxication. The toxic effects of both factors are related to mitochondrial disruption as well-given that epithelial cells treated with ExoT and ExoS-producing *P. aeruginosa* strains display enrichment of Bax and Bim proteins in the mitochondrial outer-membrane, which triggers membrane instability, cytochrome C release into the cytosol and activation of pro-apoptotic caspases 9 and 3 (37).

ExoU, a patatin-like phosphatase, and ExoY also belong to the family of T3SS effectors secreted by *P. aeruginosa* during initial infection and their expression has been linked to mortality in ICU infections (2). When translocated into its target cell, ExoU displays a strong phospholipase A2-like activity, process that interferes with immune surveillance. When injected into neutrophils, ExoU induces cell death, suppressing local activity of host defenses (38). ExoU-mediated neutrophil eradication favors extracellular bacterial replication, making ExoU a key determinant for initial infection (39). ExoU is highly immunostimulatory, triggering epithelial cell proinflammatory signaling which contributes to ongoing lung damage by inducing more neutrophil recruitment, cell death and debris (40–42). ExoY, predicted to display adenylate cyclase activity within host cells, interacts with F-actin filaments to synthesize various cyclic nucleotide monophosphates (43). The intricate role between adenylate cyclase and cytoskeleton dynamics are well-described in tissue repair (44), suggesting that ExoY might also disrupt airway parenchymal barrier function by targeting cell division and viability.

Active production of ExoS, ExoT, ExoU, and ExoY is regulated in part by ArtR, a novel and unique ABC ATPase recently discovered in *P. aeruginosa* (45). ArtR represses T3SS activities, as seen by overexpression of ExoS, ExoT, and ExoY in *artR* knockout strains. ArtR also downregulates the expression of ExsA, a member of the AraC-type DNA binding protein and transcriptional inducer of type III effectors. The relationship between type III secretion and a soluble ATPase regulator indicates a direct connection between bacterial bioenergetics and the production of virulence determinants that promote inflammation, cell death and immune deregulation.

In clinical studies analyzing the expression of T3SS by *P. aeruginosa*, between 75 to 90% of strains associated with acute pneumonia and fatalities displayed functional type III secretion systems. Of these, approximately two-thirds secreted ExoS, one-third secreted ExoU, and nearly all secrete ExoT (46, 47). In contrast, a study of 56 CF patients chronically infected with *P. aeruginosa* only 12% had isolates that secreted ExoS, ExoT but not ExoU (48). When compared with environmental, urine, endotracheal, blood and wound specimens, only CF sputum isolates of *P. aeruginosa* downregulated the expression of specific T3SS products (49). These studies clearly indicate that specific families of *P. aeruginosa* gene products, such as the effectors of the T3SS, are expressed at different times during the course of infection. Of note, downregulation of the T3SS in *P. aeruginosa* has been associated with upregulation of a different secretion machinery called the type six secretion system (T6SS) which promotes adaptation to the airway environment and chronicity (50). Strategies to block the T3SS toxins while likely effective for acute pneumonia, are unlikely to disrupt established infection as occurs in CF.

P. aeruginosa Adaptation to Immunometabolites—Formation of Biofilms in Response to Oxidant Stress

In contrast to the potent immunostimulatory capabilities seen in the clinical isolates of *P. aeruginosa* isolated from acute infections, typical of environmental and laboratory strains of *P. aeruginosa*, chronic isolates have acquired a very different immunogenic profile (**Figure 1B**). These clinical isolates have substantial decreases in the expression of components that activate the inflammasome, such as flagella, T3SS, and LPS, while up-regulating the expression of the extracellular polysaccharides that function as oxidant traps (51, 52). Similar findings have been found with other patient cohorts, where isolates from chronically infected patients with CF fail to induce inflammasome activation or IL-1β secretion due to LPS mutations or changes in T3SS toxin expression (53). The ability to follow longitudinal isolates of *P. aeruginosa* from CF patients provides insights into the process of bacterial adaptation to the inflamed airway. *P. aeruginosa*, either isolated from CF patients or simply grown in high succinate *in vitro*, have a conserved pattern of metabolic adaptation that helps them deal with the oxidant stress generated by obligate succinate metabolism.

Succinate metabolism causes sufficient oxidant stimulus to drive *P. aeruginosa* metabolic adaptation and biofilm production (54). By inducing *crc*-directed catabolite repression on glucose metabolism, succinate promotes glucose diversion into extracellular polysaccharides production (**Figure 1C**). ROS itself, as well as surface contact and its detection by WspR, are potent stimuli for the production of the master biofilm regulator cyclic-di-GMP (c-di-GMP), which drives synthesis of extracellular and anti-oxidant polysaccharides (55–57). ROS production contributes to bacterial stress, generating mutants better able to produce these biofilms (58). The diversion of a substantial amount of energy consumption to the production of extracellular polysaccharides imposes a metabolic cost upon the organism. Numerous features of biofilms enhance the persistence of bacteria that generate extracellular polysaccharides. The bacteria fall into a low replicative rate, a metabolic state that protects them against antibiotics that target bacterial division as mechanism of action. Adjacent bacteria form glycan-glycan interactions, developing a community of antibiotic resistant organisms able to evade phagocytosis. This biofilm metabolic program is much more restricted than the one used by planktonic bacteria, shutting-off ATP-dependent flagellar motility until becoming sessile (59, 60). Non-motile *P. aeruginosa* interact and form molecular bridges with nearby surfaces and other bacilli. Available succinate is preferentially consumed as regulated by the catabolite repressor locus *crc*, which obligates *P. aeruginosa* to consume succinate before any other carbon source present in the environment (21). While restricting flagellar swimming, *crc*-directed succinate assimilation augments twitching motility by *P. aeruginosa*, changes that favor bacteria-surface interactions and biofilm development (19, 20). The repression *crc* exerts on glucose catabolism leads *P. aeruginosa* to produce energy mainly from succinate oxidation, dedicating glucose monomers to the copious synthesis of extracellular polysaccharides (**Figure 1C**).

P. aeruginosa can form several distinct biopolymers that form biofilm. Alginate, a complex of O-acetylated D-mannuronate and its C5′ epimer L-guluronic acid, is responsible for the mucoid phenotype of *P. aeruginosa* typically isolated from patients with CF. Psl and Pel are associated with biofilm formation in many clinical settings, including pneumonias and CF. Psl is made of D-mannose, L-rhamnose, and D-glucose residues (51). Although Pel structures have been less studied, preliminary studies indicate that Pel is formed by acetylated galactosamine and glucosamine sugars (52). These polysaccharides act as traps for oxidant molecules, protecting *P. aeruginosa* from membrane and protein damage induced by activated phagocytes.

High levels of succinate are sufficient to stimulate the upregulation of *P. aeruginosa algD*, the gene that synthetizes the alginate precursor GDP-mannuronate (61, 62). Mucoid and small colony variants (SCV) of *P. aeruginosa* recovered from the CF airway display increased levels of *algD* that is induced by succinate (6, 54, 63–66). The biosynthesis of the precursors of the exopolysaccharides are supported through the glyoxylate shunt, an alternative to the TCA cycle that generates less oxidant stress and is upregulated in succinate-exposed *P. aeruginosa*. In *P. aeruginosa*, the glyoxylate shunt is controlled by *aceA* and *glcB*, two genes that produce glyoxylate first and then malate and succinate, respectively. The glyoxylate shunt saves two carbon atoms that are normally lost as CO_2 during the TCA cycle, which are put back into circulation as malate and succinate. Malate is a gluconeogenic precursor that replenishes the bacterial cytoplasm with glucose, a precursor for the extracellular polysaccharides (**Figure 1C**). Succinate, is an additional glyoxylate shunt byproduct, that sustains oxidative metabolism, causing a feedback response to increase the generation of pro-biofilm mutants by upregulating the same glyoxylate shunt and by generating mutations in the DNA. The oxidative metabolism of succinate accumulated in the airway both fuels *P. aeruginosa* proliferation and drives adaptive changes to mitigate the accompanying generation of oxidants.

Succinate Is Increased in Inflammation and in CF

The release of succinate by activated macrophages is a central component of the innate immune response to LPS in general and to *P. aeruginosa* specifically. Although succinate release is a consequence of excessive inflammation and a likely factor in many airway infections, it is a favored substrate for *P. aeruginosa* metabolism, preferentially utilized before other substrates (19, 21, 22, 67). The overwhelming predilection of *P. aeruginosa* for succinate utilization helps to explain the increased susceptibility of the CF airway for this specific pathogen, and not other opportunists that are not similarly hard wired to consume succinate before all other substrates (22). Associated with the diminished abundance of CFTR in epithelial and immune cell membranes, there is also decreased PTEN, the phosphatase and tensin homologue deleted on chromosome 10 (68). For normal PTEN function it must be tethered to CFTR at the cell membrane. PTEN regulates class I PI3Kα/β activity. As PTEN counterbalances PI3K activity, it is a central regulator of cellular metabolism. Impaired PTEN function, as occurs when there is insufficient binding to CFTR, results in the accumulation of succinate (54, 69, 70) (**Figure 1D**). Thus, infection in the CF airway generates even greater amounts of succinate than in normal hosts.

Not only does PTEN regulate cellular proliferation, it also induces the anti-inflammatory function of Akt and the PI3Kγ/δ subunits in phagocytes (68, 71, 72). These are proteins located in the inner leaflet of the plasma membrane during LPS-TLR4 interaction. In CF cells, the lack of the CFTR-PTEN interaction unleashes the inflammatory response, increasing NF-kB and NLRP3 activation and resulting in increased production of IL-1β and succinate (54, 68–70) (**Figure 1A**). PTEN deficiency in mitochondrial membranes further impairs *P. aeruginosa* killing and ultimately its clearance from the murine airway (68). The milieu of the CF airway, with decreased CFTR-PTEN interaction, increased succinate and oxidant generation provide an environment that favors *P. aeruginosa* proliferation and generates selective pressure for the organisms best suited for this environment, those protected from oxidants by their formation of biofilm (**Figure 1D**).

LPS Changes in Host-Adapted *P. aeruginosa*

Analysis of the genotypic and phenotypic changes found in *P. aeruginosa* strains isolated from chronic pulmonary infections provides important insights into the tremendous versatility of these strains. Host adapted bacteria alter the expression of major structural components. LPS is consistently downregulated or altered in *P. aeruginosa* from CF patients (5). Strains from chronically infected CF patients have shorter O-antigen branches compared with control laboratory strains (73), changes predicted to have an impact on the host inflammatory response (74, 75). These isolates display reduced lateral LPS ramifications, and accumulate mutations in genes that produce these changes. In *P. aeruginosa*, LPS is synthetized by several operons involved in assembly, trafficking, and anchoring of LPS on the outer-membrane (76, 77).

LPS on the cell surface provides membrane stability (78). The process of LPS exposure is well-regulated and mediated by a set of periplasmic and outer-membrane transporters within the Lpt family of proteins. LptD, the last transporter that exposes mature LPS on the cell surface (77), has been shown to be reduced and mutated in CF *P. aeruginosa* isolates (54). This has repercussions in terms of immune-activation, as LPS-deficient strains fail to induce IL-1β production and succinate release from phagocytes. As the organisms are already in a succinate-replete environment in the inflamed CF airway, positive selection for strains that do not further add to the abundance of succinate and the oxidants associated with its metabolism may help to explain the predominance of the LPS mutant strains. Similarly, selection for mutants or variants lacking immunogenic pathogen-associated molecular patterns (PAMPs), the T3SS effectors, and flagella would also substantially decrease inflammasome activation, IL-1β and further succinate release.

P. aeruginosa Modulate Host Immune Signaling

The analysis of gene expression changes in *P. aeruginosa* over the course of infection in CF, as compared with acute pneumonias has provided numerous insights into the pathogen-host dynamics. The milieu of the CF airway, with high succinate and abundant carbon sources for bacterial growth provides ample opportunity for *P. aeruginosa* colonization and adaptation, despite the presence of an immune system that functions normally in other sites. As the recruitment of phagocytes, their activation by bacterial LPS and other PAMPs induces the release of immunometabolites, such host responses drive the selection of highly adapted opportunists from the airway microbiome. These host-adapted strains suppress the expression of genes that further fuel the release of succinate, and increase the expression of extracellular polysaccharides (biofilm) to dissipate oxidant stress. In a hospital setting, with antimicrobial pressure and impaired mucociliary clearance in many hospitalized patients, these factors create conditions that favor the selection of *P. aeruginosa* and other opportunists with the metabolic flexibility to proliferate, despite the presence of an apparently robust immune response.

STAPHYLOCOCCUS AUREUS CAUSE ACUTE AND CHRONIC INFECTION

In contrast to *P. aeruginosa*, *S. aureus* are both a ubiquitous component of the commensal flora and a major cause of acute pneumonia and chronic airway infection. *S. aureus* colonize the nose in 30–40% of individuals but can cause serious infection by using numerous virulence factors and mechanisms to subvert or evade the immune system. Similar to *P. aeruginosa*, *S. aureus*, particularly methicillin-resistant strains including USA300 LAC that were especially prevalent a decade ago, are an important cause of severe acute pneumonia (79). The toxins produced by *S. aureus*, such as α-hemolysin (Hla) and PVL (Panton Valentine Leukocidin) contribute to the necrotizing pneumonias. Although substantial efforts in infection prevention and control have helped to decrease the incidence of those severe pneumonias, *S. aureus* strains, both sensitive and resistant to methicillin (MSSA and MRSA), are still frequently associated with airway infection, most often with a less fulminant course. *S. aureus* remain a major pathogen in COPD and especially in CF, where they are associated with chronic airway infection and are at least as common as *P. aeruginosa* (80, 81).

SELECTION OF SCVS IN CLINICAL SETTINGS

A clinically important adaptive change to the lung by *S. aureus* is the selection of small colony variants (SCVs) from chronically infected tissues (82). SCVs were first characterized by Proctor et al. (83) as phenotypically distinct from other *S. aureus* colonies, often with pinpoint colony size that is overlooked in clinical microbiology laboratories. Although suggested to have diminished expression of toxin genes, this may not necessarily be the case *in vivo* whereby the SCVs can revert to the WT phenotype due to availability of components they are auxotrophic for (84). SCVs have a variety of mutations typically in genes associated with electron transport chain components such as menadione, and heme (82). As a result, SCVs often have altered metabolism from normal colony variants, with decreased tricarboxylic acid (TCA cycle) activity and oxidative phosphorylation (OXPHOS) and increased glycolysis to meet their energy requirements (85). SCVs are often found within host cells or in biofilms, where they are protected from antibiotics, antibodies, complement activation, and phagocytes (**Figure 2A**). Clinical studies in CF patients indicate that their recovery correlates with poor outcomes (86), likely influenced by the antimicrobial resistance of these variants and their ability to evade immune clearance mechanisms.

S. AUREUS EVADE INFLAMMASOME—MEDIATED CLEARANCE AND INDUCE NECROPTOSIS

S. aureus are typically considered an extracellular Gram-positive pathogen. However, these pathogens can also persist within host cells, either epithelial, endothelial or immune cells. The intracellular niche provides protection for staphylococci from some antibiotics, antibody and complement, inducing the host to utilize alternative clearance mechanisms. The induction of host cell death is often beneficial as it eliminates the intracellular niche of the pathogen and triggers an innate immune response. Bacterial pathogens can either evade host cell death or benefit from it. Like *P. aeruginosa*, *S. aureus* activate the NLRP3 inflammasome using several virulence factors including pore-forming toxins and phenol-soluble modulins (PSMs) (87). This normally results in pyroptotic host cell death and the release of IL-1β and bacterial clearance in the skin (88). However, NLRP3 inflammasome signaling does not clear staphylococci from the lungs of infected mice given that WT and *Nlrp3*$^{-/-}$ mice had similar bacterial burdens following *S. aureus* intratracheal infection (89). *S. aureus*-induced NLRP3 inflammasome activation via Hla toxin prevents staphylococcal clearance by recruiting mitochondria away from phagosomes containing internalized *S. aureus* (90). In the absence of the close association of mitochondria from internalized staphylococci, macrophages were unable to effectively kill *S. aureus*. Staphyloccocal killing by co-localization with mitochondria was mediated by altered electron transport chain activity leading to ROS production, endosomal acidification and local caspase-1 activation (90).

S. aureus, like *P. aeruginosa*, undergo adaptive changes *in vivo*, such as the selection of SCVs. While suspected of deficient toxin production, the SCVs nonetheless induce robust immune signaling (84). *S. aureus* and even the *S. aureus* SCVs induce necroptosis, a caspase-independent mechanism of programmed cell death. Necroptosis is induced by the phosphorylation of the mixed lineage kinase domain-like (MLKL) protein by receptor-interacting protein kinase 3 (RIPK3) resulting in MLKL oligomerization at the plasma membrane and pore formation. Necroptosis does not efficiently clear the staphylococcal infection caused by either WT or SCV strains. A similar intracellular bacterial burden was recovered following infection of bone marrow-derived macrophages (BMDMs) from WT mice and *Mlkl*$^{-/-}$ mice that are unable to initiate necroptosis (84, 91). Furthermore, necroptosis contributes to the persistence of SCVs in a mouse model of infection; SCVs failed to establish infection in *Mlkl*$^{-/-}$ mice compared to WT mice, suggesting that necroptosis actually facilitates ongoing infection by SCVs at the expense of the integrity of the host (84). Whether this is also the case in a mouse model of pulmonary infection remains to be determined. However, *S. aureus* SCV induction of host cell death through necroptosis clearly enables the microorganisms to persist, at the expense of the integrity of the host.

S. AUREUS BIOFILM FORMATION FUNCTIONS IN THE EVASION OF INNATE CLEARANCE MECHANISMS

Wild type strains of *S. aureus* have multiple adaptive strategies to enhance persistence in the respiratory tract. *S. aureus* readily form bacterial communities encased in biofilms, a form of protection from antibiotics, antibodies, complement activation and phagocytic clearance as well as from oxidative stress. While staphylococcal biofilms are most commonly associated with infection of indwelling intravascular devices, these Gram-positive bacteria form biofilms within the airways. From the initial stages of deposition in the airway spaces, the organisms clump together forming tight bacterial clusters that are not readily dispersed (92). *S. aureus* biofilm formation can be induced via distinct pathways including via extracellular polysaccharides or the accumulation of extracellular DNA (eDNA) and proteins (93). *S. aureus* contain two gene clusters encoding enzymes essential for two distinct polysaccharides including the polysaccharide intercellular adhesin (PIA) encoded by the *icaADBC* operon (94, 95) and the capsular polysaccharide (CP) encoded by the *cap* operon (96). *S. aureus* from CF patients have been shown to be primarily positive for PIA and negative for CP (97). A link between *S. aureus* metabolic activity and subsequent biofilm formation was suggested by the observation that the mitochondrial metabolite fumarate promotes biofilm formation in clinical isolates from CF patients *in vitro* (98). However, the mechanism of action for this metabolite-driven bacterial adaptation has not yet been determined.

Biofilm formation provides substantial protection against phagocytic clearance. Neutrophils are essential in clearing *S. aureus* via the oxidative burst and through formation of antimicrobial neutrophil extracellular traps (NETs). Unlike planktonic *S. aureus*, sessile staphylococci in biofilms remain viable even after exposure to neutrophils. Of the many mechanisms to evade bacterial killing conferred by biofilm, is the elimination of neutrophils via the release of the toxins PVL and HlgAB that induce formation of NETs (99). Whilst NETs are effective at clearing planktonic bacteria, the high concentrations of NETs produced during biofilm formation instead cause neutrophil necrosis, preventing bacterial clearance (99). Macrophages, particularly the classically activated M1 macrophages, also help clear staphylococcal infections via the production of nitric oxide and ROS. Staphylococcal biofilms skew macrophage responses towards an anti-inflammatory state M2 to evade macrophage-induced killing (100). Thus, it seems likely that staphylococcal biofilm formation impacts host metabolism and the efficiency of immune clearance mechanisms that are operative in the airways.

GENOMIC CHANGES IN CLINICAL ISOLATES OF *S. AUREUS* FROM PERSISTENT INFECTION

Molecular epidemiology studies have been tremendously important in tracking *S. aureus* epidemiology, and especially the global outbreaks of MRSA infection (101, 102). Less well-studied are the changes that occur in clones that have adapted to specific sites of infection, as these can occur at the genomic, proteomic, or metabolic levels. Several studies of clinical *S. aureus* strains isolated from pneumonia, in normal hosts as well as in CF patients, indicate mutations in the *agr* locus (103). The *agr* locus divergently regulates expression of *S. aureus* toxins, including Hla and several others (104) and surface proteins, the microbial surface components recognizing adhesive matrix molecules (MSCRAMMS), including protein A (105). Hla is critical in the pathogenesis of acute pneumonia, targeting A Disintegrin and Metalloprotease 10 (ADAM-10) and initiating invasive infection (106). Hla is one of several staphylococcal pore-forming toxins, capable of inducing K^+ efflux and activating the NLRP3 inflammasome (89) to stimulate caspase-1 activation and IL-1β release. As *S. aureus* accumulate, *agr* functions in quorum sensing through the activity of small RNAs and increases Hla expression while decreasing the production of surface proteins that interact with host immune cells, such as protein A which binds both the Fc component of IgGs and the TNF receptor (107). In clinical isolates, *agr* dysfunction is associated with decreased expression of toxins, immunosuppression and staphylococcal adaptive changes to the lung.

S. AUREUS ACTIVATE AND RESPOND TO HOST METABOLISM

Genomic studies indicate that the same colonizing bacteria can cause invasive infection, indicating that host-associated factors trigger the expression of genes that promote active infection, as opposed to passive colonization. The bacteria recovered from invasive infections, such as those isolated from blood or lower airways, can also regulate their gene expression to cause chronic instead of fulminant pneumonia. While the staphylococcal genes associated with the regulation of the numerous gene products that activate host immune responses, such as *agr*, *sar*, and many others are well-characterized, much less well-understood are the host signals that trigger global changes in gene expression that promote chronic colonization vs. invasive infection. The natural history of *S. aureus* infection in CF provides an opportunity to understand how *S. aureus* changes its transcriptional program to cause chronic infection. Analysis of gene expression in longitudinal isolates of *S. aureus* from CF patients illustrates patterns that, like *P. aeruginosa*, indicate a process of adaptation to host immunometabolites and ROS (98). Just as immune cells alter their metabolism upon microbial stimulation, *S. aureus* alters its metabolic activity, often benefiting from the metabolic reprogramming of the immune cells.

METABOLIC ADAPTATION OF *S. AUREUS* TO THE LUNG

One of the strategies employed by *S. aureus* to adapt within the human host is bacterial metabolic remodeling which is driven by the host response to infection. Following invasion of human bronchial epithelial cells, *S. aureus* adapt to the intracellular environment. Internalized bacteria display population heterogeneity with one bacterial subset replicating and eventually causing host cell death whilst another subset persists by reducing growth rates (**Figure 2A**) (108). In order to survive and persist, the latter subset increases fermentation and amino acid catabolism, upregulating enzymes including 2-oxoglutarate dehydrogenase (SucA), succinyl coenzyme-A synthetase (SucC), succinate dehydrogenase (SdhA), and fumarase/fumarate hydratase (FumC), which are involved in the TCA cycle activity (**Figure 2A**, red arrows). Other

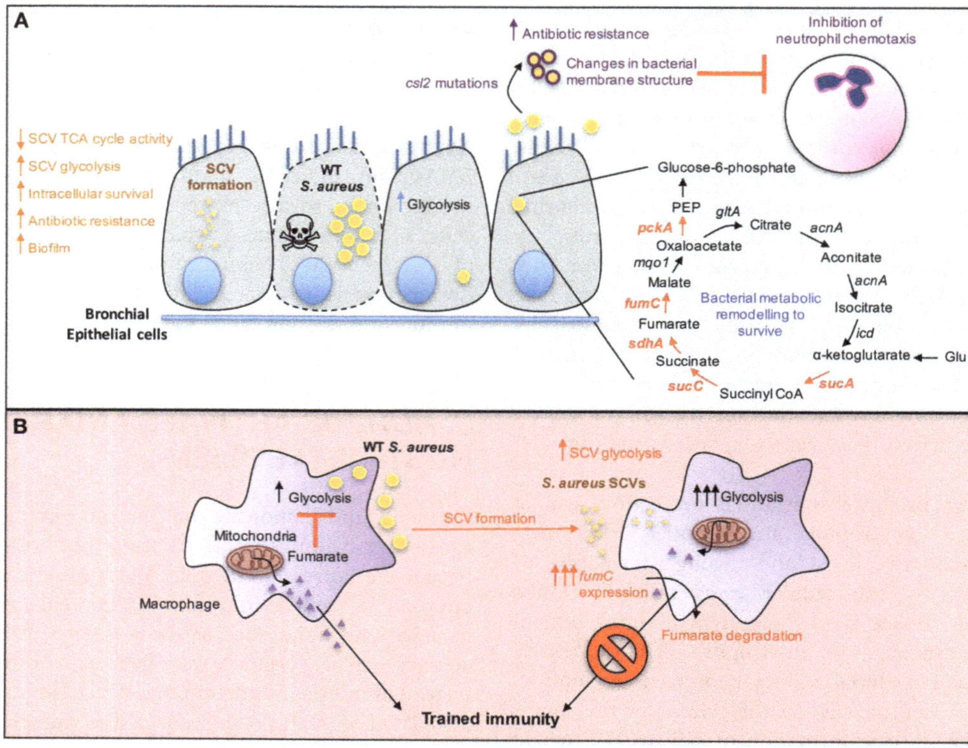

FIGURE 2 | Metabolic adaptation by *S. aureus*. **(A)** *S. aureus* acquire mutations in genes associated with terminal electron transport chain components resulting in the formation of small colony variants (SCVs) that display reduced metabolism. The decrease in TCA cycle activity from SCVs results in lower electrochemical gradient which is required for the uptake of aminoglycosides, thus rendering SCVs antibiotic resistant. In addition to their metabolic adaptation, SCVs evade the host immune system by intracellular survival and have increased biofilm forming ability that protects from oxidative stress. *S. aureus* also undergo bacterial metabolic remodeling resulting in population heterogeneity following internalization by bronchial epithelial cells. One bacterial subset replicates and induces host cell death and the other slows down its growth rate, relying on the catabolism of amino acids such as glutamate to supply oxaloacetate by fueling the TCA cycle and gluconeogenesis (red arrows). *S. aureus* also acquire mutations in the gene *csl2* that results in enhanced cardiolipin synthesis and reduced phosphatidyl glycerol, thereby altering bacterial membrane composition and impairing antibiotic penetration. The reduction in phosphatidylglycerol also leads to inhibition of neutrophil chemotaxis. **(B)** *S. aureus* SCVs, such as those auxotrophic for heme, adapt to local fumarate accumulation by overexpressing *fumC* to degrade it. This helps sustain glycolysis given the role of fumarate as a glycolytic inhibitor. Fumarate degradation is also detrimental to the host and abrogates trained immunity, promoting recurrent infections.

changes include increased levels of phosphoenolpyruvate (PEP) carboxykinase (PckA) involved in gluconeogenesis (108). Of note, the upregulation of these enzymes was previously shown to be important particularly in glutamate catabolism to supply intermediates such as oxaloacetate, α-ketoglutarate and succinyl-coenzyme-A and subsequently gluconeogenesis via PckA when glucose is depleted (**Figure 2A**) (109). This is consistent with the repression of amino acid catabolism by glucose and the inability of *S. aureus* to utilize short chain fatty acids as carbon sources, owing to the lack of β-oxidation and glyoxylate shunt pathways (109). Thus, it is important to recognize that patterns of *S. aureus* metabolism established under controlled laboratory conditions, are unlikely to accurately simulate the abundance of multiple carbon sources within the human airway. Attempts to mimic the complex milieu of the infected CF airway with "artificial sputum" provide mucins and DNA to a complex mix of amino acids and other carbon sources (110). However, even this media lacks the contribution of the immune cell metabolites and ROS that are likely to influence *S. aureus* metabolism.

METABOLIC COMPETITION BETWEEN HOST AND *S. AUREUS*

While *S. aureus* infecting the airway are adapting to the local environment, a similar process of metabolic adaptation occurs in host cells. In response to internalized staphylococci, human bronchial epithelial cells increase glucose uptake and catabolism, as well as amino acid utilization (108). These metabolic changes observed in bronchial epithelial cells upon *S. aureus* infection are reminiscent of other studies using HeLa cells and more physiologically relevant cell types, such as bone marrow-derived macrophages (BMDMs) (111) and human primary keratinocytes (112). During staphylococcal infection, HeLa cells and murine BMDMs upregulate glycolysis and glutaminolysis (111). This creates a starvation response that induces autophagy in the host cell (111). However, autophagy provides both host and pathogen with nutrients that fuel bacterial proliferation.

S. aureus infection imposes a metabolic stress on host epithelial cells by competing for glucose and O_2, which results in the activation of HIF-1α and glycolysis, as well as the many genes that are activated by this transcription factor including IL-1β (112). The *S. aureus* SCVs are especially dependent upon glycolysis, as they often lack terminal components of the electron transport chain. These SCVs associated with chronic infection substantially upregulate glycolysis in human keratinocytes and THP-1 macrophage-like immune cells (84), indicating that a hallmark of *S. aureus* infection is the induction of glucose metabolism in epithelial and immune cells. Several studies indicate that metabolically active *S. aureus* strains compete with the host for glucose to induce signaling, as opposed to non-viable organisms (112, 113), which unveils a metabolic mechanism of immune deregulation. These studies illustrate the importance of using viable bacteria for studies of host-pathogen interactions, as the metabolic signaling by both host and pathogen greatly affects immune responses.

SCV-INDUCED FUMARATE DEGRADATION INHIBITS TRAINED IMMUNITY

An example of the importance of bacterial as well as host metabolic activity in pathogenesis is the observation that *S. aureus* from clinical settings, including the SCVs, have significantly increased *fumC* activity, up to 10,000-fold as compared to a USA300 MRSA control strain (84). The ability to degrade fumarate has several benefits for the bacteria. In addition to limiting the accumulation of fumarate, which itself inhibits glycolysis (114), fumarate induces epigenetic changes in macrophages that are associated with trained immunity (115). Trained immunity refers to the increased non-specific protection against a secondary infection at the site of the primary challenge. Fumarate inhibits KDM5 histone demethylases, promoting histone modifications such as H3K4me3, at promoters of proinflammatory cytokines, serving to enhance transcription upon secondary insult (115). The importance of *fumC* expression in the persistence of SCV infection has been illustrated using a prototypic SCV, Δ*hemB* mutant that is auxotrophic for hemin (84), as well as by using *S. aureus* clinical isolates which also showed 1,000–100,000-fold *fumC* upregulation (84, 116). Fumarate catabolism correlated with the inhibition of protection from a secondary staphylococcal challenge in a mouse model of skin infection (116) and increased *fumC* activity by SCVs resulted in lower levels of fumarate during infection of human macrophage-like cells (THP-1 cells) and peripheral blood mononuclear cells (PBMCs) (84). MRSA isolated from chronically infected CF patients also exhibit significantly elevated *fumC* activity, consistent with a shared response to the host (98). The observation that *S. aureus* SCVs blunt immune memory development by depleting fumarate from the environment (**Figure 2B**) supports the idea of dynamic metabolic competition between host and pathogen.

METABOLIC CHANGES ASSOCIATED WITH *S. AUREUS* RESPIRATORY INFECTION

In addition to data accrued from laboratory constructed *S. aureus* mutants and murine models of infection, numerous adaptive changes in *S. aureus* have been identified in clinical isolates. The longitudinal sampling of *S. aureus* strains from a CF patient provides the opportunity to follow how these bacteria change in response to the conditions in the host airway. A study of CF patients with MRSA infection demonstrated that these strains undergo substantial metabolic adaptive changes, without changes in immunogenicity (98). These host-adapted strains were as immunostimulatory when incubated with human airway epithelial cells or macrophage cell lines *in vitro*, as were wild type virulent USA300 MRSA strains (98). Although genomic analyses revealed several polymorphisms in expected genes as compared with control USA300 LAC, upregulation of specific metabolic pathways such as the increased *fumC* expression was observed (98). The key role of fumarate assimilation was further confirmed, as *fumC* deletion from *S. aureus* resulted in reduced colonization from murine lungs, indicating the importance of fumarate catabolism in pulmonary colonization (98). These high *fumC*-expressing host-adapted strains also displayed abundant biofilm formation, suggesting that by consuming fumarate they not only limited the development of immune memory, as described above, but also improved community lifestyle. In addition to increasing *fumC*, other metabolic changes seen in *S. aureus* isolates from a completely different study stemmed from several non-synonymous mutations in other metabolic genes, particularly loci involved in amino acid and carbohydrate metabolism (117). This host-adapted strain from long-standing infection in CF also exhibited increased biofilm formation, changes that correlated with acquisition of stop codon mutations in the master regulator *agr* (117). The progressive acquisition of mutations in metabolic genes and upregulation of *fumC* observed in *S. aureus* isolates suggest a continual adaptation to the metabolites produced by immune and epithelial cells, changes that also favor biofilm development.

S. AUREUS METABOLIC ADAPTATION PROMOTES ANTIBIOTIC RESISTANCE

S. aureus adaptation to the host also includes the selection of antibiotic resistant strains in response to ongoing therapy. The acquisition of antibiotic resistance genes may or may not include a metabolic cost in fitness for the organisms. Isolation of *S. aureus* strains resistant to antibiotics, such as the cyclic lipopeptide and bacterial cell membrane disruptor daptomycin, are a major health concern. Recently, it has been shown that daptomycin-resistance is produced by single point mutations in the gene *csl2*, which codes for a cardiolipin synthase resulting in enhanced cardiolipin synthesis and reduced phosphatidylglycerol (118). This metabolic alteration resulted in changes in the bacterial membrane structure impairing daptomycin penetration and membrane disruption. Associated with these changes was the induction of a thwarted immune response, as strains with reduced phosphatidylglycerol promoted less neutrophil chemotaxis (**Figure 2A**). Antibiotic resistance, especially to aminoglycosides, is also exemplified by SCVs. While aminoglycosides are not first line agents for staphylococcal infection, they are frequently used in combination with cell wall active agents, and as preventative/prophylactic therapy in CF. Patients with long-term exposure to aminoglycosides have been shown to develop SCVs. The reduced susceptibility of SCVs to antibiotics is multifactorial: their intracellular location may protect them from the inhibitory concentrations, and their slow growth rate could reduce their susceptibility by non-specific mechanisms including reduced expression of pharmacological targets. Anaerobic metabolism prevents the uptake of aminoglycosides and along with reduced growth rates, OXPHOS activity and electrochemical gradients, SCVs in particular are protected from the bactericidal effects of these antibiotics (119, 120).

CONCLUSIONS

P. aeruginosa and *S. aureus* are highly successful pulmonary pathogens that are able to undergo adaptive changes to first colonize mucosal surfaces, elude mucociliary clearance to cause acute infection, and then adapt to the metabolic demands of the airway to establish chronic infection. These organisms have substantial metabolic flexibility to adapt to the environment within the host often by acquiring mutations or by changing their transcriptional profiles. While the phenotypic changes associated with adaptation to the lung, such as the expression of extracellular polysaccharides, loss of motility, or selection of small colony variants are readily apparent, most of the other adaptive changes are not. Vaccination or even therapeutic strategies to target these organisms must first consider if the intent is the prevention of colonization or suppression of organisms that have already undergone substantial adaptation to persist in the airways.

Whereas the downstream effect of these adaptive changes to establish chronic infections has been thoroughly studied, what drives these changes is less well-understood. Indeed, recent studies are focusing on the metabolic cross-talk between the host cell and the pathogen as well as the response of the pathogen to a milieu that is often filled with immunosignaling metabolites. Despite the abundance of immunometabolites, further studies are required to better understand their role in bacterial pathogenicity in physiologically relevant settings.

AUTHOR CONTRIBUTIONS

SR, TW, and AP wrote the entire manuscript and produced figures.

REFERENCES

1. Goss CH, Muhlebach MS. Review: *Staphylococcus aureus* and MRSA in cystic fibrosis. *J Cyst Fibros*. (2011) 10:298–306. doi: 10.1016/j.jcf.2011.06.002
2. Hauser AR. The type III secretion system of *Pseudomonas aeruginosa*: infection by injection. *Nat Rev Microbiol.* (2009) 7:654–65. doi: 10.1038/nrmicro2199
3. Stover CK, Pham XQ, Erwin AL, Mizoguchi SD, Warrener P, Hickey MJ, et al. Complete genome sequence of *Pseudomonas aeruginosa* PAO1, an opportunistic pathogen. *Nature*. (2000) 406:959–64. doi: 10.1038/35023079
4. Kubes JN, Fridkin SK. Factors affecting the geographic variability of antibiotic-resistant healthcare-associated infections in the United States using the CDC antibiotic resistance patient safety atlas. *Infect Control Hosp Epidemiol.* (2019) 40:597–9. doi: 10.1017/ice.2019.64
5. Winstanley C, O'Brien S, Brockhurst MA. *Pseudomonas aeruginosa* evolutionary adaptation and diversification in cystic fibrosis chronic lung infections. *Trends Microbiol.* (2016) 24:327–37. doi: 10.1016/j.tim.2016.01.008
6. Deretic V, Schurr MJ, Yu H. *Pseudomonas aeruginosa*, mucoidy and the chronic infection phenotype in cystic fibrosis. *Trends Microbiol.* (1995) 3:351–6. doi: 10.1016/S0966-842X(00)88974-X
7. Hajjar AM, Ernst RK, Tsai JH, Wilson CB, Miller SI. Human toll-like receptor 4 recognizes host-specific LPS modifications. *Nat Immunol.* (2002) 3:354–9. doi: 10.1038/ni777
8. Mills EL, Kelly B, Logan A, Costa ASH, Varma M, Bryant CE, et al. Succinate dehydrogenase supports metabolic repurposing of mitochondria to drive inflammatory macrophages. *Cell.* (2016) 167:457–70.e13. doi: 10.1016/j.cell.2016.08.064
9. Mills EL, Kelly B, O'Neill LAJ. Mitochondria are the powerhouses of immunity. *Nat Immunol.* (2017) 18:488–98. doi: 10.1038/ni.3704
10. Everts B, Amiel E, Huang SC, Smith AM, Chang CH, Lam WY, et al. TLR-driven early glycolytic reprogramming via the kinases TBK1-IKKvarepsilon supports the anabolic demands of dendritic cell activation. *Nat Immunol.* (2014) 15:323–32. doi: 10.1038/ni.2833
11. Tannahill GM, Curtis AM, Adamik J, Palsson-McDermott EM, McGettrick AF, Goel G, et al. Succinate is an inflammatory signal that induces IL-1β through HIF-1α. *Nature.* (2013) 496:238–42. doi: 10.1038/nature 11986
12. Evavold CL, Kagan JC. Inflammasomes: threat-assessment organelles of the innate immune system. *Immunity.* (2019) 51:609–24. doi: 10.1016/j.immuni.2019.08.005
13. Duncan JA, Canna SW. The NLRC4 Inflammasome. *Immunol Rev.* (2018) 281:115–23. doi: 10.1111/imr.12607
14. Guo H, Callaway JB, Ting JP. Inflammasomes: mechanism of action, role in disease, and therapeutics. *Nat Med.* (2015) 21:677–87. doi: 10.1038/nm.3893
15. He Y, Hara H, Nunez G. Mechanism and regulation of NLRP3 inflammasome activation. *Trends Biochem Sci.* (2016) 41:1012–21. doi: 10.1016/j.tibs.2016.09.002
16. Evavold CL, Ruan J, Tan Y, Xia S, Wu H, Kagan JC. The pore-forming protein gasdermin D Regulates interleukin-1 secretion from living macrophages. *Immunity.* (2018) 48:35–44.e6. doi: 10.1016/j.immuni.2017.11.013
17. Cohen TS, Prince AS. Activation of inflammasome signaling mediates pathology of acute *P. aeruginosa* pneumonia. *J Clin Invest.* (2013) 123:1630–7. doi: 10.1172/JCI66142
18. Iannitti RG, Napolioni V, Oikonomou V, De Luca A, Galosi C, Pariano M, et al. IL-1 receptor antagonist ameliorates inflammasome-dependent inflammation in murine and human cystic fibrosis. *Nat Commun.* (2016) 7:10791. doi: 10.1038/ncomms10791
19. Linares JF, Moreno R, Fajardo A, Martinez-Solano L, Escalante R, Rojo F, et al. The global regulator Crc modulates metabolism, susceptibility to antibiotics and virulence in *Pseudomonas aeruginosa. Environ Microbiol.* (2010) 12:3196–212. doi: 10.1111/j.1462-2920.2010.02292.x
20. O'Toole GA, Gibbs KA, Hager PW, Phibbs PV Jr, Kolter R. The global carbon metabolism regulator Crc is a component of a signal transduction pathway required for biofilm development by *Pseudomonas aeruginosa. J Bacteriol.* (2000) 182:425–31. doi: 10.1128/JB.182.2.425-431.2000
21. Rojo F. Carbon catabolite repression in Pseudomonas : optimizing metabolic versatility and interactions with the environment. *FEMS Microbiol Rev.* (2010) 34:658–84. doi: 10.1111/j.1574-6976.2010.00218.x
22. Gorke B, Stulke J. Carbon catabolite repression in bacteria: many ways to make the most out of nutrients. *Nat Rev Microbiol.* (2008) 6:613–24. doi: 10.1038/nrmicro1932

23. Toma I, Kang JJ, Sipos A, Vargas S, Bansal E, Hanner F, et al. Succinate receptor GPR91 provides a direct link between high glucose levels and renin release in murine and rabbit kidney. *J Clin Invest.* (2008) 118:2526–34. doi: 10.1172/JCI33293
24. Peti-Peterdi J, Gevorgyan H, Lam L, Riquier-Brison A. Metabolic control of renin secretion. *Pflugers Arch.* (2013) 465:53–8. doi: 10.1007/s00424-012-1130-y
25. Littlewood-Evans A, Sarret S, Apfel V, Loesle P, Dawson J, Zhang J, et al. GPR91 senses extracellular succinate released from inflammatory macrophages and exacerbates rheumatoid arthritis. *J Exp Med.* (2016) 213:1655–62. doi: 10.1084/jem.20160061
26. Kolb M, Margetts PJ, Anthony DC, Pitossi F, Gauldie J. Transient expression of IL-1beta induces acute lung injury and chronic repair leading to pulmonary fibrosis. *J Clin Invest.* (2001) 107:1529–36.
27. Lappalainen U, Whitsett JA, Wert SE, Tichelaar JW, Bry K. Interleukin-1beta causes pulmonary inflammation, emphysema, and airway remodeling in the adult murine lung. *Am J Respir Cell Mol Biol.* (2005) 32:311–8.
28. Gleeson LE, Sheedy FJ, Palsson-McDermott EM, Triglia D, O'Leary SM, O'Sullivan MP, et al. Cutting Edge: Mycobacterium tuberculosis induces aerobic glycolysis in human alveolar macrophages that is required for control of intracellular bacillary replication. *J Immunol.* (2016) 196:2444–9. doi: 10.4049/jimmunol.1501612
29. Deng Q, Wang Y, Zhang Y, Li M, Li D, Huang X, et al. *Pseudomonas aeruginosa* triggers macrophage autophagy to escape intracellular killing by activation of the NLRP3 inflammasome. *Infect Immun.* (2015) 84:56–66. doi: 10.1128/IAI.00945-15
30. Riffelmacher T, Richter FC, Simon AK. Autophagy dictates metabolism and differentiation of inflammatory immune cells. *Autophagy.* (2018) 14:199–206. doi: 10.1080/15548627.2017.1362525
31. Soong G, Parker D, Magargee M, Prince AS. The type III toxins of *Pseudomonas aeruginosa* disrupt epithelial barrier function. *J Bacteriol.* (2008) 190:2814–21. doi: 10.1128/JB.01567-07
32. Chesney J, Telang S. Regulation of glycolytic and mitochondrial metabolism by ras. *Curr Pharm Biotechnol.* (2013) 14:251–60. doi: 10.2174/1389201011314030002
33. Hu H, Juvekar A, Lyssiotis CA, Lien EC, Albeck JG, Oh D, et al. Phosphoinositide 3-Kinase regulates glycolysis through mobilization of aldolase from the actin cytoskeleton. *Cell.* (2016) 164:433–46. doi: 10.1016/j.cell.2015.12.042
34. Ada-Nguema AS, Xenias H, Hofman JM, Wiggins CH, Sheetz MP, Keely PJ. The small GTPase R-Ras regulates organization of actin and drives membrane protrusions through the activity of PLCepsilon. *J Cell Sci.* (2006) 119:1307–19. doi: 10.1242/jcs.03260
35. Shafikhani SH, Engel J. *Pseudomonas aeruginosa* type III-secreted toxin ExoT inhibits host-cell division by targeting cytokinesis at multiple steps. *Proc Natl Acad Sci USA.* (2006) 103:15605–10. doi: 10.1073/pnas.0605949103
36. Ritterson Lew C, Tolan DR. Targeting of several glycolytic enzymes using RNA interference reveals aldolase affects cancer cell proliferation through a non-glycolytic mechanism. *J Biol Chem.* (2012) 287:42554–63. doi: 10.1074/jbc.M112.405969
37. Kaminski A, Gupta KH, Goldufsky JW, Lee HW, Gupta V, Shafikhani SH. *Pseudomonas aeruginosa* ExoS induces intrinsic apoptosis in target host cells in a manner that is dependent on its GAP domain activity. *Sci Rep.* (2018) 8:14047. doi: 10.1038/s41598-018-32491-2
38. Sato H, Frank DW. ExoU is a potent intracellular phospholipase. *Mol Microbiol.* (2004) 53:1279–90. doi: 10.1111/j.1365-2958.2004.04194.x
39. Schulert GS, Feltman H, Rabin SD, Martin CG, Battle SE, Rello J, Hauser AR. Secretion of the toxin ExoU is a marker for highly virulent *Pseudomonas aeruginosa* isolates obtained from patients with hospital-acquired pneumonia. *J Infect Dis.* (2003) 188:1695–706. doi: 10.1086/379372
40. Saliba AM, Nascimento DO, Silva MC, Assis MC, Gayer CR, Raymond B, et al. Eicosanoid-mediated proinflammatory activity of *Pseudomonas aeruginosa* ExoU. *Cell Microbiol.* (2005) 7:1811–22. doi: 10.1111/j.1462-5822.2005.00635.x
41. Cuzick A, Stirling FR, Lindsay SL, Evans TJ. The type III pseudomonal exotoxin U activates the c-Jun NH2-terminal kinase pathway and increases human epithelial interleukin-8 production. *Infect Immun.* (2006) 74:4104–13. doi: 10.1128/IAI.02045-05
42. McMorran B, Town L, Costelloe E, Palmer J, Engel J, Hume D, et al. Effector ExoU from the type III secretion system is an important modulator of gene expression in lung epithelial cells in response to *Pseudomonas aeruginosa* infection. *Infect Immun.* (2003) 71:6035–44. doi: 10.1128/IAI.71.12.7240.2003
43. Belyy A, Raoux-Barbot D, Saveanu C, Namane A, Ogryzko V, Worpenberg L, et al. Actin activates *Pseudomonas aeruginosa* ExoY nucleotidyl cyclase toxin and ExoY-like effector domains from MARTX toxins. *Nat Commun.* (2016) 7:13582. doi: 10.1038/ncomms13582
44. Fang KM, Chen JK, Hung SC, Chen MC, Wu YT, Wu TJ, et al. Effects of combinatorial treatment with pituitary adenylate cyclase activating peptide and human mesenchymal stem cells on spinal cord tissue repair. *PLoS ONE.* (2010) 5:e15299. doi: 10.1371/journal.pone.0015299
45. Kong W, Dong M, Yan R, Liang Q, Zhang H, Luo W, et al. A unique ATPase, ArtR (PA4595), represses the type III secretion system in *Pseudomonas aeruginosa. Front Microbiol.* (2019) 10:560. doi: 10.3389/fmicb.2019.00560
46. Hauser AR, Cobb E, Bodi M, Mariscal D, Valles J, Engel JN, et al. Type III protein secretion is associated with poor clinical outcomes in patients with ventilator-associated pneumonia caused by *Pseudomonas aeruginosa. Crit Care Med.* (2002) 30:521–8. doi: 10.1097/00003246-200203000-00005
47. Roy-Burman A, Savel RH, Racine S, Swanson BL, Revadigar NS, Fujimoto J, et al. Type III protein secretion is associated with death in lower respiratory and systemic *Pseudomonas aeruginosa* infections. *J Infect Dis.* (2001) 183:1767–74. doi: 10.1086/320737
48. Jain M, Ramirez D, Seshadri R, Cullina JF, Powers CA, Schulert GS, et al. Type III secretion phenotypes of *Pseudomonas aeruginosa* strains change during infection of individuals with cystic fibrosis. *J Clin Microbiol.* (2004) 42:5229–37. doi: 10.1128/JCM.42.11.5229-5237.2004
49. Feltman H, Schulert G, Khan S, Jain M, Peterson L, Hauser AR. Prevalence of type III secretion genes in clinical and environmental isolates of *Pseudomonas aeruginosa. Microbiology.* (2001) 147:2659–69. doi: 10.1099/00221287-147-10-2659
50. Moscoso JA, Mikkelsen H, Heeb S, Williams P, Filloux A. The *Pseudomonas aeruginosa* sensor RetS switches type III and type VI secretion via c-di-GMP signalling. *Environ microbiol.* (2011) 13:3128–38. doi: 10.1111/j.1462-2920.2011.02595.x
51. Franklin MJ, Nivens DE, Weadge JT, Howell PL. Biosynthesis of the *Pseudomonas aeruginosa* extracellular polysaccharides, alginate, Pel, and Psl. *Front Microbiol.* (2011) 2:167. doi: 10.3389/fmicb.2011.00167
52. Jennings LK, Storek KM, Ledvina HE, Coulon C, Marmont LS, Sadovskaya I, et al. Pel is a cationic exopolysaccharide that cross-links extracellular DNA in the *Pseudomonas aeruginosa* biofilm matrix. *Proc Natl Acad Sci USA.* (2015) 112:11353–8. doi: 10.1073/pnas.1503058112
53. Huus KE, Joseph J, Zhang L, Wong A, Aaron SD, Mah TF, Sad S. Clinical isolates of *Pseudomonas aeruginosa* from chronically infected cystic fibrosis patients fail to activate the inflammasome during both stable infection and pulmonary exacerbation. *J Immunol.* (2016) 196:3097–108. doi: 10.4049/jimmunol.1501642
54. Riquelme SA, Lozano C, Moustafa AM, Liimatta K, Tomlinson KL, Britto C, et al. CFTR-PTEN-dependent mitochondrial metabolic dysfunction promotes *Pseudomonas aeruginosa* airway infection. *Sci Transl Med.* (2019) 11:eaav4634. doi: 10.1126/scitranslmed.aav4634
55. Chua SL, Ding Y, Liu Y, Cai Z, Zhou J, Swarup S, et al. Reactive oxygen species drive evolution of pro-biofilm variants in pathogens by modulating cyclic-di-GMP levels. *Open Biol.* (2016) 6:160162. doi: 10.1098/rsob.160162
56. McCarthy RR, Mazon-Moya MJ, Moscoso JA, Hao Y, Lam JS, Bordi C, et al. Cyclic-di-GMP regulates lipopolysaccharide modification and contributes to *Pseudomonas aeruginosa* immune evasion. *Nat Microbiol.* (2017) 2:17027. doi: 10.1038/nmicrobiol.2017.27
57. Valentini M, Filloux A. Biofilms and cyclic di-gmp (c-di-gmp) signaling: lessons from *Pseudomonas aeruginosa* and other bacteria. *J Biol Chem.* (2016) 291:12547–55. doi: 10.1074/jbc.R115.711507
58. Boles BR, Singh PK. Endogenous oxidative stress produces diversity and adaptability in biofilm communities. *Proc Natl Acad Sci USA.* (2008) 105:12503–8. doi: 10.1073/pnas.0801499105
59. Li Y, Xia H, Bai F, Xu H, Yang L, Yao H, et al. Identification of a new gene PA5017 involved in flagella-mediated motility, chemotaxis and biofilm

formation in *Pseudomonas aeruginosa*. *FEMS Microbiol Lett*. (2007) 272:188–95. doi: 10.1111/j.1574-6968.2007.00753.x

50. Conrad JC, Gibiansky ML, Jin F, Gordon VD, Motto DA, Mathewson MA, et al. Flagella and pili-mediated near-surface single-cell motility mechanisms in *P. aeruginosa*. *Biophys J*. (2011) 100:1608–16. doi: 10.1016/j.bpj.2011.02.020
51. Ahn S, Jung J, Jang IA, Madsen EL, Park W. Role of glyoxylate shunt in oxidative stress response. *J Biol Chem*. (2016) 291:11928–38. doi: 10.1074/jbc.M115.708149
52. Ha S, Shin B, Park W. Lack of glyoxylate shunt dysregulates iron homeostasis in *Pseudomonas aeruginosa*. *Microbiology*. (2018) 164:587–99. doi: 10.1099/mic.0.000623
53. Haussler S. Biofilm formation by the small colony variant phenotype of *Pseudomonas aeruginosa*. *Environ Microbiol*. (2004) 6:546–51. doi: 10.1111/j.1462-2920.2004.00618.x
54. Malone JG. Role of small colony variants in persistence of *Pseudomonas aeruginosa* infections in cystic fibrosis lungs. *Infect Drug Resist*. (2015) 8:237–47. doi: 10.2147/IDR.S68214
55. Starkey M, Hickman JH, Ma L, Zhang N, De Long S, Hinz A, et al. *Pseudomonas aeruginosa* rugose small-colony variants have adaptations that likely promote persistence in the cystic fibrosis lung. *J Bacteriol*. (2009) 191:3492–503. doi: 10.1128/JB.00119-09
56. Deretic V, Gill JF, Chakrabarty AM. Gene algD coding for GDPmannose dehydrogenase is transcriptionally activated in mucoid *Pseudomonas aeruginosa*. *J Bacteriol*. (1987) 169:351–8. doi: 10.1128/JB.169.1.351-358.1987
57. Valentini M, Lapouge K. Catabolite repression in *Pseudomonas aeruginosa* PAO1 regulates the uptake of C4 -dicarboxylates depending on succinate concentration. *Environ Microbiol*. (2013) 15:1707–16. doi: 10.1111/1462-2920.12056
58. Riquelme SA, Hopkins BD, Wolfe AL, DiMango E, Kitur K, Parsons R, et al. Cystic fibrosis transmembrane conductance regulator attaches tumor suppressor PTEN to the membrane and promotes anti *Pseudomonas aeruginosa* immunity. *Immunity*. (2017) 47:1169–81.e7. doi: 10.1016/j.immuni.2017.11.010
59. McElvaney OJ, Zaslona Z, Becker-Flegler K, Palsson-McDermott EM, Boland F, Gunaratnam C, et al. Specific inhibition of the NLRP3 Inflammasome as an anti-inflammatory strategy in cystic fibrosis. *Am J Respir Crit Care Med*. (2019) doi: 10.1164/rccm.201905-1013OC
60. Scambler T, Jarosz-Griffiths HH, Lara-Reyna S, Pathak S, Wong C, Holbrook J, et al. ENaC-mediated sodium influx exacerbates NLRP3-dependent inflammation in cystic fibrosis. *Elife*. (2019) 8:e49248. doi: 10.7554/eLife.49248.020
61. Zhang PX, Cheng J, Zou S, D'Souza AD, Koff JL, Lu J, et al. Pharmacological modulation of the AKT/microRNA-199a-5p/CAV1 pathway ameliorates cystic fibrosis lung hyper-inflammation. *Nat Commun*. (2015) 6:6221. doi: 10.1038/ncomms7221
62. Aksoy E, Taboubi S, Torres D, Delbauve S, Hachani A, Whitehead MA, et al. The p110delta isoform of the kinase PI(3)K controls the subcellular compartmentalization of TLR4 signaling and protects from endotoxic shock. *Nat Immunol*. (2012) 13:1045–54. doi: 10.1038/ni.2426
63. Kintz E, Goldberg JB. Regulation of lipopolysaccharide O antigen expression in *Pseudomonas aeruginosa*. *Future Microbiol*. (2008) 3:191–203. doi: 10.2217/17460913.3.2.191
64. Ernst RK, Yi EC, Guo L, Lim KB, Burns JL, Hackett M, Miller SI. Specific lipopolysaccharide found in cystic fibrosis airway *Pseudomonas aeruginosa*. *Science*. (1999) 286:1561–5. doi: 10.1126/science.286.5444.1561
65. Maldonado RF, Sa-Correia I, Valvano MA. Lipopolysaccharide modification in gram-negative bacteria during chronic infection. *FEMS Microbiol Rev*. (2016) 40:480–93. doi: 10.1093/femsre/fuw007
66. Sperandeo P, Martorana AM, Polissi A. The lipopolysaccharide transport (Lpt) machinery: a nonconventional transporter for lipopolysaccharide assembly at the outer membrane of gram-negative bacteria. *J Biol Chem*. (2017) 292:17981–90. doi: 10.1074/jbc.R117.802512
67. Gu Y, Stansfeld PJ, Zeng Y, Dong H, Wang W, Dong C. Lipopolysaccharide is inserted into the outer membrane through an intramembrane hole, a lumen gate, and the lateral opening of LptD. *Structure*. (2015) 23:496–504. doi: 10.1016/j.str.2015.01.001
78. Balibar CJ, Grabowicz M. Mutant alleles of lptD Increase the permeability of *Pseudomonas aeruginosa* and define determinants of intrinsic resistance to antibiotics. *Antimicrob Agents Chemother*. (2016) 60:845–54. doi: 10.1128/AAC.01747-15
79. Diekema DJ, Pfaller MA, Schmitz FJ, Smayevsky J, Bell J, Jones RN, et al. Survey of infections due to *Staphylococcus* species: frequency of occurrence and antimicrobial susceptibility of isolates collected in the United States, Canada, Latin America, Europe, and the Western Pacific region for the sentry antimicrobial surveillance program, 1997-1999. *Clin Infect Dis*. (2001) 32(Suppl. 2):S114–32. doi: 10.1086/320184
80. Limoli DH, Hoffman LR. Help, hinder, hide and harm: what can we learn from the interactions between *Pseudomonas aeruginosa* and *Staphylococcus aureus* during respiratory infections? *Thorax*. (2019) 74:684–92. doi: 10.1136/thoraxjnl-2018-212616
81. Zemanick ET, Hoffman LR. Cystic fibrosis: microbiology and host response. *Pediatr Clin North Am*. (2016) 63:617–36. doi: 10.1016/j.pcl.2016.04.003
82. Proctor RA, von Eiff C, Kahl BC, Becker K, McNamara P, Herrmann M, et al. Small colony variants: a pathogenic form of bacteria that facilitates persistent and recurrent infections. *Nat Rev Microbiol*. (2006) 4:295–305. doi: 10.1038/nrmicro1384
83. Proctor RA, van Langevelde P, Kristjansson M, Maslow JN, Arbeit RD. Persistent and relapsing infections associated with small-colony variants of *Staphylococcus aureus*. *Clin Infect Dis*. (1995) 20:95–102. doi: 10.1093/clinids/20.1.95
84. Wong Fok Lung T, Monk IR, Acker KP, Mu A, Wang N, Riquelme SA, et al. *Staphylococcus aureus* small colony variants impair host immunity by activating host cell glycolysis and inducing necroptosis. *Nat Microbiol*. (2020) doi: 10.1038/s41564-019-0597-0
85. Kriegeskorte A, Grubmuller S, Huber C, Kahl BC, von Eiff C, Proctor RA, et al. *Staphylococcus aureus* small colony variants show common metabolic features in central metabolism irrespective of the underlying auxotrophism. *Front Cell Infect Microbiol*. (2014) 4:141. doi: 10.3389/fcimb.2014.00141
86. Wolter DJ, Emerson JC, McNamara S, Buccat AM, Qin X, Cochrane E, et al. *Staphylococcus aureus* small-colony variants are independently associated with worse lung disease in children with cystic fibrosis. *Clin Infect Dis*. (2013) 57:384–91. doi: 10.1093/cid/cit270
87. Melehani JH, Duncan JA. Inflammasome activation can mediate tissue-Specific Pathogenesis or protection in *Staphylococcus aureus* infection. *Curr Top Microbiol immunol*. (2016) 397:257–82. doi: 10.1007/978-3-319-41171-2_13
88. Miller LS, Pietras EM, Uricchio LH, Hirano K, Rao S, Lin H, et al. Inflammasome-mediated production of IL-1β is required for neutrophil recruitment against *Staphylococcus aureus in vivo*. *J Immunol*. (2007) 179:6933–42. doi: 10.4049/jimmunol.179.10.6933
89. Kebaier C, Chamberland RR, Allen IC, Gao X, Broglie PM, Hall JD, et al. *Staphylococcus aureus* alpha-hemolysin mediates virulence in a murine model of severe pneumonia through activation of the NLRP3 inflammasome. *J Infect Dis*. (2012) 205:807–17. doi: 10.1093/infdis/jir846
90. Cohen TS, Boland ML, Boland BB, Takahashi V, Tovchigrechko A, Lee Y, et al. *S. aureus* evades macrophage killing through NLRP3-dependent effects on mitochondrial trafficking. *Cell Rep*. (2018) 22:2431–41. doi: 10.1016/j.celrep.2018.02.027
91. Kitur K, Wachtel S, Brown A, Wickersham M, Paulino F, Penaloza HF, et al. Necroptosis promotes *staphylococcus aureus* clearance by inhibiting excessive inflammatory signaling. *Cell Rep*. (2016) 16:2219–30. doi: 10.1016/j.celrep.2016.07.039
92. Hook JL, Islam MN, Parker D, Prince AS, Bhattacharya S, Bhattacharya J. Disruption of staphylococcal aggregation protects against lethal lung injury. *J Clin Invest*. (2018) 128:1074–86. doi: 10.1172/JCI95823
93. Dengler V, Foulston L, DeFrancesco AS, Losick R. An electrostatic net model for the role of extracellular DNA in biofilm formation by *Staphylococcus aureus*. *J Bacteriol*. (2015) 197:3779–87. doi: 10.1128/JB.00726-15
94. Mack D, Fischer W, Krokotsch A, Leopold K, Hartmann R, Egge H, et al. The intercellular adhesin involved in biofilm accumulation of *Staphylococcus epidermidis* is a linear beta-1,6-linked glucosaminoglycan: purification and structural analysis. *J Bacteriol*. (1996) 178:175–83. doi: 10.1128/JB.178.1.175-183.1996

95. Zapotoczna M, O'Neill E, O'Gara JP. Untangling the diverse and redundant mechanisms of *Staphylococcus aureus* biofilm formation. *PLoS Pathog.* (2016) 12:e1005671. doi: 10.1371/journal.ppat.1005671
96. Sau S, Sun J, Lee CY. Molecular characterization and transcriptional analysis of type 8 capsule genes in *Staphylococcus aureus. J Bacteriol.* (1997) 179:1614–21. doi: 10.1128/JB.179.5.1614-1621.1997
97. McKenney D, Pouliot KL, Wang Y, Murthy V, Ulrich M, Doring G, et al. Broadly protective vaccine for *Staphylococcus aureus* based on an *in vivo*-expressed antigen. *Science.* (1999) 284:1523–7. doi: 10.1126/science.284.5419.1523
98. Gabryszewski SJ, Wong Fok Lung T, Annavajhala MK, Tomlinson KL, Riquelme SA, Khan IN, et al. Metabolic adaptation in MRSA pneumonia. *Am J Respir Cell Mol Biol.* (2019) 61:185–97. doi: 10.1165/rcmb.2018-0389O
99. Bhattacharya M, Berends ETM, Chan R, Schwab E, Roy S, Sen CK, et al. *Staphylococcus aureus* biofilms release leukocidins to elicit extracellular trap formation and evade neutrophil-mediated killing. *Proc Natl Acad Sci USA.* (2018) 115:7416–21. doi: 10.1073/pnas.1721949115
100. Thurlow LR, Hanke ML, Fritz T, Angle A, Aldrich A, Williams SH, et al. *Staphylococcus aureus* biofilms prevent macrophage phagocytosis and attenuate inflammation *in vivo. J Immunol.* (2011) 186:6585–96. doi: 10.4049/jimmunol.1002794
101. Shopsin B, Kreiswirth BN. Molecular epidemiology of methicillin-resistant *Staphylococcus aureus. Emerging Infect Dis.* (2001) 7:323–6. doi: 10.3201/eid0702.010236
102. Hassoun A, Linden PK, Friedman B. Incidence, prevalence, and management of MRSA bacteremia across patient populations-a review of recent developments in MRSA management and treatment. *Crit Care.* (2017) 21:211. doi: 10.1186/s13054-017-1801-3
103. Smyth DS, Kafer JM, Wasserman GA, Velickovic L, Mathema B, Holzman RS, et al. Nasal carriage as a source of agr-defective *Staphylococcus aureus* bacteremia. *J Infect Dis.* (2012) 206:1168–77. doi: 10.1093/infdis/jis483
104. Jenul C, Horswill AR. Regulation of *Staphylococcus aureus* virulence. *Microbiol Spectr.* (2018) 6. doi: 10.1128/microbiolspec.GPP3-0031-2018
105. Foster TJ, Geoghegan JA, Ganesh VK, Hook M. Adhesion, invasion and evasion: the many functions of the surface proteins of *Staphylococcus aureus. Nat Rev Microbiol.* (2014) 12:49–62. doi: 10.1038/nrmicro3161
106. Bubeck Wardenburg J, Schneewind O. Vaccine protection against *Staphylococcus aureus* pneumonia. *J Exp Med.* (2008) 205:287–94. doi: 10.1084/jem.20072208
107. Gomez MI, O'Seaghdha M, Magargee M, Foster TJ, Prince AS. *Staphylococcus aureus* protein A activates TNFR1 signaling through conserved IgG binding domains. *J Biol Chem.* (2006) 281:20190–6. doi: 10.1074/jbc.M601956200
108. Palma Medina LM, Becker AK, Michalik S, Yedavally H, Raineri EJM, Hildebrandt P, et al. Metabolic cross-talk between human bronchial epithelial cells and internalized *Staphylococcus aureus* as a driver for infection. *Mol Cell Proteomics.* (2019) 18:892–908. doi: 10.1074/mcp.RA118.001138
109. Halsey CR, Lei S, Wax JK, Lehman MK, Nuxoll AS, Steinke L, et al. Amino acid catabolism in *Staphylococcus aureus* and the function of carbon catabolite repression. *MBio.* (2017) 8:e01434-16. doi: 10.1128/mBio.01434-16
110. Palmer KL, Aye LM, Whiteley M. Nutritional cues control *Pseudomonas aeruginosa* multicellular behavior in cystic fibrosis sputum. *J Bacteriol.* (2007) 189:8079–87. doi: 10.1128/JB.01138-07
111. Bravo-Santano N, Ellis JK, Mateos LM, Calle Y, Keun HC, Behrends V, et al. Intracellular *Staphylococcus aureus* modulates host central carbon metabolism to activate autophagy. *mSphere.* (2018) 3:e00374-18. doi: 10.1128/mSphere.00374-18
112. Wickersham M, Wachtel S, Wong Fok Lung T, Soong G, Jacquet R, Richardson A, et al. Metabolic stress drives keratinocyte defenses against *Staphylococcus aureus* infection. *Cell Rep.* (2017) 18:2742–51. doi: 10.1016/j.celrep.2017.02.055
113. Kremserova S, Nauseef WM. Frontline science: *Staphylococcus aureus* promotes receptor-interacting protein kinase 3- and protease-dependent production of IL-1β in human neutrophils. *J Leukoc Biol.* (2019) 105:437–47. doi: 10.1002/JLB.4HI0918-346R
114. Kornberg MD, Bhargava P, Kim PM, Putluri V, Snowman AM, Putluri N, et al. Dimethyl fumarate targets GAPDH and aerobic glycolysis to modulate immunity. *Science.* (2018) 360:449–53. doi: 10.1126/science.aan4665
115. Arts RJ, Novakovic B, Ter Horst R, Carvalho A, Bekkering S, Lachmandas E, et al. Glutaminolysis and fumarate accumulation integrate immunometabolic and epigenetic programs in trained immunity. *Cell Metab.* (2016) 24:807–19. doi: 10.1016/j.cmet.2016.10.008
116. Acker KP, Wong Fok Lung T, West E, Craft J, Narechania A, Smith H, et al. Strains of *Staphylococcus aureus* that colonize and infect skin harbor mutations in metabolic genes. *iScience.* (2019) 19:281–90. doi: 10.1016/j.isci.2019.07.037
117. Tan X, Coureuil M, Ramond E, Euphrasie D, Dupuis M, Tros F, et al. Chronic *Staphylococcus aureus* lung infection correlates with proteogenomic and metabolic adaptations leading to an increased intracellular persistence. *Clin Infect Dis.* (2019) 69:1937–45. doi: 10.1093/cid/ciz106
118. Jiang JH, Bhuiyan MS, Shen HH, Cameron DR, Rupasinghe TWT, Wu CM, et al. Antibiotic resistance and host immune evasion in *Staphylococcus aureus* mediated by a metabolic adaptation. *Proc Natl Acad Sci USA.* (2019) 116:3722–7. doi: 10.1073/pnas.1812066116
119. Eisenberg ES, Mandel LJ, Kaback HR, Miller MH. Quantitative association between electrical potential across the cytoplasmic membrane and early gentamicin uptake and killing in *Staphylococcus aureus. J Bacteriol.* (1984) 157:863–7. doi: 10.1128/JB.157.3.863-867.1984
120. Gilman S, Saunders VA. Accumulation of gentamicin by *Staphylococcus aureus*: the role of the transmembrane electrical potential. *J Antimicrob Chemother.* (1986) 17:37–44. doi: 10.1093/jac/17.1.37

16

FOXO3 Transcription Factor Regulates IL-10 Expression in Mycobacteria-Infected Macrophages, Tuning their Polarization and the Subsequent Adaptive Immune Response

Rania Bouzeyen[1,2†], Meriam Haoues[1,2†], Mohamed-Ridha Barbouche[1,2], Ramandeep Singh[3] and Makram Essafi[1,2]*

[1] Laboratory of Transmission, Control and Immunobiology of Infections (LTCII), Laboratoire de Recherche 11 (LR11), Institut Pasteur de Tunis (IPT), Tunis, Tunisia, [2] Université Tunis El Manar, Tunis, Tunisia, [3] Tuberculosis Research Laboratory, Translational Health Science and Technology Institute, NCR Biotech Science Cluster, Faridabad, India

***Correspondence:**
Makram Essafi
makram.essafi@pasteur.tn*

[†]These authors have contributed equally to this work

Alveolar Macrophages play a key role in the development of a robust adaptive immune response against the agent of Tuberculosis (TB), *Mycobacterium tuberculosis* (*M.tb*). However, macrophage response is often hampered by the production of IL-10, a potent suppressor of the host immune response. The secretion of IL-10 correlates with TB pathogenesis and persistence in host tissues. Concordantly, inhibition of IL-10 signaling, during BCG vaccination, confers higher protection against *M.tb* through a sustained Th1 and Th17 responses. Therefore, uncovering host effectors, underlying mycobacteria-induced expression of IL-10, may be beneficial toward the development of IL-10-blocking tools to be used either as adjuvants in preventive vaccination or as adjunct during standard treatment of TB. Here, we investigated the role of FOXO3 transcription factor in mycobacteria-induced secretion of IL-10. We observed that PI3K/Akt/FOXO3 axis regulates IL-10 expression in human macrophages. Knocking down of FOXO3 expression resulted in an increase of IL-10 production in BCG-infected macrophages. The gene reporter assay further confirmed the transcriptional regulation of IL-10 by FOXO3. *In silico* analysis identified four Forkhead binding motifs on the human IL-10 promoter, from which the typical FOXO3 one at position −203 was the major target as assessed by mutagenesis and CHIP binding assays. Further, we also observed a decrease in gene expression levels of the M1 typical markers (i.e., CD80 and CD86) in SiFOXO3-transfected macrophages while activation of FOXO3 led to the increase in the expression of CD86, MHCI, and MHCII. Finally, co-culture of human lymphocytes with siFOXO3-transfected macrophages, loaded with mycobacterial antigens, showed decreased expression of Th1/Th17 specific markers and a simultaneous increase in expression of IL-4 and IL-10. Taken together, we report for the first time that FOXO3 modulates IL-10 secretion in mycobacteria-infected macrophage, driving their polarization and the subsequent adaptive immune response. This work proposes FOXO3 as a potential target for the development of host-directed strategies for better treatment or prevention of TB.

Keywords: tuberculosis, macrophages, FOXO3, IL-10, M1/Th1

INTRODUCTION

Tuberculosis (TB) remains one of the top causes of death with an estimated 1.4 million deaths and 10.4 million new cases worldwide (1). The global TB burden has increased due to emergence of drug-resistant *Mycobacterium tuberculosis* (*M.tb*) strains and the limited protection conferred by *M. bovis* BCG against pulmonary TB (2). Targeting the host effectors, involved in TB immune response, has been proposed as a viable adjunct therapy for elimination of both drug-sensitive and drug-resistant TB (3) or to enhance the BCG protective efficacy (4). Therefore, there is a critical need to uncover the TB host responsive clues that might lead to the development of novel host-directed approaches for better treatment or prevention of TB.

Macrophages are major innate immune cells, which play key roles in TB infection as an intracellular niche and serve as a first line defense against *M.tb* infection (5). Phagocytosis of mycobacteria initiates a series of innate and adaptive immune responses to contain the infection (6). Importantly, macrophage-derived cytokines, such as TNF-α, IL-12, and IL-1 family members as well as chemokines and antimicrobial peptides (AMPs) are critical for host anti-mycobacterial defense and shaping the disease progression (7). However, macrophage response is often hampered by the production of IL-10, a potent suppressor of the host immune response, which was reported to be correlated with TB pathogenesis and persistent of infection in humans (8, 9). Several studies have shown that IL-10 plays an important role in shaping the initial immune response and its expression level determines the fate of mycobacterial infections. Indeed, induction of IL-10 by *M.tb*-infected macrophages and dendritic cells (DC) represents a powerful mechanism of immune evasion (10). It has been reported that *M.tb*-induced IL-10 secretion interferes with the phago-lysosome fusion, macrophage activation, and resulting in persistence of the invading bacteria (11). It has been shown that IL-10 affects antigen procession and T cells priming by downregulating the expression of the major histocompatibility complex class II, CD80, CD86, and CD11c in BCG-infected macrophages and DC (12, 13). IL-10 also inhibits the production of pro-inflammatory cytokines, and the release of reactive nitrogen and oxygen intermediates by macrophages, thereby leading to a weakened Th1/Th17 and an enhanced Th2 response (7, 14, 15). Likewise, *M.tb*-induced IL-10 promotes M2 macrophages polarization, which displays dampened anti-mycobacterial response (16).

On the other hand, IL-10 suppression promotes mycobacterial clearance by the host during the early stages of *M.tb* infection (15). IL-10 deficient mice display an enhanced Th1 immune response to aerosol challenge with *M.tb* and lower bacterial burden as compared to the wild type mice (17). In concordance, the susceptible mice strains such as the CBA/J express higher levels of IL-10 in chronic infection, while blocking of IL-10 signaling resulted in lower bacterial load and increased mice survival (18). Conversely, the artificial enhancement of IL-10 expression in a resistant mouse strain increased their susceptibility to *M.tb* infection (19). These studies suggest that IL-10 production is correlated with susceptibility to *M.tb* and suppression of the protective immune response in mice. In concordance, active TB patients present elevated levels of IL-10 in the lungs serum, sputum and bronchoalveolar lavage fluid (BAL) (20). Moreover, it has been reported that macrophages from TB patients produce higher level of IL-10 than the ones from healthy subjects (8, 21, 22). Likewise, patients with MDR-TB have an altered balance between Th1/Th2 response with decreased Th1 associated cytokines and increased IL-10 secretion (22). High level of IL-10, at the end of treatment in pulmonary TB patients, was also associated with TB recurrence (7), indicating that IL-10 plays an essential role in TB pathogenesis and disease progression. Inhibition of IL-10 signaling, during BCG vaccination, enhances antigen-specific IFN-γ and IL-17 responses and results in better protection against *M.tb* challenge (23). These findings demonstrate that modulation of IL-10 at the time of vaccination could be crucial for generating long-term protective efficacy against *M.tb* (24). Therefore, identifying host effectors that regulate mycobacteria induced IL-10 secretion might be useful for the development of host-directed therapy approaches against *M.tb*.

Previous studies have identified two important signaling cascades that control IL-10 expression in macrophages, the PI3K/Akt/GSK3b and JAK/STAT3 pathways (14). Pharmaceutical inhibition of PI3K/AKT in macrophages impairs IL-10-induced gene expression and IL-10-mediated suppression of LPS-induced pro-inflammatory gene (25). Interestingly, It has been demonstrated that BCG induces IL-10 production through PI3K/AKT signaling while prevention of IL-10 secretion and enhancement of IL-12 production is associated with a decreased Akt phosphorylation (26). In another study, it has been reported that *M.tb* evades macrophage microbicidal activity by activating the Akt/mTOR/p70S6K pathway, while inhibition of Akt phosphorylation results in reduced *M.tb* intracellular survival (27).

Forkhead box-O3 (FOXO3) protein is a transcription factor that regulates the expression of multiple genes involved in pathways such as cell-death, cell proliferation, oxidative stress resistance, inflammation, and innate immune homeostasis (28). We have previously reported that BCG-mediated apoptosis of human macrophages relies on FOXO3 activation, which is negatively regulated by the survival pathway PI3K/Akt (29). We demonstrated that BCG infection of macrophages resulted in Akt dephosphorylation and its target FOXO3. The dephosphorylated FOXO3 is subsequently translocated to the nucleus and induced the expression of the pro-apoptotic effectors NOXA and PUMA (29). In concordance, in comparison to healthy controls, low expression of FOXO3 in active TB patients is associated with a defect in monocytes apoptosis (30). The fact that high level of IL-10 expression is also a hallmark of TB pathogenesis (8, 9) suggests FOXO3 as a potential repressor of IL-10 secretion.

Here, we studied whether FOXO3 regulates IL-10 secretion in mycobacteria-infected macrophages and how this regulation would influence the adaptive immune response against mycobacterial infection. We show that FOXO3 inhibits IL-10 secretion in BCG-infected macrophage through the direct binding to and repression of IL-10 promoter, pushing the balance of the immune response toward an M1/Th1 phenotype. These observations suggest FOXO3 as a potential target to develop alternative host-directed approaches for better treatment and prevention of TB.

MATERIALS AND METHODS

Cell Culture

The THP-1 cell line (American Type Culture Collection, ATCC TIB-202) was maintained and cultured as described previously (29). Briefly cells were maintained in RPMI 1640 (Thermo Fisher, USA) supplemented with 10% fetal bovine serum (FBS) (Thermo Fisher, USA), 12 mM HEPES, 0.1 mM MEM non-essential amino acids, 1 mM Sodium Pyruvate, and 100 nM penicillin/streptomycin (Life Technologies). THP-1 monocytes were differentiated to macrophages (TDMs) with 20 ng/mL phorbol 12-myristate 13-acetate (PMA, Sigma-Aldrich, USA) for 48 h. RAW264.7 (ATCC TIB-71) and J774A.1 (ATCC TIB-67) murine macrophage cell lines were also maintained in RPMI medium. Peripheral blood mononuclear cells (PBMCs) were isolated from three healthy volunteers as approved by the institutional ethics committee of Institut Pasteur de Tunis. These donors were negative for any recent infection and had no history of TB. Briefly, cells were differentiated into macrophages derived monocytes (MDMs) and cultured as previously described (29). Macrophages were infected with a single cells suspension of BCG Pasteur strain, at a multiplicity of infection (MOI) of 1:10 for 3 h. The extracellular bacteria was removed by washing twice with 1× PBS and overlaid with medium containing inhibitors for different time points. The drugs were used at the following concentration: Wortmannin (100 nM) (Sigma-Aldrich, USA) or MK-2206 (5 μM) (Selleckchem, USA). It is worth to note that we avoided adding the inhibitors before BCG infection because PI3K/Akt pathway has been shown to control phagocytosis. Supernatants were collected 24 h post-infection and frozen at −20 until use. The cells were harvested 24 h post-infection for western blot or Real-time quantitative RT-PCR (RT-qPCR) analysis.

Cell Toxicity Assay

Cytotoxicity of the inhibitors used in this study was assessed using WST-1 kit (Sigma Aldrich, USA) as per the manufacturer's instructions. Briefly, cells (2.10^4/well in a 96-well plate) were treated with different concentrations of the inhibitors, or with equivalent volume of vehicle control. Twenty-four hours post treatment, media was removed, substrate was added and plate was further incubated at 37°C for 30 min. The optical density values were determined by a microplate reader at 450 nm and the values were normalized with those of untreated cells. All experiments were carried out in triplicates.

RNA Interference Experiments

TDMs or MDMs were transfected, using the HiPerfect Transfection reagent (Qiagen), with either 100 nM control non-silencing siRNA (SiCT), or with 50 nM FOXO3 siRNAs (siGENOME SMARTpool, Thermo Fisher Scientific) according to the manufacturer's instructions. After 48 h of transfection, cells were infected with *M. bovis* BCG at an MOI of 1:10. After 24 h of infection, cells were harvested and the knockdown of FOXO3 was verified by both Western blot and RT-qPCR analysis.

Western Blotting

For immunoblot analysis, macrophages were lysed in 1× laemmli buffer and the protein concentration was determined using Bicinchoninic Acid Protein Assay (BCA, Sigma-Aldrich). Equal amounts of protein was separated by electrophoresis on 10% SDS-PAGE gel, transferred to PVDF membrane and subsequently probed with the respective antibodies as per manufacturer recommendations. In the present study, the following primary antibodies were purchased either from Sigma Aldrich, Merck [FKHRL1-D12 (p-FOXO3^{Thr32}), FKHRL-1 (FOXO3), β-actin] or from Cell Signaling Technology, USA (Akt and p-Akt^{Ser473}). Western blots were quantified by densitometric analysis using Image J software.

Real-Time Quantitative RT-PCR

Total RNAs from treated cells were isolated using RNeasy Micro kit (Qiagen), and the cDNAs were synthesized by reverse transcriptase (RT) using the high capacity cDNA archive random priming kit (Applied Biosystems) according to the manufacturer's recommended protocol. Real-time quantitative PCR was performed using the platinum® Syber Green qPCR Supermix-UDGw/ROX (life technologies). The relative expression of the target genes was calculated using the target threshold cycle value (Ct) and the $2^{-\Delta\Delta Ct}$ method with β-actin and GAPDH as the internal loading controls. The primer sequences used for real time PCR are listed in **Tables S1, S2**.

ELISA Cytokine Assays

For cytokine assays, supernatants were collected at different time points post BCG infection and used to measure IL-10, TNF-α, IFN-γ, and IL-6 concentrations using ELISA assay kits as per manufacturer recommendations (BD Biosciences).

In silico Analysis and Gene Reporter Assay

To identify putative FOXO3 binding sites, the human IL-10 promoter region spanning from −560 to +1 was analyzed *in silico* using the MatInspector analysis tool of the Genomatix software (https://www.genomatix.de/online_help/help_matinspector/matinspector_help.html). For reporter assays, the construct pGL3-IL-10, containing the −588 IL-10 promoter sequence upstream of the luciferase transcriptional unit of the pGL3 vector was used. This construct was a gift from John W.

Steinke, Asthma and Allergic Diseases Center, Charlottesville VA, USA. Transient transfections into RAW 264.7 macrophages were performed using the Amaxa SF Cell Line 4D-nucleofector Kit (Lonza Köln, Germany) as per manufacturer recommendations. Briefly, 1×10^6 macrophages were washed and resuspended in 20 μl of transfection buffer and mixed with 1 μg of pEGFP vector, encoding for GFP or pEGFP-FOXO3TM construct, encoding for GFP-FOXOTM (constitutive active form of FOXO3 where the three Akt binding sites were mutated) along with the reporter pGL3-IL-10 construct or the pGL3 empty vector). Cells were then transfected using program Raw264.7 on Lonza 4D-nucleofector device. Cells were rapidly transferred to 37°C preheated medium and incubated for 24 h at 37°C, 5% CO_2. Twenty-four hours post-transfection, macrophages were either mock-treated or infected with BCG at an MOI of 1:10. After 6 h, macrophages were assessed for viability using Annexin-V staining and the remaining cells were harvested, lysed and luciferase activity was measured using Thermo Scientific Varioscan Flash Plate reader as per manufacturer's recommendations (Promega, Madison, WI, USA). The promoter activities are shown as relative light unit (RLU) and normalized to 100% GFP positive and viable cells (**Figure S2**) using the following equation:

$$\text{Promoter activity} = \frac{\text{RLU } x \text{ } 100}{\text{\% GFP positive and viable cells}} \quad (1)$$

Site Directed Mutagenesis of the IL-10 Promoter

The four FOXO3 binding sites in −588 IL-10 promoter construct were mutated using Quick-change XL site directed mutagenesis kit (Agilent technology) as per manufacturer's recommendations. The list of primers used to disrupt FOXO3 motifs mutagenesis is shown in **Table S3**. The mutant 1, 2, 3, and 4 were constructed by deleting CAC (position −17), GCT (position −203), AAT (position −303), and TTA (position −526), respectively. The effect of each mutation on transcriptional activity of IL-10 promoter was assessed by gene reporter assay as indicated above.

Chromatin Immunoprecipitation (CHIP)

Next, we performed CHIP assay in TDMs using the Chromatin Immunoprecipitation (CHIP) Kit (Millipore) according to the manufacturer's instructions. Briefly, macrophages were infected with BCG at an MOI of 1:10 for 2 h, washed thrice with 1× PBS and overlaid with medium containing 100 nM wortmannin for 2 h to enhance FOXO3 translocation to the nucleus. TDMs were subsequently crosslinked with 1% formaldehyde at 37°C for 10 min and quenched with 0.2 M glycine for 10 min. The crosslinked cells were washed twice and lysed in cell lysis buffer. Subsequently, chromatin was sheared by sonication at 60% power for 10 cycles, 10 s ON/1 min off, to obtain 100–1,000 bp chromatin fragments. For immunoprecipitation, the sheared chromatin was diluted 10 times, precleared with Protein A/G agarose salmon sperm DNA (Millipore) for 30 min at 4°C, then incubated with rabbit anti-FKHRL1 (FOXO3) sc-11351X, Santa cruz Biotechnology) or an equal amount of rabbit anti-IgG (sc-2027, Santa cruz Biotechnology) at 4°C overnight. The Antibody/DNA complexes were co-immunoprecipitated with protein A/G agarose at 4°C for 1 h. The immunoprecipitated DNA was eluted and crosslinking was reversed by incubation at 65°C for 4 h in 5M NaCl. The mix was later incubated with 10 mg/mL of proteinase K at 45°C for 1 h and the DNA from starting (1% input) and immunoprecipitated samples were purified by phenol-chloroform extraction and ethanol precipitation. The resulting pellets were suspended in H_2O, quantified and subjected to PCR using primers (F1 5′- CCTCTGCGCACA GAACAGCTG-3′ and R1 5′- CTAACCTCTCTAATAAACTTAG-3′) flanking the FOXO3 binding motif at −203 position.

Effect of FOXO3 on Macrophage Polarization and Adaptive Immune Response

In order to evaluate the effect of FOXO3 on macrophage polarization and adaptive immune response, human monocytes were transfected either with control or with FOXO3 specific siRNA for 48 h before the addition of autologous lymphocytes (purified after depletion of the monocytes from total PBMC) along with the mycobacterial purified protein derivative (PPD). After 96 h, secreted cytokines were quantified in supernatants by ELISA. Further, total RNA was extracted from whole cells and the gene expression profiles of M1/M2/Th1/Th2/Th17 markers were measured by qPCR. In addition, the effect of FOXO3 activation (through Akt inhibition) on macrophage polarization was also assessed in BMDMs. BMDM's were isolated from 6 to 8 weeks old female BALB/c mice as per standard protocols and resuspended in DMEM supplemented with 20% FBS, 20% L929 supernatant medium, 1% L-glutamine, 1% Pen/Strep, 1× MEM, and 1% sodium pyruvate. The BMDM's were incubated for 6 days at 37°C and 5% CO_2. For experimental setups, BMDMs were seeded in a 24 well plate at a density of 5×10^5 cells per well, infected with BCG at an MOI of 1:10 and subsequently overlaid with medium without or with 5 μM of MK-2206. Twenty-four hours post infection, BMDMs were harvested, washed and incubated for 10 min with anti-CD16/CD32 to block non-specific antibody binding. Subsequently, cells were stained with anti-CD11b (BV510), anti-CD86 (PEcy7), anti-MHC class II (PB515), anti-MHC class I (BV421) for 30 min at 4°C as per manufacturer's recommendations (BD Biosciences). The antibody-stained cells were washed twice with ice cold 1× PBS, suspended in FACS staining buffer and data was collected using flow cytometry (FACS CantoII, BD Biosciences). The acquired data was analyzed with Flow Jo software.

Statistical Analysis

Statistical analyses and generation of graphs were performed with GraphPad Prism version 7. Data are expressed as the mean ± standard error of the mean (SEM). Comparison between groups was performed by a paired t-test. Differences with a $p < 0.05$ were considered statistically significant. Data generated using blood samples from the three human volunteers were further analyzed by the one-tailed version of the Mann Whitney test, which is more suited for small-sized samples (31, 32).

RESULTS

PI3K/Akt/FOXO3 Axis Regulates IL-10 Expression in BCG-Infected Macrophages

In macrophages, IL-10 release has been shown to be dependent on PI3k/Akt activation (14). Since FOXO3 is a major target that is directly phosphorylated/inhibited by Akt (33), we sought to investigate whether the pharmacologically inhibition of PI3K/Akt signaling pathway, have an impact on FOXO3 activity and BCG-induced secretion of IL-10. To determine this, we used Wortmannin (Wort), one specific PI3K inhibitor, and MK-2206 (MK), a selective non-ATP-competitive allosteric Akt inhibitor (34). We first assessed the cytotoxicity of both inhibitors on human and murine macrophages using the WST1 test. No significant cytotoxicity was associated with different concentrations of MK-2206 in both TDMs and J774A.1 cells as >90% of both cell lines survived at concentrations lesser or equal to 5 μM (**Figure S1**). Wort treatment produced significant toxicity only at concentrations above 100 nM in TDMs cells, while, no cytotoxicity was observed in J774A.1 cells following exposure to increasing concentrations of Wort (**Figure S1**). Hence, for the subsequent experiments we used MK at a concentration of 5 μM and Wort at 100 nM.

We found that treatment of TDMs macrophages with both Wort and MK resulted in Akt dephosphorylation in both BCG-infected and non-infected cells. In concordance with our hypothesis, we also observed that treatment with these drugs resulted in FOXO3 dephosphorylation (**Figure 1A**), indicating its activation. Interestingly, MK and Wort treatment also induced a significant up-regulation of FOXO3 gene expression level in BCG-infected and non-infected TDMs and J774A.1 macrophages, indicating that PI3K/Akt pathway also inhibits FOXO3 activity by abrogating its transcription (**Figure 1B**).

Concomitantly, RT-qPCR showed that infection of macrophages with BCG increased levels of IL-10 mRNA, which were significantly abrogated upon MK and Wort treatment in both mice and human macrophages (**Figure 1C**). Consistent with RT-qPCR data, ELISA quantification revealed a significant inhibition (about 90%), by Wort ($p < 0.05$) and MK ($p < 0.001$) inhibitors of IL-10 secretion in BCG-infected TDMs. Similar results were obtained in BCG-infected mouse macrophages J774A.1 (**Figure 1C**).

These observations clearly indicates that PI3K/Akt pathway positively regulates IL-10 expression in BCG-infected macrophages and that such regulation might rely on FOXO3 inhibition. It is worth to note that we have also verified the effect of the PI3K/Akt/FOXO3 axis on the expression of TNF-α, a cytokine that plays a crucial role in TB immune response, and found that neither the used inhibitors nor the FOXO3 silencing had an effect on BCG-induced secretion of TNF-α (**Figure S3**).

To further investigate the role of FOXO3 on IL-10 expression in mycobacteria-infected macrophages, we transfected human MDMs with a pool of small interfering RNA (siRNA) targeting the endogenous expression of FOXO3. The knockdown efficiency of FOXO3 was confirmed by RT-qPCR and western blotting (**Figure 2**). We found that silencing of FOXO3 significantly enhanced the BCG-induced transcription of IL-10, compared to the scrambled Si control (SiCT)-transfected cells (**Figure 2A**), suggesting FOXO3 as an inhibitor of IL-10 transcription. In agreement, we observed an increase of BCG-induced secretion of IL-10 in SiFOXO3-transfected macrophages (**Figure 2B**). Taken together, these data suggest that FOXO3 negatively regulates IL-10 expression in BCG-infected macrophages.

FOXO3 Binds and Inhibits the Transcription From IL-10 Promoter

To evaluate whether IL-10 is subjected to direct transcriptional control by FOXO3, we performed an *in silico* analysis of the human IL-10 promoter region using the MatInspector program of the Genomatix portal (https://www.genomatix.de/online_help/help_matinspector/matinspector_help.html). Scanning for Forkhead DNA-binding elements (FKHR-DBEs) on the Genomatix-proposed IL-10 promoter sequence revealed three Forkhead putative motifs at positions −17, −303, and −526 and one typical FOXO3-response elements at position −203 (**Figure 3A** and **Table S4**). Next, we performed a gene reporter assay to understand FOXO3-mediated regulation of IL-10 promoter activity as described in methods. As shown in **Figure 3B**, we observed that infection of macrophages with BCG increased the IL-10 promoter activity by ~8.0 folds in comparison with non-infected cells ($p = 0.0010$). However, overexpression of FOXO3 almost abolished the BCG-induced IL-10 promoter activity in macrophages (**Figure 3B**, 90% inhibition, $p = 0.025$). In order to better explore the functionality of FKHR-DBEs and determine which motifs are involved in FOXO3 mediated inhibition of IL-10 promoter activity, we mutated the four putative sites and performed the luciferase assay (**Figure 4A**). We found that disruption of the FKHR binding elements at site 1 (position−17) and site 3 (position −303) partially elevated the FOXO3-mediated inhibition of IL-10 promoter activity, while the mutation of site 4 (-526) did not affect the inhibition of BCG induced IL-10 promoter activity by FOXO3. However, mutation of the typical FOXO3 motif at Site 2 (position −203) showed almost a total unleash of the FOXO3-mediated inhibition of IL-10 promoter (**Figure 4B**). These results suggest that FOXO3-mediated down regulation of IL-10 in BCG-infected macrophages mainly occurs through site 2 on which FOXO3 might bind and block the transcription.

To confirm our observation, we performed CHIP followed by a PCR using two primers flanking the −203 position, as indicated in materials and methods section. The result revealed a strong interaction between FOXO3 and the amplified region containing the motifs at −203 in non-infected cells, while BCG infection displaced FOXO3, releasing IL-10 transcription (**Figure 4C**). This data correlates with the observed higher basal activity of IL-10 promoter that bears a mutated site 2 (-203) (**Figure 4B**). Taken together, we demonstrate that FOXO3 transcription factor binds to IL-10 promoter at position −203 and negatively regulates its expression.

FOXO3 Tunes Phenotypic Maturation of Mycobacteria-Infected Macrophages

During the early phase of *M.tb* infection, the host generates the pro-inflammatory M1 type macrophages, which are associated with protection against the disease (35). As the

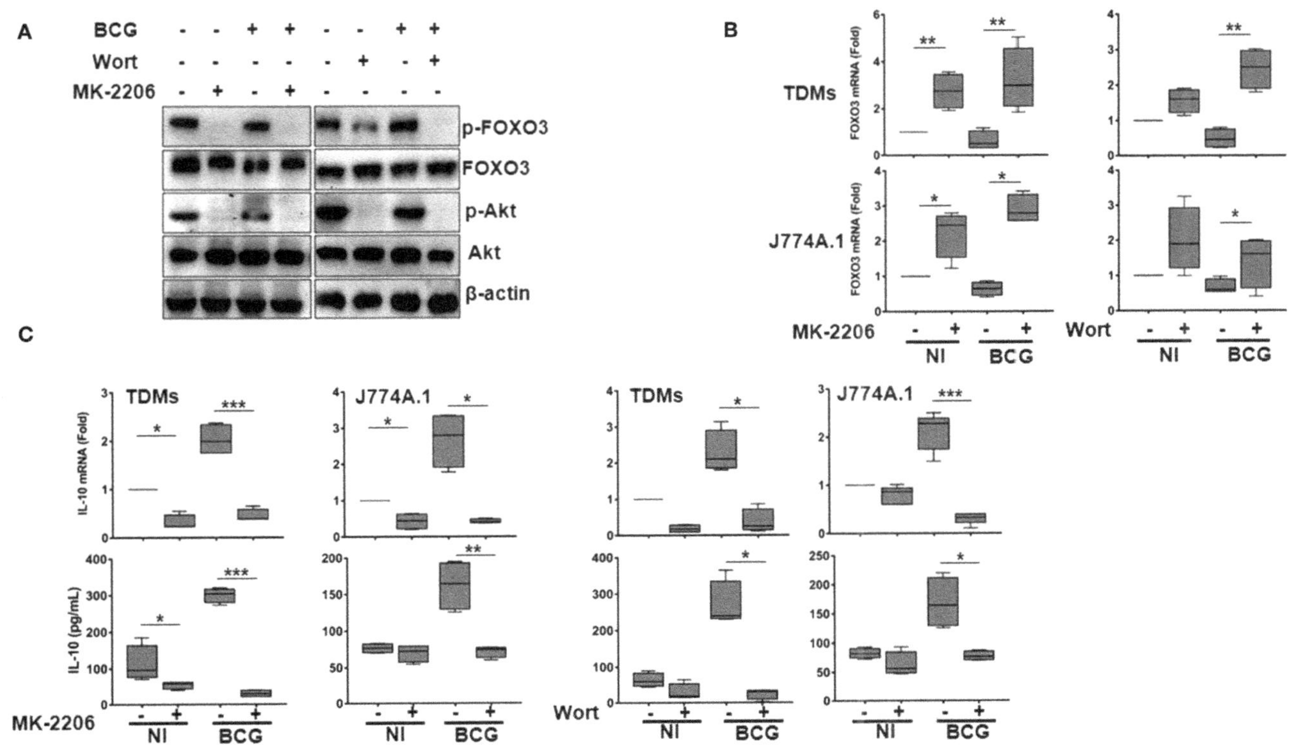

FIGURE 1 | The PI3K/Akt axis regulates BCG-induced IL-10 secretion in macrophages. Human TDMs and mice J774A.1 macrophages were mock-treated or infected with BCG at an MOI = 10 for 3 h, washed then treated or not with the PI3K inhibitor, Wortmannin (Wort, 100 nM), or with the Akt inhibitor, MK-2206 (5 μM) for 24 h. **(A)** Inactivation of PI3k/Akt axis was determined, 24 h post infection/treatment, in whole cell lysate of TDMs by western blotting using the indicated anti-phospho specific antibodies. Total Akt, FOXO3, and β-actin were used as loading controls. Shown are representative images of three independent experiments with similar results. **(B)** FOXO3 mRNA expression were quantified by qRT-PCR in both TDMs and J774A.1 macrophages. Levels of mRNA were normalized to GAPDH and fold induction was calculated relative to uninfected and untreated cells. **(C)** Assessment of IL-10 transcription and secretion levels, after the indicated treatments, were quantified by qRT-PCR and sandwich ELISA, respectively. For all panels, results are represented in box and whiskers plot format min to max and are representative of three independent experiments, each one carried out in triplicate. Asterisks indicate statistical significance (*$p < 0.05$; **$p < 0.01$; ***$p < 0.001$).

infection progresses, the pathogen induces the re-polarization of macrophages toward the immunomodulatory M2 phenotype (36). Such transition is driven by high levels of Th2 cytokines such as IL-10 and correlates with disease severity (37). In order to assess the impact of FOXO3-mediated inhibition of IL-10 expression on macrophage phenotype, we quantified the transcription levels of the two typical M1 surface markers CD80 and CD86 in PPD-treated and non-treated human macrophages, as detailed above (**Figure S4**). We found a significant decrease of the PPD-induced expression of the two studied markers after FOXO3 silencing in human macrophages, compared to the Sicontrol-transfected ones (**Figure 5A**). Conversely, pharmacological activation of FOXO3 by MK, in BCG-infected and non-infected BMDMs, resulted in the up-regulation of CD86 expression level along with the ones of MHC class II and class I, two presenting molecules and markers of M1 macrophages (**Figure 5B**). MK treatment has also significantly decreased the expression levels of the typical marker of M2 macrophages, Arg1 (**Figure 5C**). These data suggest that FOXO3-mediated inhibition of IL-10 enhances the antigen-presenting activity of macrophages and favors their polarization toward the pro-inflammatory M1 phenotype during TB immune response. We then investigated whether FOXO3 mediated inhibition of IL-10 and the subsequent activation of M1 macrophages exert a protective effect against mycobacterial infection. We examined the intracellular burden of BCG in macrophages treated with MK and found that such treatment decreased the intracellular loads of BCG by ~60% as compared to the untreated cells (**Figure 5D**), suggesting that FOXO3 activation boost the macrophage defense mechanisms against invading mycobacteria.

Silencing of FOXO3 in Macrophages Modulates Th1 Immune Response Against Mycobacterial Infection

Activated M1 macrophages are considered potent effector cells, which promote Th1 immune responses while M2 macrophages have immunoregulatory functions and participate in polarized Th2 immune responses (38–40). We then assessed the impact of FOXO3-mediated regulation of macrophage phenotype on the T cells adaptive immune response. As shown in **Figure 6**, we

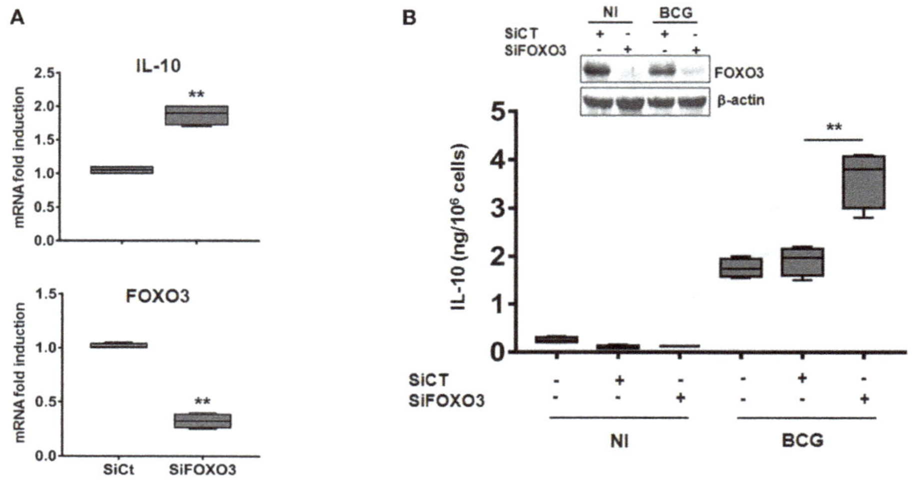

FIGURE 2 | Knockdown of FOXO3 augments IL-10 expression in BCG-infected human primary macrophages. MDMs were transfected with FOXO3 specific siRNA (SiFOXO3) or with scramble control siRNA (siCT) for 48 h and then infected with BCG for 24 h. **(A)** Fold induction levels of FOXO3 and IL-10 mRNAs were assessed by RT-qPCR in BCG-infected cells. **(B)** IL-10 secretion by the indicated treated cells was assessed in the culture supernatants by ELISA. Knocking down of FOXO3 expression was further verified by immunoblotting. Data are shown as box and whiskers (min to max values) and are representative of three independent experiments, each one carried out in triplicate ($n = 3$, $^{**}p < 0.01$).

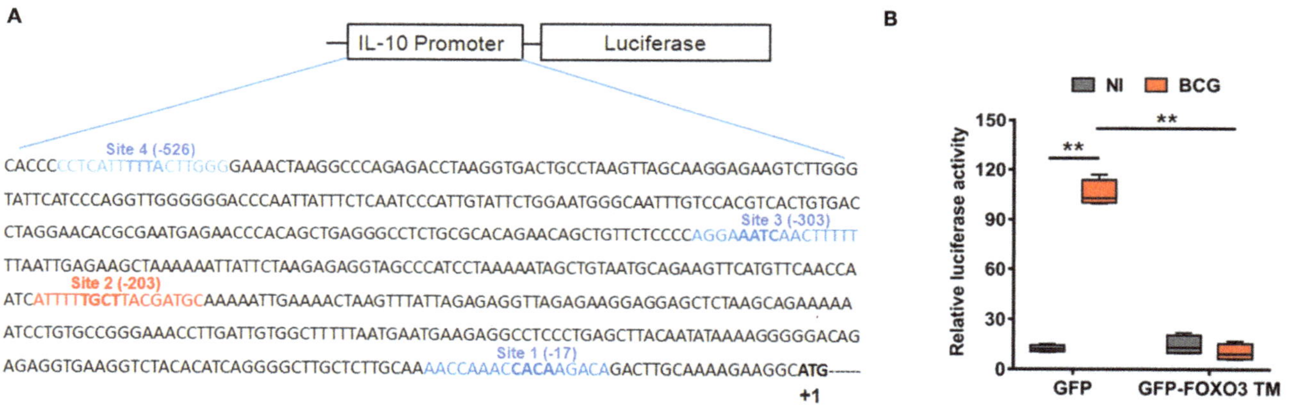

FIGURE 3 | FOXO3 inhibits IL-10 promoter activity in BCG-infected macrophages. **(A)** Schematic representation of the four putative Forkhead DNA-binding elements (FKHR-DBEs) in the proximal region of the human IL-10 promoter (-588), identified by Genomatix algorithm. The sequence in red is a typical FOXO3 binding motif. **(B)** RAW 264.7 cells were co-transfected with pGL3 plasmid containing the −588 bp IL-10 promoter region fragments plus either the GFP or GFP-FOXO3-TM-encoding vectors. Twenty-four hours later, cells were infected or not with BCG (MOI ~10) for 6 h before measuring the Luciferase activity in GFP positive alive cells. The data correspond to the mean ± SEM and correspond to a one representative of two independent experiments, each one conducted in triplicates ($n = 2$, $^{**}p < 0.01$).

found that co-culture of PPD-treated and SiFOXO3-transfected human monocytes with their autologous lymphocytes, generated significantly less IFN-γ mRNA in comparison to monocytes that were transfected with the control SiRNA ($p = 0.0030$). Quantification of IFN-γ by ELISA further corroborated this result (**Figure 6B**, $p < 0.001$). Similarly, the PPD-induced expression of IL-17 gene was significantly reduced when FOXO3 was silenced in monocytes (**Figure 6A**, $p = 0.022$). In concordance with reduced levels of Th1 cytokines, a clear reduction in PPD-induced gene expression levels of the Th1 related transcription factors RORγT ($p = 0.0074$), Tbet ($p = 0.004$), and GATA3 ($p = 0.031$) was also observed when FOXO3 level was reduced in presenting monocytes. Conversely, this transcription signature was associated with a significant increase in IL-4 ($p = 0.008$) and IL-10 ($p = 0.020$) gene expression levels and a clear reduction in PPD-induced secretion of TNF-α and IL-6 (**Figures 6A,B**). Overall, these data suggest that FOXO3 inactivation in macrophages enhances IL-10 expression, leading to a modulated M1/Th1 immune response, while active FOXO3 would enhance such immune response against mycobacterial infection, through the inhibition of IL-10 expression in macrophages (**Figure 7**).

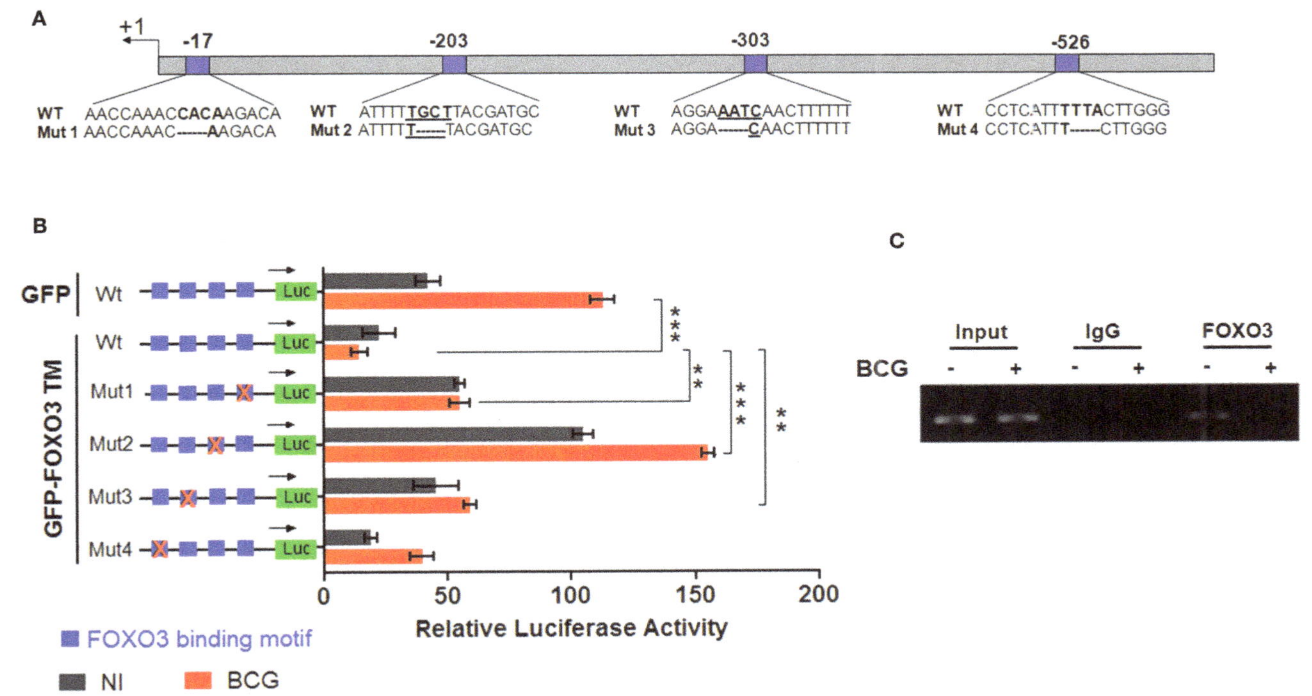

FIGURE 4 | FOXO3 binds to IL-10 promoter, inhibiting its transcriptional activity in BCG-infected cells. In order to determine the contribution of each Forkhead DNA-binding element identified *in silico*, four mutants of IL-10 promoter were generated as indicated in **(A)**. **(B)** representation of gene reporter assay performed on the wild type IL-10 promoter and the four mutants (Mut1, Mut2, Mut3, Mut4). RAW 264.7 macrophages were transfected with the indicated constructs. Twenty-four hours later, cells were infected or not with BCG and luciferase activity was measured 6 h later in GFP positive alive cells. The data correspond to the mean ± SEM of three different experiments conducted in triplicates. Asterisks indicate statistical significance ($n = 3$, ** $p < 0.01$, *** $p <$ 001). **(C)** TDMs were infected with BCG for 3 h and treated with Wort for additional 2 h. Next, CHIP assay was conducted to verify FOXO3 recruitment to the site −203 of the IL-10 promoter with either anti-FOXO3 Ab (lane 1 and 2) or anti-IgG isotype Ab (lane 3 and 4). Total input of BCG infected and non-infected cells are shown in lanes 5 and 6.

DISCUSSION

Macrophages represent the forefront of innate immune defense against *M.tb*, which response has major impact on the outcome of infection (41). However, *M.tb* has adopted remarkable strategies to circumvent host defenses. Amongst the many known evasion mechanisms, *M.tb* indeed triggers rapid induction of the anti-inflammatory cytokine IL-10. Several studies have demonstrated tight association of IL-10 secretion upon *M.tb* infection with the recurrence of the disease. Therefore, it is quiet important to understand the molecular mechanisms underlying regulation of IL-10 expression in mycobacteria-infected macrophages. In the present study, we describe the role of FOXO3 transcription factor in the regulation of IL-10 expression in mycobacteria-infected macrophages and the impact of such regulation on adaptive immune response.

Here, we first observed that IL-10 expression is positively regulated by the PI3K/Akt pathway in BCG-infected macrophages. Indeed, inhibition of either PI3K or Akt by Wort or MK, respectively abrogated the BCG-induced IL-10 production. Our findings are in accordance with a previous report showing that the inhibition of *Porphyromonas gingivalis*—mediated activation of the PI3K/Akt pathway results in an abrogation of IL-10 secretion by human monocytes (25). Further, Méndez-samperio et al., have also demonstrated that the strong BCG-induction of IL-10 expression in epithelial cells is dependent on PI3K/Akt activation (42).

FOXO3 is negatively-regulated target of PI3K/Akt pathway and we have previously reported that it is involved in BCG-induced apoptosis of human macrophages (29). Hence, we hypothesized that FOXO3 transcription factor, might act as the suppressor of IL-10 transcription in BCG-infected macrophages. In support of our hypothesis, we found that MK-mediated inhibition of IL-10 secretion was associated with FOXO3 activation at both transcriptional and protein levels. This data correlates with a previous work showing an association between FOXO3 activation and inhibition of IL-10 transcription in monocytes treated with pharmacological inhibition of Akt1/2 (43). In concordance with this, we observed that knocking-down of FOXO3 expression, using specific siRNA, resulted in a significant increase of BCG-induced transcription and secretion of IL-10. This data is in agreement with a previous study that reported a higher expression of IL-10 by neutrophils, monocytes and macrophages from FOXO3$^{-/-}$ mice infected with *Salmonella typhimurium*, as compared to non-infected mice (44). Moreover, it was shown that T cells from FOXO3$^{-/-}$ mice express higher levels of IL-10 compared to wild type ones (45). Our data also correlate with a previous study on dendritic cells

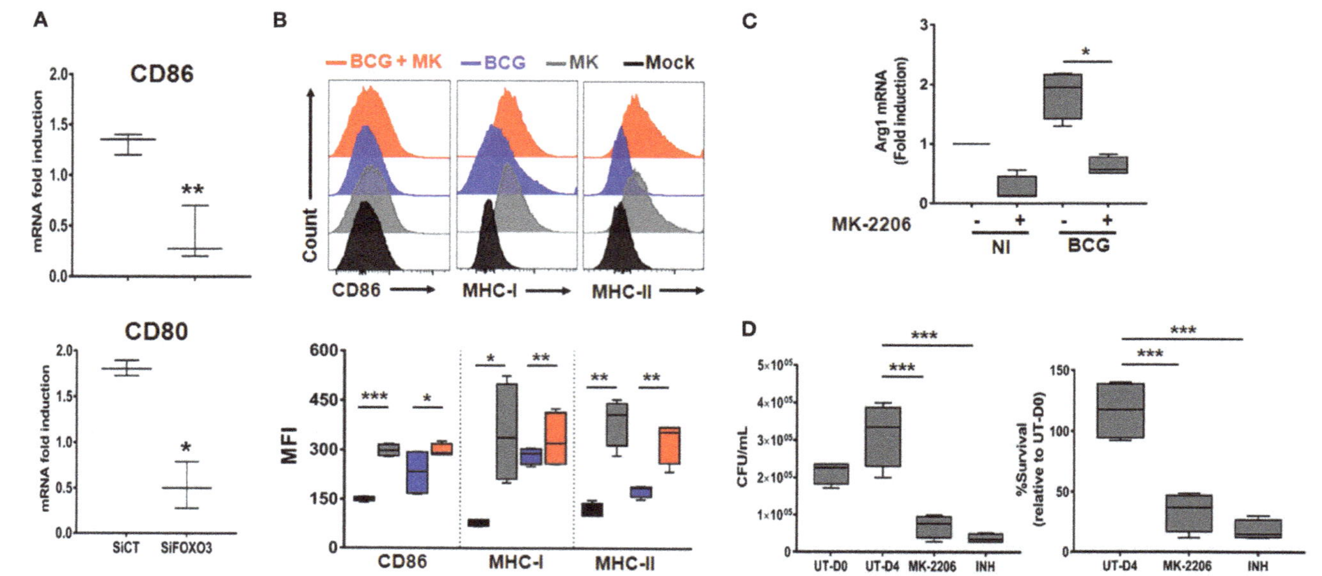

FIGURE 5 | FOXO3 tunes phenotypic maturation of mycobacteria-infected macrophages. **(A)** Human monocytes were transfected either with SiCT or SiFOXO3 for 48 h followed by PPD stimulation and incubation with the autologous lymphocytes for 4 days. Whole cells were then collected and tested for the expression levels of CD80 and CD86 by qRT-PCR. Data are presented as box and whiskers graphs (min to max) from three independent experiments (i.e., MDMs from 3 different donors), each one carried out in triplicate ($n = 3$, $^{**}p < 0.001$, $^{***}p < 0.0001$). **(B)** Non-infected or BCG-infected BMDMs were treated or not with MK-2206 (5 μM) for 24 h. The expression levels of the M1 phenotype surface markers CD86, MHC-MHC-II, and MHC-I, in $CD11b^{+}$ cells, were determined by FACS analysis using specific antibodies. FACS analysis was performed on two independent experiments and each sample was run in triplicates ($n = 2$, $^{*}p < 0.05$, $^{**}p < 0.001$, $^{***}p < 0.0001$). **(C)** J774A.1 were mock or infected with BCG at an MOI = 10 for 3 h, washed then treated or not with the Akt inhibitor MK (5 μM) for 24 h. The transcript levels of M2 marker, Arg1, was assessed by RT-PCR. Data are presented as box and whiskers (min to max) and are from two separate experiments, each one carried out in triplicate ($n = 2$, $^{*}p < 0.05$). **(D)** TDMs were infected with BCG at an MOI = 10 for 3 h. Following incubation, cells were treated with Amikacin (200 μg/ml) for 1 h to remove extracellular bacteria. The infected cells were then washed and treated with MK (5 μM) for 4 days. The antibiotic Isonicotinylhydrazide (INH) was used as positive control. Cells were lysed with sterile PBS containing 0.1% triton X100 and 10-fold serial dilutions of lysates were plated on MB7H11 for CFU Enumeration. The Intracellular colony forming units were determined at the indicated time points. UT-D0, untreated at Day 0; UT-D4, untreated at Day 4. Data are shown as box and whiskers (min to max values) and representative of two separate experiments, each one carried out in quadruplets. Asterisks indicate statistical significance ($n = 2$, $^{***}p < 0.0001$).

where FOXO1, analog of FOXO3, was found to inhibit LPS induced IL-10 production (46). Moreover, FOXO1 deletion in dendritic cells resulted in reduced DC activation and affected the adaptive immune response to bacterial challenge (47, 48). However, these studies did not investigate the mechanisms by which FOXO3 regulates IL-10 expression. We have then performed an *in silico* analysis of IL-10 promoter and identified four forkhead potential binding motifs with a typical FOXO3 binding site at −203 position. We further confirmed the negative regulation of IL-10 by FOXO3 using the reporter gene assay and highlighted the crucial role of the motif at −203 position, which directly binds to FOXO3 protein. Altogether, these data clearly show, for the first time, a negative regulation, by FOXO3, of IL-10 production in mycobacteria-infected macrophages through the direct binding to and interference with IL-10 promoter activity.

During disease progression, *M.tb* induces the re-polarization of macrophages toward the immunomodulatory M2 phenotype (36) through induction of high level of IL-10, leading to a Th2 immune response, which correlates with the severity of the disease (37). In order to assess the impact of FOXO3-mediated inhibition of IL-10 on macrophage polarization, the expression levels of the two typical M1 surface markers CD80 and CD86 was assessed, during progress of the adaptive immune response against mycobacterial antigens. As expected, we found a significant decrease of the expression levels of the two studied markers in PPD-treated and SiFOXO3-transfected macrophages, compared to the Si-control-transfected ones. Conversely, we observed that pharmacological activation of FOXO3, in BCG-infected and non-infected macrophages, resulted in the up-regulation of CD86 expression along with MHC class II and class I, two additional markers of M1 macrophages. These observations suggest that, by inhibiting the IL-10 expression in mycobacteria-infected macrophages, FOXO3 ameliorates the presenting activity and favors the polarization of host macrophages toward the pro-inflammatory M1 phenotype during TB immune response. In concordance, we observed that FOXO3 silencing in monocytes results in the modulation of Th1 related markers and the induction of a Th2 response, against mycobacterial antigens. The only discrepancy we found was the decrease in GATA3 expression associated to the upregulation of IL-4 after FOXO3 silencing in macrophages. This could be explained by the potential regulation of GATA3 transcription by FOXO3. Indeed, a previous study has proposed the positive regulation of GATA3 by FOXO1 (49),

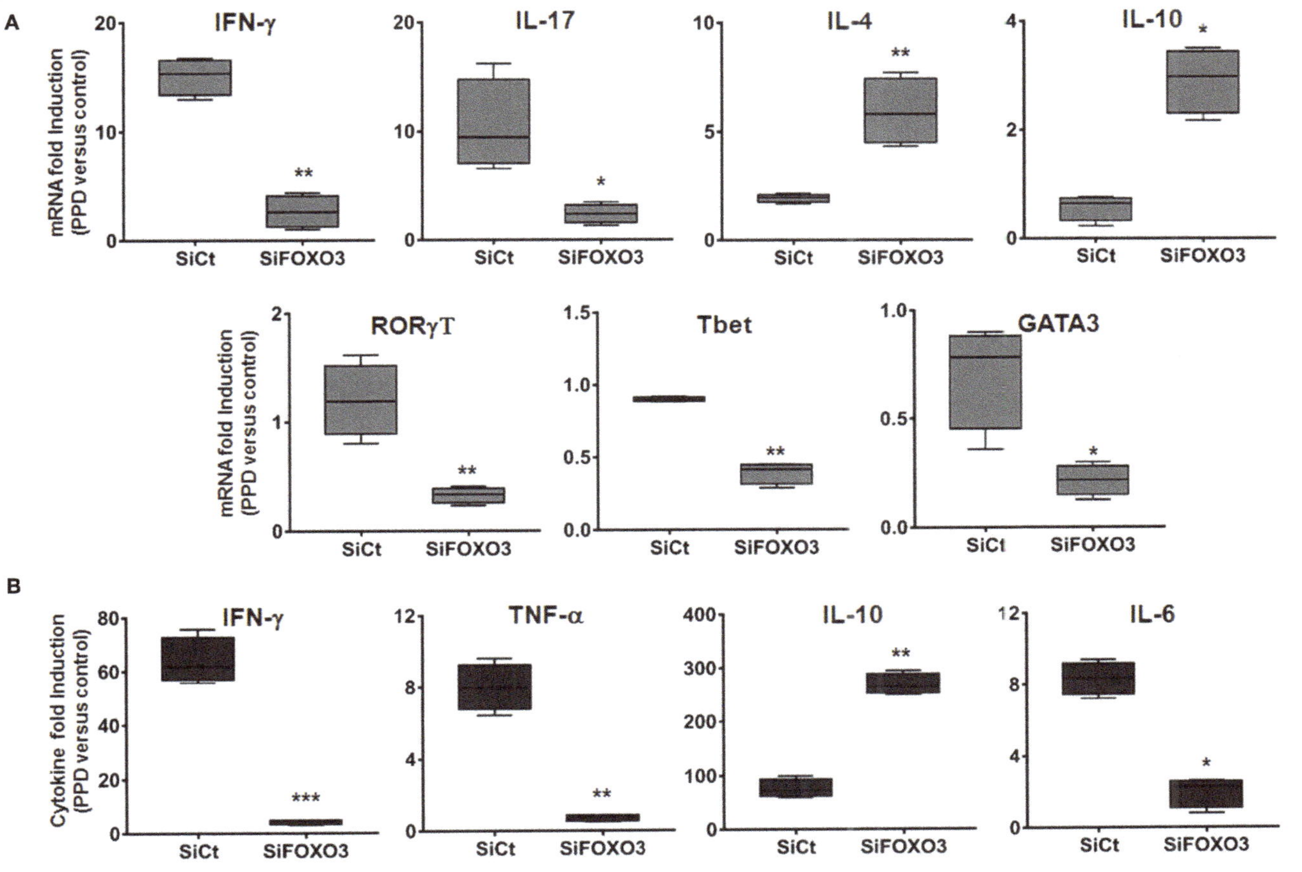

FIGURE 6 | Silencing of FOXO3 in macrophages modulates Th1 immune response against mycobacterial infection. Human monocytes were transfected either with SiCT or SiFOXO3 for 48 h followed by PPD stimulation and incubation with the autologous lymphocytes for 4 days. **(A)** Cells were then collected and tested for the expression levels of the indicated genes by qRT-PCR. **(B)** Supernatants were collected and analyzed by ELISA for IFN-γ, TNF-α, IL-10, and IL-6 secretion. The results are shown in box and whiskers (min to max values) from three independent experiments (i.e., MDMs from 3 different donors), each one carried out in triplicate. Asterisks indicate statistical significance (* $p < 0.05$, ** $p < 0.001$, *** $p < 0.0001$).

an isoform of FOXO3 with which it shares common targets (50, 51).

Taken together, our data suggest that FOXO3 acts as an inducer of a protective M1/Th1 immune response through the negative regulation of IL-10 expression in infected macrophages. Our data correlate with the previous reported protective role of FOXO3 against *Salmonella typhimurium (ST)* infection. Indeed, FOXO3 signaling inhibited IL-10 secretion with a concomitant induction of inflammatory immune responses in mice infected with ST, leading to the control of the intracellular bacteria (44). Several studies pointed that *M.tb* successfully engages activators of IL-10 transcription such as STAT3 and RelB during infection to abolish the protective response mounted by the host and ensures its survival and persistence (11, 52). Our data suggest that *M.tb* might inactivate FOXO3 as an additional mechanism to enhance IL-10 secretion in order to establish persistent infection in the host. This is in agreement with previous studies that reported an abrogation of FOXO3 expression in active TB patients, compared to healthy controls (30, 53). It has been also shown that an SNP affecting FOXO3 expression was associated with active TB in a dominant inheritance mode (54). Taken together, our study presents a strong evidence that FOXO3 constitutes a major signaling hub that is manipulated by mycobacterial species and that disruption of FOXO3 signaling might affect the regulation of anti-*M.tb* directed immune response.

In order to compromise host resistance, *M.tb* predominantly activates the pro-survival pathway PI3K/Akt to inhibit apoptosis and induce IL-10 through FOXO3 inhibition. Activated Akt will then phosphorylate the pro-apoptotic transcription factor FOXO3 at three residues, Thr32, Ser253, and Ser315, leading to its translocation to the cytosol where it is stored as a complex FOXO3/chaperone protein 14-3-3 and/or degraded by the proteasome. However, PI3K/Akt inhibition leads to activation of FOXO3, which will translocate to the nucleus and restrict

IL-10 secretion through direct binding to its proximal promoter. Inhibition of IL-10 signaling is necessary to restore the anti-mycobacterial capacity of the host and increases the polarization of macrophage toward a proinflammatory M1 phenotype, which is crucial for the shaping of an effective

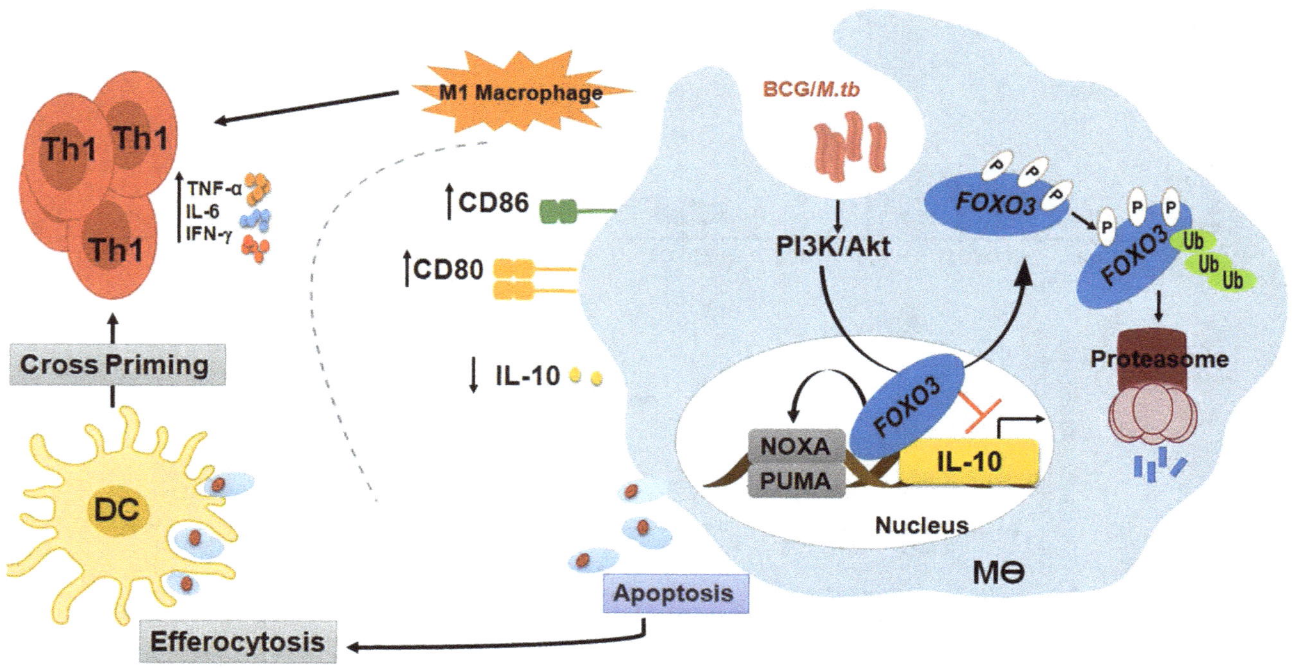

FIGURE 7 | FOXO3, a signaling hub for a protective immune response against mycobacterial infection. In order to compromise host resistance, *M.tb* predominantly activates the pro-survival pathway PI3K/Akt to inhibit apoptosis and induce IL-10 through FOXO3 inhibition. Activated Akt will then phosphorylate the pro-apoptotic transcription factor FOXO3 at three residues, Thr32, Ser253, and Ser315, leading to its translocation to the cytosol where it is stored as a complex FOXO3/chaperone protein 14-3-3 and/or degraded by the proteasome. However, PI3K/Akt inhibition leads to activation of FOXO3, which will accumulate inside the nucleus and restrict IL-10 secretion through direct binding to its proximal promoter. Inhibition of IL-10 signaling is necessary to restore the anti-mycobacterial capacity of the host and increase the polarization of macrophage toward a proinflammatory M1 phenotype, which is crucial for the shaping of an effective Th1 adaptive response against *M.tb* pathogenesis. Activation of FOXO3 would also induce the expression of PUMA and NOXA, the two effectors of macrophage apoptosis. Apoptotic bodies charged with mycobacterial antigens will be ingested by the bystander dendritic cells (DC) to better cross-prime T cells. In conclusion, activated FOXO3 in infected macrophages benefit the protection against TB in many ways. (i) Induces apoptosis of infected-macrophages and disrupts the intracellular replication of *M.tb* within the host. (ii) Inhibits IL-10 and restore the antimicrobial host responses. (iii) Boost the adaptive immune response to *M.tb*.

Th1 adaptive response against *M.tb* pathogenesis. Activation of FOXO3 would also induce macrophage apoptosis. Apoptotic bodies charged with mycobacterial antigens will be then ingested by the bystander dendritic cells (DC) to better cross-prime T cells (**Figure 7**).

The dual functions of FOXO3 as an inducer of macrophage apoptosis and inhibitor of IL-10 secretion, suggest that this factor can be proposed as a new target for host-directed therapy against Tuberculosis. Several commercially available Akt inhibitors, like the used MK2206, act through FOXO3 activation are in pre- and clinical use to treat cancers (55, 56). Based on the results obtained, we suggest that these FOXO3 activators may be used as adjunct to shorten the duration of therapy against drug-resistant TB. This may lead to enhanced repression of IL-10 secretion and higher apoptosis, thereby generating a stronger immune response and a more rapid clearance of *M.tb* infection. This hypothesis is in agreement with a previous study where authors reported that AKT1 inhibitors prevented intracellular growth of various bacteria including multi drug resistant strains of *M.tb* (57). In the other hand, targeting FOXO3 would be also useful to augment the efficacy of BCG. Indeed, activation of FOXO3 during vaccination would inhibit the BCG-induced secretion of IL-10 and enhance apoptosis of infected macrophages, leading to a stronger Th1 protective immune response against *M.tb* (**Figure 7**).

Overall, we have identified FOXO3 as a transcription factor that tunes the host inflammatory response during mycobacterial infection through the regulation of IL-10 expression. These findings advance our understanding of protective immunity to *M.tb* by revealing the importance of FOXO3 transcription factor, which deserves further investigation as it may be used as therapeutic/preventive target against TB.

ETHICS STATEMENT

The studies involving human participants were reviewed and approved by the institutional ethics committee of Institut Pasteur de Tunis. The Healthy Volunteers provided their written informed consent to participate in this study. The animal study was reviewed and approved by the Institutional animal ethics committee of THSTI, according to the control and supervision on animals (CPCSEA) guideline.

AUTHOR CONTRIBUTIONS

ME, RB, and MH conceived and designed the experiments. ME, RB, MH, and RS performed and analyzed the data, interpreted them, and wrote the paper as well. M-RB contributed with providing reagents and discussing the manuscript.

FUNDING

This work was supported by the United Nations Development Program/World Bank/World Health Organization Special Program for Research and Training in Tropical Diseases (TDR), TDR ID No. A70529 and funds from the Tunisian Ministry for Higher Education, Scientific Research and Technology (Projet Tuniso-Indien session 2013-2016). RB acknowledges Department of Science and Technology India and FICCI for providing C. V. Raman International fellowship. The authors acknowledge the funding received from Department of Biotechnology, Govt. of India (BT/IN/Indo-Tunisia/01/2014). RS is a recipient of Ramalingaswami fellowship and National Bioscience Award from Department of Biotechnology.

ACKNOWLEDGMENTS

We are grateful to Dr. John W. Steinke from the Asthma and Allergic Diseases Center, Charlottesville VA, for providing the reporter construct pGL3-IL-10 (-588). We thank Genomatix (https://www.genomatix.de) for the free 1-week trial of their software. We are also indebted to the volunteers who accepted to participate in the study along with people from the Center National de Transfusion Sanguine (Tunis, Tunisia) for their help in collecting blood samples. The authors also acknowledge Pr. Kanury Venkata Subba Rao for providing MK-2206 and the staff of Small animal facility for providing mice.

REFERENCES

1. Macneil A, Glaziou P, Sismanidis C, Maloney S, Floyd K. Global epidemiology of tuberculosis and progress toward achieving global targets — 2017. *MMWR Morb Mortal Wkly Rep.* (2019) 68:263–6. doi: 10.15585/mmwr.mm6811a3
2. Pitt JM, Blankley S, McShane H, O'Garra A. Vaccination against tuberculosis: how can we better BCG? *Microb Pathog.* (2013) 58:2–16. doi: 10.1016/j.micpath.2012.12.002
3. Wallis RS, Hafner R. Advancing host-directed therapy for tuberculosis. *Nat Rev Immunol.* (2015) 15:255–63. doi: 10.1038/nri3813
4. Li G, Liu G, Song N, Kong C, Huang Q, Su H, et al. A novel recombinant BCG-expressing pro-apoptotic protein BAX enhances Th1 protective immune responses in mice. *Mol Immunol.* (2015) 66:346–56. doi: 10.1016/j.molimm.2015.04.003
5. Sia JK, Georgieva M, Rengarajan J. Innate immune defenses in human tuberculosis: an overview of the interactions between *Mycobacterium tuberculosis* and innate immune cells. *J Immunol Res.* (2015) 2015:747543. doi: 10.1155/2015/747543
6. van Crevel R, Ottenhoff THM, van der Meer JWM. Innate immunity to *Mycobacterium tuberculosis*. *Clin Microbiol Rev.* (2002) 15:294–309. doi: 10.1128/CMR.15.2.294-309.2002
7. Domingo-gonzalez R, Prince O, Cooper A, Khader SA. Cytokines and chemokines in *Mycobacterium tuberculosis* infection. In: *Tuberculosis and the Tubercle Bacillus.* 2nd ed. Washington, DC: ASM Press (2016). p. 33–72. doi: 10.1128/microbiolspec.TBTB2-0018-2016
8. Verbon A, Juffermans N, Van deventer SJH, Speelman P, Van Deutekom H. Serum concentrations of cytokines in patients with active tuberculosis (TB) and after treatment. *Clin Exp Immunol.* (1999) 115:110–3. doi: 10.1046/j.1365-2249.1999.00783.x
9. Boussiotis VA, Tsai EY, Yunis EJ, Thim S, Delgado JC, Dascher CC, et al. IL-10 - producing T cells suppress immune responses in anergic tuberculosis patients. *J Clin Invest.* (2000) 105:1317–24. doi: 10.1172/JCI9918
10. Redpath S, Ghazal P, Gascoigne NRJ. Hijacking and exploitation of IL-10 by intracellular pathogens. *Trends Microbiol.* (2001) 9:86–92. doi: 10.1016/S0966-842X(00)01919-3
11. O'Leary S, O'Sullivan MP, Keane J. IL-10 blocks phagosome maturation in *Mycobacterium tuberculosis*-infected human macrophages. *Am J Resp Cell Mol Biol.* (2011) 45:172–80. doi: 10.1165/rcmb.2010-0319OC
12. Faulkner L, Buchan G, Baird M. Interleukin-10 does not affect phagocytosis of particulate antigen by bone marrow-derived dendritic cells but does impair antigen presentation. *Immunology.* (2000) 99:523–31. doi: 10.1046/j.1365-2567.2000.00018.x
13. Bakhru P, Sirisaengtaksin N, Soudani E, Mukherjee S, Khan A, Jagannath C. BCG vaccine mediated reduction in the MHC-II expression of macrophages and dendritic cells is reversed by activation of Toll-like receptors 7 and 9. *Cell Immunol.* (2014) 287:53–61. doi: 10.1016/j.cellimm.2013.11.007
14. Antoniv TT, Ivashkiv LB. Interleukin-10-induced gene expression and suppressive function are selectively modulated by the PI3K-Akt-GSK3 pathway. *Immunology.* (2011) 132:567–77. doi: 10.1111/j.1365-2567.2010.03402.x
15. Abdul-Aziz M, Tsolaki AG, Kouser L, Carroll MV, Al-Ahdal MN, Sim RB, et al. Complement factor H interferes with *Mycobacterium bovis* BCG entry into macrophages and modulates the pro-inflammatory cytokine response. *Immunobiology.* (2016) 221:944–52. doi: 10.1016/j.imbio.2016.05.011
16. Lopes RL, Borges TJ, Zanin RF, Bonorino C. IL-10 is required for polarization of macrophages to M2-like phenotype by mycobacterial DnaK (heat shock protein 70). *Cytokine.* (2016) 85:123–9. doi: 10.1016/j.cyto.2016.06.018
17. Cyktor JC, Carruthers B, Kominsky RA, Beamer GL, Stromberg P, Turner J. IL-10 inhibits mature fibrotic granuloma formation during *Mycobacterium tuberculosis* infection. *J Immunol.* (2013) 190:2778–90. doi: 10.4049/jimmunol.1202722
18. Beamer GL, Flaherty DK, Assogba BD, Stromberg P, Gonzalez-Juarrero M, de Waal Malefyt R, et al. Interleukin-10 promotes *Mycobacterium tuberculosis* disease progression in CBA/J mice. *J Immunol.* (2008) 181:5545–50. doi: 10.4049/jimmunol.181.8.5545
19. Redford PS, Boonstra A, Read S, Pitt J, Graham C, Stavropoulos E, et al. Enhanced protection to *Mycobacterium tuberculosis* infection in IL-10-deficient mice is accompanied by early and enhanced Th1 responses in the lung. *Eur J Immunol.* (2010) 40:2200–10. doi: 10.1002/eji.201040433
20. Redford PS, Murray PJ, O'Garra A. The role of IL-10 in immune regulation during *M. tuberculosis* infection. *Mucosal Immunol.* (2011) 4:261–70. doi: 10.1038/mi.2011.7
21. Jamil B, Shahid F, Hasan Z, Nasir N, Razzaki T, Dawood G, et al. Interferonγ/IL10 ratio defines the disease severity in pulmonary and extra pulmonary tuberculosis. *Tuberculosis.* (2007) 87:279–87. doi: 10.1016/j.tube.2007.03.004
22. Skolimowska KH, Rangaka MX, Meintjes G, Pepper DJ, Seldon R, Matthews K, et al. Altered ratio of IFN-γ/IL-10 in patients with drug resistant *Mycobacterium tuberculosis* and HIV- tuberculosis immune reconstitution inflammatory syndrome. *PLoS ONE.* (2012) 7:e46481. doi: 10.1371/journal.pone.0046481

23. Pitt JM, Stavropoulos E, Redford PS, Beebe AM, Bancroft GJ, Young DB, et al. Blockade of IL-10 signaling during bacillus calmette-guerin vaccination enhances and sustains Th1, Th17, and innate lymphoid IFN- and IL-17 responses and increases protection to *Mycobacterium tuberculosis* infection. *J Immunol.* (2012) 189:4079–87. doi: 10.4049/jimmunol.1201061
24. Dallenga T. Strategies to improve vaccine efficacy against Tuberculosis by Targeting innate immunity. *Front Immunol.* (2017) 8:1755. doi: 10.3389/fimmu.2017.01755
25. Martin M, Schifferle RE, Cuesta N, Vogel SN, Katz J, Michalek SM. Role of the phosphatidylinositol 3 kinase-Akt pathway in the regulation of IL-10 and IL-12 by Porphyromonas gingivalis lipopolysaccharide. *J Immunol.* (2003) 171:717–25. doi: 10.4049/jimmunol.171.2.717
26. Bai W, Liu H, Ji Q, Zhou Y, Liang L, Zheng R, et al. TLR3 regulates mycobacterial RNA-induced IL-10 production through the PI3K/AKT signaling pathway. *Cell Signal.* (2014) 26:942–50. doi: 10.1016/j.cellsig.2014.01.015
27. Stanley SA, Barczak AK, Silvis MR, Luo SS, Sogi K, Vokes M, et al. Identification of host-targeted small molecules that restrict intracellular *Mycobacterium tuberculosis* growth. *PLoS Pathog.* (2014) 10:e1003946. doi: 10.1371/journal.ppat.1003946
28. Hwang J-W, Rajendrasozhan S, Yao H, Chung S, Sundar IK, Huyck HL, et al. FOXO3 deficiency leads to increased susceptibility to cigarette smoke-induced inflammation, airspace enlargement, and chronic obstructive pulmonary disease. *J Immunol.* (2011) 187:987–98. doi: 10.4049/jimmunol.1001861
29. Haoues M, Refai A, Mallavialle A, Barbouche MR, Laabidi N, Deckert M, et al. Forkhead box O3 (FOXO3) transcription factor mediates apoptosis in BCG-infected macrophages. *Cell Microbiol.* (2014) 16:1378–90. doi: 10.1111/cmi.12298
30. Huang J, Jiao J, Xu W, Zhao H, Zhang C, Shi Y, et al. MiR-155 is upregulated in patients with active tuberculosis and inhibits apoptosis of monocytes by targeting FOXO3. *Mol Med Rep.* (2015) 12:7102–8. doi: 10.3892/mmr.2015.4250
31. Salkind N. *Encyclopedia of Measurement and Statistics*. Thousand Oaks, CA: SAGE Publishing (2007). doi: 10.4135/9781412952644
32. Morgan CJ. Use of proper statistical techniques for research studies with small samples. *Am J Physiol.* (2017) 313:L873–7. doi: 10.1152/ajplung.00238.2017
33. Stroeken P, Versteeg R, Koster J, Santo EE, Sluis PV, Westerhout EM. FOXO3a is a major target of inactivation by PI3K/AKT signaling in aggressive neuroblastoma. *Cancer Res.* (2013) 73:2189–98. doi: 10.1158/0008-5472.CAN-12-3767
34. Iida M, Brand TM, Campbell DA, Starr MM, Luthar N, Traynor AM, et al. Targeting AKT with the allosteric AKT inhibitor MK-2206 in non-small cell lung cancer cells with acquired resistance to cetuximab. *Cancer Biol Therapy.* (2013) 14:481–91. doi: 10.4161/cbt.24342
35. Day J, Friedman A, Schlesinger LS. Modeling the immune rheostat of macrophages in the lung in response to infection. *Proc Natl Acad Sci USA.* (2009) 106:11246–51. doi: 10.1073/pnas.0904846106
36. Refai A, Gritli S, Barbouche M, Essafi M. *Mycobacterium tuberculosis* virulent factor ESAT-6 drives macrophage differentiation toward the pro-inflammatory M1 phenotype and subsequently switches it to the anti-inflammatory M2 phenotype. (2018) 8:1–14. doi: 10.3389/fcimb.2018.00327
37. Lugo-Villarino G, Vérollet C, Maridonneau-Parini I, Neyrolles O. Macrophage polarization: convergence point targeted by *Mycobacterium tuberculosis* and HIV. *Front Immunol.* (2011) 2:43. doi: 10.3389/fimmu.2011.00043
38. Murray PJ. Macrophage polarization. *Annu Rev Physiol.* (2017) 79:541–66. doi: 10.1146/annurev-physiol-022516-034339
39. Martinez FO, Gordon S. The M1 and M2 paradigm of macrophage activation: time for reassessment. *F1000prime Rep.* (2014) 6:13. doi: 10.12703/P6-13
40. Sica A, Erreni M, Allavena P, Porta C. Macrophage polarization in pathology. *Cell Mol Life Sci.* (2015) 72:4111–26. doi: 10.1007/s00018-015-1995-y
41. Queval CJ, Brosch R, Simeone R. The macrophage: a disputed fortress in the battle against *Mycobacterium tuberculosis. Front Microbiol.* (2017) 8:2284. doi: 10.3389/fmicb.2017.02284
42. Méndez-samperio P, Trejo A, Pérez A. *Mycobacterium bovis* bacillus calmette – Guérin (BCG) stimulates IL-10 production via the PI3K/Akt and p38 MAPK pathways in human lung epithelial cells. *Cell Immunol.* (2008) 251:37–42. doi: 10.1016/j.cellimm.2008.03.002
43. Over B, Ziegler S, Foermer S, Weber ANR, Bode KA, Heeg K, et al. IRAK4 turns IL-10+ phospho-FOXO+ monocytes into pro-inflammatory cells by suppression of protein kinase B. *Eur J Immunol.* (2013) 43:1630–42. doi: 10.1002/eji.201243217
44. Joseph J, Ametepe ES, Haribabu N, Agbayani G, Krishnan L, Blais A, et al. Inhibition of ROS and upregulation of inflammatory cytokines by FoxO3a promotes survival against *Salmonella typhimurium. Nat Commun.* (2016) 7:12748. doi: 10.1038/ncomms12748
45. Lin L, Hron JD, Peng SL. Regulation of NF-κB, Th activation, and autoinflammation by the forkhead transcription factor Foxo3a. *Immunity.* (2004) 21:203–13. doi: 10.1016/j.immuni.2004.06.016
46. Chung S, Ranjan R, Lee YG, Park GY, Karpurapu M, Deng J, et al. Distinct role of FoxO1 in M-CSF- and GM-CSF-differentiated macrophages contributes LPS-mediated IL-10 : implication in hyperglycemia. *J Leukoc Biol.* (2015) 97:327–39. doi: 10.1189/jlb.3A0514-251R
47. Dong G, Wang Y, Xiao W, Pacios S, Xu F, Tian C, et al. FOXO1 regulates dendritic cell activity through ICAM-1 and CCR7. *J Immunol.* (2015) 194:3745–55. doi: 10.4049/jimmunol.1401754
48. Xiao W, Dong G, Pacios S, Alnammary M, Barger LA, Wang Y, et al. FOXO1 deletion reduces dendritic cell function and enhances susceptibility to periodontitis. *Am J Pathol.* (2015) 185:1085–93. doi: 10.1016/j.ajpath.2014.12.006
49. Wu YY, Elshimali Y, Sarkissyan M, Mohamed H, Clayton S, Vadgama J. Abstract 704: expression of FOXO1 is associated with GATA3 and Annexin-1 and predicts disease-free survival in breast cancer. *Cancer Res.* (2012) 2:704. doi: 10.1158/1538-7445.AM2012-704
50. Greer EL, Brunet A. FOXO transcription factors at the interface between longevity and tumor suppression. *Oncogene.* (2005) 24:7410–25. doi: 10.1038/sj.onc.1209086
51. Dejean AS, Hedrick SM, Kerdiles YM. Highly specialized role of forkhead Box O transcription factors in the immune system. *Antioxid Redox Signal.* (2011) 14:663–74. doi: 10.1089/ars.201 s0.3414
52. Queval CJ, Song OR, Deboosère N, Delorme V, Debrie AS, Iantomasi R, et al. STAT3 represses nitric oxide synthesis in human macrophages upon *Mycobacterium tuberculosis* infection. *Sci Rep.* (2016) 6:29297. doi: 10.1038/srep29297
53. Xi X, Zhang C, Han W, Zhao H, Zhang H, Jiao J. MicroRNA-223 is upregulated in active tuberculosis patients and inhibits apoptosis of macrophages by targeting FOXO3. *Genet Test Mol Biomark.* (2015) 19:650–6. doi: 10.1089/gtmb.2015.0090
54. Lu Y, Zhu Y, Wang X, Wang F, Peng J, Hou H, et al. FOXO3 rs12212067: T > G association with active tuberculosis in han Chinese population. *Inflammation.* (2016) 39:10–5. doi: 10.1007/s10753-015-0217-y
55. Yang J, Hung M. Molecular pathways a new fork for clinical application : T argeting forkhead T ranscription factors in cancer. *Clin Cancer Res.* (2009) 15:752–8. doi: 10.1158/1078-0432.CCR-08-0124
56. Chandarlapaty S, Sawai A, Scaltriti M, Rodrik-Outmezguine V, Grbovic-Huezo O, Serra V, et al. AKT inhibition relieves feedback suppression of receptor tyrosine kinase expression and activity. *Cancer Cell.* (2011) 19:58–71. doi: 10.1016/j.ccr.2010.10.031
57. Kuijl C, Savage NDL, Marsman M, Tuin AW, Janssen L, Egan DA, et al. Intracellular bacterial growth is controlled by a kinase network around PKB/AKT1. *Nature.* (2007) 450:725–30. doi: 10.1038/nature 06345

17

Target the Host, Kill the Bug; Targeting Host Respiratory Immunosuppressive Responses as a Novel Strategy to Improve Bacterial Clearance during Lung Infection

*Alanna M. Kelly and Rachel M. McLoughlin**

Host-Pathogen Interactions Group, School of Biochemistry and Immunology, Trinity Biomedical Sciences Institute, Trinity College Dublin, Dublin, Ireland

Correspondence:
Rachel M. McLoughlin
rachel.mcloughlin@tcd.ie

The lung is under constant pressure to protect the body from invading bacteria. An effective inflammatory immune response must be tightly orchestrated to ensure complete clearance of any invading bacteria, while simultaneously ensuring that inflammation is kept under strict control to preserve lung viability. Chronic bacterial lung infections are seen as a major threat to human life with the treatment of these infections becoming more arduous as the prevalence of antibiotic resistance becomes increasingly commonplace. In order to survive within the lung bacteria target the host immune system to prevent eradication. Many bacteria directly target inflammatory cells and cytokines to impair inflammatory responses. However, bacteria also have the capacity to take advantage of and strongly promote anti-inflammatory immune responses in the host lung to inhibit local pro-inflammatory responses that are critical to bacterial elimination. Host cells such as T regulatory cells and myeloid-derived suppressor cells are often enhanced in number and activity during chronic pulmonary infection. By increasing suppressive cell populations and cytokines, bacteria promote a permissive environment suitable for their prolonged survival. This review will explore the anti-inflammatory aspects of the lung immune system that are targeted by bacteria and how bacterial-induced immunosuppression could be inhibited through the use of host-directed therapies to improve treatment options for chronic lung infections.

Keywords: immunosuppression, lung, chronic infection, host-directed therapies, bacterial infection

INTRODUCTION

The respiratory tract is in constant contact with a myriad of bacterial species. To maintain homeostasis the healthy lung must efficiently and precisely identify friend from foe, and defend from infection without any long lasting inflammation or immunopathology occurring. The lung employs a complex network of immunosuppressive responses which are critical for maintaining a stable tolerogenic microenvironment within the tissue. However, bacterial pathogens have evolved to establish themselves within the lung by targeting this immunosuppressive arm of the immune response. In doing so bacterial species prevent appropriate clearance and create a suppressive microenvironment, facilitating their long-term survival. A better understanding of these bacterial-induced responses may aid in the development of novel host-directed therapies (HDTs) to target bacterial-induced immunosuppression. Herein we discuss how bacterial species of the lung have evolved to manipulate host immunosuppressive responses to their own advantage, hijacking important tolerogenic mechanisms to create an environment appropriate for bacterial growth. In addition we will discuss the ongoing research into HDTs and their potential for improving current treatments against bacterial lung infections.

Bacterial-induced respiratory tract infections are a major global health concern, and represent leading causes of death worldwide. These infections are of particular concern due to our dense population living habits and the growing prevalence of community-acquired pneumonia (1). The discovery and mass production of antibiotics dramatically reduced the number of mortalities associated with bacterial infection. However, with growing resistance and a lack of new discoveries, multi-drug resistance (MDR) is a huge threat to the success of antibiotics. The world health organization (WHO) has drawn up an antibiotic-resistant "priority pathogen" list classifying MDR bacteria as "critical" and "priority" depending on the threat to human health and the need for the development of novel antibiotics against these bacteria. Many of those in the "critical" group are bacteria associated with infection of the lung such as *Mycobacterium tuberculosis*, *Pseudomonas aeruginosa* and *Klebsiella pneumoniae*, with other species on the "priority" list including *Staphylococcus aureus*, *Streptococcus pneumonia* and *Haemophilus influenza*, all important bacterial species associated with invasive lung infections (2).

Our dependence on antibiotics is not sustainable and alternative therapies to current antibiotic treatments are urgently required to combat these increasingly dangerous pathogens and to prevent chronic and often fatal lung infections. As the resistance problem grows many researchers have looked into the modification of existing antibiotics to improve activity and reduce sensitivity to resistance (3). This approach has been broadly successful, however, current methods of targeting the microbe using antibiotics seem to inevitably end in resistance to the therapy in use. A potential method to overcome this may be the development of novel HDTs whereby the local host immune response during infection is targeted. Targeting host immunity can be done to either improve the immune response to infection or dampen down/disarm inappropriate immune responses, this includes strategies employed by bacteria to exploit immunosuppressive mechanisms of the host. By dampening local bacterial-induced immunosuppression it may be possible to promote a more pro-inflammatory immune response leading to improvements in bacterial killing and clearance. Achieving this however requires an in depth understanding of the intricacies of how the bacteria interact with the host to subvert immunosuppressive responses. This may reveal potential targets to intercept for the development of novel treatment modalities against intractable respiratory infections.

IMMUNE RESPONSE IN THE LUNG DURING BACTERIAL INFECTION

Pulmonary immune homeostasis is critical in maintaining a healthy lung environment and is tightly regulated by a network of tissue-resident and infiltrating immune cells that monitor the external environment continuously (4). The lung immune system has evolved to ward off pathogenic invasion while simultaneously preventing inflammation-mediated damage. An effective pro-inflammatory immune response is vital for the successful and complete elimination of bacterial pathogens. This involves a complex network of resident and infiltrating innate and adaptive inflammatory immune cells in addition to the epithelial cells lining the conducting airways and alveolar surface, which come together to orchestrate the efficient clearance of invading bacteria from the lung. These essential inflammatory immune cell responses are summarized in **Table 1**.

Once the bacterial pathogen is cleared from the respiratory tract it is vital the inflammatory immune response is quickly subdued to prevent any further tissue damage or immunopathology from occurring. The resolution of the inflammatory pulmonary immune response is an integral part of the physiological response to tissue injury and infection in the lungs. Inappropriate acute or long-term chronic inflammatory responses lead to damage of the thin-walled organ and result in impaired gas exchange and possibly life-threatening lung failure (35, 36). The termination of inflammatory immune responses is tightly regulated by a network of immunosuppressive cells including: alternatively activated alveolar macrophages (AM), myeloid-derived suppressor cells (MDSCs), tolerogenic dendritic cell (DC) subsets, IL-10-producing $CD4^{+}$ T cells, regulatory T cells (Tregs), regulatory B cells (Bregs), and lung epithelial cells (37–42), and through the release of key immunosuppressive cytokines. Immunoregulatory cells and cytokines act to prevent excessive inflammation by abrogating signaling pathways needed for inflammatory cytokine production, depleting populations of inflammatory effector cells and altering the phenotypes of leukocytes to an anti-inflammatory state (4, 43–47). In doing so, there is a return to homeostasis after a bacterial infection of the lung with minimal damage to the tissue.

MANIPULATION OF THE ANTI-INFLAMMATORY IMMUNE RESPONSES OF THE HOST LUNG

The resolution of inflammation is vital to ensure lung health, however many pulmonary bacterial pathogens have evolved to undermine these regulatory immune responses and use them against the host for their own survival.

Manipulation of Immunoregulatory Cells

Alveolar Macrophages

The plasticity of the alveolar macrophage (AM) response is critical to their role in the clearance of bacteria from the lung and the resolution of inflammation post-infection, but also makes these cells ideal targets for hijacking by many bacteria.

TABLE 1 | Important inflammatory immune responses of the lung vital for bacterial clearance.

Cell type	Function	References
Alveolar macrophage (AM)	1st line defense. Phagocytosis of infiltrating pathogens Production of inflammatory cytokines; IL-12, TNF, IL-1β, IL-8	(5–7)
Dendritic cell (DC)	Phagocytosis of pathogens & upregulation of MHC-II, presentation of bacterial antigens, and directing T effector cell differentiation. Production of inflammatory cytokines; IL-12, TNF, IL-1β	(6, 8, 9)
Neutrophil	Facilitate bacterial clearance via phagocytosis, enzymatic degradation of bacteria and NETosis	(7, 10, 11)
Natural Killer (NK) cell	Early contribution to high IFN-γ levels and promotion of Th1 responses, promote inflammatory macrophage responses	(12–14)
Innate lymphoid (ILC) cell	Contribute to the production of IL-17 and IFN-γ in the lung, leading to enhanced pro-inflammatory innate responses. Produce IL-22 promoting antimicrobial peptide production	(15–17)
Natural Killer T (NKT) cell	Contribute to high IFN-γ levels and promotion of Th1 responses, IL-17 production leading to neutrophil recruitment	(18–21)
Mucosal-associated invariant T (MAIT) cell	Contribute to IFN-γ and promotion of Th1 responses, IL-17 production resulting in neutrophil recruitment and aid in recruitment of $CD4^+$ and $CD8^+$ T cells	(22–24)
γδ T cell	Major producers of IL-17 leading to neutrophil-mediated responses. Contribute to IFN-γ production	(25, 26)
$CD4^+$ T cell	Critical contributors to the production of IL-17, IL-22 and IFN-γ, leading to enhanced innate cell activity, antimicrobial peptide production, and improved bacterial clearance	(27–31)
$CD8^+$ T cell	Contribute to IFN-γ and TNF production. Cytotoxic effects help clear infected cells and remove bacteria from the lung	(32–34)

While the prevalence of the "tissue repair" M2 phenotype is needed for resolution of inflammation, these cells represent a niche for the prolonged survival of many intracellular pathogens (48). In murine studies *M. tuberculosis* increases the expression of peroxisome proliferator-activated receptor-γ (PPAR-γ) in infected macrophages leading to an increase in anti-inflammatory "M2"-associated markers alongside reductions in respiratory burst, allowing enhanced intracellular bacterial survival (49). *Mycobacterium tuberculosis* has also been shown to induce arginase1 (Arg1) expression in infected macrophages which is associated with reduced production of reactive nitrogen intermediates and therefore enhanced survival of the bacterium (50). AMs are also polarized to an M2 phenotype during *Bordetella pertussis* intracellular infection to facilitate survival of the bacteria within these cells (51). *In vitro* studies using a THP-1 cell line demonstrated that *B. pertussis* can persist in macrophages and promote the expression of suppressor of cytokine signaling 1(SOCS1) protein, an M2-associated protein (52). The upregulation of SOCS1 promotes Arginase-1 (Arg1) activity and inhibits IFN-γ induced JAK2/STAT1 signaling and TLR/NF-kB signaling leading to reduced pro-inflammatory responses (53, 54). Similarly the bacterial toxins Pertussis toxin (Ptx) and adenylate cyclase toxin (ACT) were implicated in this macrophage phenotype switch. *In vitro* studies have demonstrated that THP-1 cells infected with strains lacking either of these toxins had lower SOCS1 expression and a decreased ability of the bacterium to survive intracellularly (51).

Dendritic Cells

Dendritic cells (DCs) have a decisive role in initiating an appropriate adaptive immune response to invading pathogens in the lung (55), while also being central to tolerogenic responses and inflammatory resolution. The induction of tolerogenic DCs is an effective method of manipulating the lung immune response employed by a number of bacterial species in order to allow the pathogen to multiply without restraint. *Yersinia pestis* promotes the expansion of tolerogenic DCs via its LcrV protein (56). *In vitro* studies using bone marrow-derived DCs (BMDCs) have shown LcrV binds TLR2/6 leading to the induction of high levels of IL-10 production by these cells which in turn promotes type 1 regulatory (Tr1) T cells and further enhanced IL-10 production (56). Similarly the induction of tolerogenic DCs were also seen during Mycobacterium *avium* subspecies *hominissuis* (MAH) co-infection (57). MAH infections are strongly associated with opportunistic co-infections by common pulmonary pathogens such as *Haemophilus influenzae*, *Staphylococcus aureus*, and *Pseudomonas aeruginosa* (57, 58). Studies using MAH-infected BMDCs stimulated with LPS, which mimicked co-infection conditions, lead to the production of high levels of TLR-mediated IL-10 alongside reduced IL-12 levels (57). *In vitro* studies of a MAH/*P. aeruginosa* co-infection showed a marked increase in IL-10-producing tolerogenic DCs. The enhanced IL-10 led to reduced MHC class II expression and antigen presentation, which eventually led to the inhibition of $CD4^+$ T cell proliferation (57). By promoting tolerogenic phenotypes of AMs and DCs in the lung bacteria can promote early IL-10 production and reduced antigen-presentation resulting in the prevention of effective protective pro-inflammatory adaptive responses leading to undisturbed bacterial growth.

Myeloid-Derived Suppressor Cells

Myeloid-derived suppressor cells (MDSCs) are emerging as key specialized suppressive cells capable of dampening inflammation to prevent tissue damage after infection (59). These cells are powerful modulators of both the innate and adaptive immune responses and in particular have potent immunosuppressive effects on T cell responses (60). These immunosuppressive innate cells have been targeted by a number of pulmonary bacteria which lead to the progression of chronic infections and these cells may be particularly important in facilitating the transition from acute to chronic infection (61–63).

MDSC are increased in the peripheral blood of patients with active tuberculosis infection (63). *In vitro* studies using a granuloma model demonstrate how MDSCs exposed to *M. tuberculosis* secrete IL-10 in abundance and upregulate their expression of PD-L1, which led to the suppression of protective T cell proliferation and promoted bacterial replication (64). The bacterium *Streptococcus pneumoniae* also has the capacity to hijack MDSCs to facilitate its persistence in the airways. Studies in mice have demonstrated a robust monocytic response in the lung following intranasal challenge with *S. pneumoniae* which was dominated by the presence of MDSCs. These cells expressed IL-10, arginase and importantly lacked phagocytic capabilities (65). This early anti-inflammatory response terminated pro-inflammatory signaling needed for clearance of the bacteria and promoted persistence in the lung. Similarly the expansion of a large population of regulatory immature myeloid cells has been described following intranasal *Francisella tularensis* infection (66). A lethal *F. tularensis* infection with a highly virulent strain, led to the recruitment of a large number of MDSC to the lungs which allowed bacterial survival and eventually resulted in host death. Interestingly, during sub-lethal infection of *F. tularensis* there was a greater recruitment of mature pro-inflammatory myeloid cells that were effective at controlling infection and clearing the bacterium (66). The depletion of the immature myeloid cells partially ameliorated mortality following lethal infection. These results indicate the lethality of *F. tularensis* infection may be through excessive MDSC recruitment which enables prolific bacterial growth within the lungs. Other bacterial species which colonize and infect the respiratory tract may also have the potential to similarly subvert the activities of MDSCs. In a systemic infection model of *S. aureus* infection, persistence of the bacterium has been shown to be associated with increased expansion of MDSCs which inhibit T cell responses (67). Similarly in a localized skin infection model *S. aureus* promotes the expansion of MDSCs leading to the upregulation of IL-10 production, which was associated with the persistence of the bacteria within the skin (68).

Treg Cells

Treg cells play a particularly important role in maintaining lung homeostasis and resolving pro-inflammatory responses promptly after pathogens have been cleared. Many pathogens that invade the lungs have the capacity to exploit the immunoregulatory function of Tregs and promote the expansion of these anti-inflammatory cells. This strategy is a direct attempt to counterbalance the pro-inflammatory effects mediated by innate cells and adaptive T cells such as Th17 cells and Th1 cells which play a particularly important role in the protective immune response to bacteria in the lung (27, 69–71). Tregs can carry out their function through the production of immunoregulatory cytokines such as IL-10 and TGF-β, via direct cell-cell contact through their immunosuppressive surface markers such as CTLA-4 or by their enhanced consumption of IL-2 which reduces effector T cell activation (72).

Peripheral blood mononuclear cells (PBMCs) from patients with active tuberculosis were shown to have raised levels of Tregs in comparison to healthy controls (73).The *ex vivo* depletion of these $CD25^+$ $FoxP3^+$ cells from PBMCs of patients led to an increased expansion of antigen-specific IFN-γ^+ T cells indicating that *M. tuberculosis*–induced Tregs were capable of suppressing these protective T cell responses. In a guinea pig model of tuberculosis it was shown that highly virulent strains induce high levels of FoxP3, IL-10, and TGF-β mRNA expression in lung tissue (74, 75). After an initial increase in mRNA expression levels of the Th1-associated cytokine IFN-γ, there was a rapid decrease in these levels and subsequent surge in Treg-associated markers and cytokines (74). It was hypothesized that highly virulent strains act as potent inducers of Tregs and that this increase in these suppressive cells enhances bacterial survival. A similar result was seen in a murine model of severe tuberculosis infection using a hyper-virulent strain HN878. An initial Th1 response was followed by a rapid increase in IL-10^+ Tregs in the lungs (76). This increase in suppressive cells enabled progression of infection which may explain the relatively short time of survival of these infected mice.

Other bacterial species such as *B. pertussis* and *S. pneumoniae* also promote Treg expansion as a means to facilitate their survival. *B. pertussis* can expand Tregs by upregulating IL-10 production by innate cells such as macrophages and DCs, which in turn directs T cell differentiation toward a regulatory phenotype (77–80). In a murine model of *S. pneumoniae* nasopharyngeal colonization it was demonstrated that Treg expansion was due to the high levels of TGF-β being produced by nasopharyngeal cells in response to the bacterium. The high levels of Treg cells promote prolonged survival of the bacteria within the host lungs while causing no damage to the host (81). The bacterium essentially goes undetected by the pro-inflammatory arm of the pulmonary immune response as it remains suppressed by the presence of high levels of TGF-β. This lack of inflammatory responses via Treg-mediated TGF-β allows bacterial survival and may lead to invasive disease.

Breg Cells

In addition to the well-characterized role of Tregs in maintaining immune homeostasis, Bregs have been shown to contribute to immune tolerance (82, 83). Their suppressive effect is mainly through IL-10 production, leading to the inhibition of Th1 and Th17 responses and the conversion of $CD4^+$ T cells into Treg cells (82, 84). The role of Bregs during pulmonary infection is not well defined, however PBMCs from patients suffering with tuberculosis were shown to contain higher numbers of Bregs compared to healthy controls (85). *In vitro* co-cultures using T cell and B cell populations isolated from patient PBMCs demonstrated that these Bregs could dampen Th17 responses (85). Bregs were also shown to have inhibitory effects on IL-22 production (86), a cytokine implicated in limiting *M. tuberculosis* intracellular survival (87, 88). More recent studies have demonstrated how circulating Bregs of active *M. tuberculosis*-infected patients were producing the immunoregulatory cytokine IL-35 (89), a potent immunosuppressive cytokine capable of suppressing effector T cell responses, promoting the expansion of Tregs and their production of IL-10 (90). Additionally, stimulating purified B cells from healthy controls with *M. tuberculosis* lysate, increased expansion of IL-35^+ Bregs (89), suggesting *M. tuberculosis* may be inducing the production of IL-35 by Bregs to enhance IL-10 production to regulate inflammatory responses. More in depth study is needed to definitively identify the function of IL-35-producing B cells in *M. tuberculosis* infection. In a murine model of *S. aureus* systemic infection a population of Bregs were expanded and acted as major producers of IL-10 (68). It is conceivable therefore that these cells also play a role in the pathology of *S. aureus* lung infection.

There are still major gaps in our understanding of how Bregs and their immunosuppressive effects are being hijacked by pulmonary bacteria, however, it seems likely that these cells are important in suppressing inflammatory immune responses in the lung through their production of the anti-inflammatory cytokines IL-10 and potentially IL-35.

Regulatory cell populations of the local respiratory immune response are key targets of bacterial pathogens. Immune cells usually central to the resolution of harmful inflammation are heavily exploited to improve bacterial survival. Bacterial-induced expansion and activation of these regulatory innate and adaptive immune cells allows the suppression of vital inflammatory responses needed for complete bacterial clearance. These cells could potentially be targeted to reduce their anti-inflammatory effects and improve infection outcome.

Manipulation of Immunosuppressive Cytokines

One of the most common survival strategies employed by bacterial species to facilitate their survival is to promote the production of various anti-inflammatory cytokines from a variety of cell types. These anti-inflammatory mediators then suppress pro-inflammatory cell populations such as innate cells and effector T cells, and reduce the production of pro-inflammatory cytokines.

IL-10

IL-10 is a key cytokine required for maintaining the steady-state within the healthy lung during infection where it inhibits the activity of many pro-inflammatory cells and prevents immunopathology. However, excessive or miss-timed IL-10 production can inhibit a protective pro-inflammatory response leading to chronic and often fatal infection (91). In a murine model of *Mycobacterium avium* infection, BALB/c mice respond with very early IL-10 production. This reduces their ability to control the pathogen compared to their C57BL/6 counterparts, which have lower IL-10 activity (92). The ablation of IL-10 signaling improved pathogen control in the BALB/c mice, highlighting the causal relationship between IL-10 and a lack of pathogen control. By limiting pro-inflammatory cell functions IL-10 can reduce immunopathology, benefitting the host. However, if produced in excess or if inappropriately timed, it can potentially dampen the protective effector immune response required for bacterial clearance.

The induction of IL-10 is a key strategy employed by *M. tuberculosis* to facilitate pathogenesis (93). The pathogen infiltrates the lung and can reside within host macrophages, here, it suppresses their pro-inflammatory function through enhanced IL-10 production via a number of mechanisms (94). The *M. tuberculosis* heat shock protein 60 (Mtbhsp60) can target TLR2 and TLR4 on macrophages leading to p30 MAPK activation and enhanced IL-10 production (95). By targeting TLR signaling *M. tuberculosis* can polarize macrophage responses to be more immunosuppressive. Das et al. identified a novel mechanism of CCR5-mediated altered cellular signaling in *M. tuberculosis* infected macrophages, leading to downstream activation of the Src kinase Lyn and the mitogen-activated protein (MAP) kinase ERK-1/2, resulting in IL-10, and also TGF-β production. The elevated IL-10 production was shown to attenuate the expression of MHC-II in the infected macrophages (94), reducing the ability of these cells to orchestrate an appropriate adaptive response. Enhanced IL-10 production from *M. tuberculosis*-infected macrophages has also been shown to inhibit phagosomal maturation which enables phagosomal escape and intracellular survival within the host lung, further contributing to impaired bacterial clearance (96–98). Furthermore, this arrest of maturation prevents appropriate presentation of antigenic peptides and subsequent induction of the adaptive immune response (99). Blocking IL-10 production *in vitro* in AMs, by pre-treating them with an anti-IL-10 antibody in advance of *M. tuberculosis* infection, was shown to improve phagosome maturation and increase killing of the internalized mycobacterium (98). Alveolar epithelial cells are also targeted by *M. tuberculosis* for IL-10 production. *Mycobacterium bovis* Bacillus Calmette Guerin (BCG) activates TLR2 and TLR4 on alveolar epithelial cells causing phosphorylation of glycogen synthase kinase-3 (GSK3) via a PI3K/Akt pathway which induces the production of IL-10 (100). *M. tuberculosis* can also manipulate IL-10 regulation at the RNA level. *M. tuberculosis* drives the anti-inflammatory microRNA (miRNA) miR-21 (101), which is one of the most highly expressed miRNAs in myeloid cells. This miRNA is induced by TLR4 signaling and limits the activity of the pro-inflammatory PDCD4 protein to promote IL-10 production (102). *M. tuberculosis* also has the capacity to activate IL-10-expressing T cells (103). T cells are the predominant producers of IL-10 later in *M. tuberculosis* infection, at ~21 days post-infection, where they contribute to impaired clearance (103).

Other bacterial species, such as *B. pertussis*, utilize a number of virulence factors to drive IL-10 production (78, 79, 104, 105). Filamentous haemaglutinin (FHA) activates TLR4 signaling in DCs and macrophages within the lung to induce IL-10 (78, 104). This increase in innate IL-10 leads to the expansion of T regulatory type 1 (Tr1) cells (78). FHA-induced IL-10 also dampens IL-12 production by DCs and leads to downregulation of protective Th17 and Th1 responses (79). However, it must be noted that more recent research has cast a question mark over the immunoregulatory role of FHA (106). The authors state that the upregulation of IL-10 may be caused by endotoxin contamination or co-purification of bacterial lipoproteins, which may contribute to FHA's cytokine inducing activity (106, 107). Adenylate cyclase toxin (ACT) of *B. pertussis* also drives IL-10 production by APCs such as DCs and macrophages (77, 108), which then further induces IL-10-secreting Treg cells (109).

Klebsiella *pneumoniae* can induce IL-10 production by macrophages in the lung (110), which enables the bacterium to inhibit inflammasome activation and pyroptotis, facilitating its' dissemination (111). Upon infection with *K. pneumoniae* strain A54970, no IL-1β production was induced in infected macrophages, suggesting a lack of inflammasome activation and associated pyroptosis (111, 112). When BMDMs from IL-10 knock-out (KO) mice were infected with the A54970 strain, these macrophages produced high levels of IL-1β and released LDH which is associated with the induction of pyroptosis, indicating that this strain was capable of inhibiting inflammasome activation and function through high induction of IL-10 (111, 113). However, the authors noted that different clinical strains investigated showed dissimilar methods of evading the host immune response. Other strains such as A28006 induced high IL-1β production and increased pyroptotic cell death in macrophages recruited to the lung (111). In a murine model of *K. pneumoniae* infection, intra-tracheal challenge with *K. pneumoniae* enhanced IL-10 mRNA expression in lung homogenates. Administration of IL-10-blocking antibodies prior to challenge was associated with an enhanced pro-inflammatory immune response, improved bacterial clearance and prolonged survival (114). It has been postulated that the capsular polysaccharide (CPS) of *K. pneumoniae* may be particularly important for the induction of IL-10 (110, 115). When mice were intranasally inoculated with a capsulated or a non-capsulated strain of *K. pneumoniae*. IL-10 levels in the bronchiolar lavage fluid (BALF) and serum of mice infected with the capsulated strain were significantly higher than those infected with the non-capsulated strain, and these mice died within 3 days of infection (110). These results suggest that the presence of CPS is inducing IL-10 production at the site of infection and may down-regulate the expression of pro-inflammatory cytokines such as TNF and IFN-γ. The multiple cellular sources of IL-10 *in vivo* and the specific signaling pathways controlling *Klebsiella*-induced IL-10 production are areas of research warranting future investigation (116).

Bacteria of the lung can also promote TLR-driven IL-10 production to facilitate their survival. Species of *Yersinia* and *S. aureus* drive IL-10 production through the exploitation of TLR2 signaling. Studies have demonstrated that *Yersinia* species upregulate host macrophage-derived IL-10 production in a TLR-2-mediated manner, resulting in suppression of pro-inflammatory cytokine production by macrophages and increased bacterial survival (117, 118). Virulence factor LcrV-induced IL-10 was shown to induce hypo-responsiveness against TLR2- or TLR4-agonists in macrophages. This hypo-responsiveness was not present in cells isolated from IL-10 KO mice (119). This result demonstrates how the bacterium is exploiting an IL-10-induced TLR tolerance mechanism of the host. Likewise, the Gram-positive bacterium *S. aureus* can drive IL-10 via TLR signaling. In addition to conventional pro-inflammatory signaling induced through TLR2 recognition of *S. aureus*, the bacteria is also capable of inducing a robust anti-inflammatory response (120). *Staphylococcus aureus*-induced TLR2 signaling in monocytes has been shown to result in PI3K/Akt signaling leading to IL-10 production, as opposed to conventional NFκB-driven TLR2 signaling which leads to pro-inflammatory cytokine production (121). The anti-inflammatory signaling response is induced independently of the pro-inflammatory response, and can be "uncoupled" from these inflammatory responses (120). It has previously been shown that *S. aureus* can induce IL-10 production in a skin infection model to promote its persistence by inhibiting effector T cells (68), suggesting that a similar mechanism may occur during *S. aureus* infection and/or colonization of the respiratory tract. *S. aureus* is a common cause of secondary pneumonia following influenza infection and Robinson et al. demonstrated a potential role for both IL-27 and IL-10 in impairing bacterial clearance in a murine model of secondary *S. aureus*-induced pneumonia (122). IL-10 KO mice cleared the bacteria from the lung more efficiently than WT mice. IL-27RA KO mice had decreased levels of IL-10 which was associated with improved bacterial clearance compared to WT counterparts (122). These results indicate that IL-10 is facilitating *S. aureus* persistence in the lung post influenza infection, and that IL-27 may have a role to play in regulating the production of IL-10 in this instance.

TGF-β

Although the induction of IL-10 represents one of the most heavily exploited immunosuppressive strategies used by bacteria to facilitate their persistence in the lung, other regulatory cytokines have also been implicated in bacterial-induced immunosuppression. Upregulation of TGF-β is commonly associated with *S. pneumoniae* carriage and lung infection. Adenoidal mononuclear cells isolated from children undergoing adenoidectomies who also tested positive for *S. pneumoniae* carriage had higher levels of TGF-β and upregulated populations of FoxP3^{+} Tregs compared to children who tested negative for the bacterium (123). It is thought that these increased immunosuppressive responses within the adenoid tissue may be facilitating chronic carriage, which is a risk factor for pneumococcal disease. It was demonstrated that the virulence factor enzyme neuraminidase A (NanA) of *S. pneumoniae* can directly activate latent TGF-β to its biologically active form by removal of sialic acids from the latency associated peptide (LAP) (124). TGF-β is associated with prolonged colonization of the nasopharynx and enhanced translocation of *S. pneumoniae* to the lower respiratory tract (125). Furthermore, *S. pneumoniae* infection of Vβ6 integrin KO mice resulted in enhanced clearance of the bacterium compared to WT mice. This was also true in the case of co-infections of influenza and *S. pneumoniae* (126). The αVβ6 integrin is expressed at low levels in healthy tissue but is upregulated in response to inflammation and injury and is the main method of activation of endogenous TGF-β in the lung (127). The complete ablation of β6 integrin from the system led to a loss of activated TGF-β which was accompanied by increased activation of AMs and type I IFN production, resulting in improved protection (126). However, other studies have shown that reduction of TGF-β during *S. pneumoniae* infection can be fatal and that the cytokine is vital in the prevention of hyper-inflammation against *S. pneumoniae* in the lung. Here, blockade of TGF-β led to the dissemination of the bacterium from the lung (128). A caveat of the β6 integrin KO model is that the β6 integrin may also regulate factors other than TGF-β1 that cause the downstream effects facilitating bacterial clearance. TGF-β is clearly critical for limiting infection-associated inflammation, but the powerful immunosuppressive effects TGF-β exerts can be exploited by pulmonary pathogens, with the timing and extent of TGF-β inhibition impacting infection outcome.

Active tuberculosis infection is also associated with the excessive production and activation of TGF-β. TGF-β has been found at high levels in the granuloma of infected patients (129). *In vitro* stimulation of human blood monocytes, with *M. tuberculosis* led to an increase in production of bioactive TGF-β (130). These cells are a likely early source of the cytokine, recruited to the lung upon infection. In a murine model of *M. bovis* pulmonary infection the inhibition of TGF-β by the administration of latency associated peptide (LAP) inhibited TGF-β activity in the lung, enhanced IFN-γ production and improved antigen-specific effector T cell responses in cells isolated from mediastinal lymph nodes of mice administered with LAP compared to PBS-treated mice. LAP treatment was also shown to reduce mycobacterium growth in the lung parenchyma and bronchiolar spaces (131).

IL-27

More recently the cytokine IL-27 has been implicated in regulation of the pulmonary immune response during infection. Insights into the function of IL-27 in the lung have primarily come from studies of viral respiratory infections where it appears to play an important role in controlling excessive inflammation. In a murine influenza model, IL-27 suppressed IL-17 production in an IL-10-dependent manner suggesting that IL-27 acts upstream of IL-10 (132). Furthermore, IL-27-mediated activation of STAT1, STAT3, or BLIMP-1 promotes IL-10 production and the generation of T regulatory type 1 (Tr1) cells, leading to the suppression of IL-17 production by $CD4^{+}$ T cells (133–136). Others have demonstrated a direct role for IL-27 in promoting maturation of Tregs during Respiratory syncytial virus (RSV) infection, which was independent of IL-10 (137). In the case of respiratory bacterial infections, IL-27 was identified as an important immune factor underlying the impaired clearance of the bacterium *P. aeruginosa*. In a murine model of *P. aeruginosa* infection this cytokine was shown to suppress the antibacterial activities of AMs (41, 138). Studies demonstrated that a secondary infection with *P. aeruginosa* in the lungs following caecal ligation and puncture (CLP)-induced sepsis in IL-27R KO mice, was associated with enhanced bacterial clearance from the lungs and improved survival rates compared to wild-type counterparts. A more rapid clearance of bacteria from the lungs of the IL-27R KO mice was associated with increased recruitment of inflammatory neutrophils to the airways (138). IL-27 seems to be directly influencing AM responses, as macrophages isolated from IL27R KO mice had enhanced co-stimulatory molecule expression and better bacterial uptake and killing compared to macrophages from wild-type mice (138). Neutralization of IL-27 was also shown to improve bacterial clearance in the lungs of septic mice infected with *P. aeruginosa* (138). Patients suffering from pulmonary infections caused by *Burkholderia pseudomallei* show elevated levels of IL-27 and *in vitro* studies demonstrated that stimulation of whole blood from healthy individuals with *B. pseudomallei* resulted in significantly increased production of IL-27 (139). The major sources of IL-27 were macrophages and neutrophils. The production of IL-27 led to enhanced bacterial survival in neutrophils which was reduced by blockade of neutrophil-derived IL-27 prior to infection (139). Taken together these results suggest that IL-27 has the potential to play an important immunosuppressive role in the lung during bacterial infection and that further studies will reveal the potential for multiple bacterial species to exploit its suppressive effects for their own advantage. One caveat to these studies is, however, the fact that mice have been shown to be capable of producing IL-27p28 in the absence of EBI3. As the subunit may be expressed on its own it is not yet clear if the reported effects of IL-27 are due to the full heterodimeric cytokine or merely to its alpha subunit. However, it has recently been reported that a transgenic mouse that can only produce IL-27p28 in the presence of EBI3 has been developed (140), which will allow for the distinct functions of IL-27 or IL-27p28 to be elucidated.

It is clear that many bacterial pathogens of the lung are profiteering from the induction of immunosuppressive cytokines. By taking advantage of their anti-inflammatory effects on the surrounding inflammatory immune response, many bacteria can survive undisturbed. There is an inextricable link between the immunoregulatory cell populations and cytokines being induced by these pathogens. By promoting the expansion of immunoregulatory cells and enhanced production of immunoregulatory cytokines bacteria can undermine the host's local inflammatory immune responses to survive within the lung (**Figure 1**).

Manipulation of Immunometabolism

Altering cell phenotype from pro- to anti-inflammatory is one of the key strategies employed by bacteria invading the lung. Metabolic re-programming is crucial for controlling the switching of cell phenotypes and their pro-inflammatory or anti-inflammatory functions (141). During infection metabolic reprogramming has implications for the production of pro-inflammatory and anti-inflammatory immune cell phenotypes and cytokines which control the ability of the host to clear the pathogen. There is emerging evidence that multiple bacteria have the potential to promote immunosuppressive cell phenotypes and cytokine production by targeting the metabolic pathways of these immune cells.

Glycolytic Reprogramming

An increase in glycolysis can be seen as a hallmark of metabolic change in immune cells undergoing activation and is associated with pro-inflammatory responses, with macrophages and DCs increasing their glycolytic metabolism when stimulated with LPS (142, 143). In DCs, this metabolic shift from oxidative phosphorylation to glycolysis upon TLR-mediated activation is antagonized by the metabolic regulator AMP kinase (AMPK), and IL-10 production was also shown to prevent this switch by partially preventing TLR-mediated AMPK hypophosphorylation (142). Bacterial-induced IL-10 production during chronic lung

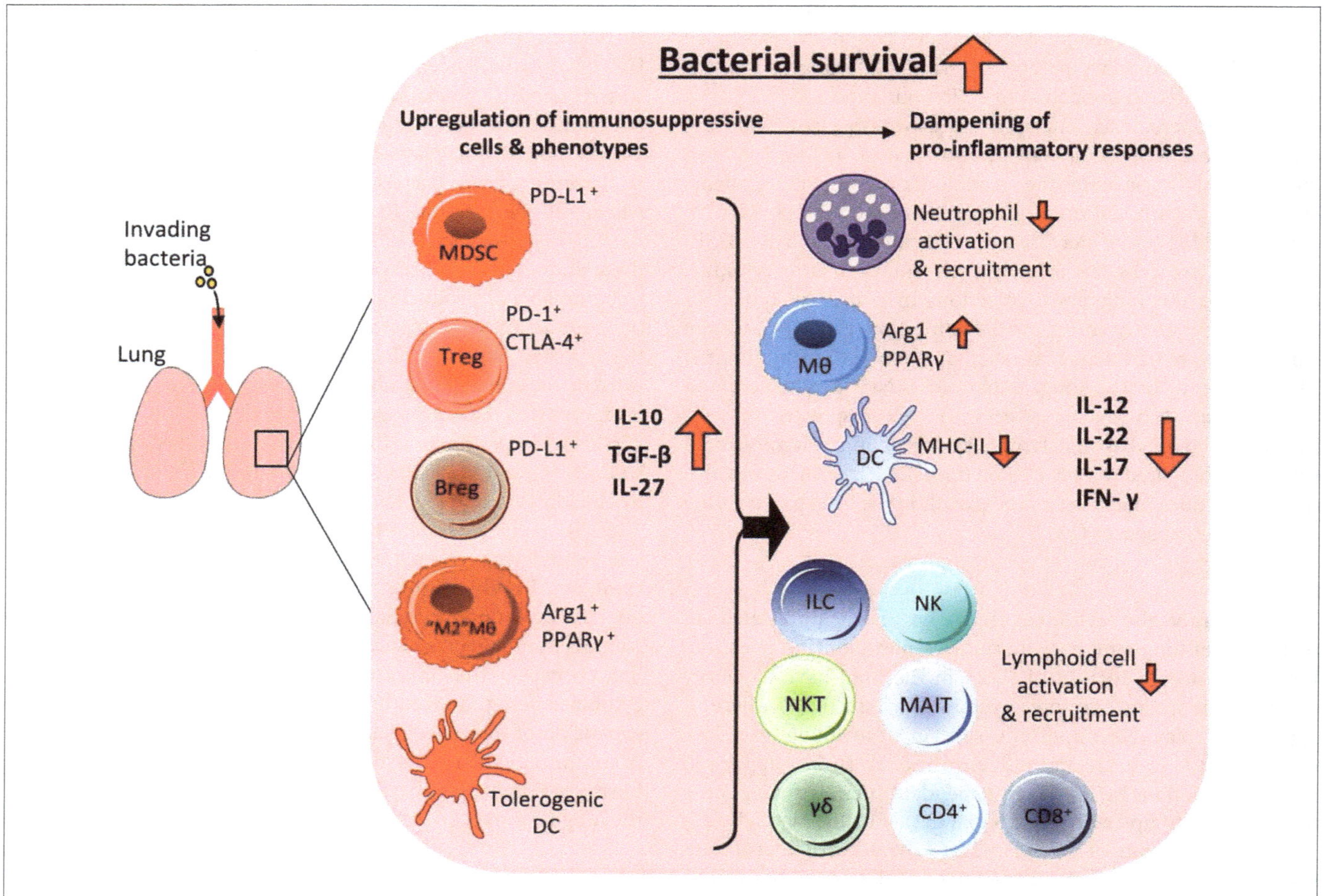

FIGURE 1 | Invading bacteria induce an immunosuppressive microenvironment in the lung resulting in bacterial persistence. To facilitate persistence during infection invading bacteria can promote immunosuppressive immune responses in the lung by targeting the anti-inflammatory arm of the host immune system. This leads to the increased production of anti-inflammatory cytokines and enhanced recruitment of anti-inflammatory cells, which together reduce pro-inflammatory cytokine production and cell populations in the airways. The bacteria can manipulate alveolar macrophages and DCs to produce high levels of regulatory cytokines such as IL-10 and IL-27. This leads to reduced recruitment and activation of inflammatory innate cells such as neutrophils, NK cells, γδ T cells, NKT cells, and MAIT cells. Impaired DC MHC-II expression and higher IL-10 production leads to reduced activation of adaptive effector T cell responses such as Th1, Th17 and cytotoxic CD8$^+$ T cells. Enhanced IL-10 production also leads to increases in Treg cell activation and recruitment. Other anti-inflammatory cell populations also undergo enhanced recruitment to the lung, such as Bregs and MDSCs. Together these anti-inflammatory cells contribute to the creation of an immunosuppressive microenvironment that is permissive to bacterial growth enabling prolonged bacterial survival within the lung without effective clearance.

infection therefore has the potential to antagonize the TLR-mediated shift to glycolysis in DCs and thus reduce pro-inflammatory adaptive responses and promote bacterial survival.

LPS-induced glucose uptake and glycolysis in macrophages is also impeded by IL-10. IL-10 inhibits glycolysis by suppressing mechanistic target of rapamycin (mTOR) activity through the induction of DDIT4, an mTOR inhibitor (113). Bone marrow-derived macrophages (BMDMs) from IL-10 KO mice stimulated with LPS were shown to have prolonged activation of mTOR complex 1 (mTORC1), of which mTOR is the catalytic subunit, while mTORC1 was quickly suppressed in macrophages of wild-type mice. The addition of exogenous IL-10 restored mTORC1 regulation in IL-10 KO macrophages (113). DDIT4 was shown to be strongly upregulated by IL-10 during LPS stimulation, indicating it was the likely candidate causing IL-10-induced mTOR suppression (113). BMDMs from Ddit4$^{-/-}$ KO mice also showed prolonged mTORC1 activity upon LPS stimulation, similar to IL-10 KO macrophages, however, treatment with exogenous IL-10 failed to inhibit mTORC1 activation suggesting that the inhibition of mTOR signaling by IL-10 is DDIT4-dependent (113). This study revealed a key role of IL-10 in controlling cellular metabolism in macrophages via inhibition of mTORC1 and suggest that high concentrations of IL-10 induced during chronic pulmonary infection could impede macrophage metabolic switching from oxidative phosphorylation to glycolysis. During active *M. tuberculosis* infection the mTOR signaling pathway is suppressed which promotes the proliferation and activation of FoxP3$^+$ Tregs cells. PBMCs isolated from patients with active tuberculosis infection showed decreased numbers of CD3$^+$ mTOR$^+$ cells and increased expression of FoxP3 compared to healthy controls. The enhanced number of Tregs in infected patients was associated with high levels of IL-10 and TGF-β (144).

Glycolytic reprogramming of macrophages is an important step in the early pulmonary defense against *M. tuberculosis* infection (145). Infection of macrophages induces a shift from oxidative phosphorylation to glycolysis which promotes phagocytosis and enhances production of protective pro-inflammatory cytokines such as IL-1β (145). However, *M. tuberculosis* induced production of IL-10 has been linked to the negative regulation of glycolysis in macrophages (113). PPAR-γ is highly upregulated in human and mouse macrophages upon mycobacterial infection (49, 146). PPAR-γ acts to regulate glucose metabolism and fatty acid storage. Increases in PPAR-γ expression leads to enhanced lipid droplet formation within macrophages, used for intracellular growth by the mycobacterium (147), increased expression of IL-10 and the downregulation of pro-inflammatory immune responses against the mycobacterium (148). *M. tuberculosis* can rewire macrophage energy metabolism to support bacterial survival by limiting ATP availability and decelerating flux through glycolysis and the tricarboxylic (TCA) cycle, increasing mitochondrial dependency on fatty acids. The deceleration of glycolysis may be via citrate, a derivative of the TCA cycle which has been seen to accumulate in monocyte-derived macrophages infected with *M. tuberculosis* (147). At high concentrations citrate can inhibit phosphofructokinase which acts as a key enzyme in glycolysis (149). One of the caveats to this work is that different metabolic outcomes occurred depending on whether BCG, heat-killed *M. tuberculosis* or live virulent *M. tuberculosis* was used during studies (147). In the case of live virulent *M. tuberculosis*, it was shown to decrease reliance on both glycolysis and oxidative phosphorylation in infected macrophages causing them to enter a state of metabolic quiescence, while also increasing mitochondrial dependency on fatty acids for survival in infected macrophages, while heat killed *M. tuberculosis* and BCG led to increases in glycolysis (147). The reduced glycolytic rate in live *M. tuberculosis*-infected macrophages indicates the mycobacterium is subverting appropriate innate immune responses. Collectively, glycolysis, and fatty acid metabolism could be potential targets for metabolic restoration during *M. tuberculosis* infection which would promote a pro-inflammatory phenotype in infected macrophages. *B. pertussis* can also promote dysregulated glucose metabolism in the host (150). A murine model of *B. pertussis* infection demonstrated insulin resistance as the bacterium negatively regulated blood glucose homeostasis (150, 151). Host immune cells depend on circulating blood glucose for their metabolic requirements, which are particularly important in responding to infection to ensure swift activation and expansion (150). The hypoglycemic state induced during *B. pertussis* infection deprives the immune system of energy needed to create an effective immune response against the bacterium.

Effects of Metabolites on Immunometabolism

Cellular metabolites which may be induced by pulmonary pathogens during infection have the potential to regulate immune cell activity. LPS-stimulated macrophages were shown to increase their production of itaconate, a cellular metabolite created by diverting aconitate from the TCA cycle during inflammatory activation of macrophages (152, 153). Itaconate has been shown to have anti-inflammatory effects on macrophages by activating the anti-inflammatory transcription factor Nrf2, and acting as a succinate dehydrogenase (SDH) inhibitor leading to reduced reactive oxygen species (ROS) production and reduced IL-12, IL-1β, and IL-6 levels (153, 154). Given that gram-negative pulmonary bacteria express high levels of LPS the induction of itaconate could be a novel method used by these bacteria during chronic infection to reduce inflammatory responses of macrophages. However, itaconate itself has been shown to have antimicrobial effects by inhibiting bacterial isocitrate lyases (ICLs), enzymes involved in bacterial metabolism of fatty acids, needed for intracellular survival for many bacteria (155). *Yersinia pestis* and *Pseudomonas aeruginosa* carry genes encoding enzymes which degrade itaconate (156). This indicates that there is a complex relationship between itaconate and bacteria, and this metabolite may play different roles during acute and chronic infection. Significant work is still needed to dissect the pathways involved in itaconate's impact during pulmonary infection.

Considering the metabolic pathways that pathogens are targeting to promote immunosuppression in the host lung could potentially reveal novel targets which would improve our ability to understand and treat a wide range of infections.

It is evident the targeting of key metabolic pathways, the expansion of regulatory immune cell populations and enhanced production of associated cytokines is an advantageous method of promoting bacterial survival within the lung. Many bacterial species which invade the lung possess a multitude of methods to skew local host immune responses toward an immunosuppressive state, enabling unperturbed survival within this tissue.

TARGETING IMMUNOSUPPRESSIVE MANIPULATION: A POTENTIAL THERAPEUTIC OPTION TO TREAT PULMONARY INFECTIONS

An improved understanding of the strategies employed by bacteria to subvert immunosuppression in the lung could open up new avenues for much needed therapeutic development. The development of HDTs represents an attractive approach that could be used as adjunct therapies to complement current antibiotics (157). By targeting the immunosuppressive responses hijacked by many pulmonary bacteria, key evasion methods are removed, allowing a more appropriate inflammatory immune response to ensue and effectively clear the infection.

Small Molecule Inhibitors-Targeting Anti-Inflammatory Responses

IL-10 Signaling

Targeting the signaling pathways of immunosuppressive cytokines using small molecule inhibitors is an effective way to dampen down their excessive inhibitory effects. In a murine model of chronic *M. tuberculosis* infection, targeting the IL-10-STAT3 signaling pathway using an aerosolized peptide inhibitor of STAT3 led to enhanced nitric oxide synthase (NOS) and NADPH oxidase activity in conjunction with reduced arginase activity in lung homogenates, resulting in improved bacterial clearance (158). In previous studies it was shown that STAT3 signaling not only increases IL-10 production but also represses NOS in human macrophages during *M. tuberculosis* infection leading to impaired T cell responses (159, 160). This study demonstrated that even without the use of antibiotics the bacterial load in the lungs could be significantly reduced using small molecule inhibitors directed against the host immune response. Similarly, the use of a selective small molecule inhibitor of IL-10Ra in a chronic *M. tuberculosis* model led to increases in lysozyme activity in the lung resulting in reduced CFUs (158). The enhanced pro-inflammatory response seen upon IL-10 blockade is likely to be partially caused by the return of normal phagosomal maturation in innate cells such as AMs. Preventing phagosomal maturation within AMs that had engulfed *M. tuberculosis* was central to bacterial intracellular survival and IL-10 blocking allowed normal maturation to occur leading to bacterial degradation and enhanced clearance of the mycobacterium (96).

Bruton's tyrosine kinase (BTK) inhibitors which are approved for treatment of B cell lymphomas have the capacity to block both BCR signaling and STAT3 activation and are capable of reducing IL-10 production and PD-L1 expression in B cells (161). The use of these inhibitors to specifically target Breg cells could potentially be used to treat infections such as *M. tuberculosis* which has been shown to subvert Breg responses (85, 89).

TGF-β Signaling

Targeting TGF-β signaling using small molecule inhibitors also holds promise for improving outcomes during pulmonary invasion. *S. pneumoniae* colonization of the nasopharynx is a major pre-requisite for invasive infection and is associated with high TGF-β levels. The administration of a small molecule inhibitor of TGF-β to mice during *S. pneumoniae* colonization enhanced neutrophil influx into the nasopharynx aiding in a profound reduction in the levels of bacterial carriage compared to control mice (81).

The regulatory cytokines IL-10 and TGF-β are both required for Treg maintenance and function (162, 163), consequently targeting these cytokines can result in the depletion of Treg cells. During *M. tuberculosis* infection inhibition of TGF-β signaling using a small molecule inhibitor which targets the TGFβ type I receptor kinase, ALK5, prevented Smad3 activation leading to reduced Treg cells and enhanced Th1 responses which promoted bacterial clearance (164). These studies demonstrate the potential for transient regulation of Tregs and their associated cytokines in improving mycobacterial clearance. In *in vitro* studies, a synthetic small peptide inhibitor of TGF-β, P17, was shown to inhibit the suppressive activities of Treg cells on effector T cells (165), indicating the potential for P17 to be used to enhance protective effector T cell responses *in vivo* during infection. Interestingly P17 was developed using a phage-displayed random peptide library. It is a useful method for high-throughput screening of protein interactions and helps in identifying bioactive peptides with high affinity ligand-binding (166, 167), a similar approach may lead to the development of small peptide inhibitors against other immunosuppressive cytokines.

Monoclonal Antibodies

Monoclonal antibodies have been in use for over four decades to treat a wide variety of human pathologies, and have revolutionized anti-cancer therapeutics (168), where these antibodies are used to target the anti-inflammatory arm of the host immune system in an attempt to promote anti-tumor immune responses. The use of monoclonal antibodies has also been investigated as method to treat infectious disease.

Blocking Immunosuppressive Cytokine Activities

In an experimental model of chronic tuberculosis infection, a monoclonal antibody targeting IL-10R was administered 90 days into the infection, as this time point was before loss of control of infection and when IL-10 levels peaked in this model, and weekly thereafter. Administration of the anti-IL-10Ra antibody led to increased numbers of $CD4^+$ and $CD8^+$ T cells infiltrating the lung and enhanced production of IFN-γ which was associated with a large reduction in bacterial burden (169). Similarly targeting TGF-β during chronic *M. tuberculosis* infection may improve effector T cell responses. *In vitro* studies using PBMCs from tuberculosis patients treated with an anti-TGF-β antibody led to reduced bacterial growth and increased IFN-γ production by these cells (170, 171). There may be a potential treatment benefit from blocking the biological functions of IL-27 in the lung post-sepsis. Cao et al. found that IL-27 regulated the increased susceptibility to secondary *P. aeruginosa* pneumonia in septic mice and promoted bacterial survival (138). During sepsis patients mount a massive inflammatory response initially. However, most patients survive the initial hyper-inflammatory period and enter into an immunosuppressed state where the individual is likely to contract and succumb to a secondary pulmonary infection (172). The inhibition of IL-27 alongside antibiotic treatment may improve survival rates. In a murine model of post-influenza secondary pneumococcal pneumonia the neutralization of IL-27 using an anti-IL-27 antibody was protective. The absence of IL-27 led to a restoration of IL-17 production from protective γδ T cells which were critical for orchestrating bacterial clearance (173).

Blocking Immunosuppressive Cells

Monoclonal antibodies have of course been used with much success to deplete specific immunosuppressive cell populations. One of the biggest success stories of monoclonal therapy is the development of immune checkpoint inhibitors for cancer immunotherapy. These antibodies target key immune regulating surface molecules on cells such as Tregs and MDSCs to impede their anti-inflammatory effects allowing for enhanced pro-inflammatory responses (174). Checkpoint inhibitor therapies in the context of treatment for pulmonary bacterial infections will be discussed in more detail below.

Checkpoint Inhibitors—Targeting Immunosuppressive Cells

Checkpoint inhibitors (CPIs) which restore pro-inflammatory T cell function have been shown to prolong survival in cancer patients with various malignancies (175, 176). CTLA-4 is constitutively expressed on Treg cells and was the first immune checkpoint protein shown to inhibit T cell proliferation (177). Following on from this other immune checkpoint mechanisms such as PDL1-PD1 interactions were identified as potential targets (176). As of 2018 six immune checkpoint inhibitors have been approved for the treatment of advanced and metastatic cancers such as advanced gastric adenocarcinoma and metastatic melanoma (178).

During an infection pathogens wish to evade detection just like cancer cells and evidence suggests that these immune checkpoint pathways may also play an important role during infection to promote regulatory immune responses (175). During active tuberculosis infection there is an increase in both CTLA-4 and PD-1 on the surface of T cells and an increase in PDL-1 expression on APCs from these patients, leading to the reduced activation of an appropriate adaptive response (179). It was shown *in vitro* that blocking PD-1 using a checkpoint inhibitor led to improved *M. tuberculosis*-specific IFN-γ^+ T cell responses (180). The blocking restored effector T cell function and reduced rates of apoptosis in these T cells (179, 180). Conflicting results were seen in PD-1 knockout mice, which had reduced survival when infected with *M. tuberculosis* (181), suggesting a possible protective role. However, it is likely complete ablation of PD-1 from the system results in an excessive inflammatory response which limits survival. During the course of *M. tuberculosis* infection there is an upregulation of PD-1. It is possible that long-term disease results in its overexpression causing the dampening of protective inflammatory immune responses (179). The short term inhibition of PD-1 during infection could improve pro-inflammatory responses while reducing the likelihood of hyper-inflammation seen in the PD-1 knockout mice. Clinical trials have been carried out using CPIs in the treatment of viral infections such as Human immunodeficiency virus (HIV) infection (182). A phase II clinical trial using anti-PD-L1 alongside anti-retroviral therapy (ART) in HIV patients was stopped early due to retinal toxicity observed in a simultaneous macaque study (183). However, two of the six patients involved in the trial showed increased antigen-specific CD4$^+$ and CD8$^+$ T cells indicating the potential for CPIs to enhance effector T cell responses during infection.

The blockade of checkpoint molecules can lead to immune-related adverse effects as these molecules are also involved in regulating immune tolerance to prevent immunopathology and autoimmunity (175). These monoclonal antibodies are used in severe cases of cancer, therefore concerns still remain over their use for infection. Further research is critical into the efficacy of CPIs as potential therapies for improving various pulmonary infection outcomes.

Targeting Metabolic Changes Induced During Infection

Metabolic reprogramming is recognized as a hallmark of cancer (184, 185) and targeting metabolic pathways has been used for the treatment of various cancers to interfere with tumor progression (184, 186). During bacterial infections of the lung the metabolic pathways of many immune cells are re-programmed to a more immunosuppressive phenotype, benefitting the bacteria and leading to chronic infection. Targeting these pathways to reverse this reprogramming has the potential to promote more pro-inflammatory responses and improve bacterial clearance.

Targeting Fatty Acid Oxidation

In murine tumor models it has been shown that tumor infiltrating MDSCs increased their fatty acid uptake and increased fatty acid oxidation (FAO) (187). Blocking FAO using the inhibitor Etomoxir, a carnitine palmitoyltransferase-1 (CPT-1) inhibitor which prevents fatty acid transport into the mitochondria for further metabolism, reduced the immunosuppressive effects of these cells leading to reductions in Treg numbers, enhanced effector T cell proliferation, and IFN-γ production which delayed tumor growth (187). FAO inhibition could also be used to directly reduce the number of Treg cells as FAO has been shown to be central to the differentiation of Treg cells (188). FAO inhibition could be an innovative approach to reduce the anti-inflammatory effects of both MDSCs and Tregs during pulmonary infection to improve bacterial clearance and current antibiotic treatments. However, it should be noted that CD8$^+$ memory T cell also use FAO as an energy source (189), the inhibition of FAO could have implications for these cells resulting in defective memory responses which could have negative impacts on infection responses.

Skewing Macrophage Phenotypes

The targeting of metabolic pathways in macrophages could also be potentially used as a therapeutic approach during pulmonary bacterial infection to skew macrophages toward a more protective M1 phenotype. Itaconate promotes macrophage switching from a pro- to an anti-inflammatory state and the metabolite is emerging as a crucial determinant in macrophage activity (190). The inhibition of itaconate may be of benefit in chronic bacterial lung infection where enhanced M1 responses could improve bacterial clearance. Irg1 signaling regulates itaconate production, the blocking of Irg1 may be a method of reducing itaconate to promote succinate dehydrogenase (SDH) activity enabling M1 responses against invading bacteria and impairing their ability to alter macrophage phenotypes to an M2 state. In a murine model of *M. tuberculosis* using Irg1$^{-/-}$ mice that do not produce itaconate, the mice exhibited an increase in neutrophil influx and pro-inflammatory cytokine production compared to WT mice (191). However, these mice succumbed due to immunopathology of excessive inflammation. It needs to be established if targeting Irg1/itaconate in a specific cell population only could prevent immunopathology.

Targeting Immunosuppressive Responses Using RNA Interference

RNA interference is a method of gene silencing mediated through the use of small interfering RNA (siRNA) or microRNA (miRNA). Studies using siRNA demonstrate how the immune response can be modified into a more pro-inflammatory phenotype during chronic *M. tuberculosis* infection (192). In mice chronically infected with *M. tuberculosis* the intrapulmonary administration of siRNA that specifically targets TGF-β leads to reduced bacterial load in the lungs and increased production of pro-inflammatory cytokines such as TNF (192). The silencing of the *tgfb1* gene directly in the lungs improves the antimicrobial capacity of the host.

Another promising method of RNA interference during bacterial infection is the use of miRNAs. The silencing of certain regulatory miRNA have the potential to improve bacterial clearance by promoting pro-inflammatory immune cell responses. The inhibition of miR-328 could improve bacterial clearance during a non-typeable *H. influenzae* (NTHi) infection (193). *In vitro* studies using murine macrophages and neutrophils demonstrated miR-328 inhibition using an antagomir of miR-328 prior to NTHi infection promoted enhanced phagocytosis, increased ROS production and improved bacterial killing in both cell types. Further *in vivo* studies found boosting miR-328 downregulation by intra-tracheal administration of the miR-328 inhibitor enhanced bacterial killing rates (193). This method of miR-328 inhibition could potentially be used during chronic pulmonary infection to remove bacterial-induced immunosuppression in innate cells such as macrophages. The use of RNA interference in the treatment of infection is an area of ongoing research.

Repurposing Chemotherapeutic Drugs to Target Immunosuppressive Responses

The repurposing of chemotherapeutic drugs developed for other diseases is an avenue of research being investigated to target regulatory immune cells induced locally during lung infection.

Targeting MDSCs

Chemotherapeutic drugs that target MDSCs could potentially be used in combination with standard antibiotic treatments to improve the immune response against chronic pulmonary bacterial infections. All-trans retinoic acid (ATRA) is an approved anti-cancer treatment, which leads to the maturation-induced ablation of MDSCs that often infiltrate tumors (194, 195). Ablation of MDSCs in a murine model of tuberculosis was carried out using ATRA treatment (196). Mice that were administered ATRA after tuberculosis infection had reduced numbers of MDSCs in their lungs, lower bacterial loads and improved effector T cell numbers (196). Sorafenib is an immunotherapeutic anti-tumor drug used against hepatocellular carcinoma (197). Sorafenib downregulates the MDSC population to promote a more pro-inflammatory anti-tumor environment (197). Drugs such as Sorafenib could potentially be used to reduce MDSCs during pulmonary infections.

Targeting Tregs

Elevated Treg levels have been associated with poor prognosis in certain types of cancer (177). Many anti-cancer therapies, such as checkpoint inhibitors mentioned earlier target Treg cells to improve outcomes in advanced cancers (178). A common chemotherapeutic used against glioblastoma is temozolimide (TMZ). In a rat glioma model, low doses of TMZ selectively inhibited the activity of Treg cells (198). In humans with advanced chemotherapy resistant cancers low iterative oral doses of cyclophosphamide resulted in a selective reduction of circulating Treg cells (199) while other T cell subset numbers and functions were preserved. It would be interesting to determine if low doses of TMZ administered to the airways during pulmonary infection could have a similar effect, selectively depleting Tregs thus promoting more pro-inflammatory responses and potentially improving rates of bacterial clearance.

The anti-cancer drug denileukin diftitox (DD) is used to treat cutaneous T cell lymphomas (200, 201). The drug is a synthetic protein that combines IL-2 and Diphtheria toxin, which acts by binding the IL-2R and delivering the diphtheria toxin to the cell resulting in cell death (201). In a murine model of tuberculosis, DD treatment during infection depleted both Treg cells and MDSCs from the lung of infected mice leading to improved bacterial clearance compared to an untreated group (202). Further investigation into the use of DD in the treatment of other chronic pulmonary bacterial infections is needed to test its efficacy. However, DD treatment is associated with adverse effects such as capillary leak syndrome, hypoalbuminemia, and visual changes which have obvious implications for the use of this treatment for infection.

The repurposing of cancer chemotherapeutics is advantageous as many of these drugs have already gone through testing, have known pharmacological properties and have reduced costs and development times compared with the production of novel antimicrobial drugs. However, because the use of chemotherapeutics to deplete immunosuppressive cell populations have the risk of promoting excessive inflammation and autoimmunity, these treatments should be approached with great caution and intensive safety testing is needed to investigate the off-target effects they may have during infection.

The ability of many lung-associated bacterial pathogens to induce immunosuppression to promote their survival can potentially be ablated by a number of HDTs targeting various aspects of the local regulatory host immune response such as regulatory cell populations, anti-inflammatory cytokines and associated metabolic signaling pathways (**Figure 2**). Combining various methods could potentially be used to improve pulmonary infection outcomes without relying on antibiotic use. The use of drugs targeting key metabolic pathways such as FAO and cellular interactions such as checkpoint molecules could drastically reduce the ability of bacterial pathogens to promote local immunosuppressive responses thus boosting protective inflammatory responses and associated bacterial elimination. The repurposing of drugs such as anti-cancer chemotherapeutics could therefore open up novel treatment options for bacterial clearance from the lung and improve MDR infections.

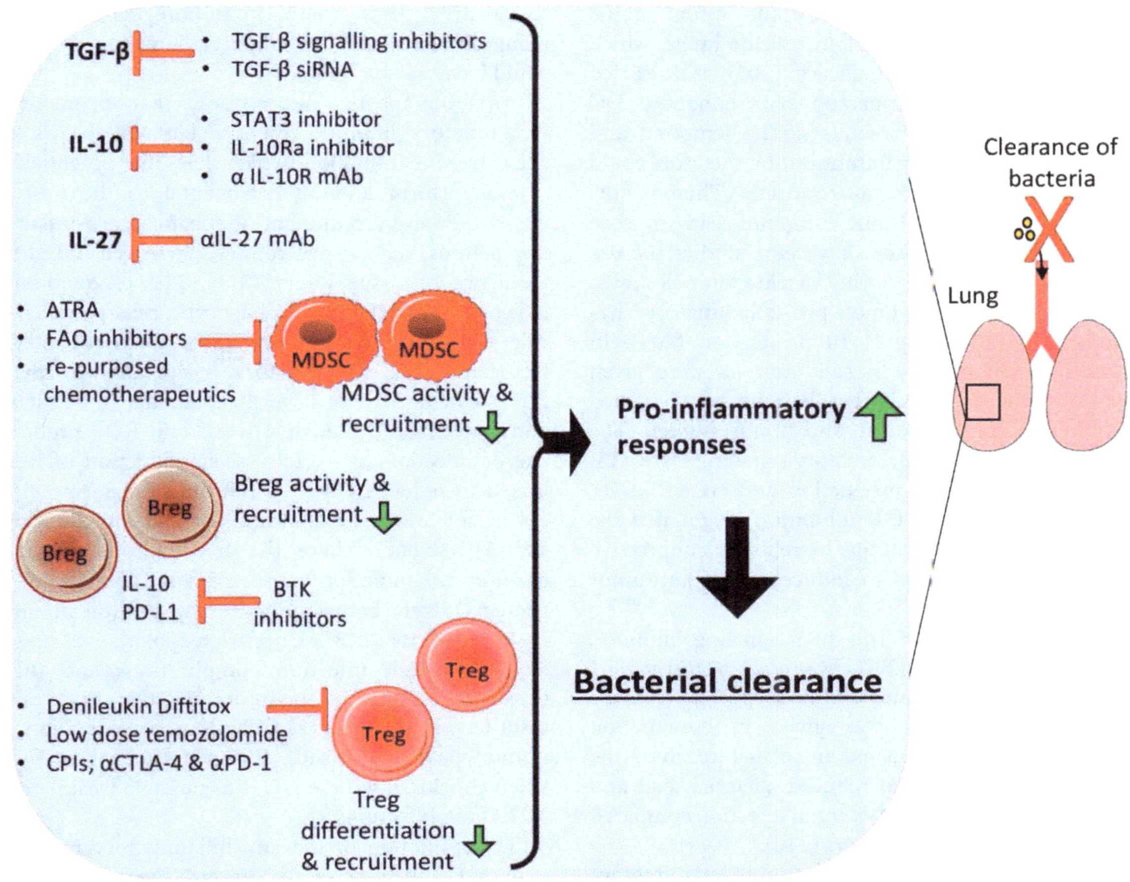

FIGURE 2 | Host-directed therapies targeting immunosuppressive responses in the lung lead to bacterial clearance. Host-directed therapies (HDTs) that target anti-inflammatory immune responses in the host lung can improve bacterial clearance and reduce chronic infection. Small molecule inhibitors of cytokine signaling pathways, monoclonal antibodies or siRNA could be used to reduce the levels of anti-inflammatory cytokines such as IL-10, TGF-β and IL-27, allowing higher pro-inflammatory cytokine production and reduced activation and expansion of anti-inflammatory cell populations. HDTs targeting specific anti-inflammatory cells could also improve infection outcome by depleting these cell populations.

TARGETING IMMUNOSUPPRESSIVE RESPONSES TO IMPROVE VACCINE EFFICACY

HDTs that specifically target the immunosuppressive arm of the pulmonary immune system during bacterial infection have the potential to undo the detrimental anti-inflammatory responses induced by bacteria, and "re-inform" the local immune response to react in a more inflammatory manner. It is possible that similar strategies could be implemented to potentially improve vaccine function by altering the immune microenvironment in which the vaccine is administered.

The BCG vaccine is currently the only available prophylactic vaccine against *M. tuberculosis*. In response to BCG vaccination there is an expansion of Treg cells and an increase in the production of IL-10 alongside the expansion of Th1 responses (203). This is likely contributing to the lack of efficacy of the BCG vaccine against pulmonary TB. In vaccination studies using IL-10 KO mice it was demonstrated that KO mice vaccinated with the BCG vaccine had enhanced DC activation and Th1 responses compared to vaccinated wild-type mice (204). DCs isolated from vaccinated IL-10 KO mice co-cultured with $CD4^+$ T cells induced significantly higher levels of IFN-γ production compared to when DCs from vaccinated WT mice were used, indicating IL-10 was suppressing these protective inflammatory responses (204). This demonstrated that IL-10 signaling was contributing to the DC dysfunction in BCG vaccination impairing these cells abilities to promote inflammatory T cell responses. Other studies showed that mice treated with IL-10R neutralizing antibodies during BCG vaccination were better protected against subsequent *M. tuberculosis* infection compared to mice who were not pre-treated with the antibody. This was due to enhanced antigen-specific IFN-γ and IL-17A responses (205, 206). These studies illustrate the potential for controlled short-term regulation of IL-10 during vaccination to establish better T cell-mediated immunity and improve vaccine efficacy.

Wu et al. demonstrated that the BCG strain of mycobacterium used in the vaccine can actually induce transcription of the immunoregulatory microRNA miR-21 in murine lungs, which may also contribute to vaccine inefficacy (207). miR-21 led to reduced IL-12 expression in macrophages, enhanced DC apoptosis, and suppressed Th1 responses. The temporal and specific blocking of miR-21 during immunization therefore could potentially improve anti-*M. tuberculosis* vaccines. There is now a growing interest in using anti-miR compounds to improve disease outcomes (208). In anti-cancer vaccine studies the use of small molecule PI3K inhibitors during vaccination was shown to improve vaccine efficacy and promote pro-inflammatory Th1-skewed responses by preventing IL-10 production (209). In a murine cancer model mice with solid tumors were given a DC vaccine consisting of DCs that had been pre-treated with a PI3K inhibitor, TLR5 agonist, and tumor antigen. The PI3K inhibitor prevented anti-inflammatory signaling from TLR activation which reduced IL-10 production and enhanced IL-12 production from the DCs. PI3K inhibition heightened the antitumor properties of the DC vaccine by relieving suppressive signals that restrict DCs abilities to induce potent antitumor T-cell responses.

The administration of an anti-TGF-βR1 signaling inhibitor, D4476, 24 h post-vaccination with BCG improved protective Th1 immune responses against subsequent pulmonary *M. tuberculosis* infection (210). This inhibitor was given in conjunction with a Th2 cell inhibitor. Vaccinated mice that received the immunomodulatory inhibitors had reduced bacterial load and better IFN-γ^+ T memory cell responses upon infection compared to mice that did not receive the inhibitors (210).

These studies indicate the inhibition of the anti-inflammatory arm of the immune response during vaccination may have the potential to improve vaccine efficacy. This method of inhibition could be used to improve current vaccines against pulmonary bacteria that exploit the anti-inflammatory immune response during infection, ensuring more pro-inflammatory responses upon exposure. Further research is needed into methods of suppressing particular cells and cytokines of the regulatory pulmonary immune response to improve vaccine outcomes against infectious disease.

CONCLUSION AND FUTURE PERSPECTIVES

The increasing incidence of multidrug resistance in pathogenic bacteria and the slow pace of novel antibiotic development threatens our ability to treat these bacterial infections effectively. Bacterial lung infections are a major concern as any damage to the lung dramatically impacts the overall health and survival of a patient. Host-directed therapeutic strategies targeting bacterial-induced anti-inflammatory immune responses must be considered as viable adjuncts to standard antimicrobial treatment. Additionally, there is the potential for targeting immunosuppression to improve vaccine efficacy for current and next-generation vaccines targeting bacterial species. However, there are challenges in bringing these new approaches to the clinic. A better understanding of the host-bacterial interaction during pulmonary infection is needed, in order to identify how these immunoregulatory responses are being induced and the impacts dampening these responses could have.

Any therapeutic intervention that promotes the pro-inflammatory immune response has a high risk of inducing excessive inflammation which has the potential to lead to cytokine storm and be detrimental to the host (157). The promotion and recruitment of enhanced pro-inflammatory cell populations, such as neutrophils, have been linked to increased incidence of tissue injury (211). The production of reactive oxygen species (ROS) by phagocytic cells plays a fundamental role in the removal of pathogens from the host. However, the dampening of regulatory responses through the use of HDTs discussed here have the potential to result in excessive and uncontrolled oxidative stress and ROS production at the site of infection (211). Excessive production of ROS has been linked to reduced CD8$^+$ T cell function during viral infection (212), and impaired immune responses in the lungs of cystic fibrosis patients where the free radicals generated during chronic inflammation cause oxidative damage of pulmonary proteins, likely contributing to the decline of lung function in CF patients (213). Unrestricted oxidative stress has been associated with infection complications and the induction of diseases such as neurodegenerative and cardiovascular disorders, and cancer (214). Serious consideration of potential immunopathological side effects must be taken into account when considering these HDTs as possible treatment options for MDR lung infections.

The inhibition of the anti-inflammatory response must be temporal and precise to prevent these hyper-inflammatory responses and off-target effects. By gaining a greater understanding of the immunoregulatory mechanisms being hijacked by pulmonary bacteria we may be able to better tailor antibacterial therapies to avoid off-target consequences. The optimal timing of when to administer these HDTs needs to be elucidated, meaning we need further investigation into how and when pulmonary bacteria are inducing these anti-inflammatory responses in order to target them at the correct point of infection. Improving delivery of anti-inflammatory inhibitors may reduce their off-target effects and could limit inhibition to certain target cells. The use of β-glucan nanoparticles, for example could be used to specifically target macrophages (215). These nanoparticles can encapsulate small molecule inhibitors or siRNA to improve their delivery into cells. The β-glucan outer shell promotes receptor-mediated uptake by phagocytic cells that express β-glucan receptors (215). This approach could be used to specifically deliver HDTs into macrophages in the lung to inhibit early immunosuppressive responses.

The study and development of novel HDTs against pathogen-induced anti-inflammatory immune responses during pulmonary infection represents a method of strategically modifying the immune response to improve current treatments and vaccine efficacy against many multidrug-resistant bacteria. In this era of re-emerging infectious diseases as a consequence of increases in antimicrobial resistance, the development of alternative antimicrobial strategies is imperative to tackle this major healthcare challenge.

AUTHOR CONTRIBUTIONS

AK and RM conceived the idea for the manuscript. AK drafted the manuscript. RM edited and added the valuable insights into the manuscript.

REFERENCES

1. Ho J, Ip M. Antibiotic-resistant community-acquired bacterial pneumonia. *Infect Dis Clin North Am.* (2019) 33:1087–103. doi: 10.1016/j.idc.2019.07.002
2. Tacconelli EN, Magrini G, Kahlmeter NS. *Global Priority List of Antibiotic-Resistant Bacteria to Guide Research, Discovery, and Development of New Antibiotics.* World Health Organization 27, 318–327. Available online at: https://www.who.int/medicines/publications/WHO-PPL-Short_Summary_25Feb-ET_NM_WHO.pdf
3. Chopra I, Hesse L, ONeill AJ. Exploiting current understanding of antibiotic action for discovery of new drugs. *J Appl Microbiol.* (2002) 92(Suppl):4S–15S. doi: 10.1046/j.1365-2672.92.5s1.13.x
4. Lloyd CM, Marsland BJ. Lung homeostasis: influence of age, microbes, and the immune system. *Immunity.* (2017) 46:549–61. doi: 10.1016/j.immuni.2017.04.005
5. Gordon SB, Read RC. Macrophage defences against respiratory tract infections. *Br Med Bull.* (2002) 61:45–61. doi: 10.1093/bmb/61.1.45
6. Guilliams M, Lambrecht BN, Hamida J. Division of labor between lung dendritic cells and macrophages in the defense against pulmonary infections. *J Mucosal immunology Hammad.* (2013) 6:464. doi: 10.1038/mi.2013.14
7. Ziltener P, Reinheckel T, Oxenius A. Neutrophil and alveolar macrophage-mediated innate immune control of legionella pneumophila lung infection via TNF and ROS. *PLoS Pathog.* (2016) 12:e1005591. doi: 10.1371/journal.ppat.1005591
8. Sertl K, Takemura T, Tschachler E, Ferrans VJ, Kaliner MA, Shevach EM. Dendritic cells with antigen-presenting capability reside in airway epithelium, lung parenchyma, and visceral pleura. *J Exp Med.* (1986) 163:436–51. doi: 10.1084/jem.163.2.436
9. Sung SS, Fu SM, Rose CE, Gaskin F, Ju ST, Beaty SR. A major lung CD103 (alphaE)-beta7 integrin-positive epithelial dendritic cell population expressing Langerin and tight junction proteins. *J Immunol.* (2006) 176:2161–72. doi: 10.4049/jimmunol.176.4.2161
10. Brinkmann V, Reichard U, Goosmann C, Fauler B, Uhlemann Y, Weiss DS, et al. Neutrophil extracellular traps kill bacteria. *Science.* (2004) 303:1532–5. doi: 10.1126/science.1092385
11. Brinkmann V, Zychlinsky A. Beneficial suicide: why neutrophils die to make NETs. *Nat Rev Microbiol.* (2007) 5:577–82. doi: 10.1038/nrmicro1710
12. Culley FJ. Natural killer cells in infection and inflammation of the lung. *Immunology.* (2009) 128:151–63. doi: 10.1111/j.1365-2567.2009.03167.x
13. Cong J, Wei H. Natural killer cells in the lungs. *Front Immunol.* (2019) 10:1416. doi: 10.3389/fimmu.2019.01416
14. Lai HC, Chang CJ, Lin CS, Wu TR, Hsu YJ, Wu TS, et al. NK cell-derived ifn-gamma protects against nontuberculous mycobacterial lung infection. *J Immunol.* (2018) 201:1478–90. doi: 10.4049/jimmunol.1800123
15. Van Maele L, Carnoy C, Cayet D, Ivanov S, Porte R, Deruy E, et al. Activation of Type 3 innate lymphoid cells and interleukin 22 secretion in the lungs during *Streptococcus pneumoniae* infection. *J Infect Dis.* (2014) 210:493–503. doi: 10.1093/infdis/jiu106
16. Xiong H, Keith JW, Samilo DW, Carter RA, Leiner IM, Pamer EG. Innate lymphocyte/Ly6C(hi) monocyte crosstalk promotes *Klebsiella pneumoniae* clearance. *Cell.* (2016) 165:679–89. doi: 10.1016/j.cell.2016.03.017
17. Cheng H, Jin C, Wu J, Zhu S, Liu YJ, Chen J. Guards at the gate: physiological and pathological roles of tissue-resident innate lymphoid cells in the lung. *Protein Cell.* (2017) 8:878–95. doi: 10.1007/s13238-017-0379-5
18. Nieuwenhuis EE, Matsumoto T, Exley M, Schleipman RA, Glickman J, Bailey DT, et al. CD1d-dependent macrophage-mediated clearance of *Pseudomonas aeruginosa* from lung. *Nat Med.* (2002) 8:588–93. doi: 10.1038/nm0602-588
19. Michel ML, Keller AC, Paget C, Fujio M, Trottein F, Savage PB, et al. Identification of an IL-17-producing NK1.1(neg) iNKT cell population involved in airway neutrophilia. *J Exp Med.* (2007) 204:995–1001. doi: 10.1084/jem.20061551
20. Paget C, Trottein F. Role of type 1 natural killer T cells in pulmonary immunity. *Mucosal Immunol.* (2013) 6:1054–67. doi: 10.1038/mi.2013.59
21. Crosby CM, Zbigniew M, Kronenberg M. NKT cell subsets involved in host defense from pulmonary *Streptococcus pneumoniae* infection. *Am Assoc Immnol.* (2017) 198(1 Supplement)131.24.
22. Le Bourhis L, Martin E, Peguillet I, Guihot A, Froux N, Core M, et al. Antimicrobial activity of mucosal-associated invariant T cells. *Nat Immunol.* (2010) 11:701–8. doi: 10.1038/ni.1890
23. Hartmann N, Harriff MJ, McMurtrey CP, Hildebrand WH, Lewinsohn DM, Kronenberg M. Role of MAIT cells in pulmonary bacterial infection. *Mol Immunol.* (2018) 101:155–9. doi: 10.1016/j.molimm.2018.06.270
24. Trottein F, Christophe J. Natural killer T cells and mucosal-associated invariant T cells in lung infections. *Front Immunol Paget.* (2018) 9:1750. doi: 10.3389/fimmu.2018.01750
25. Cheng M, Hu S. Lung-resident gammadelta T cells and their roles in lung diseases. *Immunology.* (2017) 151:375–84. doi: 10.1111/imm.12764
26. Simonian PL, Roark CL, Wehrmann F, Lanham AM, Born WK, OBrien RL, et al. IL-17A-expressing T cells are essential for bacterial clearance in a murine model of hypersensitivity pneumonitis. *J Immunol.* (2009) 182:6540–9. doi: 10.4049/jimmunol.0900013
27. Ross PJ, Sutton CE, Higgins S, Allen AC, Walsh K, Misiak A, et al. Relative contribution of Th1 and Th17 cells in adaptive immunity to *Bordetella pertussis*: towards the rational design of an improved acellular pertussis vaccine. *PLoS Pathog.* (2013) 9:e1003264. doi: 10.1371/journal.ppat.1003264
28. Mills KH, Barnard A, Watkins J, Redhead K. Cell-mediated immunity to *Bordetella pertussis*: role of Th1 cells in bacterial clearance in a murine respiratory infection model. *Infect Immun.* (1993) 61:399–410. doi: 10.1128/IAI.61.2.399-410.1993
29. Chen K, McAleer JP, Lin Y, Paterson DL, Zheng M, Alcorn JF, et al. Th17 cells mediate clade-specific, serotype-independent mucosal immunity. *Immunity.* (2011) 35:997–1009. doi: 10.1016/j.immuni.2011.10.018
30. Chen K, Kolls JK. T cell-mediated host immune defenses in the lung. *Annu Rev Immunol.* (2013) 31:605–33. doi: 10.1146/annurev-immunol-032712-100019
31. Valeri M, Raffatellu M. Cytokines IL-17 and IL-22 in the host response to infection. *Pathog Dis.* (2016) 74:ftw111. doi: 10.1093/femspd/ftw111
32. Woodworth JS, Behar SM. *Mycobacterium tuberculosis*-specific CD8+ T cells and their role in immunity. *Crit Rev Immunol.* (2006) 26:317–52. doi: 10.1615/CritRevImmunol.v26.i4.30
33. Weber SE, Tian H, Pirofski LA. CD8+ cells enhance resistance to pulmonary serotype 3 *Streptococcus pneumoniae* infection in mice. *J Immunol.* (2011) 186:432–42. doi: 10.4049/jimmunol.1001963
34. Prezzemolo T, Guggino G, La Manna MP, Di Liberto D, Dieli F, Caccamo N. Functional signatures of human CD4 and CD8 T cell responses to *Mycobacterium tuberculosis*. *Front Immunol.* (2014) 5:180. doi: 10.3389/fimmu.2014.00180
35. Levy BD, Serhan CN. Resolution of acute inflammation in the lung. *Annu Rev Physiol.* (2014) 76:467–92. doi: 10.1146/annurev-physiol-021113-170408
36. Moldoveanu B, Otmishi P, Jani P, Walker J, Sarmiento X, Guardiola J, et al. Inflammatory mechanisms in the lung. *J Inflamm Res.* (2009) 2:1–11. doi: 10.2147/JIR.S4385

37. de Heer HJ, Hammad H, Soullie T, Hijdra D, Vos N, Willart MA, et al. Essential role of lung plasmacytoid dendritic cells in preventing asthmatic reactions to harmless inhaled antigen. *J Exp Med.* (2004) 200:89–98. doi: 10.1084/jem.20040035
38. Strickland DH, Stumbles PA, Zosky GR, Subrata LS, Thomas JA, Turner DJ, et al. Reversal of airway hyperresponsiveness by induction of airway mucosal CD4+CD25+ regulatory T cells. *J Exp Med.* (2006) 203:2649–60. doi: 10.1084/jem.20060155
39. Hintzen G, Ohl L, del Rio ML, Rodriguez-Barbosa JI, Pabst O, Kocks JR, et al. Induction of tolerance to innocuous inhaled antigen relies on a CCR7-dependent dendritic cell-mediated antigen transport to the bronchial lymph node. *J Immunol.* (2006) 177:7346–54. doi: 10.4049/jimmunol.177.10.7346
40. Lo B, Hansen S, Evans K, Heath JK, Wright JR. Alveolar epithelial type II cells induce T cell tolerance to specific antigen. *J Immunol.* (2008) 180:881–8. doi: 10.4049/jimmunol.180.2.881
41. Branchett WJ, Lloyd CM. Regulatory cytokine function in the respiratory tract. *Mucosal Immunol.* (2019) 12:589–600. doi: 10.1038/s41385-019-0158-0
42. Dai YC, Zhong J, Xu JF. Regulatory B cells in infectious disease (Review). *Mol Med Rep.* (2017) 16:3–10. doi: 10.3892/mmr.2017.6605
43. Denney L, Byrne AJ, Shea TJ, Buckley JS, Pease JE, Herledan GM, et al. Pulmonary epithelial cell-derived cytokine tgf-beta1 is a critical cofactor for enhanced innate lymphoid cell function. *Immunity.* (2015) 43:945–58. doi: 10.1016/j.immuni.2015.10.012
44. Li MO, Richard A. TGF-β: a master of all T cell trades. *J Cell Flavell.* (2008) 134:392–404. doi: 10.1016/j.cell.2008.07.025
45. Travis MA, Sheppard D. TGF-beta activation and function in immunity. *Annu Rev Immunol.* (2014) 32:51–82. doi: 10.1146/annurev-immunol-032713-120257
46. Fiorentino DF, Zlotnik A, Mosmann T, Howard RM, OGarra A. IL-10 inhibits cytokine production by activated macrophages. *J Immunol.* (1991) 147:3815–22.
47. Macatonia SE, Doherty TM, Knight SC, OGarra A. Differential effect of IL-10 on dendritic cell-induced T cell proliferation and IFN-gamma production. *J Immunol.* (1993) 150:3755–65.
48. Allard B, Panariti A, Martin JG. Alveolar macrophages in the resolution of inflammation, tissue repair, and tolerance to infection. *Front Immunol.* (2018) 9:1777. doi: 10.3389/fimmu.2018.01777
49. Rajaram MV, Brooks MN, Morris JD, Torrelles JB, Azad AK, Schlesinger LS. *Mycobacterium tuberculosis* activates human macrophage peroxisome proliferator-activated receptor gamma linking mannose receptor recognition to regulation of immune responses. *J Immunol.* (2010) 185:929–42. doi: 10.4049/jimmunol.1000866
50. El Kasmi KC, Qualls JE, Pesce JT, Smith AM, Thompson RW, Henao-Tamayo M, et al. Toll-like receptor-induced arginase 1 in macrophages thwarts effective immunity against intracellular pathogens. *Nat Immunol.* (2008) 9:1399–406. doi: 10.1038/ni.1671
51. Valdez HA, Oviedo JM, Gorgojo JP, Lamberti Y, Rodriguez ME. *Bordetella pertussis* modulates human macrophage defense gene expression. *Pathog Dis.* (2016) 74:ftw073. doi: 10.1093/femspd/ftw073
52. Wilson HM. SOCS proteins in macrophage polarization and function. *Front Immunol.* (2014) 5:357. doi: 10.3389/fimmu.2014.00357
53. Ryo A, Suizu F, Yoshida Y, Perrem K, Liou YC, Wulf G, et al. Regulation of NF-kappaB signaling by Pin1-dependent prolyl isomerization and ubiquitin-mediated proteolysis of p65/RelA. *Mol Cell.* (2003) 12:1413–26. doi: 10.1016/S1097-2765(03)00490-8
54. Yoshimura A, Naka T, Kubo M. SOCS proteins, cytokine signalling and immune regulation. *Nat Rev Immunol.* (2007) 7:454–65. doi: 10.1038/nri2093
55. Cook PC, MacDonald AS. Dendritic cells in lung immunopathology. *Semin Immunopathol.* (2016) 38:449–60. doi: 10.1007/s00281-016-0571-3
56. Depaolo RW, Tang F, Kim I, Han M, Levin N, Ciletti N, et al. Toll-like receptor 6 drives differentiation of tolerogenic dendritic cells and contributes to LcrV-mediated plague pathogenesis. *Cell Host Microbe.* (2008) 4:350–61. doi: 10.1016/j.chom.2008.09.004
57. Kim WS, Yoon JH, Shin MK, Shin SJ. Infection of dendritic cells with *Mycobacterium avium* subspecies hominissuis exhibits a functionally tolerogenic phenotype in response to toll-like receptor agonists via IL-10/Cox2/PGE2/EP2 axis. *Front Microbiol.* (2019) 10:1795. doi: 10.3389/fmicb.2019.01795
58. Wickremasinghe M, Ozerovitch LJ, Davies G, Wodehouse T, Chadwick MV, Abdallah S, et al. Non-tuberculous mycobacteria in patients with bronchiectasis. *Thorax.* (2005) 60:1045–51. doi: 10.1136/thx.2005.046631
59. Medina E, Hartl D. Myeloid-derived suppressor cells in infection: a general overview. *J Innate Immun.* (2018) 10:407–13. doi: 10.1159/000489830
60. Gabrilovich DI, Srinivas J. Myeloid-derived suppressor cells as regulators of the immune system. *Nat Rev Immunol.* (2009) 9:162. doi: 10.1038/nri2506
61. Magcwebeba T, Dorhoi A, du Plessis N. The emerging role of myeloid-derived suppressor cells in tuberculosis. *Front Immunol.* (2019) 10:917. doi: 10.3389/fimmu.2019.01528
62. Pawelec G, Chris PV, Suzanne J, Rosenberg O. Myeloid-derived suppressor cells: not only in tumor immunity. *Front Immunol.* (2019) 10:1099. doi: 10.3389/fimmu.2019.01099
63. du Plessis N, Loebenberg L, Kriel MF, Groote-Bidlingmaier V, Ribechini E, Loxton AG, et al. Increased frequency of myeloid-derived suppressor cells during active tuberculosis and after recent *Mycobacterium tuberculosis* infection suppresses T-cell function. *Am J Respir Crit Care Med.* (2013) 188:724–32. doi: 10.1164/rccm.201302-0249OC
64. Agrawal N, Streata I, Pei G, Weiner J, Kotze L, Bandermann S, et al. Human monocytic suppressive cells promote replication of *Mycobacterium tuberculosis* and alter stability of in vitro generated granulomas. *Front Immunol.* (2018) 9:2417. doi: 10.3389/fimmu.2018.02417
65. Ahn D, Penaloza H, Wang Z, Wickersham M, Parker D, Patel P, et al. Acquired resistance to innate immune clearance promotes *Klebsiella pneumoniae* ST258 pulmonary infection. *JCI Insight.* (2016) 1:e89704. doi: 10.1172/jci.insight.89704
66. Periasamy S, Avram D, McCabe A, MacNamara KC, Sellati TJ, Harton JA. An immature myeloid/myeloid-suppressor cell response associated with necrotizing inflammation mediates lethal pulmonary tularemia. *PLoS Pathog.* (2016) 12:e1005517. doi: 10.1371/journal.ppat.1005517
67. Tebartz C, Horst SA, Sparwasser T, Huehn J, Beineke A, Peters G, et al. A major role for myeloid-derived suppressor cells and a minor role for regulatory T cells in immunosuppression during *Staphylococcus aureus* infection. *J Immunol.* (2015) 194:1100–11. doi: 10.4049/jimmunol.1400196
68. Leech JM, Lacey KA, Mulcahy ME, Medina E, McLoughlin RM. IL-10 plays opposing roles during *Staphylococcus aureus* systemic and localized infections. *J Immunol.* (2017) 198:2352–65. doi: 10.4049/jimmunol.1601018
69. Shen H, Chen ZW. The crucial roles of Th17-related cytokines/signal pathways in *M. tuberculosis* infection. *Cell Mol Immunol.* (2018) 15:216–25. doi: 10.1038/cmi.2017.128
70. Lyadova IV, Panteleev AV. Th1 and Th17 cells in tuberculosis: protection, pathology, and biomarkers. *Mediators Inflamm.* (2015) 2015:854507. doi: 10.1155/2015/854507
71. Ferraro A, Buonocore SM, Auquier P, Nicolas I, Wallemacq H, Boutriau D, et al. Role and plasticity of Th1 and Th17 responses in immunity to *Staphylococcus aureus*. *Hum Vaccin Immunother.* (2019) 15:1–13. doi: 10.1080/21645515.2019.1613126
72. Sabbagh P, Karkhah A, Nouri HR, Javanian M, Ebrahimpour S. The significance role of regulatory T cells in the persistence of infections by intracellular bacteria. *Infect Genet Evol.* (2018) 62:270–4. doi: 10.1016/j.meegid.2018.05.001
73. Guyot-Revol V, Innes JA, Hackforth S, Hinks T, Lalvani A. Regulatory T cells are expanded in blood and disease sites in patients with tuberculosis. *Am J Respir Crit Care Med.* (2006) 173:803–10. doi: 10.1164/rccm.200508-1294OC
74. Shang S, Harton M, Tamayo MH, Shanley C, Palanisamy GS, Caraway M, et al. Increased Foxp3 expression in guinea pigs infected with W-Beijing strains of *M. tuberculosis*. *Tuberculosis.* (2011) 91:378–85. doi: 10.1016/j.tube.2011.06.001
75. Cardona P, Cardona PJ. Regulatory T cells in *Mycobacterium tuberculosis* infection. *Front Immunol.* (2019) 10:2139. doi: 10.3389/fimmu.2019.02139
76. Ordway D, Henao-Tamayo M, Harton M, Palanisamy G, Troudt J, Shanley C, et al. The hypervirulent *Mycobacterium tuberculosis* strain HN878 induces a potent TH1 response followed by rapid down-regulation. *J Immunol.* (2007) 179:522–31. doi: 10.4049/jimmunol.179.1.522
77. Ross PJ, Lavelle EC, Mills KH, Boyd AP. Adenylate cyclase toxin from *Bordetella pertussis* synergizes with lipopolysaccharide to

promote innate interleukin-10 production and enhances the induction of Th2 and regulatory T cells. *Infect Immun.* (2004) 72:1568–79. doi: 10.1128/IAI.72.3.1568-1579.2004

78. McGuirk P, McCann C, Mills KH. Pathogen-specific T regulatory 1 cells induced in the respiratory tract by a bacterial molecule that stimulates interleukin 10 production by dendritic cells: a novel strategy for evasion of protective T helper type 1 responses by *Bordetella pertussis*. *J Exp Med.* (2002) 195:221–31. doi: 10.1084/jem.20011288
79. Higgs R, Higgins SC, Ross PJ, Mills KH. Immunity to the respiratory pathogen *Bordetella pertussis*. *Mucosal Immunol.* (2012) 5:485–500. doi: 10.1038/mi.2012.54
80. Coleman MM, Finlay CM, Moran B, Keane J, Dunne PJ, Mills KH. The immunoregulatory role of CD4(+) FoxP3(+) CD25(-) regulatory T cells in lungs of mice infected with *Bordetella pertussis*. *FEMS Immunol Med Microbiol.* (2012) 64:413–24. doi: 10.1111/j.1574-695X.2011.00927.x
81. Neill DR, Coward WR, Gritzfeld JF, Richards L, Garcia-Garcia FJ, Dotor J, et al. Density and duration of pneumococcal carriage is maintained by transforming growth factor beta1 and T regulatory cells. *Am J Respir Crit Care Med.* (2014) 189:1250–9. doi: 10.1164/rccm.201401-0128OC
82. Blair PA, Norena LY, Flores-Borja F, Rawlings DJ, Isenberg DA, Ehrenstein MR, et al. CD19(+)CD24(hi)CD38(hi) B cells exhibit regulatory capacity in healthy individuals but are functionally impaired in systemic lupus erythematosus patients. *Immunity.* (2010) 32:129–40. doi: 10.1016/j.immuni.2009.11.009
83. Mauri C, Menon M. Human regulatory B cells in health and disease: therapeutic potential. *J Clin Invest.* (2017) 127:772–9. doi: 10.1172/JCI85113
84. Flores-Borja F, Bosma A, Ng D, Reddy V, Ehrenstein MR, Isenberg DA, et al. CD19+CD24hiCD38hi B cells maintain regulatory T cells while limiting TH1 and TH17 differentiation. *Sci Transl Med.* (2013) 5:173ra23. doi: 10.1126/scitranslmed.3005407
85. Zhang M, Zheng X, Zhang J, Zhu Y, Zhu X, Liu H, et al. CD19(+)CD1d(+)CD5(+) B cell frequencies are increased in patients with tuberculosis and suppress Th17 responses. *Cell Immunol.* (2012) 274:89–97. doi: 10.1016/j.cellimm.2012.01.007
86. Zhang M, Zeng G, Yang Q, Zhang J, Zhu X, Chen Q, et al. Anti-tuberculosis treatment enhances the production of IL-22 through reducing the frequencies of regulatory B cell. *Tuberculosis.* (2014) 94:238–44. doi: 10.1016/j.tube.2013.12.003
87. Zeng G, Chen CY, Huang D, Yao S, Wang RC, Chen ZW. Membrane-bound IL-22 after de novo production in tuberculosis and anti-*Mycobacterium tuberculosis* effector function of IL-22+ CD4+ T cells. *J Immunol.* (2011) 187:190–9. doi: 10.4049/jimmunol.1004129
88. Dhiman R, Indramohan M, Barnes PF, Nayak RC, Paidipally P, Rao LV, et al. IL-22 produced by human NK cells inhibits growth of *Mycobacterium tuberculosis* by enhancing phagolysosomal fusion. *J Immunol.* (2009) 183:6639–45. doi: 10.4049/jimmunol.0902587
89. Dai YC, Wang WD, Zhang JA, Chen C, Luo HL, Xu H, et al. MTB driven B cells producing IL-35 and secreting high level of IL-10 in the patients with active pulmonary tuberculosis. *Mol Immunol.* (2019) 112:175–81. doi: 10.1016/j.molimm.2019.05.004
90. Olson BM, Sullivan JA, Burlingham WJ. Interleukin 35: a key mediator of suppression and the propagation of infectious tolerance. *Front Immunol.* (2013) 4:315. doi: 10.3389/fimmu.2013.00315
91. Couper KN, Blount DG, Riley EM. IL-10: the master regulator of immunity to infection. *J Immunol.* (2008) 180:5771–7. doi: 10.4049/jimmunol.180.9.5771
92. Roque S, Nobrega C, Appelberg R, Correia-Neves M. IL-10 underlies distinct susceptibility of BALB/c and C57BL/6 mice to *Mycobacterium avium* infection and influences efficacy of antibiotic therapy. *J Immunol.* (2007) 178:8028–35. doi: 10.4049/jimmunol.178.12.8028
93. Redford PS, Murray PJ, OGarra A. The role of IL-10 in immune regulation during *M. tuberculosis* infection. *Mucosal Immunol.* (2011) 4:261–70. doi: 10.1038/mi.2011.7
94. Das S, Banerjee S, Majumder S, Chowdhury BP, Goswami A, Halder K, et al. Immune subversion by *Mycobacterium tuberculosis* through CCR5 mediated signaling: involvement of IL-10. *PLoS ONE.* (2014) 9:e92477. doi: 10.1371/journal.pone.0092477
95. Parveen N, Varman R, Nair S, Das G, Ghosh S, Mukhopadhyay S. Endocytosis of *Mycobacterium tuberculosis* heat shock protein 60 is required to induce interleukin-10 production in macrophages. *J Biol Chem.* (2013) 288:24956–71. doi: 10.1074/jbc.M113.461004
96. Ehrt S, Schnappinger D. Mycobacterial survival strategies in the phagosome: defence against host stresses. *Cell Microbiol.* (2009) 11:1170–8. doi: 10.1111/j.1462-5822.2009.01335.x
97. Armstrong JA, Arcy PD. Response of cultured macrophages to *Mycobacterium tuberculosis*, with observations on fusion of lysosomes with phagosomes. *J Exp Med Hart.* (1971) 134:713–40. doi: 10.1084/jem.134.3.713
98. OLeary S, OSullivan MP, Keane J. IL-10 blocks phagosome maturation in *Mycobacterium tuberculosis*-infected human macrophages. *Am J Respir Cell Mol Biol.* (2011) 45:172–80. doi: 10.1165/rcmb.2010-0319OC
99. Pauwels AM, Trost M, Beyaert R, Hoffmann E. Patterns, receptors, and signals: regulation of phagosome maturation. *Trends Immunol.* (2017) 38:407–22. doi: 10.1016/j.it.2017.03.006
100. Lutay N, Hakansson G, Alaridah N, Hallgren O, Westergren-Thorsson G, Godaly G. *Mycobacteria bypass* mucosal NF-kB signalling to induce an epithelial anti-inflammatory IL-22 and IL-10 response. *PLoS ONE.* (2014) 9:e86466. doi: 10.1371/journal.pone.0086466
101. Sheedy FJ. Turning 21: induction of miR-21 as a key switch in the inflammatory response. *Front Immunol.* (2015) 6:19. doi: 10.3389/fimmu.2015.00019
102. Sheedy FJ, Palsson-McDermott E, Hennessy EJ, Martin C, OLeary JJ, Ruan Q, et al. Negative regulation of TLR4 via targeting of the proinflammatory tumor suppressor PDCD4 by the microRNA miR-21. *Nat Immunol.* (2010) 11:141–7. doi: 10.1038/ni.1828
103. Moreira-Teixeira L, Redford PS, Stavropoulos E, Ghilardi N, Maynard CL, Weaver CT, et al. T cell-derived IL-10 impairs host resistance to *Mycobacterium tuberculosis* infection. *J Immunol.* (2017) 199:613–23. doi: 10.4049/jimmunol.1601340
104. McGuirk P, Mills KH. Direct anti-inflammatory effect of a bacterial virulence factor: IL-10-dependent suppression of IL-12 production by filamentous hemagglutinin from Bordetella pertussis. *Eur J Immunol.* (2000) 30:415–22. doi: 10.1002/1521-4141(200002)30:2<415::AID-IMMU415>3.0.CO;2-X
105. Dirix V, Mielcarek N, Debrie AS, Willery E, Alonso S, Versheure V, et al. Human dendritic cell maturation and cytokine secretion upon stimulation with *Bordetella pertussis* filamentous haemagglutinin. *Microbes Infect.* (2014) 16:562–70. doi: 10.1016/j.micinf.2014.04.003
106. Villarino Romero R, Hasan S, Fae K, Holubova J, Geurtsen J, Schwarzer M, et al. *Bordetella pertussis* filamentous hemagglutinin itself does not trigger anti-inflammatory interleukin-10 production by human dendritic cells. *Int J Med Microbiol.* (2016) 306:38–47. doi: 10.1016/j.ijmm.2015.11.003
107. Wakelin SJ, Sabroe I, Gregory CD, Poxton IR, Forsythe JL, Garden OJ, et al. Dirty little secrets–endotoxin contamination of recombinant proteins. *Immunol Lett.* (2006) 106:1–7. doi: 10.1016/j.imlet.2006.04.007
108. Bagley KC, Abdelwahab SF, Tuskan RG, Fouts TR, Lewis GK. Pertussis toxin and the adenylate cyclase toxin from *Bordetella pertussis* activate human monocyte-derived dendritic cells and dominantly inhibit cytokine production through a cAMP-dependent pathway. *J Leukoc Biol.* (2002) 72:962–9. Available online at: https://www.jlb.onlinelibrary.wiley.com/doi/full/10.1189/jlb.72.5.962
109. Hickey FB, Brereton CF, Mills KH. Adenylate cycalse toxin of *Bordetella pertussis* inhibits TLR-induced IRF-1 and IRF-8 activation and IL-12 production and enhances IL-10 through MAPK activation in dendritic cells. *J Leukoc Biol.* (2008) 84:234–43. doi: 10.1189/jlb.0208113
110. Yoshida K, Matsumoto T, Tateda K, Uchida K, Tsujimoto S, Yamaguchi K. Induction of interleukin-10 and down-regulation of cytokine production by *Klebsiella pneumoniae* capsule in mice with pulmonary infection. *J Med Microbiol.* (2001) 50:456–61. doi: 10 1099/0022-1317-50-5-456
111. Codo AC, Saraiva AC, Dos Santos LL, Visconde MF, Gales AC, Zamboni DS, et al. Inhibition of inflammasome activation by a clinical strain of *Klebsiella pneumoniae* impairs efferocytosis and leads to bacterial dissemination. *Cell Death Dis.* (2018) 9:1182. doi: 10.1038/s41419-018-1214-5
112. Martín-Sánchez F, Diamond C, Marcel Zeitler AI, Gomez A, Baroja-Mazo J, Bagnall D, et al. Inflammasome-dependent IL-1 β release depends upon membrane permeabilisation. *Cell Death Mortellaro Different.* (2016) 23:1219–31. doi: 10.1038/cdd.2015.176

113. Ip WKE, Hoshi N, Shouval DS, Snapper S, Medzhitov R. Anti-inflammatory effect of IL-10 mediated by metabolic reprogramming of macrophages. *Science.* (2017) 356:513–9. doi: 10.1126/science.aal3535
114. Greenberger MJ, Strieter RM, Kunkel SL, Danforth JM, Goodman RE, Standiford TJ. Neutralization of IL-10 increases survival in a murine model of *Klebsiella pneumonia. J Immunol.* (1995) 155:722–9.
115. Lawlor MS, Handley SA, Miller VL. Comparison of the host responses to wild-type and cpsB mutant *Klebsiella pneumoniae* infections. *Infect Immun.* (2006) 74:5402–7. doi: 10.1128/IAI.00244-06
116. Bengoechea JA, Sa Pessoa J. *Klebsiella pneumoniae* infection biology: living to counteract host defences. *FEMS Microbiol Rev.* (2019) 43:123–44. doi: 10.1093/femsre/fuy043
117. Sing A, Rost D, Tvardovskaia N, Roggenkamp A, Wiedemann A, Kirschning CJ, et al. Yersinia V-antigen exploits toll-like receptor 2 and CD14 for interleukin 10-mediated immunosuppression. *J Exp Med.* (2002) 196:1017–24. doi: 10.1084/jem.20020908
118. Overheim KA, Depaolo RW, Debord KL, Morrin EM, Anderson DM, Green NM, et al. LcrV plague vaccine with altered immunomodulatory properties. *Infect Immun.* (2005) 73:5152–9. doi: 10.1128/IAI.73.8.5152-5159.2005
119. Reithmeier-Rost D, Bierschenk S, Filippova N, Schroder-Braunstein J, Sing A. Yersinia V antigen induces both TLR homo- and heterotolerance in an IL-10-involving manner. *Cell Immunol.* (2004) 231:63–74. doi: 10.1016/j.cellimm.2004.12.003
120. Peres AG, Stegen C, Li J, Xu AQ, Levast B, Surette MG, et al. Uncoupling of pro- and anti-inflammatory properties of *Staphylococcus aureus. Infect Immun.* (2015) 83:1587–97. doi: 10.1128/IAI.02832-14
121. Frodermann V, Chau TA, Sayedyahossein S, Toth JM, Heinrichs DE, Madrenas J. A modulatory interleukin-10 response to staphylococcal peptidoglycan prevents Th1/Th17 adaptive immunity to *Staphylococcus aureus. J Infect Dis.* (2011) 204:253–62. doi: 10.1093/infdis/jir276
122. Robinson KM, Lee B, Scheller EV, Mandalapu S, Enelow RI, Kolls JK, et al. The role of IL-27 in susceptibility to post-influenza *Staphylococcus aureus* pneumonia. *Respir Res.* (2015) 16:10. doi: 10.1186/s12931-015-0168-8
123. Jiang XL, Zhang GL, Yang T, Yang BH, Wang LJ, Wang QH, et al. Association of pneumococcal carriage and expression of Foxp3+ regulatory T cells and Th17 cells in the adenoids of children. *Respiration.* (2015) 90:25–32. doi: 10.1159/000381724
124. Gratz N, Loh LN, Mann B, Gao G, Carter R, Rosch J, et al. *Pneumococcal neuraminidase* activates TGF-beta signalling. *Microbiology.* (2017) 163:1198–207. doi: 10.1099/mic.0.000511
125. Orihuela CJ, Gao G, Francis KP, Yu J, Tuomanen EI. Tissue-specific contributions of pneumococcal virulence factors to pathogenesis. *J Infect Dis.* (2004) 190:1661–69. doi: 10.1086/424596
126. Meliopoulos VA, Van de Velde LA, Van de Velde NC, Karlsson EA, Neale G, Vogel P, et al. An epithelial integrin regulates the amplitude of protective lung interferon responses against multiple respiratory pathogens. *PLoS Pathog.* (2016) 12:e1005804. doi: 10.1371/journal.ppat.1005804
127. Breuss JM, Gallo J, DeLisser HM, Klimanskaya IV, Folkesson HG, Pittet JF, et al. Expression of the beta 6 integrin subunit in development, neoplasia and tissue repair suggests a role in epithelial remodeling. *J Cell Sci.* (1995) 108(Pt 6):2241–51.
128. Neill DR, Fernandes VE, Wisby L, Haynes AR, Ferreira DM, Laher A, et al. T regulatory cells control susceptibility to invasive pneumococcal pneumonia in mice. *PLoS Pathog.* (2012) 8:e1002660. doi: 10.1371/journal.ppat.1002660
129. Aung H, Toossi Z, McKenna SM, Gogate P, Sierra J, Sada E, et al. Expression of transforming growth factor-beta but not tumor necrosis factor-alpha, interferon-gamma, and interleukin-4 in granulomatous lung lesions in tuberculosis. *Tuber Lung Dis.* (2000) 80:61–7. doi: 10.1054/tuld.2000.0235
130. Aung H, Wu M, Johnson JL, Hirsch CS, Toossi Z. Bioactivation of latent transforming growth factor beta1 by *Mycobacterium tuberculosis* in human mononuclear phagocytes. *Scand J Immunol.* (2005) 61:558–65. doi: 10.1111/j.1365-3083.2005.01623.x
131. Wilkinson KA, Martin TD, Reba SM, Aung H, Redline RW, Boom WH, et al. Latency-associated peptide of transforming growth factor beta enhances mycobacteriocidal immunity in the lung during *Mycobacterium bovis* BCG infection in C57BL/6 mice. *Infect Immun.* (2000) 68:6505–8. doi: 10.1128/.68.11.6505-6508.2000
132. Liu FD, Kenngott EE, Schroter MF, Kuhl A, Jennrich S, Watzlawick R, et al. Timed action of IL-27 protects from immunopathology while preserving defense in influenza. *PLoS Pathog.* (2014) 10:e1004110. doi: 10.1371/journal.ppat.1004110
133. Stumhofer JS, Laurence A, Wilson EH, Huang E, Tato CM, Johnson LM, et al. Interleukin 27 negatively regulates the development of interleukin 17-producing T helper cells during chronic inflammation of the central nervous system. *Nat Immunol.* (2006) 7:937–45. doi: 10.1038/ni1376
134. Stumhofer JS, Silver JS, Laurence A, Porrett PM, Harris TH, Turka LA, et al. Interleukins 27 and 6 induce STAT3-mediated T cell production of interleukin 10. *Nat Immunol.* (2007) 8:1363–71. doi: 10.1038/ni1537
135. Yoshimura T, Takeda A, Hamano S, Miyazaki Y, Kinjyo I, Ishibashi T, et al. Two-sided roles of IL-27: induction of Th1 differentiation on naive CD4+ T cells versus suppression of proinflammatory cytokine production including IL-23-induced IL-17 on activated CD4+ T cells partially through STAT3-dependent mechanism. *J Immunol.* (2006) 177:5377–85. doi: 10.4049/jimmunol.177.8.5377
136. Pot C, Apetoh L, Awasthi A, Kuchroo VK. Induction of regulatory Tr1 cells and inhibition of T(H)17 cells by IL-27. *Semin Immunol.* (2011) 23:438–45. doi: 10.1016/j.smim.2011.08.003
137. Pyle CJ, Uwadiae FI, Swieboda DP, Harker JA. Early IL-6 signalling promotes IL-27 dependent maturation of regulatory T cells in the lungs and resolution of viral immunopathology. *PLoS Pathog.* (2017) 13:e1006640. doi: 10.1371/journal.ppat.1006640
138. Cao J, Xu F, Lin S, Song Z, Zhang L, Luo P, et al. IL-27 controls sepsis-induced impairment of lung antibacterial host defence. *Thorax.* (2014) 69:926–37. doi: 10.1136/thoraxjnl-2014-205777
139. Rinchai D, Khaenam P, Kewcharoenwong C, Buddhisa S, Pankla R, Chaussabel D, et al. Production of interleukin-27 by human neutrophils regulates their function during bacterial infection. *Eur J Immunol.* (2012) 42:3280–90. doi: 10.1002/eji.201242526
140. Muller SI, Friedl A, Aschenbrenner IJ, von Bieren, E, Zacharias M, Devergne O, et al. A folding switch regulates interleukin 27 biogenesis and secretion of its alpha-subunit as a cytokine. *Proc Natl Acad Sci USA.* (2019) 116:1585–90. doi: 10.1073/pnas.1816698116
141. ONeill LA, Kishton RJ, Rathmell J. A guide to immunometabolism for immunologists. *Nat Rev Immunol.* (2016) 16:553–65. doi: 10.1038/nri.2016.70
142. Krawczyk CM, Holowka T, Sun J, Blagih J, Amiel E, DeBerardinis RJ, et al. Toll-like receptor-induced changes in glycolytic metabolism regulate dendritic cell activation. *Blood.* (2010) 115:4742–9. doi: 10.1182/blood-2009-10-249540
143. Rodriguez-Prados JC, Traves PG, Cuenca J, Rico D, Aragones J, Martin-Sanz P, et al. Substrate fate in activated macrophages: a comparison between innate, classic, and alternative activation. *J Immunol.* (2010) 185:605–14. doi: 10.4049/jimmunol.0901698
144. Zhang X, Huang T, Wu Y, Peng W, Xie H, Pan M, et al. Inhibition of the PI3K-Akt-mTOR signaling pathway in T lymphocytes in patients with active tuberculosis. *Int J Infect Dis.* (2017) 59:110–7. doi: 10.1016/j.ijid.2017.04.004
145. Gleeson LE, Sheedy FJ, Palsson-McDermott EM, Triglia D, OLeary SM, OSullivan MP, et al. Cutting Edge: *Mycobacterium tuberculosis* induces aerobic glycolysis in human alveolar macrophages that is required for control of intracellular bacillary replication. *J Immunol.* (2016) 196:2444–9. doi: 10.4049/jimmunol.1501612
146. Almeida PE, Silva AR, Maya-Monteiro CM, Torocsik D, DAvila H, Dezso B, et al. *Mycobacterium bovis* bacillus Calmette-Guerin infection induces TLR2-dependent peroxisome proliferator-activated receptor gamma expression and activation: functions in inflammation, lipid metabolism, and pathogenesis. *J Immunol.* (2009) 183:1337–45. doi: 10.4049/jimmunol.0900365
147. Cumming BM, Addicott KW, Adamson JH, Steyn AJ. *Mycobacterium tuberculosis* induces decelerated bioenergetic metabolism in human macrophages. *Elife.* (2018) 7:e39169. doi: 10.7554/eLife.39169

148. Mahajan S, Dkhar HK, Chandra V, Dave S, Nanduri R, Janmeja AK, et al. *Mycobacterium tuberculosis* modulates macrophage lipid-sensing nuclear receptors PPARgamma and TR4 for survival. *J Immunol.* (2012) 188:5593–603. doi: 10.4049/jimmunol.1103038
149. Usenik A, Matic L. Evolution of allosteric citrate binding sites on 6-phosphofructo-1-kinase. *J PLoS ONE.* (2010) 5:15447. doi: 10.1371/journal.pone.0015447
150. Freyberg Z, Harvill ET. Pathogen manipulation of host metabolism: a common strategy for immune evasion. *PLoS Pathog.* (2017) 13:e1006669. doi: 10.1371/journal.ppat.1006669
151. Furman BL, Sidey FM, Wardlaw AC. Role of insulin in the hypoglycaemic effect of sublethal *Bordetella pertussis* infection in mice. *Br J Exp Pathol.* (1986) 67:305–12.
152. Hooftman A, ONeill LAJ. The immunomodulatory potential of the metabolite itaconate. *Trends Immunol.* (2019) 40:687–98. doi: 10.1016/j.it.2019.05.007
153. Lampropoulou V, Sergushichev A, Bambouskova M, Nair S, Vincent EE, Loginicheva E, et al. Itaconate links inhibition of succinate dehydrogenase with macrophage metabolic remodeling and regulation of inflammation. *Cell Metab.* (2016) 24:158–66. doi: 10.1016/j.cmet.2016.06.004
154. Mills EL, Dylan G, Hiran A, Prag D, Dikovskaya DM. Itaconate is an anti-inflammatory metabolite that activates Nrf2 via alkylation of KEAP1. *Nature.* (2018) 556:113. doi: 10.1038/nature25986
155. McKinney JD, Honer zu Bentrup K, Munoz-Elias EJ, Miczak A, Chen B, Chan WT, et al. Persistence of Mycobacterium tuberculosis in macrophages and mice requires the glyoxylate shunt enzyme isocitrate lyase. *Nature.* (2000) 406:735–8. doi: 10.1038/35021074
156. Sasikaran J, Ziemski MŁ, Zadora PK, Fleig A, Ivan AB. Bacterial itaconate degradation promotes pathogenicity. *Nat Chem Biol.* (2014) 10:371. doi: 10.1038/nchembio.1482
157. Chiang CY, Uzoma I, Moore RT, Gilbert M, Duplantier AJ, Panchal RG. Mitigating the impact of antibacterial drug resistance through host-directed therapies: current progress, outlook, and challenges. *MBio.* (2018) 9:e01932–17. doi: 10.1128/mBio.01932-17
158. Upadhyay R, Sanchez-Hidalgo A, Wilusz CJ, Lenaerts AJ, Arab J, Yeh J, et al. Host directed therapy for chronic tuberculosis via intrapulmonary delivery of aerosolized peptide inhibitors targeting the IL-10-STAT3 pathway. *Sci Rep.* (2018) 8:16610. doi: 10.1038/s41598-018-35023-0
159. Queval CJ, Song OR, Deboosere N, Delorme V, Debrie AS, Iantomasi R, et al. STAT3 represses nitric oxide synthesis in human macrophages upon *Mycobacterium tuberculosis* infection. *Sci Rep.* (2016) 6:29297. doi: 10.1038/srep29297
160. Harling K, Adankwah E, Guler AA, Afum-Adjei A, Adu-Amoah L, Mayatepek E, et al. Constitutive STAT3 phosphorylation and IL-6/IL-10 co-expression are associated with impaired T-cell function in tuberculosis patients. *Cell Mol Immunol.* (2018) 16:275–87. doi: 10.1038/cmi.2018.5
161. Li L, Zhang J, Chen J, Xu-Monette ZY, Miao Y, Xiao M, et al. B-cell receptor-mediated NFATc1 activation induces IL-10/STAT3/PD-L1 signaling in diffuse large B-cell lymphoma. *Blood.* (2018) 132:1805–17. doi: 10.1182/blood-2018-03-841015
162. Hsu P, Santner-Nanan B, Hu M, Skarratt K, Lee CH, Stormon M, et al. IL-10 potentiates differentiation of human induced regulatory T cells via STAT3 and Foxo1. *J Immunol.* (2015) 195:3665–74. doi: 10.4049/jimmunol.1402898
163. Saito A, Horie M, Nagase T. TGF-beta signaling in lung health and disease. *Int J Mol Sci.* (2018) 19:2460. doi: 10.3390/ijms19082460
164. Bhattacharya D, Dwivedi VP, Maiga M, Maiga M, Van Kaer L, Bishai WR, et al. Small molecule-directed immunotherapy against recurrent infection by *Mycobacterium tuberculosis. J Biol Chem.* (2014) 289:16508–15. doi: 10.1074/jbc.M114.558098
165. Gil-Guerrero L, Dotor J, Huibregtse IL, Casares N, Lopez-Vazquez AB, Rudilla F, et al. *In vitro* and *in vivo* down-regulation of regulatory T cell activity with a peptide inhibitor of TGF-beta1. *J Immunol.* (2008) 181:126–35. doi: 10.4049/jimmunol.181.1.126
166. Dotor J, Lopez-Vazquez AB, Lasarte JJ, Sarobe P, Garcia-Granero M, Riezu-Boj JI, et al. Identification of peptide inhibitors of transforming growth factor beta 1 using a phage-displayed peptide library. *Cytokine.* (2007) 39:106–15. doi: 10.1016/j.cyto.2007.06.004
167. Wu CH, Liu IJ, Lu RM, Wu HC. Advancement and applications of peptide phage display technology in biomedical science. *J Biomed Sci.* (2016) 23:8. doi: 10.1186/s12929-016-0223-x
168. Elgundi Z, Reslan M, Cruz E, Sifniotis V, Kayser V. The state-of-play and future of antibody therapeutics. *Adv Drug Deliv Rev.* (2017) 122:2–19. doi: 10.1016/j.addr.2016.11.004
169. Beamer GL, Flaherty DK, Assogba BD, Stromberg P, Gonzalez-Juarrero MR, Waal Malefyt D, et al. Interleukin-10 promotes *Mycobacterium tuberculosis* disease progression in CBA/J mice. *J Immunol.* (2008) 181:5545–50. doi: 10.4049/jimmunol.181.8.5545
170. Hirsch CS, Hussain R, Toossi Z, Dawood G, Shahid F, Ellner JJ. Cross-modulation by transforming growth factor beta in human tuberculosis: suppression of antigen-driven blastogenesis and interferon gamma production. *Proc Natl Acad Sci USA.* (1996) 93:3193–8. doi: 10.1073/pnas.93.8.3193
171. Hirsch CS, Ellner JJ, Blinkhorn R, Toossi Z. *In vitro* restoration of T cell responses in tuberculosis and augmentation of monocyte effector function against *Mycobacterium tuberculosis* by natural inhibitors of transforming growth factor beta. *Proc Natl Acad Sci USA.* (1997) 94:3926–31. doi: 10.1073/pnas.94.8.3926
172. Hotchkiss RS, Coopersmith CM, McDunn JE, Ferguson TA. The sepsis seesaw: tilting toward immunosuppression. *Nat Med.* (2009) 15:496–7. doi: 10.1038/nm0509-496
173. Cao J, Wang D, Xu F, Gong Y, Wang H, Song Z, et al. Activation of IL-27 signalling promotes development of postinfluenza pneumococcal pneumonia. *EMBO Mol Med.* (2014) 6:120–40. doi: 10.1002/emmm.201302890
174. Haanen JB, Robert C. Immune checkpoint inhibitors. *Prog Tumor Res.* (2015) 42:55–66. doi: 10.1159/000437178
175. Abers MS, Lionakis MS, Kontoyiannis DP. Checkpoint inhibition and infectious diseases: a good thing? *Trends Mol Med.* (2019) 25:1080–93. doi: 10.1016/j.molmed.2019.08.004
176. Azoury SC, Straughan DM, Shukla V. Immune checkpoint inhibitors for cancer therapy: clinical efficacy and safety. *Curr Cancer Drug Targets.* (2015) 15:452–62. doi: 10.2174/156800961506150805145120
177. Tanaka A, Sakaguchi S. Regulatory T cells in cancer immunotherapy. *Cell Res.* (2017) 27:109–18. doi: 10.1038/cr.2016.151
178. Hargadon KM, Johnson CE, Williams CJ. Immune checkpoint blockade therapy for cancer: an overview of FDA-approved immune checkpoint inhibitors. *Int Immunopharmacol.* (2018) 62:29–39. doi: 10.1016/j.intimp.2018.06.001
179. Singh A, Mohan A, Dey AB, Mitra DK. Inhibiting the programmed death 1 pathway rescues *Mycobacterium tuberculosis*-specific interferon gamma-producing T cells from apoptosis in patients with pulmonary tuberculosis. *J Infect Dis.* (2013) 208:603–15. doi: 10.1093/infdis/jit206
180. Day CL, Abrahams DA, Bunjun R, Stone L, de Kock M, Walzl G, et al. PD-1 expression on *Mycobacterium tuberculosis*-specific CD4 T cells is associated with bacterial load in human tuberculosis. *Front Immunol.* (2018) 9:1995. doi: 10.3389/fimmu.2018.01995
181. Lazar-Molnar E, Chen B, Sweeney KA, Wang EJ, Liu W, Lin J, et al. Programmed death-1 (PD-1)-deficient mice are extraordinarily sensitive to tuberculosis. *Proc Natl Acad Sci USA.* (2010) 107:13402–7. doi: 10.1073/pnas.1007394107
182. Wykes MN, Lewin SR. Immune checkpoint blockade in infectious diseases. *Nat Rev Immunol.* (2018) 18:91–104. doi: 10.1038/nri.2017.112
183. Gay CL, Bosch RJ, Ritz J, Hataye JM, Aga E, Tressler RL, et al. Clinical trial of the Anti-PD-L1 antibody BMS-936559 in HIV-1 infected participants on suppressive antiretroviral therapy. *J Infect Dis.* (2017) 215:1725–33. doi: 10.1093/infdis/jix191
184. Smith LK, Rao AD, McArthur GA. Targeting metabolic reprogramming as a potential therapeutic strategy in melanoma. *Pharmacol Res.* (2016) 107:42–7. doi: 10.1016/j.phrs.2016.02.009
185. Yoshida GJ. Metabolic reprogramming: the emerging concept and associated therapeutic strategies. *J Exp Clin Cancer Res.* (2015) 34:111. doi: 10.1186/s13046-015-0221-y

186. Castro I, Sampaio-Marques B, Ludovico P. Targeting metabolic reprogramming in acute myeloid leukemia. *Cells.* (2019) 8:967. doi: 10.3390/cells8090967

187. Hossain F, Al-Khami AA, Wyczechowska D, Hernandez C, Zheng L, Reiss K, et al. Inhibition of fatty acid oxidation modulates immunosuppressive functions of myeloid-derived suppressor cells and enhances cancer therapies. *Cancer Immunol Res.* (2015) 3:1236–47. doi: 10.1158/2326-6066.CIR-15-0036

188. Michalek RD, Gerriets VA, Jacobs SR, Macintyre AN, MacIver NJ, Mason EF, et al. Cutting edge: distinct glycolytic and lipid oxidative metabolic programs are essential for effector and regulatory CD4+ T cell subsets. *J Immunol.* (2011) 186:3299–303. doi: 10.4049/jimmunol.1003613

189. Lochner M, Berod L, Sparwasser T. Fatty acid metabolism in the regulation of T cell function. *Trends Immunol.* (2015) 36:81–91. doi: 10.1016/j.it.2014.12.005

190. Yu XH, Zhang DW, Zheng XL, Tang CK. Itaconate: an emerging determinant of inflammation in activated macrophages. *Immunol Cell Biol.* (2019) 97:134–41. doi: 10.1111/imcb.12218

191. Nair S, Huynh JP, Lampropoulou V, Loginicheva E, Esaulova E, Gounder AP, et al. Irg1 expression in myeloid cells prevents immunopathology during *M. tuberculosis* infection. *J Exp Med.* (2018) 215:1035–45. doi: 10.1084/jem.20180118

192. Rosas-Taraco AG, Higgins DM, Sanchez-Campillo J, Lee EJ, Orme IM, Gonzalez-Juarrero M. Local pulmonary immunotherapy with siRNA targeting TGFbeta1 enhances antimicrobial capacity in *Mycobacterium tuberculosis* infected mice. *Tuberculosis.* (2011) 91:98–106. doi: 10.1016/j.tube.2010.11.004

193. Tay HL, Kaiko GE, Plank M, Li J, Maltby S, Essilfie AT, et al. Antagonism of miR-328 increases the antimicrobial function of macrophages and neutrophils and rapid clearance of non-typeable Haemophilus influenzae (NTHi) from infected lung. *PLoS Pathog.* (2015) 11:e1004549. doi: 10.1371/journal.ppat.1004549

194. Kusmartsev S, Cheng F, Yu B, Nefedova Y, Sotomayor E, Lush R, et al. All-trans-retinoic acid eliminates immature myeloid cells from tumor-bearing mice and improves the effect of vaccination. *Cancer Res.* (2003) 63:4441–9. Available online at: https://cancerres.aacrjournals.org/content/63/15/4441.short

195. Dorhoi A, Glaria E, Garcia-Tellez T, Nieuwenhuizen NE, Zelinskyy G, Favier B, et al. MDSCs in infectious diseases: regulation, roles, and readjustment. *Cancer Immunol Immunother.* (2019) 68:673–85. doi: 10.1007/s00262-018-2277-y

196. Knaul JK, Jorg S, Oberbeck-Mueller D, Heinemann E, Scheuermann L, Brinkmann V, et al. Lung-residing myeloid-derived suppressors display dual functionality in murine pulmonary tuberculosis. *Am J Respir Crit Care Med.* (2014) 190:1053–66. doi: 10.1164/rccm.201405-0828OC

197. Cao M, Xu Y, Youn JI, Cabrera R, Zhang X, Gabrilovich D, et al. Kinase inhibitor Sorafenib modulates immunosuppressive cell populations in a murine liver cancer model. *Lab Invest.* (2011) 91:598–608. doi: 10.1038/labinvest.2010.205

198. Banissi C, Ghiringhelli F, Chen L, Carpentier AF. Treg depletion with a low-dose metronomic temozolomide regimen in a rat glioma model. *Cancer Immunol Immunother.* (2009) 58:1627–34. doi: 10.1007/s00262-009-0671-1

199. Ghiringhelli F, Menard C, Puig PE, Ladoire S, Roux S, Martin F, et al. Metronomic cyclophosphamide regimen selectively depletes CD4+CD25+ regulatory T cells and restores T and NK effector functions in end stage cancer patients. *Cancer Immunol Immunother.* (2007) 56:641–8. doi: 10.1007/s00262-006-0225-8

200. Kaminetzky D, Hymes KB. Denileukin diftitox for the treatment of cutaneous T-cell lymphoma. *Biologics.* (2008) 2:717–24. doi: 10.2147/BTT.S3084

201. Negro-Vilar AZ, Dziewanowska ES, Groves V, Stevens JK, Zhang M, Prince A, et al. Efficacy and safety of denileukin diftitox (Dd) in a phase III, double-blind, placebo-controlled study of CD25+ patients with cutaneous T-cell lymphoma *(CTCL). J Clin Oncol Sterry.* (2007) 25:8026–6. doi: 10.1200/jco.2007.25.18_suppl.8026

202. Gupta S, Cheung L, Pokkali S, Winglee K, Guo H, Murphy J, et al. Suppressor cell-depleting immunotherapy with denileukin diftitox is an effective host-directed therapy for tuberculosis. *J Infect Dis.* (2017) 215:1883–87. doi: 10.1093/infdis/jix208

203. Akkoc T, Aydogan M, Yildiz A, Karakoc-Aydiner E, Eifan A, Keles S, et al. Neonatal BCG vaccination induces IL-10 production by CD4+ CD25+ T cells. *Pediatr Allergy Immunol.* (2010) 21:1059–63. doi: 10.1111/j.1399-3038.2010.01051.x

204. Xu H, Jia Y, Li Y, Wei C, Wang W, Guo R, et al. IL-10 dampens the Th1 and Tc activation through modulating DC functions in BCG vaccination. *J Mediat Inflamm.* (2019) 2019:1–10. doi: 10.1155/2019/8616154

205. Schaible UE, Linnemann L, Redinger N, Patin EC, Dallenga T. Strategies to improve vaccine efficacy against tuberculosis by targeting innate immunity. *Front Immunol.* (2017) 8:1755. doi: 10.3389/fimmu.2017.01755

206. Pitt JM, Stavropoulos E, Redford PS, Beebe AM, Bancroft GJ, Young DB, et al. Blockade of IL-10 signaling during bacillus Calmette-Guerin vaccination enhances and sustains Th1, Th17, and innate lymphoid IFN-gamma and IL-17 responses and increases protection to *Mycobacterium tuberculosis* infection. *J Immunol.* (2012) 189:4079–87. doi: 10.4049/jimmunol.1201061

207. Wu Z, Lu H, Sheng J, Li L. Inductive microRNA-21 impairs anti-mycobacterial responses by targeting IL-12 and Bcl-2. *FEBS Lett.* (2012) 586:2459–67. doi: 10.1016/j.febslet.2012.06.004

208. van Rooij E, Purcell AL, Levin AA. Developing microRNA therapeutics. *Circ Res.* (2012) 110:496–507. doi: 10.1161/CIRCRESAHA.111.247916

209. Marshall NA, Galvin KC, Corcoran AM, Boon L, Higgs R, Mills KH. Immunotherapy with PI3K inhibitor and Toll-like receptor agonist induces IFN-gamma+IL-17+ polyfunctional T cells that mediate rejection of murine tumors. *Cancer Res.* (2012) 72:581–91. doi: 10.1158/0008-5472.CAN-11-0307

210. Bhattacharya D, Dwivedi VP, Kumar S, Reddy MC, Van Kaer L, Moodley P, et al. Simultaneous inhibition of T helper 2 and T regulatory cell differentiation by small molecules enhances Bacillus Calmette-Guerin vaccine efficacy against tuberculosis. *J Biol Chem.* (2014) 289:33404–11. doi: 10.1074/jbc.M114.600452

211. Mittal M, Siddiqui MR, Tran K, Reddy SP, Malik AB. Reactive oxygen species in inflammation and tissue injury. *Antioxid Redox Signal.* (2014) 20:1126–67. doi: 10.1089/ars.2012.5149

212. Lang PA, Xu HC, Grusdat M, McIlwain DR, Pandyra AA, Harris IS, et al. Reactive oxygen species delay control of lymphocytic choriomeningitis virus. *Cell Death Differ.* (2013) 20:649–58. doi: 10.1038/cdd.2012.167

213. Starosta V, Rietschel E, Paul K, Baumann U, Griese M. Oxidative changes of bronchoalveolar proteins in cystic fibrosis. *Chest.* (2006) 129:431–7. doi: 10.1378/chest.129.2.431

214. Deramaudt TB, Dill C, Bonay M. Regulation of oxidative stress by Nrf2 in the pathophysiology of infectious diseases. *Med Mal Infect.* (2013) 43:100–7. doi: 10.1016/j.medmal.2013.02.004

215. Soto ER, Caras AC, Kut LC, Castle MK, Ostroff GR. Glucan particles for macrophage targeted delivery of nanoparticles. *J Drug Deliv.* (2012) 2012:143524. doi: 10.1155/2012/143524

Permissions

All chapters in this book were first published by Frontiers; hereby published with permission under the Creative Commons Attribution License or equivalent. Every chapter published in this book has been scrutinized by our experts. Their significance has been extensively debated. The topics covered herein carry significant findings which will fuel the growth of the discipline. They may even be implemented as practical applications or may be referred to as a beginning point for another development.

The contributors of this book come from diverse backgrounds, making this book a truly international effort. This book will bring forth new frontiers with its revolutionizing research information and detailed analysis of the nascent developments around the world.

We would like to thank all the contributing authors for lending their expertise to make the book truly unique. They have played a crucial role in the development of this book. Without their invaluable contributions this book wouldn't have been possible. They have made vital efforts to compile up to date information on the varied aspects of this subject to make this book a valuable addition to the collection of many professionals and students.

This book was conceptualized with the vision of imparting up-to-date information and advanced data in this field. To ensure the same, a matchless editorial board was set up. Every individual on the board went through rigorous rounds of assessment to prove their worth. After which they invested a large part of their time researching and compiling the most relevant data for our readers.

The editorial board has been involved in producing this book since its inception. They have spent rigorous hours researching and exploring the diverse topics which have resulted in the successful publishing of this book. They have passed on their knowledge of decades through this book. To expedite this challenging task, the publisher supported the team at every step. A small team of assistant editors was also appointed to further simplify the editing procedure and attain best results for the readers.

Apart from the editorial board, the designing team has also invested a significant amount of their time in understanding the subject and creating the most relevant covers. They scrutinized every image to scout for the most suitable representation of the subject and create an appropriate cover for the book.

The publishing team has been an ardent support to the editorial, designing and production team. Their endless efforts to recruit the best for this project, has resulted in the accomplishment of this book. They are a veteran in the field of academics and their pool of knowledge is as vast as their experience in printing. Their expertise and guidance has proved useful at every step. Their uncompromising quality standards have made this book an exceptional effort. Their encouragement from time to time has been an inspiration for everyone.

The publisher and the editorial board hope that this book will prove to be a valuable piece of knowledge for researchers, students, practitioners and scholars across the globe.

List of Contributors

Shugang Qin
Department of Biomedical Sciences, School of Medicine and Health Sciences, University of North Dakota, Grand Forks, ND, United States
State Key Laboratory of Biotherapy, West China Hospital, Sichuan University, Chengdu, China

Jiaxin Li
Department of Biomedical Sciences, School of Medicine and Health Sciences, University of North Dakota, Grand Forks, ND, United States
Department of Liver Surgery, West China Hospital, Sichuan University, Chengdu, China

Chuanmin Zhou, Breanna Privratsky, Jacob Schettler and Min Wu
Department of Biomedical Sciences, School of Medicine and Health Sciences, University of North Dakota, Grand Forks, ND, United States

Yong Zeng and Hong Wu
State Key Laboratory of Biotherapy, West China Hospital, Sichuan University, Chengdu, China

Xin Deng and Zhenwei Xia
Department of Pediatrics and Department of Pulmonary & Critical Care Medicine, Ruijin Hospital Affiliated to Shanghai Jiao Tong University School of Medicine, Shanghai, China

Lokesh Sharma, Clemente J. Britto and Charles S. Dela Cruz
Section of Pulmonary, Critical Care and Sleep Medicine, Yale University School of Medicine, New Haven, CT, United States

Jingjing Feng
Section of Pulmonary, Critical Care and Sleep Medicine, Yale University School of Medicine, New Haven, CT, United States
Department of Respiratory Medicine, The Fifth People's Hospital of Shanghai, Fudan University, Shanghai, China

Hagyu Kim and Sung Jae Shin
Department of Microbiology, Institute for Immunology and Immunological Diseases, Brain Korea 21 Program for Leading Universities and Students (PLUS) Project for Medical Science, Yonsei University College of Medicine, Seoul, South Korea

Dahee Shim
Department of Microbiology, Institute for Immunology and Immunological Diseases, Brain Korea 21 Program for Leading Universities and Students (PLUS) Project for Medical Science, Yonsei University College of Medicine, Seoul, South Korea
Department of Life Science, Research Institute for Natural Sciences, College of Natural Sciences, Hanyang University, Seoul, South Korea

Ethan S. FitzGerald, Nivea F. Luz and Amanda M. Jamieson
Division of Biology and Medicine, Department of Molecular Microbiology and Immunology, Brown University, Providence, RI, United States

Jieling Lim, Vanessa Hui Qi Koh, Sharol Su Lei Cho, Maurizio Vacca and Sylvie Alonso
Department of Microbiology and Immunology, Yong Loo Lin School of Medicine, National University of Singapore, Singapore, Singapore
Immunology Programme, Life Sciences Institute, National University of Singapore, Singapore, Singapore

Balamurugan Periaswamy, Dawn Poh Sum Choi and Paola Florez De Sessions
Genome Institute of Singapore, Agency for Science, Technology and Research (A*STAR), Singapore, Singapore

Pavol Kudela and Werner Lubitz
Biotech Innovation Research Development & Consulting (BIRD-C), Vienna, Austria

Giorgia Pastorin
Department of Pharmacy, Faculty of Science, National University of Singapore, Singapore, Singapore

Julio Sempere, Fernando González-Camacho and Mirian Domenech
Centro Nacional de Microbiología, Instituto de Salud Carlos III, Madrid, Spain

Sara de Miguel
Servicio de Epidemiología de la Comunidad de Madrid, Dirección General de Salud Pública, Madrid, Spain

José Yuste
Centro Nacional de Microbiología, Instituto de Salud Carlos III, Madrid, Spain
Centro de Investigación Biomédica en Red de Enfermedades Respiratorias (CIBERES), Madrid, Spain

Alicia K. Wooten, Emad I. Arafa and Matthew R. Jones
Pulmonary Center, Boston University School of Medicine, Boston, MA, United States
Department of Medicine, Boston University School of Medicine, Boston, MA, United States

Anukul T. Shenoy and Ian M. C. Martin
Pulmonary Center, Boston University School of Medicine, Boston, MA, United States

Hisashi Akiyama and Suryaram Gummuluru
Department of Microbiology, Boston University School of Medicine, Boston, MA, United States

Lee J. Quinton
Pulmonary Center, Boston University School of Medicine, Boston, MA, United States
Department of Medicine, Boston University School of Medicine, Boston, MA, United States
Department of Microbiology, Boston University School of Medicine, Boston, MA, United States
Department of Pathology and Laboratory Medicine, Boston University School of Medicine, Boston, MA, United States

Guangchun Bai
Department of Immunology and Microbial Disease, Albany Medical College, Albany, NY, United States

Joseph P. Mizgerd
Pulmonary Center, Boston University School of Medicine, Boston, MA, United States
Department of Medicine, Boston University School of Medicine, Boston, MA, United States
Department of Microbiology, Boston University School of Medicine, Boston, MA, United States
Department of Biochemistry, Boston University School of Medicine, Boston, MA, United States

Nastaran Mues and Hong Wei Chu
Department of Medicine, National Jewish Health, Denver, CO, United States

Changhoon Oh, Ambika Verma and Youssef Aachoui
Department of Microbiology and Immunology, Center for Microbial Pathogenesis and Host Responses, University of Arkansas for Medical Sciences, Little Rock, AR, United States

Silke Niemann, Jannik Schlagowski and Claudia Neumann
Institute of Medical Microbiology, University Hospital Münster, Münster, Germany

Susann Herzog, Felix Dach and Barbara C. Kahl
Interdisciplinary Center for Clinical Research, Münster, Germany

Nicole de Buhr and Maren von Köckritz-Blickwede
Institute of Physiological Chemistry, University of Veterinary Medicine Hannover, Hanover, Germany

Diego Chaves-Moreno and Dietmar H. Pieper
Helmholtz Center for Infection Research, Helmholtz Association of German Research Centers (HZ), Brunswick, Germany

Jonas Goretzko and Ursula Rescher
Center for Molecular Biology of Inflammation (ZMBE), Institute of Medical Biochemistry, University of Münster, Münster, Germany

Vera Schwierzeck and Alexander Mellmann
Institute of Hygiene, University Hospital Münster, Münster, Germany

Angelika Dübbers
Department of Pediatrics, University Hospital Münster, Münster, Germany

Peter Küster and Holger Schültingkemper
Department of Pediatrics, Clemenshospital, Münster, Germany

M. Kinnersley and Lia A. Michaels
Division of Biological Sciences, University of Montana, Missoula, MT, United States

Patrick R. Secor
Division of Biological Sciences, University of Montana, Missoula, MT, United States
Center for Translational Medicine, University of Montana, Missoula, MT, United States
Center for Biomolecular Structure and Dynamics, University of Montana, Missoula, MT, United States

Laura K. Jennings and Valery Roman-Cruz
Division of Biological Sciences, University of Montana, Missoula, MT, United States
Center for Translational Medicine, University of Montana, Missoula, MT, United States

Elizabeth B. Burgener
Department of Pediatrics, Center for Excellence in Pulmonary Biology, Stanford University, Stanford, CA, United States
Division of Infectious Diseases and Geographic Medicine, Department of Medicine, Stanford University, Stanford, CA, United States

Carlos E. Milla
Department of Pediatrics, Center for Excellence in Pulmonary Biology, Stanford University, Stanford, CA, United States

Medeea Popescu, Jonas D. Van Belleghem, Naomi Haddock, Christiaan R. de Vries, Qingquan Chen, Julie Pourtois and Paul L. Bollyky
Division of Infectious Diseases and Geographic Medicine, Department of Medicine, Stanford University, Stanford, CA, United States

Travis J. Wheeler
Center for Biomolecular Structure and Dynamics, University of Montana, Missoula, MT, United States
Department of Computer Science, University of Montana, Missoula, MT, United States

Conner Copeland
Department of Computer Science, University of Montana, Missoula, MT, United States

Woosuk Choi, Shawn Choe and Gee W. Lau
Department of Pathobiology, University of Illinois at Urbana-Champaign, Urbana, IL, United States

Zyanya Lucia Zatarain-Barrón, Octavio Ramos-Espinosa, Brenda Marquina-Castillo, Jorge Barrios-Payán, Camilo Molina-Romero, Dulce Adriana Mata-Espinosa and Rogelio Hernández-Pando
Experimental Pathology Laboratory, Department of Pathology, Instituto Nacional de Ciencias Médicas y Nutrición "Salvador Zubirán", Mexico City, Mexico

Fernanda Cornejo-Granados, Gamaliel López-Leal and Adrián Ochoa-Leyva
Departamento de Microbiología Molecular, Instituto de Biotecnología, Universidad Nacional Autónoma de México, Cuernavaca, Mexico

Otoniel Maya-Lucas
Department of Genetics and Molecular Biology, Centro de Investigaciones y de Estudios Avanzados (CINVESTAV), Mexico City, Mexico

Richard M. Anthony and Dick van Soolingen
Tuberculosis Reference Laboratory, National Institute for Public Health and the Environment (RIVM), Bilthoven, Netherlands

Inti Alberto De La Rosa-Velázquez and Rosa Gloria Rebollar-Vega
Genomics Laboratory, Red de Apoyo a la Investigación (RAI), Universidad Nacional Autónoma de México – Instituto Nacional de Ciencias Médicas y Nutrición "Salvador Zubirán", Mexico City, Mexico

Robin M. Warren
Division of Molecular Biology and Human Genetics, Department of Biomedical Sciences DST/NRF Centre of Excellence for Biomedical Tuberculosis Research, MRC Centre for Molecular and Cellular Biology, Faculty of Health Sciences, Stellenbosch University, Tygerberg, South Africa

Sivasami Pulavendran, Maram Prasanthi, Akhilesh Ramachandran, Rezabek Grant, Timothy A. Snider, Jerry R. Malayer and Narasaraju Teluguakula
College of Veterinary Medicine, Oklahoma State University, Stillwater, Oklahoma, OK, United States

Vincent T. K. Chow
Department of Microbiology and Immunology, School of Medicine, National University of Singapore, National University Health System, Singapore, Singapore

Sebastián A. Riquelme, Tania Wong Fok Lung and Alice Prince
Department of Pediatrics, Columbia University Medical Center, New York, NY, United States

Rania Bouzeyen, Meriam Haoues, Mohamed-Ridha Barbouche and Makram Essafi
Laboratory of Transmission, Control and Immunobiology of Infections (LTCII), Laboratoire de Recherche 11 (LR11), Institut Pasteur de Tunis (IPT), Tunis, Tunisia
Université Tunis El Manar, Tunis, Tunisia

Ramandeep Singh
Tuberculosis Research Laboratory, Translational Health Science and Technology Institute, NCR Biotech Science Cluster, Faridabad, India

Alanna M. Kelly and Rachel M. McLoughlin
Host-Pathogen Interactions Group, School of Biochemistry and Immunology, Trinity Biomedical Sciences Institute, Trinity College Dublin, Dublin, Ireland

Index

www.ingramcontent.com/pod-product-compliance
Lightning Source LLC
LaVergne TN
LVHW082152200926
84844LV00008B/2144
9798887405827